ATOMIC FORCE MICROSCOPY INVESTIGATIONS INTO BIOLOGY – FROM CELL TO PROTEIN

Edited by **Christopher L. Frewin**

Atomic Force Microscopy Investigations into Biology – From Cell to Protein
Edited by Christopher L. Frewin

Published by InTech
Janeza Trdine 9, 51000 Rijeka, Croatia

Publishing Process Manager Oliver Kurelic

Technical Editor Teodora Smiljanic

Cover Designer InTech Design Team

Additional hard copies can be obtained from orders@intechopen.com

Atomic Force Microscopy Investigations into Biology – From Cell to Protein,
Edited by Christopher L. Frewin
p. cm.
ISBN 978-953-51-0114-7

For EU product safety concerns:
IN TECH d.o.o., Prolaz Marije Krucifikse Kozulić 3, 51000 Rijeka, Croatia,
info@intechopen.com or visit our website at intechopen.com.

Meet the editor

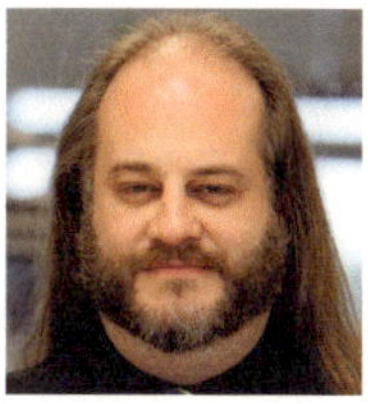

Dr. Christopher L. Frewin is a National Institute of Health Ruth L. Kirschstein National Research Service Post Doctoral Fellow in the Department of Molecular Pharmacology and Physiology at the University of South Florida. He began as materials scientist. He designed and generated a chemical vapor deposition reactor for the heteroepitaxial growth of cubic silicon carbide (3C-SiC). He used the AFM at Max-Planck-Institut für Festkörperforschung, Stuttgart, Germany to evaluate topographic changes in the etched surfaces of SiC. He employed AFM techniques to characterize his 3C-SiC crystals grown in the CVD reactor. During his Ph.D. candidacy, he switched focus from materials science to bioengineering by characterizing the in vitro biocompatibility of 3C-SiC and diamond to neural cells. The key of this investigation centered on living cell AFM measurements which were used to assess cellular lamellipodia/ filopodia permissiveness. Currently he is developing 3C-SiC implantable neural prosthetics for brain machine interface devices.

Contents

Preface

Atomic force microscopy, AFM, is a modern technique for generating high resolution surface topography images and can image many orders of magnitude below the optical diffraction limit. It uses a principal similar to the one used by the phonograph developed by Thomas Alva Edison. Essentially, the phonograph has a sharp object which is dragged across a moving surface, and the tip is deformed by the features it encounters. The AFM uses this principal as well, with the AFM tip generating a physical deflection in the cantilever according to Hooke's law, but unlike the phonograph, the AFM can capitalize on a wider variety of forces generated between the sharp tip and the scanned surface. The AFM cantilever deflection is quantified through the use of a laser reflected off of the back of the cantilever onto an array of photodiodes. Of course, as was seen with Edison's original invention, scanning an object at a constant height presents the danger of a collision with the surface. With this problem in mind, the AFM cantilever is mounted onto a piezoelectric column commonly called a head stage, which moves the cantilever to maintain constant force according to feedback from the measured deflection. The combination of all of these components can be recorded and produces a topographical image of the surface with nanoscale resolution. This measurement technique has also been used to develop a method of force spectroscopy which measures the force between the tip and the sample as a function of distance. However, this technique is not the only measurement these devices can produce.

The AFM is not limited to only one operating mode, but has a second distinctive mode, which itself has been developed into another mode of operation. The previous mode we discussed is known as contact or static mode, and the next mode we will briefly introduce is called non-contact, or dynamic, mode. In this mode, the tip is oscillated near its natural resonance, and brought close to the surface. As the tip approaches the surface, the interaction between the surface and tip forces generates a change in the natural resonance of the cantilever. The feedback circuit is used to reestablish the original oscillation set point by changing the distance between the sample and the tip. The difference that the cantilever moves can be recorded and compiled to produce topographical images. Oscillation differences can be detected as a function of amplitude or frequency. Detections of changes in the frequency of oscillation produce very high-resolution measurements. Through the measurement of changes in amplitude, non-contact mode becomes the third main mode, known as tapping or intermittent mode. In tapping mode, the physical distance of the amplitude of oscillation is large enough to produce brief contact with the surface. This contact leads to changes the amplitude which is measured by the feedback circuit. The head stage moves the cantilever to maintain constant amplitude, and once again can be used to generate topographical images. Changes in the phase of oscillations can also be measured in this mode and is useful in detecting differences in surface friction or between different materials.

The AFM is a very dynamic measurement tool and provides many methods to quantitatively measure a wide range of physical, electromagnetic, and atomic forces. However, the one aspect of this device is that puts it in a class by itself among nanoscale microscopy is the fact that AFM can be used in almost any environment. Vacuum, air, and liquid are not a barrier for this measurement style, and because of this, the AFM lends itself very well for biological investigations where environmental factors can influence biological reactions. This book was developed to showcase the growing use of AFM techniques and methodologies in the investigation of many different aspects of biological and medical sciences. Another, less known advantage for the use of biological AFM is it can be used to investigate structures as large as a whole cell down to the very proteins which constitute the cells themselves. Another advantage is this measurement technique does not require complicated, invasive, and often permanent sample preparation like that required for other microscopy techniques.

Personally, I was unknowledgeable about this fantastic device until I was almost a senior in college. Even further from my expectations is that I never thought I would have used AFM as a tool to investigate biology, specifically neurological cells and their properties. After taking undergraduate physics, and influenced greatly by my childhood idol Nikola Tesla, I wanted to explore the mysteries of electricity and magnetism, so I chose electrical engineering. As with most students, I entered college with preconceptions as to what I would be exposed to within this field, but I found that my expectations were not in line with reality. I thought that I would learn about electrical circuits, power transfer, and communications and then go out into the world and work in some job designing these things, but in the beginning of my junior year, I was fortunate to be able to join, Professor Stephen E. Saddow, in his silicon carbide (SiC) laboratory. Little did I know it at the time, but Dr. Saddow would become my Ph.D. mentor. At first, like many undergraduates, I was just amazed to be in a real research laboratory, but became slightly disillusioned with research due to my preconceptions. My new lab was focused on materials research, which seemed more like chemistry and only seemed connected to electrical engineering due to the fact that crystalline SiC is a semiconductor. As time moved on, I slowly began to understand the importance of this research as educational maturity set in. Finally I was able to look past the chemistry and see a material which could withstand almost every base or acid compound, conduct large amounts of electricity, dissipate heat as well as copper, and even emit visible light from yellow to blue. I began to become intrigued with the possibilities, and wanted to build electrical devices with this wonderful material.

After redesigning the control system for Professor Saddow's SiC reactor, I was teamed with one of his graduate students, Dr. Camilla Coletti, who was studying the surface effects of hydrogen etching on SiC in collaboration with Dr Ulrich Starke of the Max-Planck-Institut für Festkörperforschung in Stuttgart, Germany. Thanks to the graciousness of both Professor Saddow and Dr. Starke, I was able to study at the Institut for a month so that I could gather some data for Dr. Coletti. Here it was that I had my first "hands on" exposure to AFM. It was an experience I will never forget as we immediately got off the plane, drove to the institute, and after introductions to Dr. Starke's group, Prof. Saddow trained me on how to operate the AFM. In a laboratory where there were many complicated, large, ultra-high vacuum instruments, like time-of-flight secondary ion mass spectrometry (ToF-SIMS) and scanning tunneling microscopy (STM) systems, the small, blue can-like system sitting on a floating table seemed almost out of place and ineffectual for surface science. However, I was amazed to find that such a simple machine could be used to examine so many different properties. I imaged the surfaces of the SiC materials we had hydrogen etched in the CVD reactor back in Florida, and Dr. Colletti was able to answer some issues she had concerning the etching process.

I found that AFM was an invaluable tool in not only examining etched SiC surfaces, but also in the development of an improved heteroepitaxial growth process for cubic silicon carbide (3C-SiC) on silicon substrates, as many of the defects at the hetero-epitaxial interface are transferred to the 3C-SiC film surface. AFM proved to be a fast and efficient method, especially when compared to instruments like transmission electron microscopy (TEM) and X-ray Diffraction (XRD), to perform quick analysis of the crystal film so one could determine what growth parameters needed to be adjusted for the reduction of defects. AFM reduced the amount of empirical experimentation involved in SiC heteroepitaxial growth, and reduced the analysis workload by allowing us to only analyze our best materials using more time and preparation intensive methods, like TEM and XRD.

Of course, this is not a book about the use of AFM in materials science, as it is a mainstay in that field, but about the use of AFM in applications within biological sciences. Personally, the experience once again began with Professor Saddow, who saw the potential of SiC for use in medical technology. His group began in earnest to examine SiC biocompatibility using the AFM, starting with Dr. Coletti, continuing with myself, and now with Alexandra Oliveros, a current PhD candidate in his group, to this day. Dr. Saddow purchased a Park Systems XE-100 AFM system because it not only could examine dry materials, but with a removable liquid cell would allow us to examine the interaction of living cells on our materials. During my early graduate experience, I was exposed to many biological science techniques through Dr. Coletti. Her methods included chemical assays to examine cellular proliferation, fluorescent microscopy to examine cellular morphology, and AFM to examine fixed cells on our novel materials. During my Ph.D., I came across a difficulty that stemmed from many optical microscopes used for biology. Although 3C-SiC is translucent, our films are on silicon, which is opaque. The fluorescent optical microscopes I had available to me at the time were all inverted; illuminating the sample from the base and collecting the transmitted light from optics placed above the sample, making live examination of the cells difficult at best. The AFM provided the ideal solution in that we could look at the interaction between our novel materials and living cell concurrently. I also found that AFM easily visualized the protrusions of many motile cells, the lamellipodia and filopodia, and we monitored changes in these protrusions to get an insight into surface permissiveness. AFM also was able to image in great detail paraformaldehyde fixed cells. The AFM is a crucial tool in the exploration of both materials properties as well as biological processes on novel materials in Professor Saddow's research. He is just one of many researchers the world over who are finding out that this tool can assist them with specific biological issues.

The book is divided into five sections. It begins with a section which gives an overview of the AFM, its measurement modes, and techniques associated with the device. This section would be a good starting point for readers unfamiliar with this type of microscopy, but it also contains a good deal of information on image artifacts and difficulties associated with the AFM. The next four sections are divided by the objects being investigated. The second section investigates measurements concerning the smallest biological particles, proteins and amino acid molecules, with each subsequent section growing in biological complexity. The book ends with a section dedicated to the examination of cells, starting with sections of cells, then whole cells, then matrices of several fibers from cells.

The first section, General Techniques, begins with an overview by Dr. Michele Giocondo, *et al.*, which details AFM functional modes, the physics behind AFM functionality, and general examples of AFM applications for biological materials. This is followed by an excellent chapter by Dr. Egor Ukraintsev, *et al.* which details something that has plagued me personally, and I expect many others who have performed AFM at one time or another have seen as well: AFM artifacts. The final part of the section, by Dr. Nadine Mourougou-Candoni, not only examines the use of the tapping mode in liquid, but also gives an excellent assessment of the methods used to prepare biological materials for AFM investigation.

Section two of the book investigates small (10^{-9} m) particles which either are components for larger, more complex structures, or are engineered by man to interact or visualize biological processes at this scale. Prof. Loredana Latterini and L. Tarpani report their utilization of AFM to examine interactions between engineered and industrial particulates with proteins and DNA to gain a better understanding of toxicity related to the workplace. The second chapter, by Dr. Taiji Ikawa, details his process to capture biological molecules within a matrix of azobenzene-containing polymers isomirized through photo-illumination so they can be more easily examined with the AFM. Professor Borut Božič, *et al.* detail the increasingly complex stages of their *in vitro* study which models interactions between a phospholipid membrane, proteins, and antibody-antigen interactions and is measured through the use of AFM. The last chapter in the section, by Dr. Dong Mingdong, *et al.*, details investigation of various natural and artificial amyloid fibers, and provides as a bonus a detailed explanation of the method of using AFM as a force spectroscope.

The biological complexity increases within the third section of the book, which is dedicated to the AFM methodologies for examining deoxyribonucleic acid (DNA), chromatin, and biological membranes. Professor Yong Jiang and Yuan Yin have generated AFM methods to quantitatively identify and examine DNA, and substantiate their results using gel electrophoresis. The next chapter, by Dr. Yamini Dalal, *et al.*, increases the level of complexity and examines chromatins and related DNA transcriptional pathways through functionalized AFM tips. This chapter also provides an interesting comparison between many traditional biological analytical methodologies. Dr. György Váró and Zsolt Szegletes detail in the final chapter of the section the process for generating artificial and natural lipid membranes to allow for the examination of individual membrane proteins, like bacteriorhodopsin, with AFM techniques.

The next section leaves the realm of the nanostructure and examines AFM for virology. Dr. Benjamín Pineda, *et al.*, details virology basics and how AFM can be used to identify virus particles efficiently and quickly during the initial stages of an epidemic. The second chapter of this last section, by M.Sc. Luis Cuellar Jose, *et al.*, uses the AFM in force spectroscopy mode to quantify and model viral shells and capsids as well as investigate viral receptor pathways through the functionalization of an AFM tip.

The final section of the book focuses on cellular components and processes, either through examination of different parts of a cell as a whole, or using the AFM to measure a whole cell and its functionality. Although the first chapter of the section does not examine cells per se, it exemplifies the spirit of the section in that Dr. David J. Burritt, *et al.* are fractionalizing plant cell walls in order to study their structure and composite materials. Their development AFM force mapping simulation is very interesting and could be applied to study structures *in situ*. The next section, by Professor Stephen E. Saddow, *et al.*, combines both principals of using the AFM to examine novel materials and whole cell AFM to investigate aspects of neural permissiveness on a substrate as well as the effects of self assembled monolayers on cellular behavior. Dr. Irina V. Ogneva and Igor B. Ushakov end the section and the book by demonstrating how the AFM can be used to quantitatively measure the material properties of transversal stiffness and Young's modulus in rat and gerbil skeletal muscle fibers.

In closing I would like to give each of the authors and the people that assisted them in gathering the data and analysis for each of these chapters a great deal of thanks. These chapters show that there is not only a broad range of research that the AFM can be used for, but there are a lot of creative people who are moving the edge of science forward. The use of AFM in biology is clearly growing by leaps and bounds, as is seen by companies like Bruker and Park Systems making specific systems which combine fluorescent or confocal microscopes with the power of AFM. The wide variety of the subjects in this book shows that in the next decade will have AFM increase in popularity and utility within biological research. It is my hope that many of the readers of this book who are unfamiliar with the AFM technique will see the utility of this measurement and will be able to use it to perform investigations of their own. Lastly, I hope that you the reader will find that this book is interesting and informative.

Christopher L. Frewin
University of South Florida
USA

Part 1

General Techniques

1

Atomic Force Spectroscopies: A Toolbox for Probing the Biological Matter

Michele Giocondo et al.*
CNR-IPCF, Institute for Chemical and Physical Processes, National Research Council
Italy

1. Introduction

Since its introduction in the early 1980's (Binnig et al., 1986), scanning probe microscopy (SPM) has shown its huge potential for the investigation of the matter at the micro- and nano- scale. In the following years, many variants have been introduced, exploiting electrostatic, magnetic or van der Waals-like forces acting between the sample surface and the probe. In the present chapter, we will be concerned with the latter, also known as atomic force microscopy (AFM). The heart of an atomic force microscope is a sharp tip attached to the extremity of a flexible cantilever, that interacts with the sample surface while the sample is scanned under the tip. The interaction forces between the tip and the sample cause the bending of the cantilever. When the sample is scanned under the tip, the tiny movements of the cantilever are detected by an optical lever system (a device for magnifying small angular displacements of a rotating body, exploiting the reflection of a fixed laser beam over a small mirror attached to the body) producing a spot of light whose position is measured, and they are used as the basis to reconstruct a pseudo-3D image of the sample surface. An atomic force microscope offers the possibility to operate in many different modes (namely: contact, non-contact and intermittent-contact modes), making this technique extremely versatile as it can be adapted to many classes of materials, from the solid state to the biological molecules. According to the sample stiffness, one can adopt the most suitable operating mode in order to reduce or even prevent any damage of the observed specimen.

Nowadays, AFM has proven as an essential tool for the analysis of microbial systems. Emerging methods have rapidly been implemented to make them available to biologists and there exists a great potential for future applications of this technique to biological systems. At the level of the whole cell, AFM has provided an integrated analysis of how the microbial cell exploits its environment through the cell surface. At the macromolecular level, AFM investigation into the properties of surface macromolecules and the energies associated with

*Said Houmadi[1], Emanuela Bruno[1,2], Maria P. De Santo[1,2], Luca De Stefano[3], Emmanuelle Lacaze[4], Sara Longobardi[5] and Paola Giardina[5]
[1]*CNR-IPCF, Institute for Chemical and Physical Processes, National Research Council, Italy*
[2]*Department of Physics, Università della Calabria, Italy*
[3]*CNR-IMM Institute for Microelectronics and Microsystems, National Research Council, Italy*
[4]*CNRS-INSP Institute of Nano-Sciences National Scientific Research Council, France*
[5]*Dept. of Organic Chemistry and Biochemistry, University of Naples "Federico II", Italy*

their conformation and functionality has helped unravel the complex interactions of microbial cells (Casuso et al., 2011; Wright et al., 2010). AFM has been used for the characterization of marine gel network and marine biopolymers self-assembly, which are not accessible by other techniques (Radic et al., 2011). Moreover, submolecular details of protein surfaces can be identified and conformational changes visualized. It allows visualization of macromolecules without labelling, and provides information on the sizes and forms of protein complexes (Baclayon et al., 2010). Indeed AFM is now recognized as the tool of choice for studying biomolecular machines at work, allowing direct observation of function-related structural changes induced by variation of temperature, pH, ionic strength.

Probably the most striking results have been obtained on membrane proteins using contact mode imaging (Muller et al., 2011). The case of membrane proteins is particularly interesting because they are, due to their amphiphilic character, inherently difficult to study with other techniques. Not only can membrane protein surfaces be imaged in their native environment and their oligomeric states resolved, but conformational changes can be visualized, and the forces dictating protein folding in the presence or absence of ligands can be assessed. Moreover, unlike other local probe microscopy such as scanning tunneling microscopy (STM), the AFM offers the possibility to investigate any type of samples (conductor, semiconductor, insulator, inorganic and organic) but also can work under controlled conditions like ultra-high vacuum (UHV) or under physiological liquid environments like the ones required in biological membrane domain. This makes it a very useful instrument for probing these kind of samples.

AFM techniques are normally used for surface imaging. Length and height measurements for surface features can be easily performed on micrometric and nanometric scale and statistically analyzed (roughness, size dispersion). Nevertheless, beyond the bare surface imaging, an AFM can perform much more sophisticated analyses based on the possibility to measure the forces acting between the probing tip and the sample surface, or some other quantities strictly connected to the interaction force details such as the cantilever resonance frequency shift or/and the phase lag between the driving signal and the cantilever response, when in non-contact or intermittent-contact mode. These operating modes are grouped under the common hat of atomic force spectroscopy (AFS). Thanks to the very accurate positioning allowed by the piezoelectric scanners and to the closed-loop feedback control, it is possible to perform the sampling of the interaction forces as a function of the tip-sample gap. These forces can be measured in a static mode, the "so-called" repulsive or contact mode, or in a more indirect manner in the dynamical regime, occurring in the non-contact mode, exploiting the attractive region of the interaction force, and the tapping mode that in rough can be considered as a combination of the remaining.

Because of the extreme weakness of the measurable forces, and the related possibility to tune the sample perturbation, AFS is a powerful tool to probe fragile samples, such as biological molecules like proteins in particular. Many nanoscopic features can be revealed by this technique, ranging from hydropathy to visco-elasticity. Moreover, sample patterning in the physical-chemical properties can be revealed by the combined use of AFS with AFM topographic imaging.

This chapter is devoted to a review of the available atomic force spectroscopic modes and their application to the biological matter. Section 2 is devoted to a short introduction to the

AFM fundamentals; in Section 3 the theoretical basis of AFM is presented; finally, in Section 4 applications of force spectroscopy to biological and soft materials are presented along with experimental details and a discussion of some relevant experiments.

2. AFM fundamentals

It is appropriate to give in this section a short description about the fundamentals and the operation modes of an AFM. The starting point is the Lennard-Jones interaction between a microscopic particle and a surface, shown in Fig. 1.

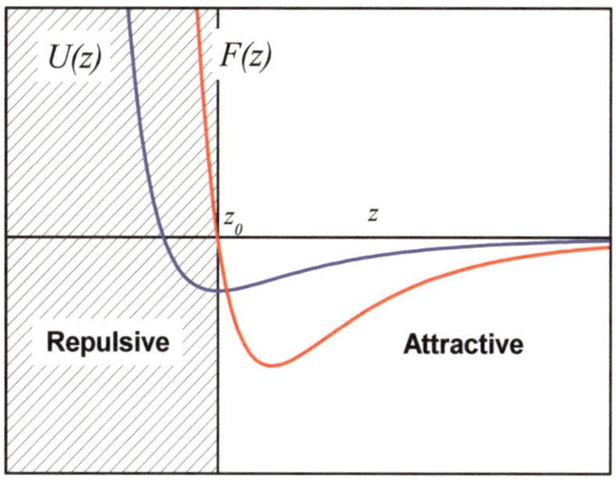

Fig. 1. Lennard-Jones potential $U(z)$ (blue) and the related force $F(z)$ (red).

Let us recall that the force, $F(z)$, depends on the potential, $U(z)$, by the relationship:

$$F(z) = -\nabla U(z) = -\frac{dU(z)}{dz}. \tag{1}$$

Therefore, in Fig. 1 we can distinguish two different regimes, separated by z_0, the distance corresponding to a stationary point for the potential, $U(z)$, and hence to $F(z_0) = 0$. For z values larger than z_0, the particle will experience an attractive force, whereas for z values smaller that z_0, the force will be repulsive. As the force is the derivative of the potential, we can deduce that, because of the difference in the potential slope of the two regimes, the attractive forces will be considerably weaker than the repulsive ones, as Fig. 1 shows.

An AFM is essentially made of a micro/nanoscopic probe tip flying over the specimen under investigation, at a distance spanning in the Nanometers range. In the following, we will show that the tip "flying altitude" setting is essential for discriminating the interaction character, attractive or repulsive, between the probe and the sample surface.

2.1 Scanner and optical lever

As shown in Fig. 2, the sample is fixed on the top of a 3-axes piezoelectric stage in a typical AFM that moves the sample under the tip. During the image acquisition, the movements X, Y are controlled by the computer that generates two synchronized voltage ramps, allowing for the scanning of the chosen sample area, whereas the movement of the Z piezo is controlled by the feedback circuit.

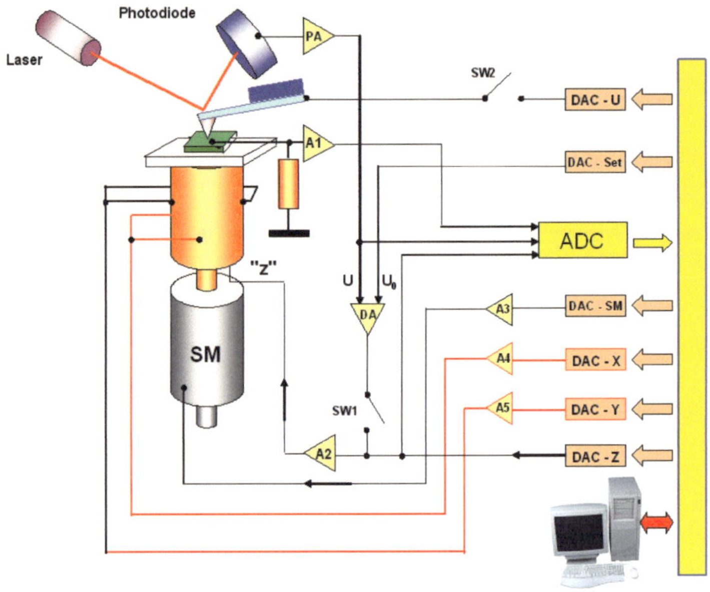

Fig. 2. AFM scheme.

Fig. 3 shows the raster pattern of the scanner. It moves the sample along the fast scan direction by steps of length L/N, where L is the linear dimension of the scanned area and N is the total number of points that are acquired for each line (Hartmann, 2005). At each step the specimen z-height is sampled and in this way the first array of heights is acquired. At the end of the first line, the controller will move the piezo stage one step in the slow scan direction and the acquisition restarts. Nevertheless, most AFM microscopes allow to acquire both the trace and the retrace pathways before the next step in the slow scan direction. This process will be iterated N times, in order to acquire a N x N matrix in which each element corresponds to a point on the sampled area, and its value is the height of that point.

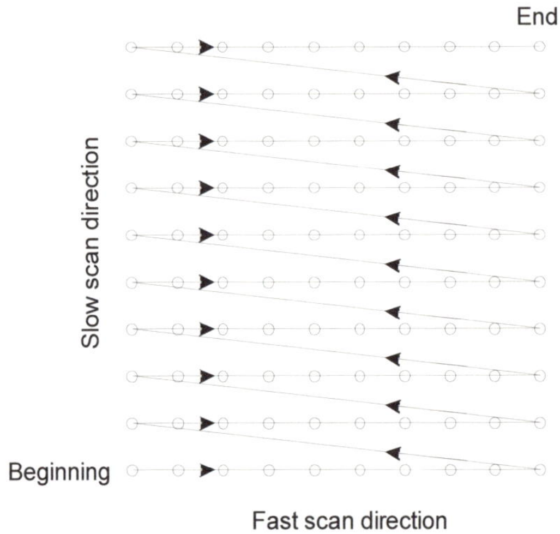

Fig. 3. Scanning raster pattern.

In short, there are three operating modes in SFM: contact, non-contact, and tapping (also called intermittent contact) mode. The coarse positioning is accomplished by step motors that are driven by the control system, allowing the automatic approach of the tip to the sample. The same software allows for the acquisition of multiple images of the sample area at high resolution, particularly useful for imaging living tissues. The AFM head stage contains the optical system, consisting of the laser and photodiode, for the detection of the micro lever deflection (Fig. 2).

The cantilever bends up and down when the sample is scanned under the tip due to the interaction forces between the tip and the sample, providing information on the sample height. Depending on the sample roughness, the movement of the cantilever can be very small, less than 1 nm. A detection system that is able to record such tiny variation in the cantilever bending is required. The system is also known as optical lever and it is composed by a laser diode and a two or a four segments photodiode. The laser diode is equipped with a lens that provides a spot size in the order of a few microns. The laser is fixed at the top of the head through a plate that can be adjusted across two micrometric screws, in order to focus the spot on the cantilever. The beam reflected by the cantilever is directed towards the centre of a two or four quadrants photodetector; the last can record simultaneously the vertical and horizontal displacement of the spot. The optical system (Fig. 4) can thus measure two quantities: the deflection of the cantilever due to the attractive or repulsive force, F_z, (topography) and the torsion of the cantilever due to the lateral component of the interaction force, F_L, of the tip-surface force (friction force).

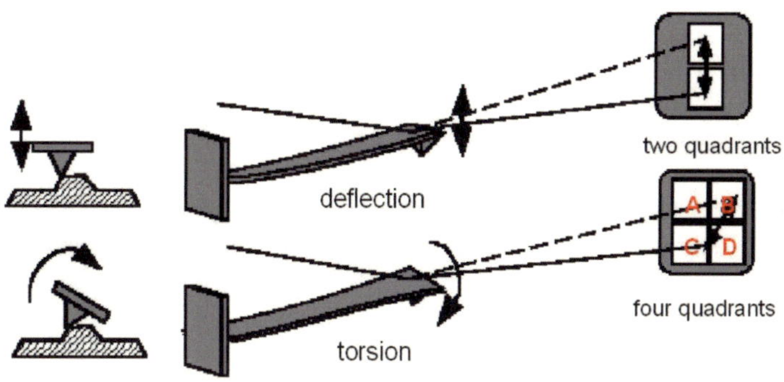

Fig. 4. Optical detection scheme of the cantilever deflection.

The deflection in either the vertical or lateral direction is determined by suitably combining the four quadrants output, i.e. (A + B) : (C + D) or (A + C) : (B + D), where A, B, C, and D are the respective output voltages proportional to the beam intensity on each quadrant. (Bhushan, 2003)

2.2 AFM operating modes

In describing the operating AFM modes usually we refer to the main interaction forces between the tip and the sample, coming from the Lennard-Jones interaction. In Fig. 5 it is depicted the potential and the related force acting between the tip and the sample as a function of the distance z.

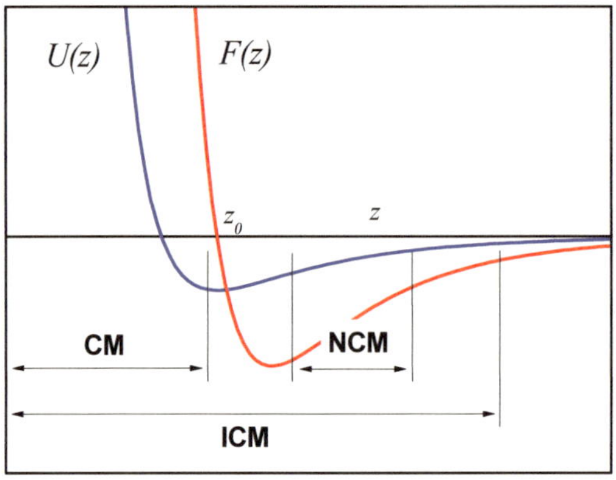

Fig. 5. Distance dependence of Lennard-Jones potential and force vs. tip-surface separation. The tip-surface separation ranges in the contact mode (CM), non-contact mode (NCM), intermittent contact mode (ICM) are highlighted.

2.2.1 Contact mode

Contact mode imaging is so called because the probe remains "in contact" with the sample all the time. Historically, the atomic force microscope was designed to exploit the strong short-range repulsive forces between a probing tip and the sample surface. The probe (tip) is brought into contact with the surface (hence the name) and repulsive forces result in the deflection of the cantilever.

In contact mode the sample surface can be scanned at constant force or at constant tip-sample distance. In the first case the AFM feed-back loop keeps the cantilever deflection, and hence the force between the tip and the sample, constant. Before the scan starts, a setpoint, i.e. a deflection value of the lever that we want to keep constant during the imaging, is chosen. If the tip encounters a feature on the sample surface, the repulsive force varies, causing a bending of the lever. The feedback system compares the actual bending with the setpoint; if they do not coincide, the control system modulates the signal applied to the piezo so that the scanner retracts or extends in order to bring the deflection back to the setpoint. It is important to stress that, in this case, for the aim of sample topography reconstruction, the exact knowledge of the cantilever features is not necessary. In fact, the cantilever bending is measured in an indirect way, "measuring" instead the piezo displacement necessary to recover the initial position of the reflected beam over the photodetector. Therefore, topographical data are derived from the z-axis piezo voltage.

In the constant height mode the feedback system is switched off, so that z-height remains constant during the X-Y scanning, the photodetector output signal is converted in z values. This mode can be used only on samples which are relatively flat and smooth but, for surfaces to which it is applicable, it can provide images with a sharper resolution and in a shorter time compared to the constant force mode.

2.2.2 Non-contact mode

In the non-contact mode the cantilever is never in contact with the sample, and the tip-sample forces are attractive. In this case the involved forces are much weaker than the contact mode case, and hence a more sensitive and sophisticated detection technique, instead of the bare cantilever displacement, is required.

The non-contact mode is one of the two oscillating AFM modes. The cantilever is forced to oscillate through a bimorph that is placed at the base of the cantilever holder. The resonance curve of the cantilever in the free space is shown in fig. 6 (red curve). While the tip approaches the surface, the cantilever vibration regime is affected by the presence of the interaction forces between the tip and the sample. This causes a shift in the resonance curve that will be discussed in more detail in the following sections. In non-contact mode the oscillation frequency is locked to a value slightly larger than the resonance frequency.

When the tip approaches the sample, a reduction in the amplitude of vibration occurs (Fig. 6). During the image acquisition the feedback circuit attempts to restore the amplitude of vibration toward the setpoint slightly larger than the natural resonance. If the tip gets too close or too far to/from the sample the cantilever oscillation amplitude varies and, analogously to the previous case, the feedback system modulates the signal applied to the piezo-scanner so that it either retracts or extends in order to bring the cantilever oscillation amplitude back to the set point.

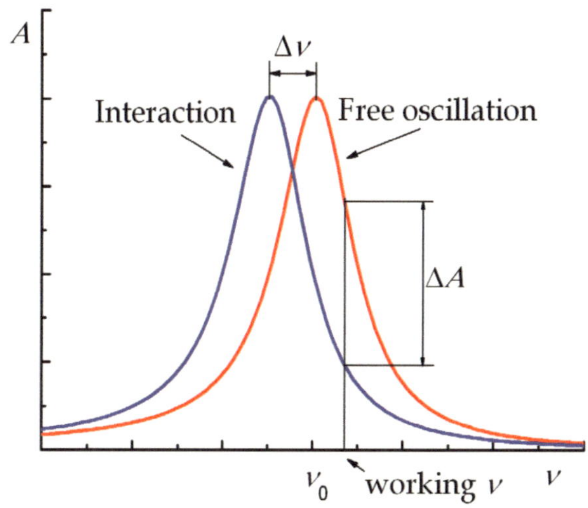

Fig. 6. Calculated cantilever resonance curve in the free oscillation regime (red curve) and in presence of interaction (blue curve).

The cantilevers used in the non-contact mode are stiffer than those used in the contact mode to prevent the cantilever to get pulled into the sample.

2.2.3 Intermittent or tapping mode

Intermittent, or tapping, mode is similar to non-contact mode in many ways, but the cantilever is vibrating 1÷10 nm above the sample with a larger amplitude so that the tip hits the sample at the lowest point of each oscillation cycle.

In this operating mode, the cantilever is excited at a frequency slightly lower than the mechanical resonance, and the topographical features are extracted using the amplitude modulation due to the forces generated by the intermittent interaction between the AFM tip and the sample. Tapping mode is possible at ambient temperature; however, the non-contact and intermittent modes of operation are easier in vacuum where the damping of cantilever oscillations is negligible, allowing for a much sharper resonance peak of the cantilever and hence higher sensitivity while measuring the shift in resonance frequency (Gauthier & Tsukada, 1999; Gauthier et al., 2001; Gauthier & Pérez, 2002; Giessibl, 1997, Giessibl & Bielefeldt 2000, Hong et al., 1999; Jarvis et al., 2001; Martìnez & Garcia., 2006; Matsushige, 2001). Tapping mode is the most used operating mode in biology. It is not disruptive for fragile samples since it eliminates completely friction forces between the tip and the sample that are dominant in contact mode. At the same time its resolution is better than in the no contact mode, in which the tip is in average farer from the sample.

3. AFM spectroscopic modes

Spectroscopy in AFM, in both static and dynamic modes, is a powerful technique to reach a deep insight in the properties of the sample surfaces beyond topography, as it allows the measurement of forces in the nN range. There are several theories describing the interaction between a tip and a sample surface that become very refined when they go to dynamic modes. Here we will introduce the main interaction forces between a tip and a sample and how they can be visualized in the static and dynamic AFM modes.

3.1 Interaction between microscopic bodies: A spherical tip and a flat surface

When describing the interaction between a tip and a sample the best starting point is the interaction between two atoms or small molecules. Usually, we refer to van der Waals interaction that is made of three main contributions: the Keesom interaction (between existing dipoles), the Debye interaction (between dipole-induced dipole), and the London interaction (dispersion forces of quantum mechanical nature). van der Waals interaction is long ranged ($r > 10$ nm) and can be expressed as:

$$w_{vdW} = -\frac{C}{r^6} = -\frac{C_{dip} + C_{ind} + C_{disp}}{r^6} \tag{2}$$

Where C is a constant that takes into account the polarization properties of the two atoms or small molecules. At very small molecular separations, the electronic clouds of atoms overlap, giving rise to very strong repulsive forces.

The potential that better describes the interaction between two atoms or small molecules, including also the attractive van der Waals interaction, was proposed in 1931 by John Lennard-Jones:

$$w(r) = 4\varepsilon\left[\left(\frac{\sigma}{r}\right)^{12} - \left(\frac{\sigma}{r}\right)^{6}\right] \tag{3}$$

where ε is the minimum energy and σ is the diameter of a sphere approximating the atom or molecule. When calculating the interaction between microscopic bodies, other forces have to be taken into account together with the afore mentioned van der Waals forces, i.e. electrostatic, adhesion and capillary forces.

We can calculate the van der Waals attractive force between macroscopic bodies in vacuum, under proper approximations, taking into account the densities and the shapes of the two bodies. For example, the interaction energy between a flat surface and a tip, approximated by a sphere of radius R, can be obtained adding up the pairwise interactions between all the molecules in the tip and in the surface, and be expressed as (Israelachvili, 1992):

$$F = -\frac{HR}{6(d + a_0)^2} \tag{4}$$

H is the Hamaker constant that accounts for the material density and polarizability, featuring a typical value of 10^{-19} J for the condensed phase in vacuum. d is the distance between the tip and the sample and a_0 is an intramolecular distance introduced to avoid the force divergence at the contact. For a tip with a curvature radius R = 10 nm, d = 3Å and H = 10^{-19} J, van der Waals forces are about F = 1.9 nN.

As mentioned above, other forces are involved in the interaction between a tip and a flat surface. As an example, electrostatic forces can be very strong and long ranged, and their intensity depends on how charges are positioned in the media involved in the interaction. Fortunately, in air the electrostatic interaction forces can be minimized with proper experimental devices as, for example, grounding the tip.

During the contact between the tip and the surface, adhesion forces play an important role. We introduce a few fundamental concepts on adhesion. We define "work of adhesion" as the free energy exchange needed to separate two unit areas, 1 and 2, from the contact, and bring them to an infinite distance. For two different media this energy is called work of adhesion W_{12}, while for identical media the energy is called work of cohesion W_{11}. The surface energy or surface tension γ_1 is the energy necessary to increase the body surface of one unit area. The process of creation of a unit area can be seen as the energy necessary to separate two half areas from the contact then, the work of cohesion is related to the surface tension as $\gamma_1 = W_{11}/2$. For solid media γ_1 is denoted as γ_S while for liquid media $\gamma_1 = \gamma_L$. When the surfaces are immersed in a third medium such as water vapor, few water molecules can be adsorbed on the surfaces causing the surface tension to lowers to new values γ_{SV} or γ_{LV}.

In the interaction between the tip and the sample the surface deformation due to the mechanical contact between the two surfaces must be taken into account. This deformation depends on the applied force and on the material properties. There are several models that describe this phenomenon. In particular, Johnson-Kendall-Roberts (JKR) and Derjaguin-Muller-Toporov (DMT) have provided analytical relationships between deformation and applied force. These models are used as standard models for tribology studies using AFM. The JKR model describes the contact between two surfaces with relatively low stiffness and high adhesion forces. The adhesion force magnitude is calculated as:

$$F_a = \frac{9}{8}\frac{HR}{6a_0^2} \tag{5}$$

Nevertheless, real surfaces are never completely rigid and can deform under the influence of attractive forces, giving rise to finite contact area even if no external loads are applied. In JKR theory, the contact area between a spherical surface of radius R and a flat surface, with elastic modulus K, more deformable than the sphere, is expressed as:

$$a^2 = \frac{R}{K}\left[F + 3\pi R W_{12} + \sqrt{6\pi W_{12} F + (3\pi R W_{12})^2}\right] \tag{6}$$

Unlike the JKR model, the DMT model describes the contact between rigid surfaces in the case of low adhesion forces and small tip radii. The contact force is calculated using the relationship:

$$F_{ts}(d) = \frac{4E^* \sqrt{R}}{3 - 3v_s^2}(a_0 - d)^{\frac{3}{2}}, \quad d \le a_0 \tag{7}$$

where:

$$\frac{1}{E^*} = \frac{1 - v_t^2}{E_t} + \frac{1 - v_s^2}{E_s} \tag{8}$$

E and v are respectively the Young modulus and the Poisson coefficient. The subscripts t and s are related respectively to the tip and the surface.

However, these models have some limitations. They suppose the surfaces to be completely flat. As a matter of fact, real surfaces have some roughness that has to be considered in the calculation of the adhesion force. When working in air, small amounts of water vapor in the atmosphere can capillary condense in the contact points, causing an additional attractive force between surfaces. If we consider a sphere of radius R and a flat surface separated by a distance d, the capillary force that is applied in the contact points is given by:

$$F_C = \frac{4\pi R(\gamma_L \cos\theta)}{\left(1 + \frac{d}{D}\right)} \tag{9}$$

where D is the height of the tip immersed in the water meniscus, and θ is the contact angle.

3.2 Spectroscopy mode in static AFM: Force vs. distance curves

Force spectroscopy is a technique to measure forces acting between a tip and a sample surface (Cappella &. Dietler, 1999). It is performed with the tip held in a fixed position in the plane parallel to the sample surface while, in the perpendicular direction, the sample moves by gradually approaching to or retracting from the tip. This results in a force vs. distance curve. To obtain quantitative data from force vs. distance curve measurements, important details must be respected. To accurately measure the deflection of the cantilever, a force curve between the tip and a hard substrate is used to determine the cantilever sensitivity, which relates the cantilever deflection to the voltage of the z-piezo stage. After this calibration the laser alignment has to be kept unchanged. The next step is to convert the deflection into a force using the force constant of the selected cantilever. This value, together with the resonance frequency, is specified by the manufacturer, but generally for each cantilever there can be a quite large difference between the real value and those declared by the manufacturer. Therefore, to ensure the ability to collect data accurately, direct determination of the force constant is advised. Different methods to measure the force constant can be used (Cleveland et al., 1993; Torii et al., 1996). Perhaps the most accessible calibration technique is the thermal noise method (Hutter & Bechhoefer 1993).

During the acquisition of a force vs. distance curve the sample is approached to the tip while the cantilever deflection, δ_c, is recorded. The cantilever bending force is given by the well-known Hooke law:

$$F_c = -k\delta_c \tag{10}$$

During the measurement, the AFM controls z, i.e. the distance between the sample surface and the tip rest position (Fig. 7). d and z are related to the cantilever deflection δ_c and the sample deformation, δ_s, as follows:

$$d = z - (\delta_c + \delta_s) \tag{11}$$

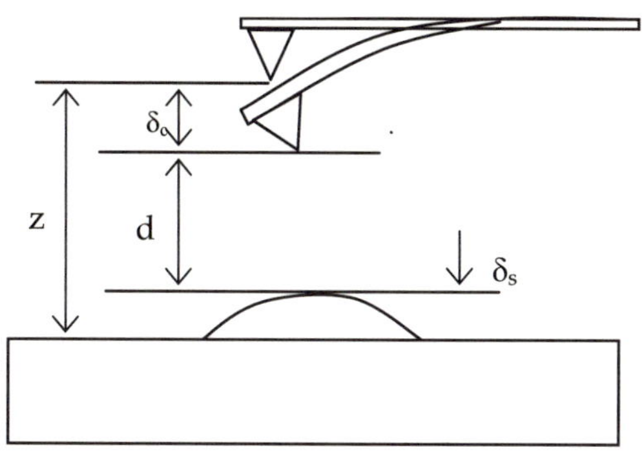

Fig. 7. Tip–sample distance.

The AFM static mode force-distance curve is the result of the balance between two forces: the tip-sample interaction force and the elastic force of the cantilever (Butt et al, 2005; Seo et al., 2008). Fig. 8b shows the typical tip-sample force curve, which takes into account the long-range van der Waals force and the short-range repulsive forces, as a function of the tip-sample gap, z.

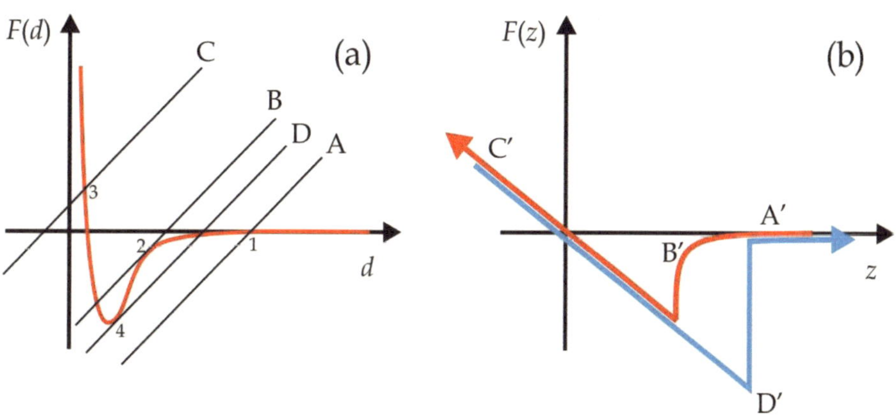

Fig. 8. (a) Force between the tip and the sample as a function of distance. (b) Force vs. z curve acquired by AFM.

In Fig. 8a, lines A, B, C, D represent the elastic force of the cantilever. At each given distance between the tip and the sample, to reach the equilibrium state the cantilever bends until the elastic force equals the tip-sample interaction force. The force values at the equilibrium are given by the intersections 1, 2, 3 and 4 between the lines A, B, C, D and the *F*(*d*) curve respectively. When the tip is far from the sample (line A) no force is detected (branch A′ in 8b). As the tip approaches to the sample (line B) the force experienced by the tip is attractive. At point 2 a change occurs, the tip jumps to contact with the sample surface, *jump-in* point, and the force starts to raise (branch B′ in 8b). At point 3 the force is repulsive. If we assume the surface very stiff, the force curve is close to a straight line (branch C′ in 8b). When the tip retracts from the sample (line D), at the *jump-off* point a sudden separation of the tip from the sample surface occurs (branch D′ in 8b). The hysteresis loop A′B′D′ in Fig 8b is the signature of adhesion effects between the tip and the sample. They may originate from specific tip-sample interactions, or from capillary forces due to the atmospheric water vapor condensation. In performing experiments the choice of the most suitable cantilever stiffness is of crucial importance and it should be adapted to the mechanical properties of the sample. In the following pictures (Fig. 9) the approach and the retract curves for a soft sample (notice the smooth raising for small distances), presenting two adhesion points, are shown.

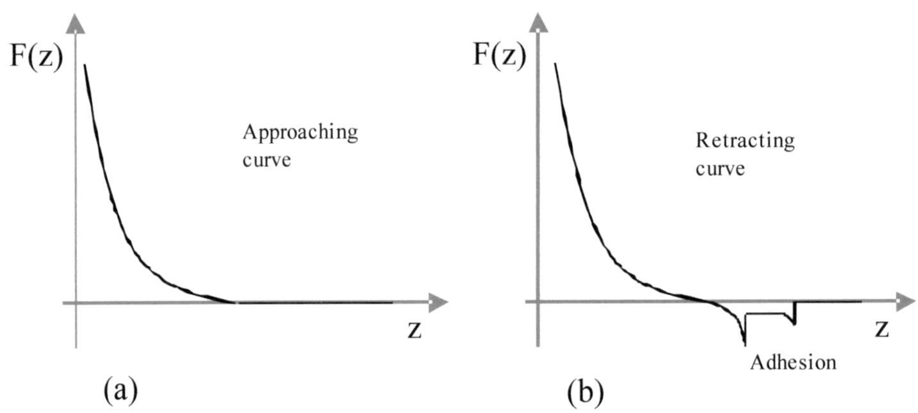

Fig. 9. Approaching (a) and retracting (b) force vs. distance curves on a soft sample in presence of adhesion forces. In (b) two jump-off points are visible.

Using AFM in contact mode, the mechanical properties of samples at the nano-scale such as elastic modulus, strength, adhesion, and friction can be measured. Indeed, different materials with reduced dimensions have been investigated by AFM, and their mechanical properties have been accurately determined by the force-distance curve measurements, including inorganic nanocoils (Qin, et al., 2010), metallic nanowires (Wu et al., 2005, 2006) and biological fibrils (Yang et al., 2008; Smith et al., 2006). However, in many cases, because of the damage that contact mode AFM may cause on the soft materials, the dynamic mode should be preferred, instead, in order to minimize the sample damage.

3.3 Dynamics of an oscillating tip in proximity of a surface

As mentioned above, force spectroscopy can also be performed with a vibrating tip approaching the sample surface. Before describing the tip-sample interaction in this peculiar case we will introduce few concepts on the dynamics of a vibrating lever. The forces acting on a vibrating lever are basically three: its weight (a force that is distributed along the lever), the weight of the tip attached to the lever (which represents a concentrated force at one point) and the external force that acts between the tip and the surface as if it was concentrated in one point. Every point in the lever oscillates with a harmonic motion with the exception of its support and the nodal points which are stationary. The lever dynamics in the free space (i.e., far from the surface where the tip-sample force is null) can be approximated to that of a forced-damped harmonic oscillator and hence described through the related well known equation:

$$m\frac{d^2x}{dt^2} = -kx - c\frac{dx}{dt} + F \tag{12}$$

where $c\ dx/dt$ is the viscous term proportional to the lever velocity, $c = m\Gamma$, where Γ is the damping coefficient, m the mass of the lever and $k = m\omega_0^2$ is the elastic constant of the lever with ω_0 its angular resonance frequency. If we assume that the external driving force is an oscillating one $F(t) = F_0 \cos\omega t$, trivial calculations show that the lever oscillates with a certain amplitude proportional to the modulus of F multiplied by a factor ρ and that the lever does not oscillate in phase with the applied force but the phase is shifted of an angle φ (Fig. 10):

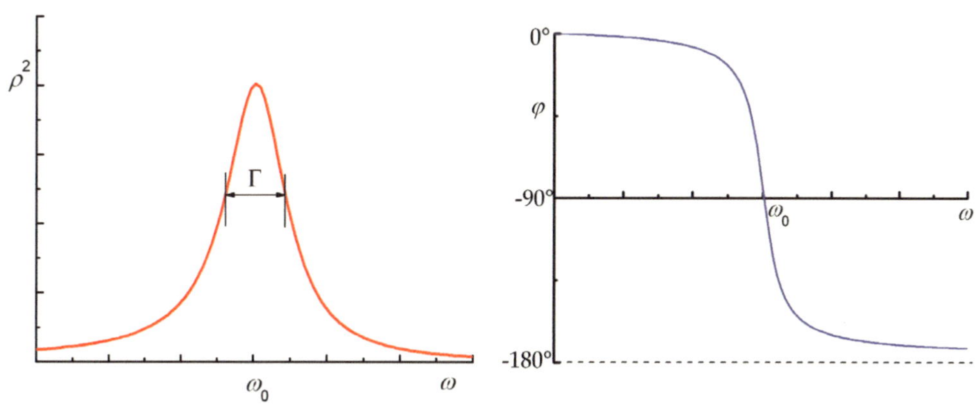

Fig. 10. (left) ρ^2 as a function of frequency; (right) phase shift as a function of frequency

$$\rho^2 = \frac{1}{m^2[(\omega^2 - \omega_0^2)^2 + \Gamma^2\omega^2]} \tag{13}$$

$$\tan\varphi = -\frac{\Gamma\omega}{(\omega_0^2 - \omega^2)} \tag{14}$$

The phase shift can be expressed as a function of the quality factor, $Q = \omega_0/\Gamma$, of the spring. This is a dimensionless factor that describes the degree of damping of an oscillator. In general, Q is defined as the ratio between the energy stored in the oscillator and the energy dissipated in a cycle. A high Q means a low energy loss during the lever oscillation with respect to the one stored in the system. Using Q the phase shift can be expressed as:

$$\tan\varphi = -\frac{m\omega\omega_0}{Q(k - m\omega^2)} \tag{15}$$

So far we are referring to a lever vibrating in the free space. When the tip is brought close to the sample surface, its oscillation regime changes due to the tip-sample interactions. Magonov in 1997 (Magonov et al., 1997) studied experimentally how the amplitude and phase of the cantilever oscillation vary according to the tip-sample distance. If we vibrate the tip in the free space at its resonance frequency, as shown in the figure above, the phase angle is 90° and the amplitude is at its maximum value. When the tip starts to interact with the sample surface, experiencing attractive forces, the resonance peak shifts towards lower frequencies and the phase angle at ω_0 becomes larger than 90°. Decreasing the distance between the tip and the sample, then increasing the repulsive interaction, the resonance peak shifts towards higher frequencies and the phase angle becomes smaller than 90°. Fig. 11 elucidates this behaviour.

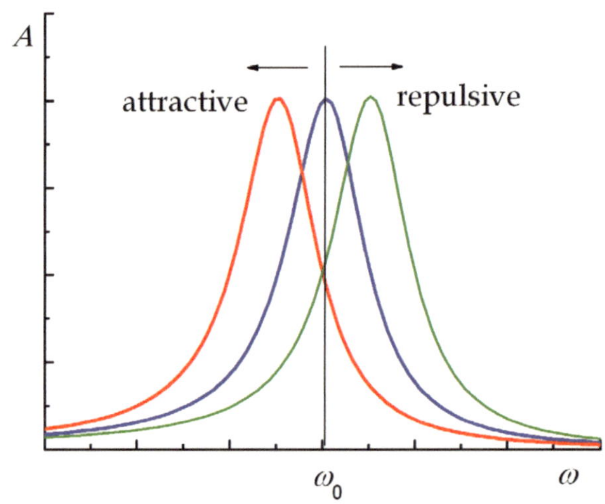

Fig. 11. Variation of the amplitude curves vs. frequency as a function of the forces between the tip and the sample. The cantilever resonance frequency in the free space (blue line) is lowered (red line) or increased (green line) when attractive or repulsive forces, respectively, are present.

In a first approximation the consequence of the tip-sample interaction is to change the elastic constant of the cantilever to a new effective value:

$$k_{eff} = k + \sigma \tag{16}$$

Where σ represents the sum of the derivatives of the external forces acting on the tip:

$$\sigma = \sum_i \frac{\partial F_i}{\partial z} \tag{17}$$

In this formula, z represents the relative displacement between the tip and the sample. Then the phase angle φ, can be expressed through the relationship:

$$\tan(\varphi) = -\frac{m\omega\omega_0}{Q(k+\sigma-m\omega^2)} \tag{18}$$

This expression is useful to relate the phase to the oscillation frequency.

To quantitatively describe the cantilever movement when the oscillating tip approaches the sample surfaces we need to go back to the expression for the damped harmonic oscillator, introducing new terms. When the tip hits the sample, it experiences van der Waals forces, but if the sample is soft and has viscoelastic properties, as often happens with polymers and biological materials, there is also a dissipation of part of the energy stored in the oscillator through the sample, then a viscous damping has to be taken into account. The cantilever motion can then be described through the following equation:

$$m\frac{d^2x}{dt^2} = -kx - c\frac{dx}{dt} + F + F_{ts} + F_v \tag{19}$$

where F_v represents the viscous response of the sample to the tip movement and is given by:

$$F_v = -\eta\sqrt{R\delta}\frac{dz}{dt} \tag{20}$$

where η is the sample viscosity, R is the tip radius and δ the sample deformation. In this model the sample is characterized by its elastic and viscosity coefficients. Interaction forces, as previously described, can be described by the modified DMT mechanics that takes into account adhesion forces:

$$F_{ts} = \begin{cases} F_{vdW} = -\dfrac{HR}{6z^2}, & z > a_0 \\ F_{DTM} = \dfrac{4E^*\sqrt{R}}{3-3v_S^2}(a_0 - z)^{\frac{3}{2}} - \dfrac{HR}{6a_0}, & z \le a_0 \end{cases} \tag{21}$$

Analogously, if capillary forces are not negligible, a further term has to be added to the force expression.

3.4 Spectroscopy mode in dynamic AFM mode: Phase vs. distance curves

Garcia and colleagues (Garcia & Perez, 2002; Tamayo & Garcia, 1996, 1997) numerically approached the problem of the cantilever motion, obtaining a trend for the phase of the oscillation as a function of the distance between the tip and the sample. In Fig. 12 experimental results are reported (only the approach curve is shown). For large separations ($z > 60$ nm) the phase is 90°, as expected, and no appreciable shifts are observed. When the tip gets closer to the sample surface, an increase of the phase is observed. There, the interaction potential is dominated by attractive forces. The positive gradient of the force shifts the cantilever resonance frequency to lower values. This, in turn, shifts the phase upwards. While approaching closer to the surface, when in the tip-sample interaction repulsive contributions dominate, the phase shift decreases with decreasing separation due to the negative gradient of the interaction force.

Phase vs. distance curves are particularly useful for the information they can provide on the energy dissipated in the sample, helping in assessing the visco-elastic properties of the material.

In Fig.12, the difference between the tip interacting with a hard surface, mica, and a soft polymeric one, polypropylene, is shown. Three major differences between the mica and the PP curves are observed.

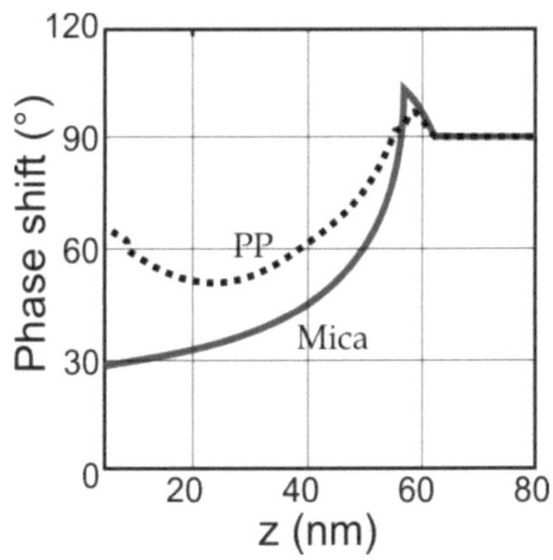

Fig. 12. Phase vs. distance curves for a hard material (solid line) and a soft one (dashed line)

1. The transition between non-contact and intermittent contact produces a sudden decrease of the phase for mica, while in the polymer there is a smooth variation.
2. The phase shift between the starting and final position is larger for mica than for polymer.
3. The polymer also shows an increase of the phase for tip–sample equilibrium separations smaller than 20 nm.

These results underline the complex behavior of phase shifts in dynamic force microscopy where elastic and inelastic processes alike may be involved. Cleveland and his colleagues (Cleveland et al., 1998) studied a model for the interaction in terms of power dissipated by the cantilever. At equilibrium, the average energy that is supplied to the cantilever must be equal to the average energy that is dissipated by the cantilever itself and by the tip during a cycle. Cleveland splits the power dissipated in two parts:

$$P_{in} = P_0 + P_{tip} \tag{22}$$

where P_{in} is the average power provided to the lever, P_0 is the power dissipated by the body of the lever in air and can be modeled by viscous damping, while P_{tip} takes into account all the possible dissipations due to the interaction between tip and sample. P_{in} and P_0 can be calculated and this leads to an expression for the power dissipated by the tip as a function of the phase φ when the cantilever oscillates close to its resonance frequency:

$$P_{tip} = \frac{1}{2}\frac{kA^2\omega_0}{Q}\left[\left(\frac{A_0}{A}\right)\sin\varphi - 1\right] \tag{23}$$

where A_0 is the oscillation amplitude in the free space.

4. Applications to biological samples

4.1 Single Molecule Force Spectroscopy

During recent years single molecule force spectroscopy (SMFS) methods have been developed to perform mechanical experiments with single molecules on generic surfaces under ambient conditions and within liquid electrolytes. Single molecule experiments allow the precise measurement of inter- and intra-molecular forces, providing the experimental platform for understanding, at a molecular level, adhesion and de-adhesion processes. In SMFS experiments force is applied to molecules by stretching them between the sample surface and the tip of an AFM cantilever featuring a typical spring constant in the 10-100 pN/nm range. Molecules are attached to the AFM tip by covalent bonding or through antibodies at specific sites (Zheng et al., 2011). Often, in order to address proteins specifically, force measurements are performed using functionalized tips.

Early experiments were concerned in the interaction between pairs molecules, such as the ligand-receptor pair biotin-avidin (Florin et al., 1994), complementary strands of DNA (Lee et al., 1994) or an antibody-antigen (Dammer et al., 1996).

The same technique allows for investigating the unfolding/refolding process in proteins and other biological molecules, such as force measurements on single molecules, and involves the rupture of single chemical bonds and the stretching of polymer chains. The first AFM-based SMFS unfolding and refolding experiments were performed in the 1997 (Rief et al., 1997) on the sarcomeric protein of striated muscle, the titin (Lange et al., 2006). In that paper, native titin molecules were allowed to adsorb from solution onto a gold surface. Then, the AFM tip was put in contact with the surface in order to allow the protein to adsorb onto the tip. Thereafter, upon the tip retraction, the force vs. distance curve is acquired, featuring a characteristic sawtooth profile consistent with the sequential unfolding of individual titin domains (Fig. 13).

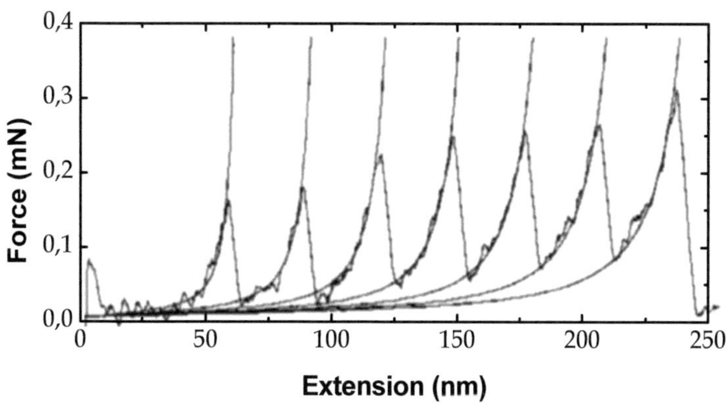

Fig. 13. Titin unfolding force-distance curve (courtesy of H. Gaub).

This force behaviour is well described by chain models: the worm-like chain (WLC) (Bustamante et al., 1994), the freely jointed chain (FJC) (Smith et al., 1992), and the freely rotating chain (FRC) (Hugel et al., 2005; Livadoru et al., 2003). When force is applied to the chain an initial uncoherent stretching is observed, until the "unfolding threshold force" is attained, and molecular bond breaks or a structural element unfolds, resulting in a sudden increase in contour length and in a drop in force (see Fig. 13). Another interesting feature of the curve force is the increasing in the peaks maxima with the increasing extension. This behavior is ascribed to the circumstance that the weakest domains unfold first and the strongest last.

Experiments were also performed on reconstituted and native membrane proteins (Kedrov et al., 2005; Oesterhelt et al., 2000; Preiner et al., 2007), and on cells (Alsteens et al., 2009). When the chain stretching starts by increasing the external force below the unfolding threshold, the energy barrier between the folded and unfolded states lowers, making the system more sensitive to other experimental parameters such as pulling speed (Dudko et al., 2008; Evans et al., 1997) or temperature (Schlierf & Rief, 2005). Under these conditions, a fluctuation can push the system to overcome the unfolding barrier, entering in the model as stochastic contributions.

Following the results of Evans & Ritchie in 1997, the unfolding force could not be considered as a constant parameter, because the faster the molecule is pulled, the higher the unfolding force measured (Fig. 14). Therefore, dynamic force spectroscopy was introduced, allowing for the varying of the pulling rate in order determine the unfolding potential. (Rief et al., 1998).

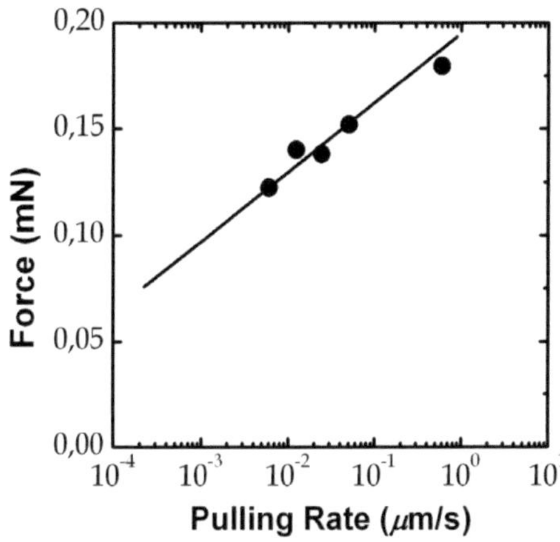

Fig. 14. Titin domain unfolding force versus pulling rate graph.

The maximum load rate allowed by a commercial AFM is determined by the characteristics of the scanner piezo tube which, at the same time, must fulfill the general requirement of the greatest accuracy in the positioning. Therefore, the range of the accessible loading rates for commercial AFM is in the range of 10-100 Hz, resulting in separation rates smaller than 50 μm/s.

This technique has been enhanced through the modification of a commercial AFM (Ptak et al., 2006) by adding an extra z piezo-actuator capable of up 50 kHz loading rates, components for data processing, and special AFM cantilevers featuring high resonance frequency, in the order of a few hundreds kHz, and low spring constant (<1N/m). In this experiment, the direct comparison between the signal driving, the additional piezo element, and the one resulting from the cantilever deflection, gives straightforward informations on the load applied on the sample, on the loading rate and on the adhesion strength (Fig. 15).

Thereafter, the "force clamp" was introduced. In this technique, the molecule is tethered between the tip and the surface and the deflection of the cantilever (i.e. the force) is kept

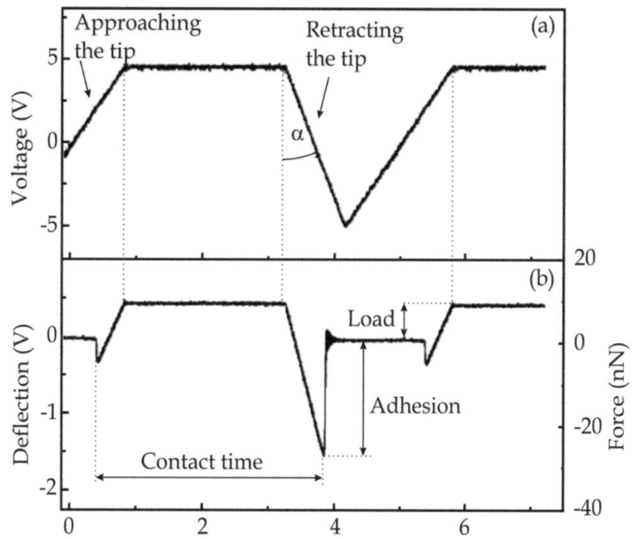

Fig. 15. Examples of input (a) and output (b) signals. Loading rate is proportional to cot(α). (b) Deflection of the cantilever during approach and retraction of the AFM tip. (Reprinted with permission from Ptak, Kappl, Butt, *APL*, Vol. 88, No. 26, Article Number: 263109. (2006). Copyright 2006, American Institute of Physics.)

constant during each experiment run. The separation increases when a domain unfolds, allowing for the measurement of the lifetime of a domain under a certain force-load value (Fig. 16) (Oberhauser et al., 2001).

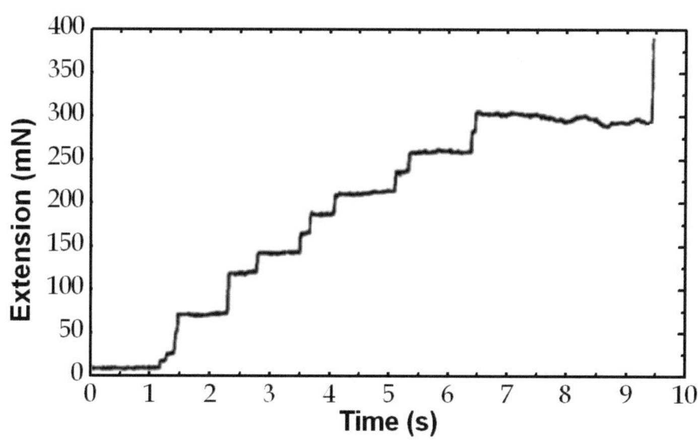

Fig. 16. Titin molecule tethered between tip and surface in a force clamp experiment.

In more recent experiments the force clamp technique has been useful for detecting the "catch" bond behavior between receptor-ligand pairs. Such bonds mediate cell adhesion and their dissociation occurs via modulating off-rates. Off-rates control how long receptor-ligand bonds last and how much force they withstand. The off-rates derived from forced dissociation data depend both on the force and on the history of force application (Kong et al., 2009; Marshall et al., 2005).

4.2 Viscoelasticity and adhesion forces measurements

Contact mode force spectroscopy is based on the detection of the static or quasi-static cantilever bending. Here, "quasi-static" has to be read in terms of relatively slow oscillations, well below the cantilever resonance. In such cases, informations are extracted directly and only from the cantilever deflection that "measures" the applied force.

Dynamic mode AFM allows one to go further into the tip-sample interaction details and, in addition, the oscillation amplitude and the phase shift can be recorded simultaneously, offering further "probes" for detecting different sample properties. In AFM dynamic modes, both non-contact (NC) and intermittent contact (IC), the cantilever is excited to oscillate at or close to the resonance; nevertheless, in the IC mode, oscillation amplitudes are larger, spanning between the attractive and the repulsive part of the tip-sample interaction potential. The result is an intermittent contact between the tip and the sample, whose dynamics are influenced by the sample properties such as adhesion, elasticity, or visco-elasticity. All these features can be revealed by the analysis of the amplitude-phase-distance (APD) curves, where the amplitude and the phase of the oscillating cantilever are recorded as a function of the average tip-sample distance.

Tamayo & Garcia (1996), proposed a model in which viscoelasticity and adhesion forces are considered as possible sources of phase contrast. When large oscillation amplitudes are used, the amplitude-distance curves feature discontinuities connected to the transition from the purely attractive regime, to the repulsive interaction occurring close to the lower inflection point of the vibrating cantilever (Anczykowski et al., 1996). In this work, a comparison between experimental results and computer simulations has been performed, considering different oscillatory regimes (above, below and at the resonance), and they display evidence of the role of contamination layers in the discontinuities in the phase curves. More recently Garcia & San Paulo (1999) demonstrated that the attractive to repulsive regime transition has a clear signature in the phase vs. distance curve, where a net phase φ jump from values above 90° to values below 90°, discriminates the two regimes: in the repulsive regime is always $\varphi < 90°$, whereas the attractive regime is characterized by phase shifts $\varphi > 90°$.

When oscillating a tip, the attractive–repulsive regime transition can be influenced by the presence of an adsorbed water film. This aspect has been faced by Zitzler et al. (2002), who measured the critical oscillation amplitude for which the attractive/repulsive transition occurs vs. the Relative Humidity (RH). They demonstrate that, for both hydrophilic tip and sample, there is an increasing in the critical amplitude when increasing the RH value. On the contrary, this effect is not observed in the case of hydrophobic sample/hydrophilic tip for which the critical amplitude is practically independent on RH. In practice, the forces connected to the cyclic formation-rupture of a capillary neck enter in the dynamical model with the role of an attractive contribution, affecting possible quantitative, or even qualitative, measurements of local adhesion, elastic or visco-elastic properties of the sample.

As a consequence, force spectroscopy experiments in dynamic AFM mode should be carried out under controlled humidity and temperature, in order to discriminate the effect of capillary condensation. These techniques are becoming relatively popular for high resolution imaging of soft materials in tapping mode (Thomson, 2005). Nevertheless, the effect of the water film, or of the inhomogeneities in the physical properties, can severely affect the topographic image of heterogeneous samples, featuring areas with different physical-chemical properties, as micro- or nano- composites. This influence can result in wrong height measurements and in some extreme cases even contrast inversion can be observed (Kopp-Marsaudon et al., 2000; Palacios-Lidon et al., 2010). The possibility to investigate physical and chemical properties at the nano-scale in some cases has been used to reveal structural features or conformational properties of complex molecules and aggregates. In literature a reduced number of papers devoted to this subject can be found, essentially devoted to polymers studies(Zhuang et al., 2005).

In a recent paper, phase vs. distance measurements in controlled humidity were exploited to investigate the structural properties of the class I Vmh-2 hydrophobin protein aggregates (Houmadi et al., 2011). In that paper, hydrophobin samples were obtained by Langmuir techniques under the form of monolayer and bilayers, and their properties were compared with those of the rod-like assemblies (rodlets) that are typical of class I hydrophobins. More in detail, Langmuir-Blodgett (LB) monolayers were transferred on hydrophilic SiO_2 substrates, whereas Langmuir-Schaefer (LS) monolayers were transferred on SiO_2 substrates made hydrophobic by a silane layer. The considered bilayers were made by subsequent depositions LB+LS and LS+LB. The analysis of the phase vs. distance curves (Fig. 17) revealed the viscoelastic behavior of the LB sample, ascribed to the large flexible β-loop typical of class I hydrophobins. This behavior was not observed in the remaining samples, included the rod-like self assemblies, allowing for the conclusions that the β-loop is directly involved in the aggregation process.

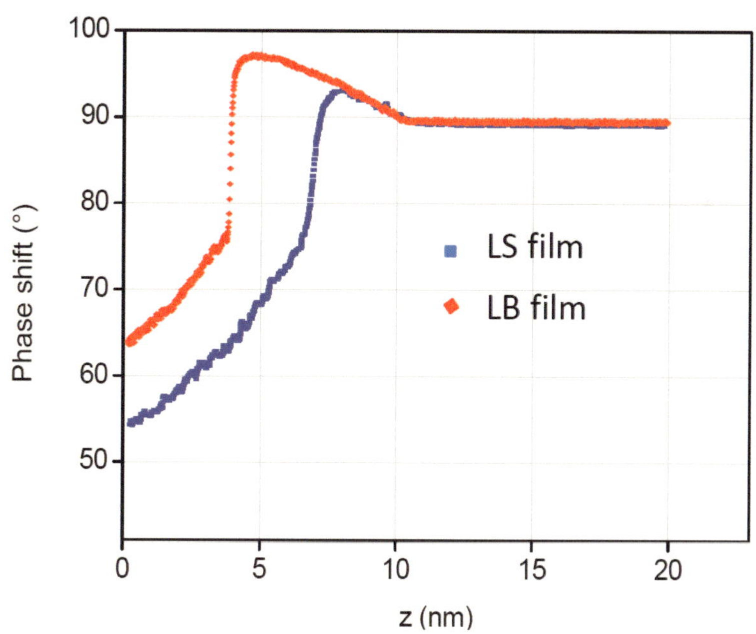

Fig. 17. Phase vs. tip-sample separation curves performed on Vmh-2 hydrophobin monolayers: LS film (blue dots) and LB film (red dots). The measurements were performed in dry atmosphere in order to eliminate capillary adhesion effects. The difference in the phase jump is due to the different viscoelastic properties between the LB ("more viscoelastic") and LS monolayers.

5. Conclusion

In this chapter, we have described various applications for the AFM, and have explained some possibilities offered by this technique for the samples investigation, in particular for biological matter. We have emphasized the possibility to obtain three-dimensional images with a high resolution in various AFM modes, but also discussed how to obtain information beyond the topography, including surface roughness, mechanical and other structural sample properties. Due to advantages that the AFM technique offers, it is extensively used in several domains, varying from physics, to biology, to polymer sciences. However, there is still room for improvement of this technique. Indeed, the development of commercial instruments continues, in order to increase the ability to acquire images in a much shorter time. This will play an important role in the field of bio-nanotechnology.

6. References

Alsteens, D.; Dupres, V.; Klotz, S. A.; Gaur, N. K.; Lipke, P. N. & Dufrêne, Y. F. (2009). Unfolding individual Als5p adhesion proteins on live cells. *ACS Nano*, Vol. 3, No. 7, pp. 1677–1682.

Anczykowski, B.; Kruger, D. & Fuchs, H. (1996). Cantilever dynamics in quasinoncontact force microscopy: Spectroscopic aspects. *PHYSICAL REVIEW B*, Vol. 53, No. 23, pp. 15485-15488

Baclayon, M.; Roos, W. H. & Wuite, G. J. L. (2010) Sampling Protein Form and Function with the Atomic Force Microscope. *MOLECULAR & CELLULAR PROTEOMICS*, Vol. 9, No. 8, pp. 1678-1688

Bhushan, B. (2003). *Handbook of Nanotechnology* (2nd Edition). Springer, ISBN 978-3-642-02524-2.

Binnig, G.; Quate, C. F. & Gerber, Ch. (1986). Atomic Force Microscope. *Phys. Rev. Lett.*, Vol. 56, 930

Bustamante, C.; Marko, J. F.; Siggia, E.D. & Smith, S. (1994). Entropic elasticity of lambda-phage DNA. *Science*, 1994, Vol. 265, pp. 1599-1600.

Butt, H.J.; Cappella, B. & Kappl, M. (2005). Force measurements with the atomic force microscope: Technique, interpretation and applications. *SURFACE SCIENCE REPORTS*, Vol. 59, pp. 1–152.

Cappella, B. & Dietler G. (1999). Force-distance curves by atomic force microscopy, *Surf. Sci. Rep.*, Vol. 34, No. 1-3, pp. 1-104.

Casuso, I.; Rico, F. & Scheuring, S. (2011) Biological AFM: where we come from - where we are - where we may go. *JOURNAL OF MOLECULAR RECOGNITION*, Vol. 24, No. 3, pp. 406-413

Cleveland, J.P.; Anczykowski, B.; Schmid, A.E. & Elings V.B. (1998). Energy dissipation in tapping-mode atomic force microscopy. *APPLIED PHYSICS LETTERS*, Vol.72, pp.2613-2615.

Cleveland, J.P.; Manne, S.; Bocek, D. & Hansma, P.K. (1993). A non-destructive method for determining the spring constant of cantilevers for scanning force microscopy. *REVIEW OF SCIENTIFIC INSTRUMENTS*, Vol. 64, No. 2, pp. 403-405.

Dammer, U.; Hegner, M.; Anselmetti, D.; Wagner, P.; Dreier, M.; Huber, W. & Güntherodt, H. J. (1996). Specific antigen/antibody interactions measured by force microscopy. *Biophys. J.*, Vol. 70, No. 5, pp. 2437–2441.

Dougan, L.; Feng, G.; Lu, H. & Fernandez, J. M. (2008). Solvent molecules bridge the mechanical unfolding transition state of a protein. *Proc. Natl. Acad. Sci. USA*, Vol. 105, pp. 3185-3190.

Dudko, O. K.; Hummer, G. & Szabo, A. (2008). Theory, analysis, and interpretation of single-molecule force spectroscopy experiments. *Proc. Natl. Acad. Sci. USA*, Vol. 105, pp. 15755-15760.

Evans, E. & Ritchie, K.; (1997). Dynamic strength of molecular adhesion bonds. *Biophys J*, Vol. 72, pp. 1541-1555.

Florin, E-L., Moy, V. T. & Gaub H. E. (1994). Adhesion forces between individual ligand-receptor pairs. *Science*, Vol. 264, pp. 415–417.

Garcia, R. & San Paulo, A. (1999). Attractive and repulsive tip-sample interaction regimes in tapping-mode atomic force microscopy. *PHYSICAL REVIEW B*, Vol. 60, No. 7, pp. 4961-4967

Garcia, R. & Perez, R. (2002). Dynamic atomic force microscopy methods. *SURFACE SCIENCE REPORTS*, Vol. 47, pp. 197-301.

Gauthier, M. & Tsukada, M. (1999). Theory of noncontact dissipation force microscopy. *Physical Review B*, Vol. 60, No. 16, pp. 11716-11722.

Gauthier, M.; Sasaki, N. & Tsukada, M. (2001). Dynamics of the cantilever in noncontact dynamic force microscopy: The steady-state approximation and beyond. *Physical Review B*, vol.64, pp. 085409.

Gauthier, M.; Pérez, R.; Arai, T.; Tomitori, M. & Tsukada, M. (2002). Interplay between Nonlinearity, Scan Speed, Damping, and Electronics in Frequency Modulation Atomic-Force Microscopy. *Physical Review Letters*, Vol. 89, No. 14, Article number 146104.

Giessibl, F. J. (1997). Forces and frequency shifts in atomic-resolution dynamic-force microscopy. *Physical Review B*, Vol. 56, No. 24, pp. 16010-16015.

Giessibl, F. J. & Bielefeldt, H. (2000). Physical interpretation of frequency-modulation atomic force microscopy, *PHYSICAL REVIEW B*, Vol. 61, No. 15, pp. 9968-9971

Hartmann, U. (n.d.). An Elementary Introduction to Atomic Force Microscopy and Related Methods. Jul. 10, 2011, <http://www.uni-saarland.de/fak7/hartmann/files/docs/pdf/download/IntroductionAfm.pdf>

Hong, J.W.; Park, S.I. & Khim, Z.G. (1999). Measurement of hardness, surface potential, and charge distribution with dynamic contact mode electrostatic force microscope. *Review of Scientific Instruments*, Vol. 70, No. 30, pp. 1735-1739.

Houmadi, S.; Rodriguez R. D.; Longobardi, S.; Giardina, P.; Fauré M. C.; Giocondo, M. & Lacaze, E. (2011). Self-assembly of hydrophobin protein rodlets studied with atomic force spectroscopy in dynamic mode. (In press on Langmuir, Manuscript Number: la2028093, DOI: http://dx.doi.org/10.1021/la2028093).

Hugel, T.; Rief, M.; Seitz, M.; Gaub, H. E. & Netz R. R. (2005). Highly stretched single polymers: atomic-force-microscope experiments versus ab-initio theory. *Phys Rev Lett*, Vol. 94 pp. 048301.

Hutter, J.L. & Bechhoefer, J. (1993). Calibration of atomic-force microscope tips. *REVIEW OF SCIENTIFIC INSTRUMENTS*, Vol. 64, No. 7, pp. 1868-1873.

Israelachvili, J. N. (1992), *Intermolecular and Surface Forces*. (2nd edition), Academic Press Inc, 978-0123751812.

Jarvis, M. R.; Pérez,R. & Payne, M. C. (2001). Can Atomic Force Microscopy Achieve Atomic Resolution in Contact Mode?. *Physical Review Letters*, vol. 86, No. 7, pp. 1287-1290.

Kedrov, A.; Krieg, M.; Ziegler, C.; Kuhlbrandt, W. & Muller, D. J. (2005). Locating ligand binding and activation of a single antiporter. *EMBO Rep*. Vol. 6, No. 7, pp. 668–674.

Kong, F.; Garcia, A. J.; Mould, A. P.; Humphries, M. J. & Zhu, C. (2009). Demonstration of catch bonds between an integrin and its ligand. *J. Cell Biol.*, Vol. 185, No. 7, pp. 1275–1284.

Kopp-Marsaudon, S.; Leclere, P.; Dubourg, F.; et al. (2000). Quantitative measurement of the mechanical contribution to tapping-mode atomic force microscopy images of soft materials. *LANGMUIR*, Vol. 16, No. 22, pp. 8432-8437

Lange, S.; Ehler, E. & Gautel, M. (2006). From A to Z and back? Multicompartment proteins in the sarcomere, *TRENDS IN CELL BIOLOGY*, Vol. 16, No. 1, pp. 11-18

Lee, G.U.; Chrisey, L.A. & Colton, R. J. (1994). Direct measurements of the forces between complementary strands of DNA. *Science*, Vol. 266, pp. 771–773.

Livadaru, L.; Netz, R. R. & Kreuzer, H. J. (2003). Stretching response of discrete semiflexible polymers. *Macromolecules*, Vol. 36, pp. 3732-3714.

Magonov, S.N.; Elings, V. & Whangbo, M.H. (1997). Phase imaging and stiffness in tapping mode atomic force microscopy. *SURFACE SCIENCE*, Vol. 375, pp. L385-L391.

Marshall, B. T.; Sarangapani, K. K.; Lou, J. H.; McEver, R. P. & Zhu, C. (2005). Force history dependence of receptor-ligand dissociation. *Biophys. J.*, Vol. 88, No. 2, pp. 1458–1466.

Martìnez, N. F. & Garcìa, R. (2006). Measuring phase shifts and energy dissipation with amplitude modulation atomic force microscopy. *Nanotechnology*, Vol. 17, pp. S167–S172.

Matsushige, K.; Kobayashi, K.; Yamada, H.; Itoh, H. & Horiuchi, T. (2001). *Review of Scientific Instruments*, vol. 72, No. 12, pp. 4383-4387.

Mueller, S.A.; Mueller, D.J. & Engel, A. (2011) Assessing the structure and function of single biomolecules with scanning transmission electron and atomic force microscopes. *MICRON*, Vol. 42, No. 2, pp. 186-195

Oberhauser, A. F.; Hansma, P. K.; Carrion-Vazquez, M. & Fernandez, J. M. (2001). Stepwise unfolding of titin under force-clamp atomic force microscopy. *Proc. Natl. Acad. Sci. USA*, Vol. 98, No. 2, pp. 468–472.

Oesterhelt, F.; Oesterhelt, D.; Pfeiffer, M.; Engel, A.; Gaub, H. E. & Mueller D. J. (2000). Unfolding pathways of individual bacteriorhodopsins. *Science*, Vol. 288, No. 5463, pp. 143–146.

Palacios-Lidon, E.; Munuera, C.; Ocal, C.; et al. (2010). Contrast inversion in non-contact Dynamic Scanning Force Microscopy: What is high and what is low? *ULTRAMICROSCOPY*, Vol. 110, No. 7, pp. 789-800

Preiner, J.; Janovjak, H.; Rankl, C.; Knaus, H.; Cisneros, D. A.; Kedrov, A.; Kienberger, F.; Muller, D. J. & Hinterdorfer, P. (2007). Free energy of membrane protein unfolding derived from single-molecule force measurements. *Biophys. J.*, Vol. 93, No. 3, pp. 930–937.

Ptak, A.; Kappl, M. & Butt, H. J. (2006). Modified atomic force microscope for high-rate dynamic force spectroscopy. *APPLIED PHYSICS LETTERS*, Vol. 88, No. 26, Article Number: 263109.

Qin, Y.; Kim, Y.; Zhang, L.; Lee, S.-M.; Yang, R.B.; Pan, A.L.; Mathwig, K.; Alexe, M.; Gösele, U. & Knez, M. (2010). Preparation and elastic properties of helical nanotubes obtained by atomic layer deposition with carbon nanocoils as templates. *SMALL*, Vol. 6, No. 8, pp. 910–914.

Radic, T. M.; Svetlicic, V.; Zutic, V.; et al. (2011). Seawater at the nanoscale: marine gel imaged by atomic force microscopy. *JOURNAL OF MOLECULAR RECOGNITION*, Vol. 24, No. 3, pp.: 397-405

Rief, M.; Gautel, M.; Oesterhelt, F.; Fernandez, J. M. & Gaub, H. E. (1997). Reversible Unfolding of Individual Titin Immunoglobulin Domains by AFM, *Science*, Vol. 16, pp. 1109-1112.

Rief, M.; Gautel, M.; Schemmel, A. & Gaub, H. E. (1998). The mechanical stability of immunoglobulin and fibronectin III domains in the muscle protein titin measured by atomic force microscopy. *Biophys. J.*, Vol. 75, pp. 3008–3014.

Schlierf, M. & Rief, M. (2005). Temperature softening of a protein in singlemolecule experiments. *J Mol Biol*, Vol. 354, pp. 497-503.

Seo, Y. & Jhe, W. (2008). Atomic force microscopy and spectroscopy. *REPORTS ON PROGRESS IN PHYSICS*, Vol. 71, 016101, 24pp.

Smith, S. B.; Finzi, L. & Bustamante, C. (1992). Direct mechanical measurements of the elasticity of single DNA-molecules by using magnetic beads. *Science*, Vol. 258, pp. 1122-1126.Wright, C. J.; Shah, M. K.; Powell, L. C.; et al. (2010). Application of AFM From Microbial Cell to Biofilm. *SCANNING* Vol. 32, No. 3, pp. 134-149

Smith, J.F.; Knowles, T.P.J.; Dobson, C.M.; MacPhee, C.E. & Welland, M.E. (2006). Characterization of the nanoscale properties of individual amyloid fibrils. *PROCEEDINGS OF THE NATIONAL ACADEMY OF SCIENCES OF THE UNITED STATES OF AMERICA*, Vol. 103, No. 44, pp. 15806-15811.

Tamayo, J. & Garcia, R. (1996). Deformation, contact time, and phase contrast in tapping mode scanning force microscopy. *LANGMUIR*, Vol. 12, No. 18, pp. 4430-4435

Tamayo, J. & Garcia, R. (1997). Effects of elastic and inelastic interactions on phase contrast images in tapping-mode scanning force microscopy. *APPLIED PHYSICS LETTERS*, Vol. 71, No. 16, pp. 2394-2396.

Thomson, N. H. (2005). The substructure of immunoglobulin G resolved to 25 kDa using amplitude modulation AFM in air. *ULTRAMICROSCOPY*, Vol. 105, No. 1-4 pp. 103-110

Torii, A.; Sasaki, M.; Hane, K. & Okuma, S. (1996). A method for determining the spring constant of cantilevers for atomic force microscopy. *MEASUREMENT SCIENCE & TECHNOLOGY*, Vol. 7, No. 2, pp. 179-184.

Wu, B.; Heidelberg, A. & Boland, J.J. (2005). Mechanical properties of ultrahigh-strength gold nanowires. *NATURE MATERIALS*, Vol. 4, No. 7, pp.525-529.

Wu, B.; Heidelberg, A.; Boland, J.J; Sader J.E.; Sun, X.M. & Li, Y.D. (2006). Microstructure-hardened silver nanowires. *NANOLETTERS*, Vol. 6, No. 3, pp. 468-472.

Yang, L.; Van der Werf, K.O.; Fitié, C.F.C.; Bennink, M.L.; Dijkstra, P.J.; Feijen, J. (2008). Mechanical properties of native and cross-linked type I collagen fibrils. *BIOPHYSICAL JOURNAL*, Vol. 94, No. 6, pp. 2204–2211

Zheng, P.; Cao, Y. & Li H. (2011). Title: Facile Method of Constructing Polyproteins for Single-Molecule Force Spectroscopy Studies. *LANGMUIR*, Vol. 27, No. 10, pp. 5713-5718.

Zhuang, W.; Ecker, C.; Metselaar, G. A.; et al. (2005). SFM characterization of poly(isocyanodipeptide) single polymer chains in controlled environments: Effect of tip adhesion and chain swelling. *MACROMOLECULES*, Vol. 38, No. 2, pp. 473-480

Zitzler, L.; Herminghaus, S. & Mugele, F. (2002). Capillary forces in tapping mode atomic force microscopy. *PHYSICAL REVIEW B*, Vol. 66, No. 15, Article Number: 155436

2

Artifacts in Atomic Force Microscopy of Biological Samples

E. Ukraintsev, A. Kromka, H. Kozak, Z. Remeš and B. Rezek
Institute of Physics, Academy of Sciences of the Czech Republic, Prague 6
Czech Republic

1. Introduction

Atomic force microscopy (AFM) is a frequently used method applicable also to biological studies due to its capability of measuring in native environment. Sharp Si, Si_3N_4 or C (carbon nanotubes, diamond, diamond coated) cantilevers repeatedly touching a sample are used in this method as sensitive probes. It is possible to control the interaction between the tip and the sample in order to make less invasive measurements or, conversely, to modify the sample. However, AFM images often contain features which are not present on the sample in reality, but are a direct result of the measurements itself. Such structures or features are denoted as artifacts. The artifacts arise from various reasons. Some of them can be avoided during measurements, other ones are inherent. The artifacts shown in this chapter are divided into several categories based on the part of AFM which is responsible for them. Examples of many artifacts are presented and their reasons are explained. This chapter will be helpful for AFM users who observe strange effects, presumably related to the AFM technique, but do not know their reason. This chapter can also answer questions about the validity of imaged features as well as their accuracy.

AFM is commonly used in biology to study proteins (Ukraintsev et al., 2007; Ukraintsev et al., 2009; Rezek et al., 2009), peptides (Kransnoslobodtsev et al., 2005), DNA (Hamon et al., 2007), tissues (Graham et al., 2010), viruses (Kuznetsov et al., 2003) and living cells (H. X. You & Yu, 1999). The possibility to perform such measurements *in situ* is the main advantage of this technique. On the other hand, optical and electron microscopy are not so often used for environmental examination in biology. More specifically, optical and fluorescence microscopy are usually applied on stained cells because non-stained cells are practically transparent. Scanning electron microscope (SEM) measurements are usually performed on dried samples with a few exceptions employing environmental SEM (Hawkes, 1988). Another important factor is high spatial resolution; for example, AFM can resolve individual spread molecules of ssDNA (Klinov et al., 2009) or even the morphology of upright dsDNA molecules (Rezek et al., 2006; Rezek, Shin & Nebel, 2007).

In situ studies of soft matter in a solution can reveal different protein conformations, which are not detectable in air (Moreno-Herrero et al., 2004; Rezek et al. 2009, Rezek et al., 2011). Besides, cell morphology in an air and in a medium is different. However, AFM imaging in solution can be difficult since the tip-molecule interaction must be tuned to be weaker than the molecule-substrate interaction. Van der Waals forces are screened off in liquids, making molecule-substrate interaction weak. For this reason, the AFM imaging technique must be chosen in a way which minimizes intrusiveness (Moreno-Herrero et al., 2004).

Using AFM, one can *in situ* study not only cell morphology (H. X. You & Yu, 1999), but also mechanical properties of an individual cell (Müller et al., 2009). For cells attached to a sample, the force scanning method produces high-resolution spatial modulus map (Darling, 2011) and force spectroscopy reveals elastic and adhesive properties of cell membranes (Volle et al., 2008; Kwon et al., 2009). For cells attached to a cantilever, the force spectroscopy method gives information about the interaction between cells and diamond surfaces with different chemistry (Chong et al., 2007; Helenius et al., 2008).

However, AFM has some disadvantages. First of all, it is an invasive method (H. X. You & Yu, 1999) with a few exceptions like non-contact mode measurements in vacuum (Maeda et al., 1999) and in solution (Checco et al., 2006). Usually, the influence is undesirable, but in some cases it has potential. For example, AFM tip can be used as a "nanoscalpel" or "nanoneedle" for surgery of biological cells (Beard, Gordeev & Guy, 2011) or as a spade to remove proteins from the surface (Rezek et al., 2009). Second, it is a slow method. Nevertheless, it is possible to measure much faster using either a small cantilever (Crampton et al., 2007), spiral scanning (Mahmood & Moheimani, 2009) or contact mode (CM) with controllable force (Choi et al., 2008). Third, an AFM image does not always correspond to real morphology (Ricci & Braga, 2003; Su, Wei & Liu, 2005; Eaton, 2010). One can even postulate that the real morphology always differs from the shape measured by AFM.

AFM is a commonly used technique with applications in different fields; however, only a limited number of articles has been published about AFM artifacts (Kühle et al., 1998; Ricci & Braga, 2003; Velegol et al., 2003; Eaton, 2010; Rezek, Ukraintsev & Kromka, 2011). A number of artifacts related to the study of cells were analyzed and the influence of different AFM parameters (scanning mode, tip shape) on measured parameters (cellular volume, particles height) were discussed (Wu et al., 2008). Artificially formed features can be divided into four categories: artifacts related to the tip, to the scanner, to the sample and artifacts related to the interaction between them.

For example, an artifact related to the tip is the so-called double tip (Y. Chen et al., 2004). A finite tip radius and a pyramidal tip shape causes broadening of the image (Klinov et al., 2009) and shadows around high objects, respectively (Velegol et al., 2003). Piezoelectric creep, thermal drift and scanner-induced vibrations are the main problems associated with the scanner. They can cause the distortion of the image and additional noise (Mahmood & Moheimani, 2009). The sample can be too sticky or too soft. In this case, artifacts due to multiple probe-sample contact points occur (Morton et al., 2003; Sokolov, 2007). AFM image of a charged nonconductive sample may not correspond to topography. Charge distribution measured by AFM may not fully correspond to the real charge distribution (Lambert, Guthmann & Saint-Jean, 2003). A "contrast reversal" artifact is an effect which causes wrong height determination. It is related to the tip-sample interaction and to the switching between attractive and repulsive regimes (Kühle et al., 1998).

Sometimes researchers publish articles about new effects and others claim that the observed effects are due to AFM-related artifacts. For example, Azulay and coworkers presented the "comprehensive local probe study", which, from their point of view, "clearly indicates that the dominant transport route in undoped μc-Si:H is in the disordered tissue that encapsulates the crystallites columns"(Azulay et al., 2005). But Vetushka and coworkers state "a completely different origin of the higher conductivity at the grain boundaries, namely, the influence of surface oxidation induced by the tip when the sample is positively biased" (Vetushka et al., 2010), i.e. they claim that the observed effect is due to local anodic oxidation, an artifact of Kelvin force microscopy. Another example is the work of Sajanlal and Pradeep, who presented the formation of well-aligned gold nanotriangle arrays on indium tin oxide substrate (Sajanlal & Pradeep, 2008), but Diao with coworkers state that those triangles are tip artifacts (Diao et al., 2009). The purpose of this chapter is to show different AFM artifacts relevant to biological specimens, explain their reasons and present a way to avoid them.

2. Materials and methods

In this section our biological specimens as well as measurement methods are described. As our substrate of choice for biological studies, we use the monocrystalline diamond (MCD) as it is a well-defined and chemically tailorable substrate (Rezek et al., 2007; Rezek et al., 2010).

Bulk MCD was prepared by chemical vapor deposition and chemically cleaned in acids (97.5 % H_2SO_4 + 99 % powder KNO_3) at 200 °C for 30 minutes. The surface was then hydrogenated at 800 °C for 10 minutes. The MCD substrates were lithographically processed to generate alternating H- and O-terminated patterns of 30 μm widths. A positive photoresist ma-P 1215 (micro resist technology GmbH, Germany) was applied. The MCD substrates with lithography mask were treated in oxygen radio-frequency plasma (300W power, 1 minute process time) to oxidize the surface and hence to generate hydrophilic patterns. Then the sample was rinsed in acetone, photoresist stripper, de-ionized water and dried by air blow. This process minimized possible surface contamination (Rezek & Nebel, 2006). The H-/O-termination quality was proved by a scanning electron microscope (SEM; JEOL Superprobe 733). Electronic measurements detected a surface conductivity of 10^{-5} S/sq on the H-terminated surfaces (Kozak et al., 2009). Surfaces with O-termination were highly resistive. The H-terminated diamond is a hydrophobic surface, contact angle ~ 80-100 °. The O-terminated diamond has hydrophilic properties, contact angle ~ 5-20 °.

Proteins were adsorbed on the MCD substrates from 15 % fetal bovine serum (FBS) solution (PAA) in McCoy's 5A medium with stable Glutamine without Phenolred (BioConcept). The serum contains several proteins, usually bovine serum albumin, fibronectin and vitronectin. FBS is heat inactivated (56 °C, 25 min) to destroy the immunological components yet to preserve the proteins. 1 ml of this solution was applied on a diamond surface and in-situ measurements were performed. All experiments were performed at room temperature.

As a common bio-linker, an organosilane layer containing amino-groups (-NH2) was adsorbed on the O-terminated MCD substrate from an organosilane coupling agent N-(6-aminohexyl) aminopropyl trimethoxysilane (AHAPS, purchased in liquid form from Gelest Ltd., UK). The O-terminated MCD substrate was placed into a quartz cuvette filled with AHAPS solution diluted with absolute toluene and left in dark (chemical method) or exposed to UV irradiation (photochemical method) (Kozak et al., 2011). Both methods of MCD amination were performed for 3 hours at room temperature.

AFM devices from diverse manufactures were used for the study of proteins and the AHAPS layers on the diamond substrates. NTEGRA (NT-MDT) and Dimension (Veeco) AFMs were used, both in tapping mode (TM) and CM as well as in air and in solution. Different types of cantilevers were used, ranging from very soft (k = 0.06 N/m) to very stiff (k = 120 N/m). Ordinary cantilevers with tips $r \sim 10$ nm (Multi75Al, NSG, CSG) and ultrasharp tips (NTI Europe) were employed.

A critical parameter for any AFM measurement is a set point. The set point value (*SP*) is the ratio between the amplitude of oscillation during scanning A and the free oscillation amplitude near the surface A_0. Let us define also SP_0 value as a maximal value of *SP* which can be used to observe a normal ("true") image. If $SP > SP_0$, cantilever will lose contact. The *SP* value for noninvasive measurements should be slightly lower than SP_0. If $SP \ll SP_0$ and $SP \sim 0$, the force applied to the tip makes this TM similar to CM in terms of applied force. Set point ratio of $SP \sim 0.5$-0.7 was used for most of the images unless specified otherwise. Usually, for studies in solution, the SP_0 value for Multi75Al tip is around $SP_0 = 0.6$-0.7, and $SP = 0.5$ gives stable image for several scans. After several scans, the tip can adsorb something from the surface (Eaton, 2010) and it is sometimes necessary to recalibrate the frequency and amplitude.

The amplitude of oscillations in TM AFM is another critical parameter. In our study the oscillation amplitude of 20-800 nm was used in air. The amplitude in liquid was in the range of 10-60 nm. Feedback gain (*FB*) is an important parameter which shows how quickly piezotube will respond to changes in morphology. It is different in different AFM systems. Usually in Ntegra AFM with P8 controller $FB \sim 0.1$-0.5 was used to prevent oscillations and achieve fast enough piezo-response. The scanned area was as large as 135x135 μm for an overall image to check homogeneity. Small 1x1 μm areas were scanned for high resolution images.

3. Examples of different artifacts

In this section, a comprehensive set of experiments illustrating diverse AFM artifacts is provided. The main focus is on organic and biological specimens on diamond substrates. Hard substrates such as diamond can increase the possibility of damaging the tip, yet they provide sound background with tailorable properties for studies of molecules and organic specimens in general (Rezek, Ukraintsev & Kromka, 2011; Hoffmann et al., 2011).

3.1 Artifacts related to the AFM tip and cantilever

The first group of artifacts concerns tip-related artifacts. The AFM sensing element is a cantilever (a flexible plate with force constant k, resonance frequency f and quality factor Q) with a tip (a sharp probe usually with pyramidal shape and radius of curvature r). All these parameters (k, f, Q and r) are important for the measurements.

An AFM image is inherently a convolution of the imaging tip shape with the actual shape of the imaged object (Allen et al., 1992). Thus, whatever is the sharpness of the tip, one will observe broadening of the sample features. For example, the diameter of DNA (2 nm) (Klinov et al., 2009) is much smaller than the tip radius r for ordinary cantilevers (10 nm). Obtained width values are 10-20 nm for dsDNA studied by normal tip (Maeda, Matsumoto & Kawai, 1999), and 2.7-5 nm studied by ultrasharp tips (Klinov et al., 2009).

There is a possibility how to get round this problem, for example one can use ultrasharp tips with tip radii ~ 1-2 nm. Some of those tips are based on carbon nanotubes (CNT) (Zhao et al., 2008) or diamond-like needles grown under conditions of low temperature plasma in an atmosphere of $CH_4/H_2O/Ar$ (Klinov et al., 2009). So far, ultrasharp tips cannot be used in liquid because of their relatively high force constant. The development of soft and sharp tips for imaging in liquid would be very helpful for this type of structural analysis (Moreno-Herrero et al., 2004). It was shown that it is possible to make soft AFM cantilevers with a CNT tip, which may be used in liquid, but only measurements in air in CM were shown as an example (I.-C. Chen et al., 2007). There are sharp silicon probes attached to silicon nitride cantilevers which can operate in liquid, but their tip radii r are still about 8 nm (Shekhawat et al., 2009).

Another possibility to reduce the effect of broadening of the picture is to apply the deconvolution procedure to the image (Moreno-Herrero et al., 2004). The deconvolution procedure estimates the tip shape and subtracts it from the topography image. There are two methods how to do it: using a test sample or "blind" mathematical restoration (Keller & Franke, 1993; Dongmo, 1996). Measurements of test samples are useful to estimate real tip shape; however, the resolution of this method is limited to the radius of "tips" on the grating. Moreover, during such procedure, the AFM tip can be damaged. There are several ways how to perform "blind" mathematical restoration. A dilation and an erosion are non-linear mathematical operations consisting in an over- and under-estimation of the tip broadening effect which may help to estimate real object's shape. There were made several attempts to use other deconvolution methods and find the "real" topography based on AFM image, for example using similar angle identification (Bernardes-Filho & Assis, 2005).

In addition to a simple feature broadening, the AFM tip may have several protrusions, the so called double tip. Double tip is a common effect; it can be divided into double-probe, double-tip, triple-tip effect and so on (Y. Chen et al., 2004). We illustrate this effect on the AHAPS layer on the MCD surface. A periodical structure with the period of $d = 20$ nm on AHAPS layer on MCD was observed using a new (out of the box) cantilever (Multi75Al, Budget Sensors) (see Fig. 1a). The first step to check if this is an artifact or not is to change the scan size and scan position. On two consecutive scans, the same periodical structure was observed. But the next scan on a different place without additional changes in scanning parameters didn't reveal periodical structure (see Fig. 1c). Ultrasharp tips were used on both NTEGRA and Veeco AFM to check that indeed there is no periodical structure. Therefore, we can claim that such periodical structure is an artifact. Hence, even if AFM image is clear and detailed, it still can be an artifact due to tip properties.

For instance, if the tip is damaged during approach or during measurements, one will see repetitive features on the image. The AFM image may contain many triangular features, pairs of features with similar shape and ghost objects (Y. Chen et al., 2004). During approach on AFM in TM, the amplitude of the cantilever oscillations may became zero or much lower than the Set Point value (see Fig. 2). The curves were obtained using NTEGRA AFM, but this effect occurs generally. After approach, the piezotube oscillations can cause oscillations. The optimization of scanning parameters (feedback value, close loop parameters) usually takes some time and during this process oscillations are a common effect. The AFM tip can be damaged during this process.

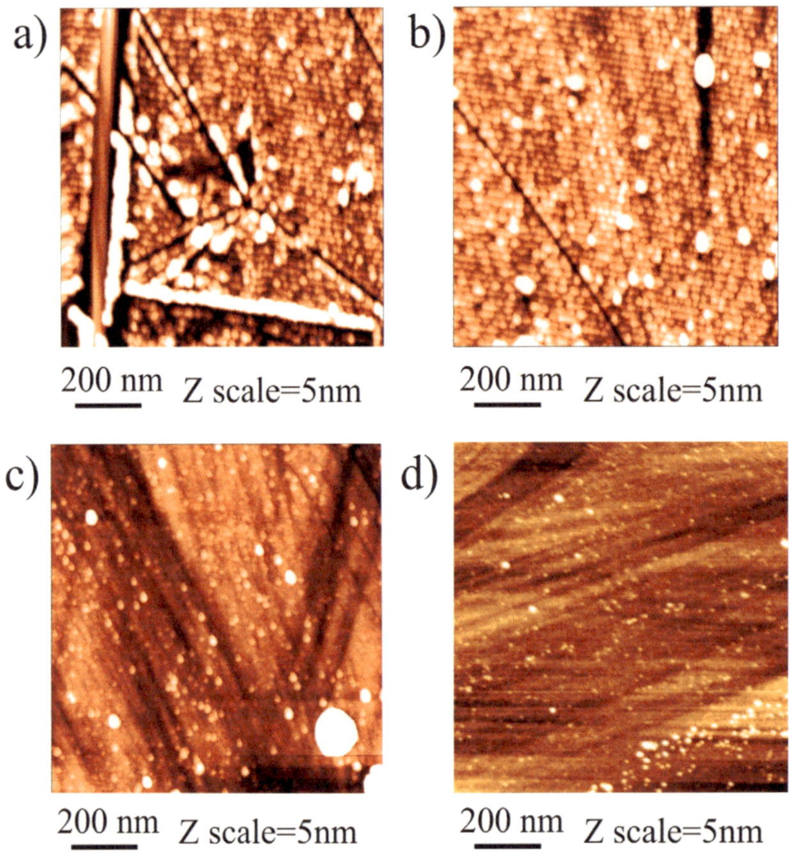

Fig. 1. AFM topography images (1×1 μm) of organosilane layer chemically grafted to O-terminated monocrystalline diamond using Multi75Al cantilever and NTEGRA AFM a) just after approach, b) second scan, c) after several scans; d) The image of AHAPS layer on MCD using ultrasharp tip and Veeco AFM. The images were observed in air.

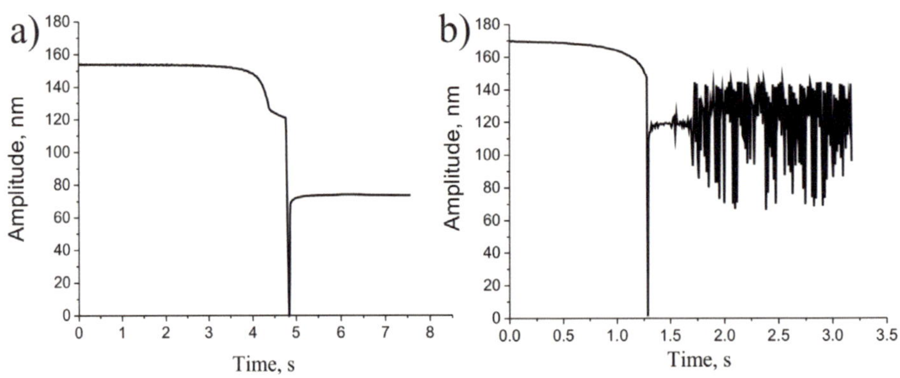

Fig. 2. a) The approach curve on NTEGRA AFM. The amplitude became zero when cantilever touched the surface. b) After the approach, oscillations occur.

During scanning, the tip can be changed due to collisions on the surface. If a scan size is large or the tip does not get blunt after such event, there is no visible change in the topography image, yet big changes in the phase image and even change of the sign can be observed as shown in Fig. 3.

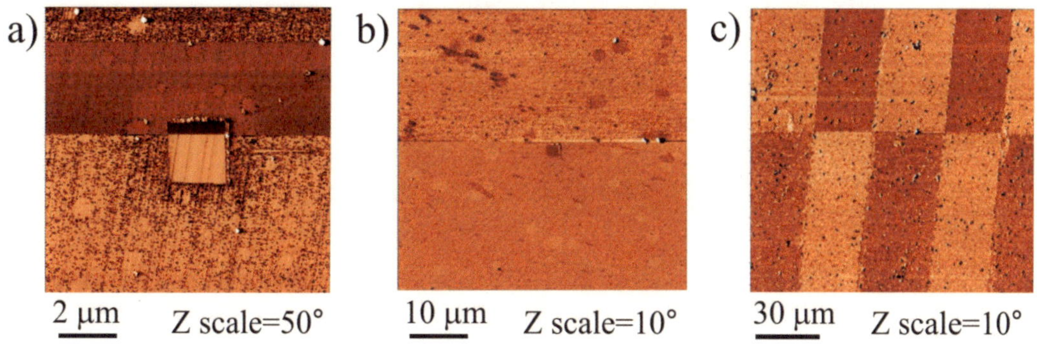

Fig. 3. Phase images were obtained in air and in solution. There is one collision event in each image, which causes some changes in phase image. a) The central 2x2 μm area was nanoshaved in CM. During 10x10 μm overscan in TM, the phase contrast changed to the opposite. b) A large scan (50x50 μm) was made to check the homogeneity of the FBS on MCD sample. At some point, the tip hit something on the surface and the phase contrast changed. c) A 135x135 μm scan was made across 30 μm wide hydrogen and oxygen stripes on MCD with FBS layer on it. At some point, the phase contrast was reversed.

If the object height is large enough (for example bigger than several micrometers) the artifact due to the pyramidal shape of the tip can appear as shadows (Hyde, Jacobs & Compton, 2004). Shadows in AFM images of *Escherichia coli* K12 were oriented in parallel lines 27° from the direction of the cantilever tilt, regardless of the scan direction (Velegol et al., 2003). As another example, Fig. 4 shows the topography of organosilane layer photochemically grafted to O-terminated monocrystalline diamond. This image contains shadows near each cluster and the globular particles do not look like a sphere but rather like facetted crystals.

We have seen that feature width is inherently overestimated in AFM. On the other hand, the height of the soft object is usually underestimated (Rezek, Shin & Nebel, 2007) (0.7 nm for dsDNA (Maeda et al., 1999) or 1.2 nm (Klinov et al., 2009)). This is due to the force which is applied to the sample even during TM scanning which results in elastic deformation of DNA and other polymers.

The force constant of the cantilever *k* plays an important role in such studies. For stiffer cantilevers, the compression is usually higher than for a soft cantilever. For the lower set point value (*SP*), the compression is usually higher than for higher *SP*. In non-contact AFM, lower forces are applied than in TM. This method gives better vertical resolution than TM AFM (Maeda et al., 1999). In this method, AFM tip oscillates near the surface and "the cantilever/tip ensemble is maintained within the long range tail of the attractive surface potential" (Checco et al., 2006). Nowadays, jumping mode AFM (Moreno-Herrero et al., 2004) can be used to diminish the problem of sample deformation and achieve even better resolution, for example DNA height of 1.7 ± 0.3 nm was measured (Moreno-Herrero et al., 2004). This value is close to the real one (2 nm), yet it is still smaller. In jumping mode AFM, force versus distance curves

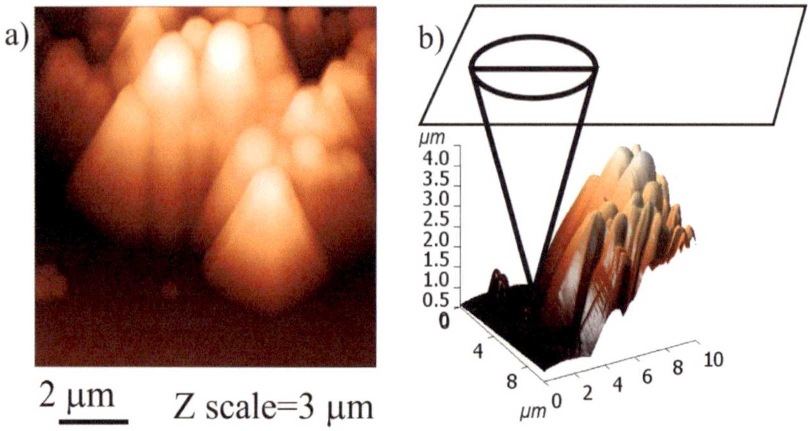

Fig. 4. a) The two-dimensional AFM topography image (10×10 µm) of the organosilane layer photochemically grafted to O-terminated monocrystalline diamond. b) The same data presented in a 3D image with a model of AFM cantilever with finite cone angle. Images were made using Multi75Al cantilever and NTEGRA AFM.

are measured at each point of the measured surface with applied feedback in between. The non-contact and jumping mode AFM are technically challenging methods compared to tapping or contact mode and they are not generally applicable.

Also the resonance frequency of a cantilever plays an important role. Steps in height up to 200 nm were observed at a boundary of H- and O-terminated surface region on MCD in solution using soft cantilever CSG01 oscillated in TM (Rezek, Ukraintsev & Kromka, 2011). This is artificial as the real height difference between H/O surfaces is smaller than 1 nm, as obtained using medium frequency NSG01 and Multi75Al cantilevers both in CM and TM. For soft cantilevers such as CSG01 (which properly work in air at $f \sim 30$ kHz), measurements in TM in solution are not recommended, because oscillations at the first resonance frequency become small and measurements at the second harmonic may cause incorrect height determination (Rezek, Ukraintsev & Kromka, 2011). Nevertheless, higher harmonic oscillations can be used to study stiffness of the material (Sahin et al., 2004).

New AFM methods may appear in the nearest future, for example based on very soft polymers cantilevers (Calleja et al., 2005). True atomic resolution imaging of muscovite mica by a frequency modulated atomic force microscopy (FM-AFM) in water was recently demonstrated using a low noise all-fiber interferometer as the deflection sensor (Rasool et al., 2010). Contact resonance imaging (force modulation mode) is applicable for measurements of soft and sticky samples because in this case the sample and the tip are always in contact (Wadu-Mesthrige et al., 2001). Combined frequency and force modulated AFM was suggested but not tried yet (Solares, 2007). Amplitude-modulated AFM was used to determine the morphology and the compositional variations of surfaces in their natural environment. The applications in biology, polymer science and microelectronics illustrate the potential of phase-imaging force microscopy for nanoscale analysis (Rezek, Shin & Nebel, 2007; Garfias-García et al., 2008). Magnetic alternating current mode AFM is a very useful tool to image soft materials in liquid, where ordinary TM is difficult due to poor resonance of the cantilever (Ge et al., 2007).

The AFM cantilever can cause artifacts not only due to the tip shape and force constant, but also due to the lever shape and the laser light position. For example, experimental results show a nonlinear relationship between the detected signal and the actual deflection of the cantilever. There are at least 8 possible sources for such nonlinearity, but the main reason of this artifact is the shape and intensity distribution of the laser light hitting the detector (Thormann, Pettersson & Claesson, 2009). If the sample is too bright and the laser spot is too large, one can see laser interference patterns. Readjusting the laser or using low-coherence laser sources can reduce this problem (Eaton, 2010).

3.2 Artifacts related to the AFM scanner

Another group of artifacts are those related to a piezoscanner that moves the tip and/or sample in AFM. The piezoelectric creep and edge overshoot are well known artifacts (Eaton, 2010). For example, just after setting up the tip, adjusting laser, setting sample and approaching the tip to the sample one can observe piezoelectric creep and changes in the oscillation amplitude of the tip. The best way to solve these problems is to wait for some time (up to 30 min). After reaching equilibrium, these problems will disappear in most cases. These problems are smaller, yet still present with an active closed loop scanner system. The active closed loop can also cause additional piezotube oscillations, which sometimes makes it impossible to use high feedback values needed for efficiently fast tracking of the surface and therefore should be switched off in such cases.

In the case of a commonly employed piezotube scanner, the piezoelectric tube bends during measurements and this effect causes z position error and introduces background curvatures. For flat samples, it is easy to correctly subtract the artificial curvatures, but for patterned structures with big feature height it is very difficult. The degree of curvature depends not only on the scan size and scan speed, but also on the x-y offset and z position, making it impossible to correctly subtract the curvatures.

When scanning feedback gains are too high, the scanner can oscillate, generating high-frequency periodic noise in the image, which is sometimes even audible. This may occur throughout the image or be localized to features with steep slopes. However, when feedback gains are too low, the tip cannot track the surface, and features will be distorted and smeared out (Ricci & Braga, 2003). With a low feedback value and quite fast scanning speed, the piezotube response in z-direction is not fast enough, so one can observe different object shapes depending on the scanning directions.

An example of this problem is presented in Fig. 5, where oscillations at $FB = 0.1$ are clearly visible and they do not disappear after lowering the feedback to $FB = 0.05$. At this value, the feedback does not follow the surface well. So, no good image can be obtained in such conditions.

Other effects from this group are thermal drift and hysteresis nonlinearity. AFM with three dimensional feedback control loops are able to minimize these effects, but these feedback controllers are often not designed to deal with the highly resonant nature of an AFM's scanner nor with the cross coupling between various axes (Mahmood & Moheimani, 2009). The extension of features in the scanning direction, positive and negative noise peaks, positive and negative sticking effects were presented (Gainutdinov & Arutyunov, 2001).

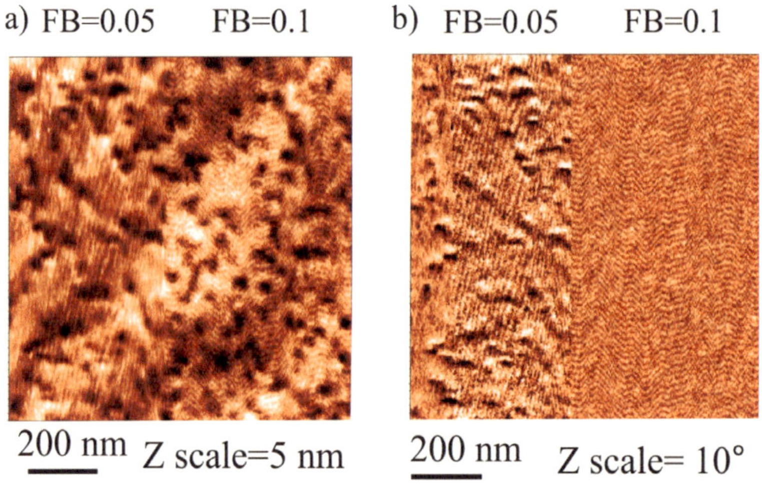

Fig. 5. The AFM image of FBS layer on MCD surface was measured in solution using Multi75Al cantilever and NTEGRA AFM. At $FB = 0.1$ oscillations, which reduce the quality of the image, were clearly visible. At $FB = 0.05$, the oscillations were still visible, and features were distorted. a) topography image, b) phase image.

3.3 Artifacts related to the sample properties

The next group of artifacts appears due to specific properties of a sample. For example, the sample can drift in one direction even if it is well attached to the sample holder. If this drift is due to thermal drift, one can reduce it by stabilizing the temperature. If it is due to other reasons, one can scan faster (Eaton, 2010). If the sample is too sticky or too soft, an artifact due to multiple probe-sample contact points occurs (Morton et al., 2003; Sokolov, 2007). This problem is highly relevant to cells studies (Touhami, Jericho & Beveridge, 2004). If the sample is nonconductive, electrostatic charge can be stored and generate long range forces, and the AFM image may thus not correspond to topography (Miyazaki et al., 2000; Verveniotis et al., 2011). Note that the charge distribution measured by Kelvin force microscopy may not fully correspond to real charge distribution (Lambert et al., 2003).

3.4 Artifacts related to the interaction between tip and sample

The last group of artifacts is related to the interaction between the tip and the sample. One such well known effect is a "contrast reversal" artifact. The artifact occurs when the oscillating cantilever is in an attractive or repulsive mode according to the dominant tip-sample interaction mechanism (Kühle et al., 1998). If during scanning the attractive regime switches to the repulsive one, one can observe strange contours, unexpected height shifts, and changes of the apparent resolution in the acquired images. Contact resonance imaging (Wadu-Mesthrige et al., 2001) may be a good replacement of TM in that case.

Fig. 6 shows an example of the "contrast reversal" artifact during measurements of the AHAPS layer on the MCD surface using an ultrasharp AFM tip and very soft tapping mode ($SP = 0.98*SP_0$). It looks like there are holes in the center of high objects. The explanation is that in some points AFM changes regimes from a repulsive to an attractive one and then back again to the repulsive. SP/SP_0 may differ across the sample, thus this artifact may be present only in one part of the image.

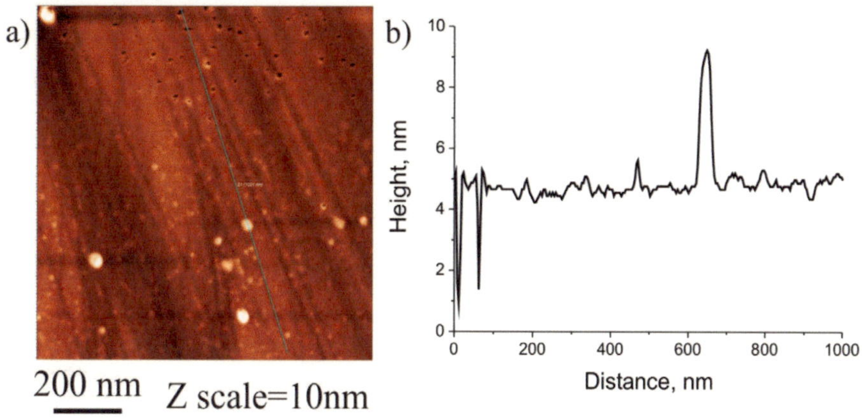

Fig. 6. The AFM image of the AHAPS layer on the MCD surface was observed using ultrasharp tip (NTI Europe). At the top part, a lot of 5 nm objects look like 2-3 nm holes on the surface. This artifact is due changes from repulsive to attractive regime. Usually conditions for such effect are $SP_0 \sim SP$, $SP > SP_0$ at the top part and $SP < SP_0$ at the bottom part.

Another example was observed on the FBS layer on the MCD sample as shown in Fig. 7. At the bottom part of the image, SP is setup a bit lower than SP_0 and the measurements are carried out well. But during scanning the tip accumulates something on it and gets heavier. This causes a drop in A_0 and, therefore, increase in SP. Fig. 7 illustrates the frequency shift and amplitude reduction during measurements. ΔA indicates a drop in the amplitude of oscillations due to the adsorption of material on the tip. Eventually, SP will be equal to SP_0 and the image will be blurred or even the intermittent contact will be lost. This means that one should change SP value correspondingly to changes in SP_0. Such artifacts may appear during AFM study especially when measurements are performed in liquid, where the Q factor of cantilever is low, and on a soft material, which can be easily removed by tip.

The contamination of the tip should be considered in nanoshaving experiments that are used to study thin protein layers (Rezek et al., 2009). In this method, the first image is made in CM, and second is made in TM. One can obtain deep hole in the layer, but if one continues to perform TM measurements, one will observe the reduction of the layer height due to the tapping mode nanoshaving (Rezek, Ukraintsev & Kromka, 2011). If the bottom surface is not very clean or well visible, one can think that the hole is filled with proteins. Only larger overview scan can prove that there is no such effect. The easiest way to define the layer height and get around this problem with tapping mode nanoshaving is to use a single TM scan with small amplitude.

The tapping mode nanoshaving effect can also cause blurring of the topography images. In this case, the layer is partially destroyed during the first TM scan. Tapping mode nanoshaving leads to blurring of the image.

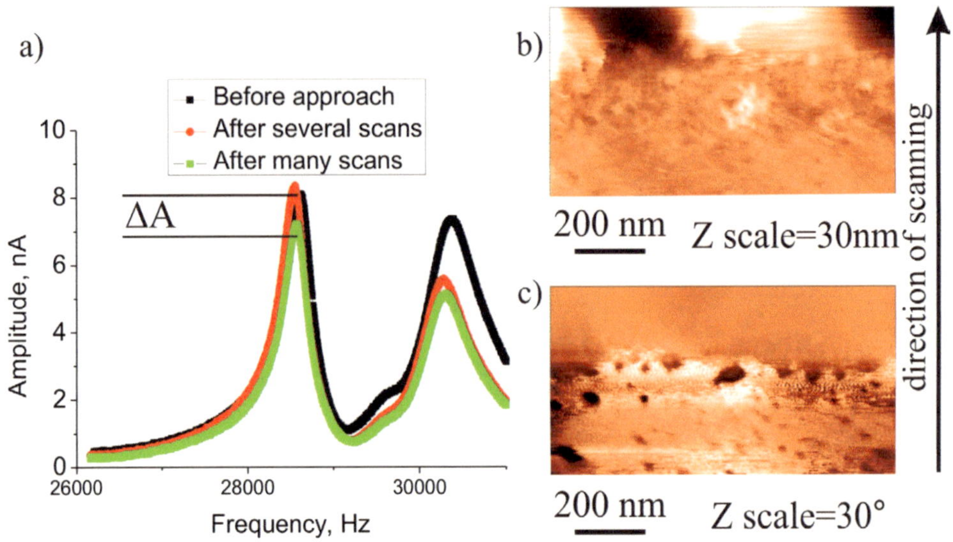

Fig. 7. The AFM morphology of the FBS layer on the MCD surface measured in solution. a) The frequency shift for Multi75Al cantilever for imaging in solution. b) The tip loses contact due to decrease of the oscillation amplitude. The topography image became blurred. c) The phase image illustrates loss of the phase contrast after *SP* reached SP_0.

It is important to make a high resolution scan before making an overall image, because the tip may become blunt during the overall scan. The proper order is to make two high resolution images on two differently terminated areas of the surface, for example H- and O-terminated diamond surfaces, and then to define the position of those areas using the big scan. The problem which usually occurs is that it is not possible to find out where the initial fine scans were made, because positions of fine scans were too close to the H/O-border.

A very important factor for AFM imaging is also the tip surface chemistry. If the tip is not contaminated, but its surface has been modified, for example with liquid 1-decanethiol, this tip will not work the same way as a clean tip (Nie & McIntyre, 2007). It was observed that in this case the cantilever amplitude will be unstable and AFM images become noisy. Under such conditions, the amplitude change is dominated by the extra forces induced by the active material loaded on the tip apex, overwhelming the amplitude change caused by the geometry of the sample surface, thus resulting in noise in the image (Nie & McIntyre, 2007).

In the case of tip contaminations, the debris particles may partially detach from the tip and may, during the scan, leave a diagonal track in the image that could be erroneously interpreted as a surface feature. Telltale signs in this case are the instabilities and glitches in the feedback signal that occur each time the particle is dragged along (Ricci & Braga, 2003). Fig. 8 is an example of such an effect. In this case, dust particles were moved on the MCD surface during a measurement. Traces of the dragged particles are clearly visible in the phase image (Fig. 8b), in contrast to the topography image (Fig. 8a).

During scanning one should keep *SP* a bit lower than SP_0 to obtain good contact and to avoid high pressure. However, SP_0 is often much lower than the recommended *SP* value for scanning, e.g. with ultrasharp tips (NTI Europe) and NTEGRA AFM (NT-MDT) $SP_0 = 0.7$, while recommended $SP=0.95$. This means that one may break the ultrasharp tip even before getting the image. Blurred images may be obtained with high *SP* ratio (recommended value) and increased interaction between the tip and the surface will break the very tip.

One of the most important artifacts related to the tip-sample interaction is the flying tip artifact (Eaton, 2010). In this case feedback loop is not adequate and the tip does not follow the sample. Usually increase in feedback gain, reduction of the setpoint and slowing down the scanning speed helps. But if not, which is often the case when studying soft protein layers, there is no straightforward solution to this problem. For example, it is difficult to obtain good images of weakly attached cells due to the interaction between the cantilever and the cell membrane. Another possible reason for bad contact between the tip and the sample is the electrostatic interaction between the tip and the sample, as in the case of charged sample which was described in Section 3.3. The grounding of both conductive and not conductive samples usually helps in this situation.

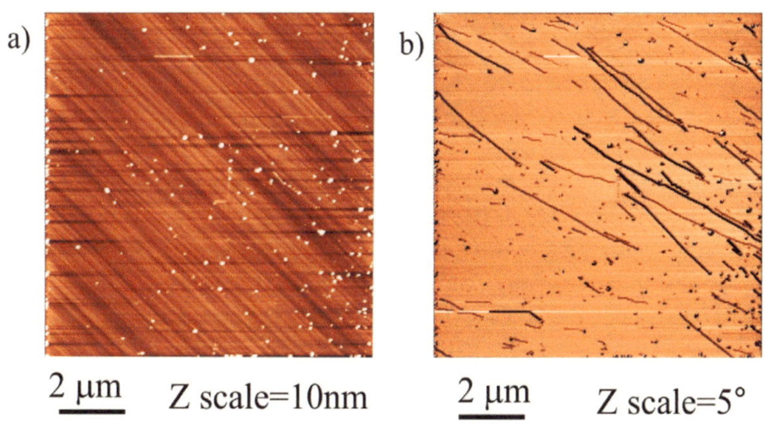

Fig. 8. AFM micrographs of the MCD surface which was dirty after insufficient cleaning. The dust was easily moveable on the surface when using TM AFM. The linear traces are observed in the phase image (b), but not in the topography (a).

3.5 Artifact related to the interference between specimen grating and the scan raster of AFM

AFM artifacts can usually be easily discerned in the images. But sometimes, well looking AFM images may be an artifact as described in Section 3.1. For example, there are a lot of publications where images with moiré - interference between the specimen grating and the scan raster of the AFM (Su et al., 2005) - are shown and ways to remove them are proposed. In this case, the topography image does not correspond to the real topography of the specimen.

An example of the moiré artifact on MCD surface measured in TM is presented in Fig. 9. This wave structure is not reproducible and direction of waves depends on scanning parameters. Therefore we can claim that this wave structure is the moiré artifact, not topography.

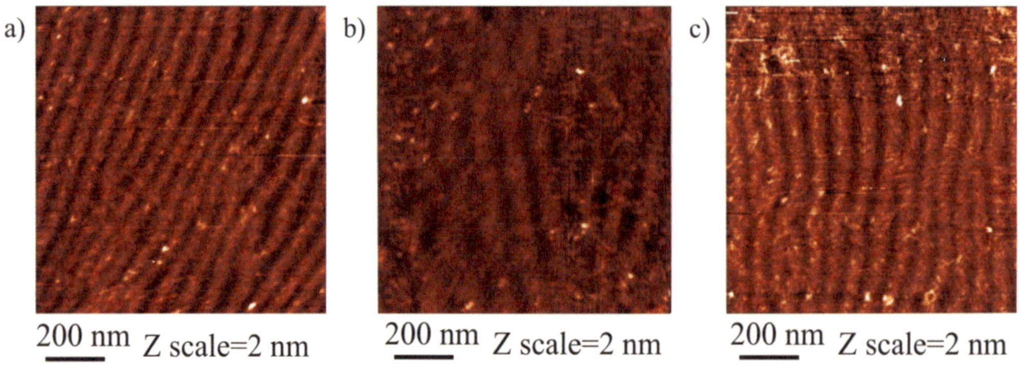

Fig. 9. The MCD surface was measured in TM with different parameters: a) horizontal scan, $SP = 0.69$, b) vertical scan, $SP = 0.69$, c) horizontal scan, $SP = 0.65$.

4. Solutions how to avoid artifacts

4.1 The tip shape

The first step which one has to do to obtain an AFM image is to approach the surface. This initial tip approach to the surface must be performed carefully as the approach itself may "crash" the tip even in TM (see Fig. 10). One should monitor the amplitude during the approach so that it does not drop to 0. Fig. 2a shows that the amplitude of oscillations drops to 0 and the tip runs into surface. If the feedback value is too high during approach, the tip will start to oscillate immediately after the tip-surface interaction is established ("contact") (see Fig. 2b). These oscillations may damage the tip as well. After these events, the tip may become blunt. To estimate the force which is applied to the tip during this event one can assume that the tip is pressed against the surface for a distance equal to the expected amplitude. Roughly, this corresponds to the force which is applied to the cantilever during CM measurements, for example ~ 600 nN for NSG cantilevers.

The best way to get around this problem is to do approach in several steps. First, a fast approach with $SP > SP_0$ for ordinary cantilevers should be made. At this point, the cantilever starts to feel the surface and its resonance frequency changes. After that, it is important to make tuning of the cantilever again to adjust the amplitude and the frequency and make the approach again with the required set point and lower speed. "Safe" approach on the final step is also recommended. Contact mode approach is not recommended because of the high force applied to the tip during the first contact with the surface.

Tapping and contact mode approaches can be less destructive for the tip if used in the "safe" approach mode, where, after each step made by the motor, the piezotube extends and shrinks back and the software checks whether the set point is already reached and only after that if it is safe for the tip the next step by motor is made. Although safe for the cantilever, it is a slow way to approach the surface.

Just after approach, the tip quality is usually the best and therefore the image quality is the best one can achieve with that particular tip. This means that the first images are the most important. For example the result presented in Fig. 1 shows a periodical structure which was observed during the first and the second scan. That periodical structure maybe a real

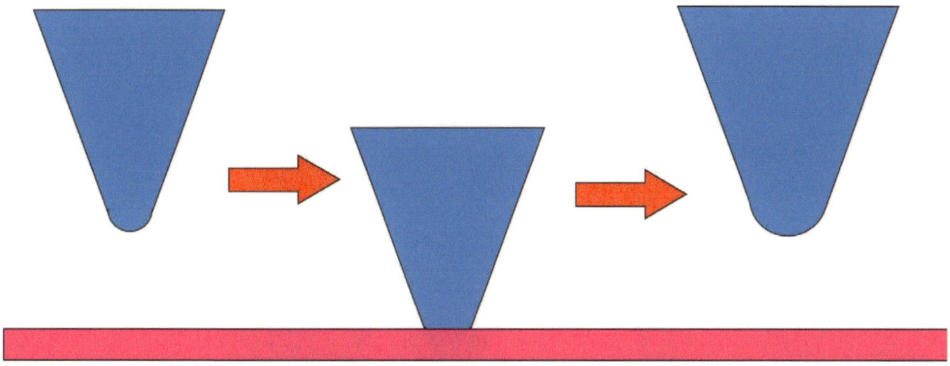

Fig. 10. A cantilever runs into surface during approach. After such event, it may get blunt.

structure and the tip has a needle which was extremely sharp (Fig. 11a), but since neither an ultrasharp tip (NTI Europe) using both NTEGRA AFM (Fig. 1c) and Veeco (Fig. 1d) later could see such periodicity, nor SEM resolved it, we have concluded that this structure is an artifact. Moreover, features are not duplicated and this periodical structure disappears after several images yet the quality of the image was quite good, i.e. the tip did not become blunt. Therefore, this should be an artifact of the tip. The main reason for such an effect may be a doubled tip, but this case is more complicated, because there is a fine scratch (black line) which is not doubled and there are also a lot of AHAPS clusters which are single. Fig. 11 illustrates two models which may explain such a periodical structure with single line. There is small probability that the Multi75Al tip was very sharp ($r \sim 1$ nm) after approach and there is such fine structure on the surface. After several scans tip radius increased up to $r \sim 10$ nm and periodical structure became invisible. But most probable version is that the tip had two or four sharp needles and after several scans one of them broke.

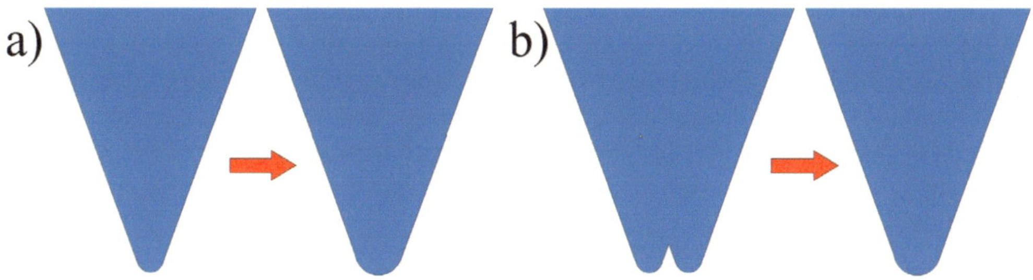

Fig. 11. Two models which may explain periodical structure. a) The extremely sharp tip Multi75Al (nominal $r = 10$ nm) which is sharper than ultrasharp tip (NTI Europe) became normal tip ($r = 10$ nm) after collision. b) Double tip with sharp needles became normal tip after collision.

The changes in tip's shape during measurements are very important to watch for. In Fig. 3 several phase images with collision event are shown. Such events usually occur when the tip hits a high object on the surface. When the tip hits such an object, it can become blunt or it can dislodge particles from the surface and these particles can become attached to the tip (see Fig. 12). In this case, the mass of the tip is changed, leading to changes in the resonance frequency and the amplitude of oscillation and, therefore, to offset in phase shift between

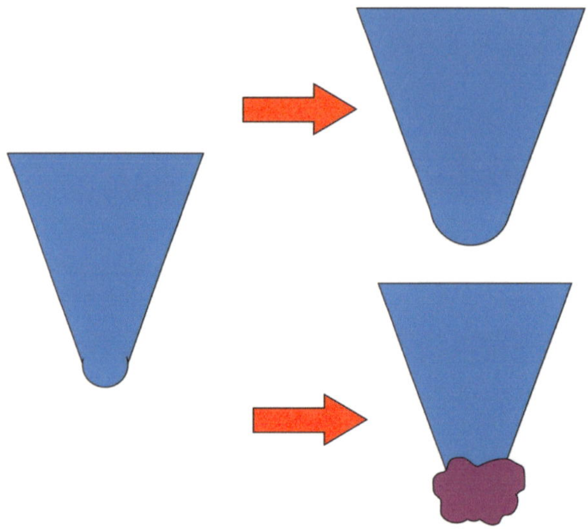

Fig. 12. Collision events, which can cause some changes in phase image. The tip can become blunt or it can dislodge particles from the surface and these particles can become attached to the tip.

the resonance and the driving frequency. The changes in surface chemistry (e.g. protein on the tip surface) can cause different energy dissipation and, therefore, changes in the interaction between the tip and the surface and also changes in the phase contrast. On the other hand, if the tip does not become too blunt or the scan size is quite large, no changes in the topography will be observed. There is no general way how to avoid such effects, except for avoiding sharp and/or hard features on the surface.

As the changes in the tip shape can cause reversal of phase contrast, it is important to somehow calibrate the phase contrast during the measurements. One possibility is to have standard objects on the surface with a known phase contrast and measure them before and after the experiment. Another possibility is to use the same tip for all the measurements and monitor whether the tip has changed or not. Since after several images the tip may get blunt, it is better to use diamond or diamond-coated tips to control the phase contrast.

If the tip radius is bigger than the object size, the tip broadening effect will occur and the object will appear bigger than it is (Rezek, Ukraintsev & Kromka, 2011). If the tip radius is bigger than the distance between the nearest objects, the tip does not touch the substrate between the two objects and, therefore, both objects will be recognized as one bigger object (see Fig. 13b). The best way to avoid this artifact is to use sharp tips with *r* lower than the average feature size.

There are two main parameters which define the tip shape: the tip radius and the pyramidal or cone shape of the tip. The latter can cause an artifact when the tip is used to study high features. In Fig. 4, one can see that different objects have similar edge shape. The main reason for this effect is the tip shape, i.e. that the cone angle is not zero (see Fig. 14). The best way to avoid this artifact is to use cantilever with aspect ratio as high as possible.

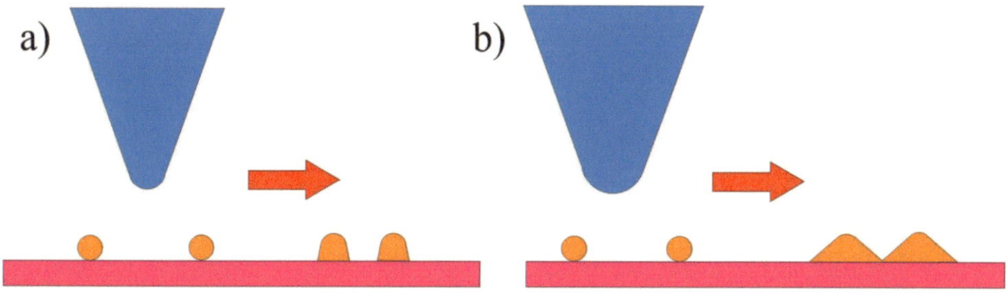

Fig. 13. The tip broadening artifact. a) In case of a sharp tip, the object looks slightly bigger than it is. b) In case of a blunt tip, objects look much bigger than they are, two objects may look like one large object.

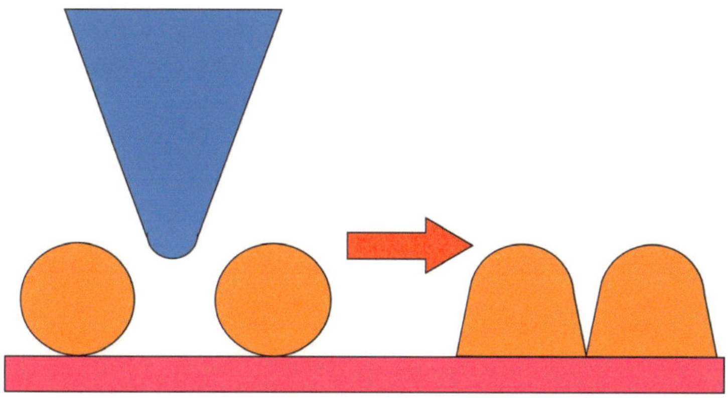

Fig. 14. The model which described edge shape of high object based on tip shape and finite cone angle.

It was shown that the tip is the main part of AFM which determines the image quality. The sharpest tips are seemingly the best choice, but they have a lot of disadvantages in particular for studies in biology. For example, most of the ultrasharp tips cannot work in solution. NP-STT cantilevers from Veeco have a second, shorter tip which is also formed near the main tip as result of the process used to create the sharper tip. Those cantilevers should be used for flat samples otherwise one will observe "twins" due to the double tip. For ultrasharp cantilevers used in air in tapping mode, $SP \sim 0.95$ should be used, so the strength of the tip does not allow any measurements in CM and nanoshaving. If the radius of the tip is small, it can penetrate the cell membrane (H. You, 2000). Ultrasharp cantilevers are also significantly more expensive than ordinary cantilevers.

There are several methods that can improve the tip quality. When the tip is hit against the surface it becomes better (sharper, without double tip, etc.) or it will become blunt. The easiest way to hit the surface is to cause strong tip oscillation close to the surface for example by increasing feedback gain (FB = 2-10). To improve the quality of a contaminated tip one can use UV-light treatment that produces ozone and removes organic debris (Thundat et al., 1993), piranha solution (mixture of sulfuric acid and hydrogen peroxide) (Lo et al., 1999), hydrogen, oxygen and argon plasma etching (Chapman, 1980) or CO_2 snow which removes organic debris from the surface because of a transient formation of liquid CO_2 (Hills, 1995).

4.2 The cantilever spring constant *k*

The choice of a cantilever spring constant depends on a particular system under study. For various applications cantilevers with different spring constants should be used. One can use very soft cantilevers ($k << 0.01$ N/m), sometimes made from polymers, for biosensor applications (Calleja et al., 2005). Usually those cantilevers do not have any tip. The working part of the cantilever is its whole surface, which can be modified and used as a sensor for example to study the interaction between lysozyme molecules (Ukraintsev et al., 2007).

Soft cantilevers ($k = 0.06$ N/m) are typically used for force spectroscopy measurements (Kransnoslobodtsev et al., 2005). When these cantilevers are used to study topography several artifacts can appear. Due to low resonance frequency, these cantilevers have low quality factor Q, especially in solution, so these cantilevers do not oscillate well on the first resonance frequency and one has to use the second harmonic, which causes an improper height determination (Rezek, Ukraintsev & Kromka, 2011). For samples with properties similar in every point it usually does not cause any problem and even higher resolution can be achieved than when measuring on higher harmonic (Giessibl, 2006), but for samples with different surface chemistry it may not work. To avoid such artifacts, stiffer cantilevers should be used.

The cantilevers with spring constant $k \sim 1$ N/m can be used to study living cells in-situ (P. Chen et. al, 2009). Such tips are often the best choice for nanoshaving experiments on biological samples.

The stiff cantilevers with high spring constant ($k = 40$ N/m) are usually used in air for most of the studies. Sometimes they are too stiff and easily penetrate protein layer or cell (Kwon et al., 2009).

The even stiffer cantilevers ($k = 120$ N/m), for example made from diamond, can be used on hard samples or for cutting of biological material (H. X. You & Yu, 1999). Such tips are often the best choice for nanoshaving experiments on chemically synthesized samples with high layer rigidity, on which the interaction between the layer and the substrate is much higher than for biological samples.

The pressure applied to the sample depends on the applied force and the active surface area, i.e. the tip shape. One needs to take care of the tip shape, because blunt tips will change the forces and pressures needed for cell penetration.

The stiffer the cantilever, the more energy injects the tip to the sample during each approach cycle. This energy is equal to $\Delta E = 2\pi^2 c_t A^2 f$, where c_t is the total damping coefficient, A – the amplitude, and f – the frequency (S.-M. Lin & C.-C. Lin, 2009). The total energy of the tip is $E = ½kA^2$. Q factor is defined as $Q = 2\pi E/\Delta E$ and drastically depends on a medium due to changes in c_t and depends on the distance between the tip and the surface (Naik, 2003). In liquid, usually $Q<10$, but if only part of the tip is inside the liquid, Q may reach 100 (LeDue et al., 2009). The decrease in frequency and Q factor is typical for cantilevers in liquid compared to vacuum or air (Reed et al., 2009).

For example, cantilever with $k \sim 3$ N/m and $A \sim 60$ nm has energy $E \sim 10^{-15}$ J and therefore injects $\Delta E \sim 10^{-16}$-10^{-15} J per cycle. If energy E is high enough (for example $E \sim 10^{-15}$ J for an

FBS layer or weakly attached cells) to move objects on the surface, this cantilever will remove the protein layer or move the weakly attached cell. In air, Q is higher and ΔE is lower than in liquid. This means that stiff and very stiff cantilevers ($k \sim 40$ N/m) may be used in air, but not in liquid for soft matter on hard surfaces.

4.3 The amplitude of cantilever oscillation *A*

If the amplitude of cantilever oscillation A is increased the quality factor of cantilever oscillation Q is also increased. This is very important when study is performed in liquid ($Q < 10$). With low amplitude ($A \sim 10$ nm), it is difficult to get stable performance of AFM and make a good image. The increase in amplitude will lead to better resolution and lower noise, but will also increase the size of the smallest object which can be observed. This is the reason why all studies on subnanometer scale are performed with very low amplitude and often in UHV. In some cases, the RMS signal instead of the MAG signal for feedback signal in TM allows one to obtain a better image.

Measurements with high amplitude may result in tapping mode nanoshaving (Ukraintsev et al., 2009). To avoid this artifact, softer cantilevers or smaller amplitude should be used. But softer cantilevers may cause the "contrast reversal" artifact, and smaller amplitude may reduce the resolution of the image. Hence, a compromise must be found in each specific case. For protein-diamond samples studied in solution, cantilevers with $k \sim 3$ N/m and the amplitude of oscillation 10-60 nm are the optimal choice.

4.4 The set point value *SP* and the feedback value *FB*

Small changes in the AFM set point can dramatically change the acquired image due to changes between the attractive and repulsive modes, i.e. the "contrast reversal" artifact. To avoid this artifact, one should use a lower SP value. On the other hand, a switching vibrating cantilever mode was proposed to enhance the contrast on flat multi-phase samples as switching depends on the difference in the material properties of the phases (Kühle et al., 1998). A switching vibrating cantilever mode is similar to jumping mode AFM (Sotres et al., 2007). It is based on placing the feedback set point in the repulsive electrical double-layer curve just before the mechanical instability occurs, i.e. there is no mechanical contact between the tip and the sample at any time. This method was used to image single biomolecules in aqueous media (Sotres et al., 2007).

It is often recommended to use a set-point value as high as possible (close to SP_0), but this is relevant only for the measurement on "clean" samples, from which nothing can become attached to the tip. When measuring in solution on soft matter, the best way to avoid this effect is to use $SP \sim 0.9 * SP_0$ and slightly reduce SP if image gets blurred. It is not recommended to use very low SP value because in this case the imaging is invasive and image gets blurred due to the interaction with tip.

It is also important to choose the appropriate scanning feedback value. This is not straightforward, because the reduction of the FB value may cause blurring of the topography image, but increasing may lead to oscillations and additional noise on the topography image and even to loss of the contrast in phase image.

4.5 Measurements of tall features

The scanning range, the image mode and the tip shape influence such cell characteristics as cellular volume and ultrastructural roughness (Wu et al., 2008). True morphology can be partially reconstructed using procedures based on tip shape estimation (Keller & Franke, 1993). In many cases the simple mathematical procedure such as subtraction of the smoothed data from the original data greatly improves the image contrast and quality (Kienberger et al., 2006). This method is applicable not only for tall objects, but also for small particles on a flat surface.

For measurements of tall features with height close to the range of the Z-scanner piezotube, one can use the following technique. Usually AFM is adjusted to the middle of the Z-scanner range after the tip is approached to the surface. For flat and leveled samples this means that only half of the range of the piezotube is available for height measurements. For tall objects, it is thus better to level the sample first and then to approach so that the whole range of piezotube can be used to measurements.

5. Conclusions

Various AFM methods and literature data relevant to the characterization of biological specimens were reviewed in this chapter. Diverse AFM artifacts that arise during AFM characterization of such soft matter samples were illustrated by measurements of FBS proteins and AHAPS linker molecules on diamond substrates. The artifacts were divided into four categories: artifacts related to the tip, to the scanner, to the sample and artifacts related to the interaction between them. Various effects in AFM morphology and AFM phase data were demonstrated and their physical origins were explained based on the schematic models.

Possible artifacts related to feature height and other specific structural, chemical, and electronic properties of the samples were considered. Sub-nanometer roughness of monocrystalline diamond substrates provided well-defined background for the AFM study of organic molecules. Moreover, the possibility of tailoring diamond surface properties by modifying surface atoms and linking molecules (for example AHAPS with NH_2 groups) opens prospects for broader applications in biological studies.

The influence of the tip shape, cantilever spring constant, amplitude of tip oscillations, feedback and set point values on the reliability of AFM characterization were also discussed. We showed how to choose a proper cantilever depending on the specific sample and characteristics of interest. Every cantilever has its own application area. In summary, soft cantilevers ($k \sim 0.06$ N/m) are the best choice for force spectroscopy measurements and stiffer cantilevers (1-120 N/m) should be used for nanoshaving experiments on biological and chemically synthesized samples. Cantilevers with $k \sim 3$ N/m are the most suitable for *in-situ* measurements of proteins (Rezek, Ukraintsev & Kromka, 2011). Several further guidelines how to obtain reliable AFM characteristics of molecules and cells were presented. Different ways to avoid artifacts such as tapping mode nanoshaving, negative contrast, or image blurring were described. The presented work may thus help researchers to optimize and better understand AFM measurements and to avoid incorrect conclusions.

6. Acknowledgements

We would like to acknowledge a kind assistance of V. Jurka with photolithography, Z. Poláčková with chemical treatment, O. Babchenko and J. Potměšil with hydrogen plasma treatment, and M. Kalbacova for protein donation. This research was financially supported by AV0Z10100521, research projects KAN400100701 (ASCR), LC06040 (MŠMT), LC510 (MŠMT), and the Fellowship J. E. Purkyně (ASCR).

7. References

Allen, M.; Hud, N.; Balooch, M.; Tench, R.; Siekhaus, W. & Balhorn, R. 1992. Tip-radius-induced artifacts in AFM images of protamine-complexed DNA fibers. *Ultramicroscopy*, 42-44: 1095-1100.

Azulay, D.; Balberg, I.; Chu, V.; Conde, J. P. & Millo O. 2005. Current routes in hydrogenated microcrystalline silicon. *Physical review B* 71, 113304.

Beard, J. D.; Gordeev, S. N. & Guy, R. H. 2011. AFM Nanotools for Surgery of Biological Cells. *Journal of Physics: Conference Series*: 012003.

Bernardes-Filho, R. & Assis, O. B. G. de. 2005. Development of an algorithm for tip-related artifacts identification in AFM biological film imaging. *Brazilian Archives of Biology and Technology*, 48(4): 667-674.

Calleja, M.; Nordström, M.; Alvarez, M.; Tamayo, J.; Lechuga, L. M. & Boisen, A. 2005. Highly sensitive polymer-based cantilever-sensors for DNA detection. *Ultramicroscopy*, 105(1-4): 215–222.

Crampton, N.; Yokokawa, M.; Dryden, D. T.; Edwardson, J. M.; Rao, D. N.; Takeyasu, K.; Yoshimura S.H.; Henderson R.M. 2007. Fast-scan atomic force microscopy reveals that the type III restriction enzyme EcoP15I is capable of DNA translocation and looping. *Proceedings of the National Academy of Sciences*, 104(31): 12755.

Darling, E. M. 2011. Force scanning: a rapid, high-resolution approach for spatial mechanical property mapping. *Nanotechnology*, 22(17): 175707.

Diao, P.; Zhang, D, Guo, M. & Zhang Q. 2009. „Comments on 'Electric-Field-Assisted Growth of Highly Uniform and Oriented Gold Nanotriangles on Conducting Glass Substrates'". *Advanced Materials*, 21 (13): 1317-1319. doi:10.1002/adma.200801390.

Dongmo, S. 1996. Blind restoration method of scanning tunneling and atomic force microscopy images. *Journal of Vacuum Science & Technology B: Microelectronics and Nanometer Structures*, 14(2): 1552.

Eaton, P. 2010. *Atomic force microscopy*. Oxford; New York: Oxford University Press.

Gainutdinov & Arutyunov. 2001. Artifacts in Atomic Force Microscopy, *Russian Microelectronics*, 30(4): 219-224.

Garfias-García, E.; Romero-Romo, M.; Ramírez-Silva, M. T.; Morales, J. & Palomar-Pardavé, M. 2008. Mechanism and kinetics of the electrochemical formation of polypyrrole under forced convection conditions. *Journal of Electroanalytical Chemistry*, 613(1): 67-79.

Ge, G.; Han, D.; Lin, D.; Chu, W.; Sun, Y.; Jiang, L.; Ma W.; Wang C. 2007. MAC mode atomic force microscopy studies of living samples, ranging from cells to fresh tissue. *Ultramicroscopy*, 107(4-5): 299–307.

Giessibl, F. J. 2006. Higher-harmonic atomic force microscopy. *Surface and Interface Analysis*, 38(12-13): 1696-1701.

Graham, H. K.; Hodson, N. W.; Hoyland, J. A.; Millward-Sadler, S. J.; Garrod, D.; Scothern, A. et al. 2010. Tissue section AFM: In situ ultrastructural imaging of native biomolecules. *Matrix Biology*, 29(4): 254–260.

Hamon, L.; Pastré, D.; Dupaigne, P.; Breton, C. L.; Cam, E. L. & Piétrement, O. 2007. High-resolution AFM imaging of single-stranded DNA-binding (SSB) protein—DNA complexes. *Nucleic acids research*, 35(8): e58.

Hawkes, P. 1988. *Advances in electronics and electron physics*. Boston: Academic Press.

Helenius, J.; Heisenberg, C.-P.; Gaub, H. E. & Muller, D. J. 2008. Single-cell force spectroscopy. *Journal of Cell Science*, 121(11): 1785-1791.

Hills, M. M. 1995. Carbon dioxide jet spray cleaning of molecular contaminants. *Journal of Vacuum Science & Technology A: Vacuum, Surfaces, and Films*, 13(1): 30.

Hoffmann R.; Kriele A.; Obloh H.; Tokuda N.; Smirnov W.; Yang N. & Nebel C.E. 2011. The creation of a biomimetic interface between boron-doped diamond and immobilized proteins.*Biomaterials*, 32, 7325-7332.

Hyde, M. E.; Jacobs, R. M. J. & Compton, R. G. 2004. An AFM Study of the Correlation of Lead Dioxide Electrocatalytic Activity with Observed Morphology. *The Journal of Physical Chemistry B*, 108(20): 6381-6390.

Chapman, B. Glow discharge processes: Sputtering and Plasma Etching, *John Wiley & Sons*, New York (1980).

Checco, A.; Cai, Y.; Gang, O. & Ocko, B. M. 2006. High resolution non-contact AFM imaging of liquids condensed onto chemically nanopatterned surfaces. *Ultramicroscopy*, 106, (8-9): 703-708.

Chen, I.-C.; Chen, L.-H.; Orme, C. A. & Jin, S. 2007. Control of Curvature in Highly Compliant Probe Cantilevers during Carbon Nanotube Growth. *Nano Letters*, 7(10): 3035-3040.

Chen, P.; Dong, H.; Chen, L.; Sun, Q. & Han, Dong. 2009. Application of atomic force microscopy to living samples from cells to fresh tissues. *Chinese Science Bulletin*, 54(14): 2410-2415.

Chen, Y.; Cai, J.; Liu, M.; Zeng, G.; Feng, Q. & Chen, Z. 2004. Research on double-probe, double-and triple-tip effects during atomic force microscopy scanning. *Scanning*, 26(4): 155–161.

Choi, I.; Kim, Y.; Kim, J. H.; Yang, Y. I.; Lee, J.; Lee, S.; Hong, S. & Yi, J. 2008. Fast image scanning method in liquid-AFM without image distortion. *Nanotechnology*, 19: 445701.

Chong, K. F.; Loh, K. P.; Vedula, S. R. K.; Lim, C. T.; Sternschulte, H.; Steinmüller, D.; et al. 2007. Cell Adhesion Properties on Photochemically Functionalized Diamond. *Langmuir*, 23(10): 5615-5621.

Keller, D. & Franke, F. 1993. Envelope reconstruction of probe microscope images. *Surface Science*, 294(3): 409-419.

Kienberger, F.; Pastushenko, V. P.; Kada, G.; Puntheeranurak, T.; Chtcheglova, L.; Riethmueller, C.; Rankl, C.; Ebner & A.; Hinterdorfer, P. 2006. Improving the contrast of topographical AFM images by a simple averaging filter. *Ultramicroscopy*, 106(8-9): 822–828.

Klinov, D. V.; Neretina, T. V.; Prokhorov, V. V.; Dobrynina, T. V.; Aldarov, K. G. & Demin, V. V. 2009. High-resolution atomic force microscopy of DNA. *Biochemistry (Moscow)*, 74(10): 1150-1154.

Kozak, H.; Kromka, A.; Ledinsky, M. & Rezek, B. 2009. Enhancing nanocrystalline diamond surface conductivity by deposition temperature and chemical post-processing. *Phys. Stat. Sol. (a)* 206, 276–280.

Kozak, H.; Remes, Z.; Kromka, A. & Ledinsky, M. 2011. Optical characterisation of organosilane-modified nanocrystalline diamond films. *Chemical Papers*, 65 (1): 36-41.

Kransnoslobodtsev, A. V.; Shlyakhtenko, L. S.; Ukraintsev, E.; Zaikova, T. O.; Keana, J. F. W. & Lyubchenko, Y. L. 2005. Nanomedicine and protein misfolding diseases. *Nanomedicine: Nanotechnology, Biology and Medicine*, 1(4): 300-305.

Kühle, A.; Sorensen, A. H.; Zandbergen, J. B. & Bohr, J. 1998. Contrast artifacts in tapping tip atomic force microscopy. *Applied Physics A: Materials Science & Processing*, 66(7): S329-S332.

Kuznetsov, Y. G.; Victoria, J. G.; Robinson Jr, W. E. & McPherson, A. 2003. Atomic force microscopy investigation of human immunodeficiency virus (HIV) and HIV-infected lymphocytes. *Journal of virology*, 77(22): 11896.

Kwon, E.-Y.; Kim, Y.-T. & Kim, D.-E. 2009. Investigation of penetration force of living cell using an atomic force microscope. *Journal of Mechanical Science and Technology*, 23(7): 1932-1938.

Lambert, J.; Guthmann, C. & Saint-Jean, M. 2003. Relationship between charge distribution and its image by electrostatic force microscopy. *Journal of Applied Physics*, 93(9): 5369.

LeDue, J. M.; Lopez-Ayon, M.; Burke, S. A.; Miyahara, Y. & Grütter, P. 2009. High *Q* optical fiber tips for NC-AFM in liquid. *Nanotechnology*, 20(26): 264018.

Lin, S.-M. & Lin, C.-C. 2009. Phase shifts and energy dissipations of several modes of AFM: Minimizing topography and dissipation measurement errors. *Precision Engineering*, 33(4): 371-377.

Lo, Y.-S.; Huefner, N. D.; Chan, W. S.; Dryden, P.; Hagenhoff, B. & Beebe, T. P. 1999. Organic and Inorganic Contamination on Commercial AFM Cantilevers. *Langmuir*, 15(19): 6522-6526.

Maeda, Y.; Matsumoto, T. & Kawai, T. 1999. Observation of single-and double-stranded DNA using non-contact atomic force microscopy. *Applied surface science*, 140(3-4): 400–405.

Mahmood, I. A. & Moheimani, S. O. R. 2009. Making a commercial atomic force microscope more accurate and faster using positive position feedback control. *Review of Scientific Instruments*, 80(6): 063705.

Shimizu N.; Ikeda M.; Yoshida E.; Murakami H.; Miyazaki S. & Hirose M. 2000. Charging states of Si quantum dots as detected by AFM/Kelvin probe technique. *Jpn. J. Appl. Phys.*, 39, 2318-2320.

Moreno-Herrero, F.; Colchero, J.; Gómez-Herrero, J. & Baró, A. 2004. Atomic force microscopy contact, tapping, and jumping modes for imaging biological samples in liquids. *Physical Review E*, 69(3).
http://link.aps.org/doi/10.1103/PhysRevE.69.031915, 2011.

Morton, D. N.; Roberts, C. J.; Hey, M. J.; Mitchell, J. R.; Hipkiss, J. & Vercauteren, J. 2003. Surface Characterization of Caramel at the Micrometer Scale. *Journal of Food Science*, 68(4): 1411-1415.

Müller, D. J.; Helenius, Jonne, Alsteens, D. & Dufrêne, Y. F. 2009. Force probing surfaces of living cells to molecular resolution. *Nature Chemical Biology*, 5(6): 383-390.

Naik, T. 2003. Dynamic response of a cantilever in liquid near a solid wall. *Sensors and Actuators A: Physical*, 102(3): 240-254.

Nie, H.-Y. & McIntyre, N. S. 2007. Unstable amplitude and noisy image induced by tip contamination in dynamic force mode atomic force microscopy. *Review of Scientific Instruments*, 78(2): 023701.

Rasool, H. I.; Wilkinson, P. R.; Stieg, A. Z. & Gimzewski, J. K. 2010. A low noise all-fiber interferometer for high resolution frequency modulated atomic force microscopy imaging in liquids. *Review of Scientific Instruments*, 81(2): 023703.

Reed, J.; Schmit, J.; Han, S.; Wilkinson, P. & Gimzewski, J. 2009. Interferometric profiling of microcantilevers in liquid. *Optics and Lasers in Engineering*, 47(2): 217-222.

Rezek, B.; Shin, D.; Nakamura, T. & Nebel, C. E. 2006. Geometric Properties of Covalently Bonded DNA on Single-Crystalline Diamond. *Journal of the American Chemical Society*, 128: 3884-3885.

Rezek, B.; Nebel, C.E. 2006. Electronic properties of plasma hydrogenated diamond surfaces: a microscopic study. *Diamond Relat. Mater.* 15, 1374 - 1377.

Rezek, B., Shin, D. & Nebel, C. E. 2007. Properties of hybridized DNA arrays on single-crystalline undoped and boron-doped (100) diamonds studied by atomic force microscopy in electrolytes. *Langmuir* 23(14): 7626-7633.

Rezek, B.; Shin, D.; Uetsuka, H. & Nebel, C. E. 2007. Microscopic diagnostics of DNA molecules on mono-crystalline diamond. *Physica status solidi (a)*, 204(9): 2888-2897.

Rezek, B.; Ukraintsev, E.; Michalíková, L.; Kromka, A.; Zemek, J. & Kalbacova, M. 2009. Adsorption of fetal bovine serum on H/O-terminated diamond studied by atomic force microscopy. *Diamond and Related Materials*, 18(5-8): 918-922.

Rezek, B.; Ukraintsev, E.; Kromka, A.; Ledinský, M.; Brož, A.; Nosková, L.; Hartmannova, H. & Kalbacova, M. 2010. Assembly of osteoblastic cell micro-arrays on diamond guided by protein pre-adsorption. *Diamond and Related Materials*, 19(2-3): 153-157.

Rezek, B.; Krátká, M.; Ukraintsev, E.; Babchenko, O.; Kromka, A.; Brož, A.; Kalbacova M. Diamond as functional material for bioelectronics and biotechnology In: *"New Perspectives in Biosensors Technology and Applications"* Intech 2011, pp. 177-196, ISBN 978-953-307-448-1.

Rezek, B.; Ukraintsev, E. & Kromka, A. 2011. Optimizing atomic force microscopy for characterization of diamond-protein interfaces. *Nanoscale research letters*, 6(1): 1–10.

Ricci, D. & Braga, P. C. 2003. Recognizing and Avoiding Artifacts in AFM Imaging. *Atomic Force Microscopy*: 25-38. http://www.springerlink.com/openurl.asp?genre=book&id=doi:10.1385/1-59259-647-9:25, 2011, New Jersey: Humana Press.

Sahin, O.; Quate, C.; Solgaard, O. & Atalar, A. 2004. Resonant harmonic response in tapping-mode atomic force microscopy. *Physical Review B*, 69(16). http://link.aps.org/doi/10.1103/PhysRevB.69.165416, 2011.

Sajanlal, P. R. & Pradeep, T. 2008. Electric-Field-Assisted Growth of Highly Uniform and Oriented Gold Nanotriangles on Conducting Glass Substrates. *Advanced Materials*, 20(5): 980-983.

Shekhawat, G. S.; Lambert, M. P.; Sharma, S.; Velasco, P. T.; Viola, K. L.; Klein, W. L. & Dravid V.P. 2009. Soluble state high resolution atomic force microscopy study of Alzheimer's β-amyloid oligomers. *Applied Physics Letters*, 95(18): 183701.

Sokolov, I. 2007. Atomic force microscopy in cancer cell research. *Cancer Nanotechnology. Valencia, CA: American Scientific Publishers*, 1–17.

Solares, S. D. 2007. Frequency and force modulation atomic force microscopy: low-impact tapping-mode imaging without bistability. *Measurement Science and Technology*, 18: L9.

Sotres, J.; Lostao, A.; Gomezmoreno, C. & Baro, A. 2007. Jumping mode AFM imaging of biomolecules in the repulsive electrical double layer. *Ultramicroscopy*, 107(12): 1207-1212.

Su, F.; Wei, J. & Liu, Y. 2005. Removal of AFM moiré measurement errors due to non-linear scan and creep of probe. *Nanotechnology*, 16: 1681.

Thormann, E.; Pettersson, T. & Claesson, P. M. 2009. How to measure forces with atomic force microscopy without significant influence from nonlinear optical lever sensitivity. *Review of Scientific Instruments*, 80(9): 093701.

Thundat, T.; Zheng, X.-Y.; Chen, G. Y.; Sharp, S. L.; Warmack, R. J. & Schowalter, L. J. 1993. Characterization of atomic force microscope tips by adhesion force measurements. *Applied Physics Letters*, 63(15): 2150.

Touhami, A.; Jericho, M. H. & Beveridge, T. J. 2004. Atomic force microscopy of cell growth and division in Staphylococcus aureus. *Journal of bacteriology*, 186(11): 3286.

Ukraintsev, E. V.; Kiselev, G. A.; Kudrinskii, A. A.; Lisichkin, G. V. & Yaminskii, I. V. 2007. Formation of lysozyme fibrils on a solid support. *Polymer Science Series B*, 49(1-2): 6-9.

Ukraintsev, E.; Rezek, B.; Kromka, A.; Broz, A. & Kalbacova, M. 2009. Long-term adsorption of fetal bovine serum on H/O-terminated diamond studied *in situ* by atomic force microscopy. *physica status solidi (b)*, 246(11-12): 2832-2835.

Velegol, S. B.; Pardi, S.; Li, X.; Velegol, D. & Logan, B. E. 2003. AFM Imaging Artifacts due to Bacterial Cell Height and AFM Tip Geometry. *Langmuir*, 19(3): 851-857.

Verveniotis, E.; Kromka, A.; Ledinský, M.; Čermák, J. & Rezek, B. 2011. Guided assembly of nanoparticles on electrostatically charged nanocrystalline diamond thin films. *Nanoscale Research Letters*, 6: 144.

Vetushka, A.; Fejfar, A.; Ledinský, M.; Rezek, B.; Stuchlík, J. & Kočka J. 2010. Comment on "Current routes in hydrogenated microcrystalline silicon". *Physical review* B 81, 237301.

Volle, C. B.; Ferguson, M. A.; Aidala, K. E.; Spain, E. M. & Nuñez, M. E. 2008. Quantitative Changes in the Elasticity and Adhesive Properties of *Escherichia coli* ZK1056 Prey Cells During Predation by *Bdellovibrio bacteriovorus* 109J. *Langmuir*, 24(15): 8102-8110.

Wadu-Mesthrige, K.; Amro, N. A.; Garno, J. C.; Cruchon-Dupeyrat, S. & Liu, G. Y. 2001. Contact resonance imaging–a simple approach to improve the resolution of AFM for biological and polymeric materials. *Applied surface science*, 175: 391–398.

Wu, Y.; Hu, Y.; Cai, J.; Ma, S.; Wang, X. & Chen, Y. 2008. The analysis of morphological distortion during AFM study of cells. *Scanning*, 30(5): 426-432.

You, H. 2000. Atomic force microscopy imaging of living cells: a preliminary study of the disruptive effect of the cantilever tip on cell morphology. *Ultramicroscopy*, 82(1-4): 297-305.

You, H. X. & Yu, L. 1999. Atomic force microscopy imaging of living cells: progress, problems and prospects. *Methods in cell science*, 21(1): 1–17.

Zhao, M.; Sharma, V.; Wei, H.; Birge, R. R.; Stuart, J. A.; Papadimitrakopoulos, F. & Huey B.D. 2008. Ultrasharp and high aspect ratio carbon nanotube atomic force microscopy probes for enhanced surface potential imaging. *Nanotechnology*, 19(23): 235704.

3

Tapping Mode AFM Imaging for Functionalized Surfaces

Nadine Mourougou-Candoni
CNRS, Aix-Marseille University, CINaM
France

1. Introduction

The tapping mode in Atomic Force Microscopy (AFM) is a key advance in AFM technology for functionalized surface imaging. In fact, the basic technique of AFM, which is contact AFM, is not well adapted to examine such surfaces due to problems of friction and adhesion. Therefore, the tapping mode of operation was developed to overcome drawbacks of contact mode (Binnig et al, 1986). This mode uses oscillation of the cantilever tip at or near its natural resonant frequency while allowing the cantilever tip to impact the target sample for a minimal amount of time. This intermittent contact lessens the damage done to the soft surface and to the tip, compared to the amount done in contact. Thus, the tapping mode is the method of choice for imaging functionalized surfaces. A functionalized surface is a solid surface where molecules have been adsorbed leading to various patterns, from isolated molecules dispersed on the surface to homogeneous films. The patterns provide ideal platforms for the immobilization or recognition and specific interaction of biomolecules. In the preparation of functionalized surfaces, the first process consists in understanding the mechanism of adsorption. The aim is to yield good orientation and stability of the immobilized molecules, thus leading to high-functionality of the surface for applications, such as biosensors.

The purpose of this chapter is to highlight potentialities of AFM in the tapping mode, for imaging functionalized surfaces in air. Therefore, we explore quantitative and qualitative information given by AFM during processes of functionalization of substrates by molecules. For the substrate, the surface must be as flat as possible in order to reach high resolution imaging. Indeed, a molecule of a diameter of a few nm placed on a surface of a roughness of a few nm would not be visible in an AFM height image as it would be "hidden" by the surface topography. Thus, we focus on mica which presents a surface with atomically flat terraces. Concerning molecules, they range from more or less modified alkane chains to derivatives of DNA. Hence, we study the immobilization of single molecules and the formation of self-assembled monolayers (SAMs) and polymerized films. In the resulting pattern, molecules either adsorb by physical binding, e.g. via counter ions or hydrophobic interaction, or form covalent bonds on the surface.

We start with a brief description of the topographical mode of tapping AFM. Then, various illustrations of surface functionalization are investigated by AFM imaging. In the last part, we present improvements on conventional AFM in tapping mode.

2. Topographical imaging with AFM taping mode

2.1 Principle of AFM in tapping mode

In tapping mode, the AFM scans the sample surface with a very tiny and sharp tip mounted at the end of a flexible cantilever. The tip is oscillated and moved towards the sample (Binnig et al., 1986). Only intermittently touching or "tapping" occurs on the sample. Hence the dragging forces during scanning are greatly reduced (Tamayo & Garcia, 1996). Moreover, during oscillation, the tip goes through both the attractive and the repulsive regions of the tip-sample force field. In case of functionalized surfaces, AFM parameters are selected to minimize modification of the surface caused by moving or removing molecules which are loosely bound to the surface and easily damageable.

The cantilever is mounted to a piezoelectric actuator (figure 1). A position sensitive photo detector receives a laser beam reflected off the end-point of the beam to provide cantilever deflection feedback. During the scan of the tip over the sample surface with feedback mechanisms, PZT scanners enable to maintain the tip at a constant force or a constant height. The operation mode called constant force is the most common in tapping AFM. Thus, the tip is moved up and down with the contour of the surface and the laser beam deflected from the cantilever provides measurements of the difference in light intensities between the upper and lower photo detectors.

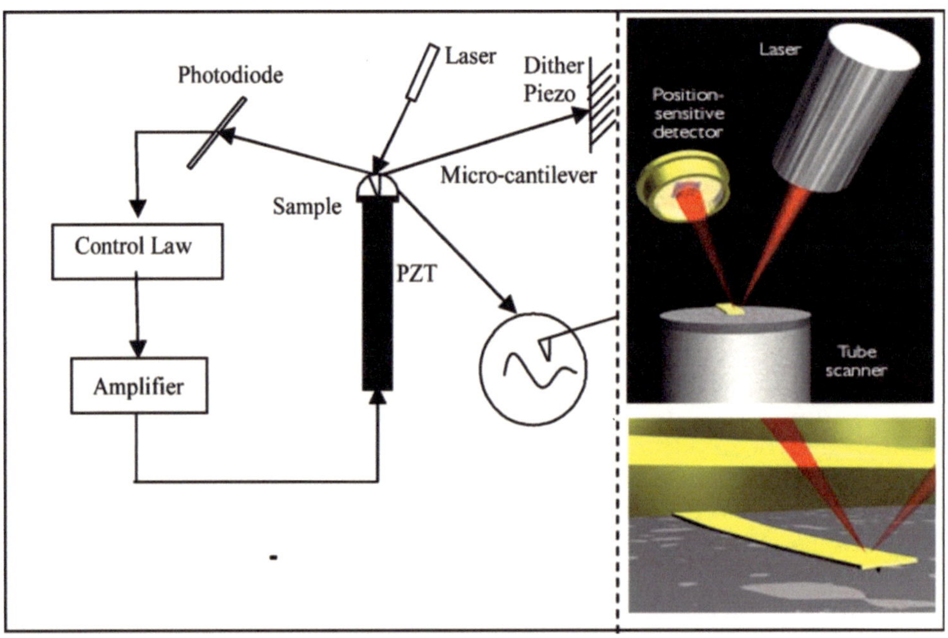

Fig. 1. Schematic of basic AFM operation (left), real micro-cantilever and components (right) (Jalili & Laxminarayana, 2004).

The PZT actuator applies a force on the cantilever base and makes the cantilever tip vibrate. The frequency of oscillation is fixed near the resonance of the tip and the oscillation amplitude is monitored. Starting from free oscillation amplitude, the sample is approached to the tip until its amplitude is reduced to the set point value, which is selected to reduce damage to the sample. When the tip-sample gap is in the nanometer range, the oscillation amplitude is damped by tip-sample repulsive interactions that occur each cycle, due to energy loss (figure 2). Then the oscillation amplitude is kept at the set point by adjusting the vertical (z-axis) position of the tip with a piezoelectric drive. Therefore, the vertical motion is controlled by the feedback mechanism, which allows the adjustment of the signal to keep the amplitude constant. The variations of the z-position of the tip during scanning are plotted as a function of the xy position of the tip to create the height image, in which gray or color contrast is used to show the z-variations. Thus, the reduction of the oscillation amplitude due to interactions with molecules of the surface is generally used to identify and measure surface topographic features.

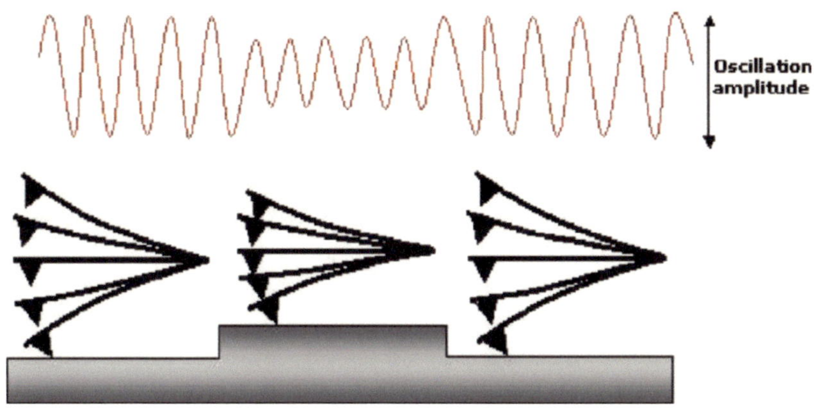

Fig. 2. Schematic representation of an AFM tips operating in the tapping mode (Alessandrini & Facci, 2005).

2.2 Parameters influencing topographic imaging

In topographic imaging, the lateral resolution is given by the radius of curvature of the tip. However, using commercial cantilevers with a 10 to 50 nm radius of curvature for the tip, surprisingly permits to acquire (sub)-nanometer resolution on reconstituted surface. In fact, the resolution is higher than that expected on the basis of radius of curvature, due to the presence of nano-scale asperities extending irregularly from the tip. In this case, the asperities may play the role of the true imaging tip (Müller et al., 1999). Moreover the shape of the tip also plays an important role in the resolution. A common source of artifacts appears when height variations are in the range of the tip's radius of curvature, i.e. 10 to 50 nm. Then, the sample interacts with the sides of the probe. The resulting image is a combination of the real sample topography and the tip geometry, hence broadening the surface features. Another common problem is the shadowing or multiplication of small structures produced by multiple probe effects. These are due to the presence of multiple asperities on the tip apex, which usually originate from contamination.

Another important parameter influencing image resolution is the type of sample. The sample preparation procedure must be chosen so as molecule-surface interaction is always stronger than tip-molecules interaction. In fact, the spatial resolution increases with hardness and flatness of the sample. This is due to long-range forces, which play a significant role. They involve a huge number of atoms contributing to the contrast formation mechanism, even if true atomic resolution images have been obtained by the AFM on layered samples (Ohnesorge & Binnig, 1993). In the case of soft or damageable functionalized surfaces, the resolution crucially depends on the softness of the sample. Hence, cell membranes induce a resolution in the range of a few tens of nanometers. For isolated molecules like proteins, the resolution can be improved to few nanometers. Concerning the choice of the substrate, popular substrates are glass, silicon or mica. We have selected mica because it exhibits the smoothest surface. In addition, thanks to the crystallographic structure of mica, a clean and very flat surface can be easily obtained by peeling off the outer leaflet of the surface using a simple cellophane tape. The smoothness of mica subsists when we cover it with gold by evaporation.

3. Imaging isolated molecules

In the case of functionalization with single molecules, we have been interested by oligonucleotides, i.e. pieces of single-stranded DNA. The functionalization of surface with these oligonucleotides is of great interest for the development of DNA chips, which are based on the capacity of oligonucleotides to recognize and to hybridize with their complementary strand. This method is widely used for the detection and characterization of genetic material for both clinical and environmental analysis. One critical aspect for the synthesis of such chips is the immobilization of oligonucleotides on the device surface. In fact, oligonucleotides must be available to hybridization without displaying rapid removal under hybridization or washing conditions.

3.1 Preparation of the substrate

Generally, the immobilization of oligonucleotides is achieved by covalent coupling with the surface. It requires activation with a cross-linking reagent and/or modification of the oligonucleotide with a reactive group. Several studies have been carried out on Si/SiO_2 surfaces (Chrisey et al., 1996; Cloarec et al., 1999), on gold surfaces (Herne & Tarlov, 1997; Steel et al., 1998; Kelley et al., 1998; Lisdat et al., 1999; Huang E. et.al, 2001) or on mica (Hansma et al., 1996; Shlyakhtenko et al., 1999). Among these substrates, we have chosen mica for its flatness and we have covered it with gold in order to adsorb thiol-functionalized oligonucleotides via gold-sulfur bond. In fact, this linkage allows configurational freedom for oligonucleotides to form a double helix with the complementary molecule. Therefore, mica is covered with gold by evaporation in an UHV chamber at a rate of 1-2 Å s^{-1} for a surface temperature of 460 °C, the film thickness being monitored by a quartz microbalance (Klein et al., 2000). In figure 3, AFM images of Au (111) surface shows atomically flat terraces of 500 nm (figure 3a) and presence of atomic steps (figure 3b). It must be pointed out that these terraces and steps correspond to the structure of mica.

3.2 Functionalization with isolated molecules

Previous works on the adsorption of thiolated oligonucleotides on gold substrates used surface chemical analysis techniques such as Surface Plasmon Resonance (SPR) (Herne & Tarlov, 1997), X-ray Photoelectron Spectroscopy (XPS) (Levicky et al., 1998), neutron reflectivity (Steel et al., 1998) or electrochemical quantitation (Peterlinz et al., 1997). However these techniques give only the average structure of the oligonucleotide. The

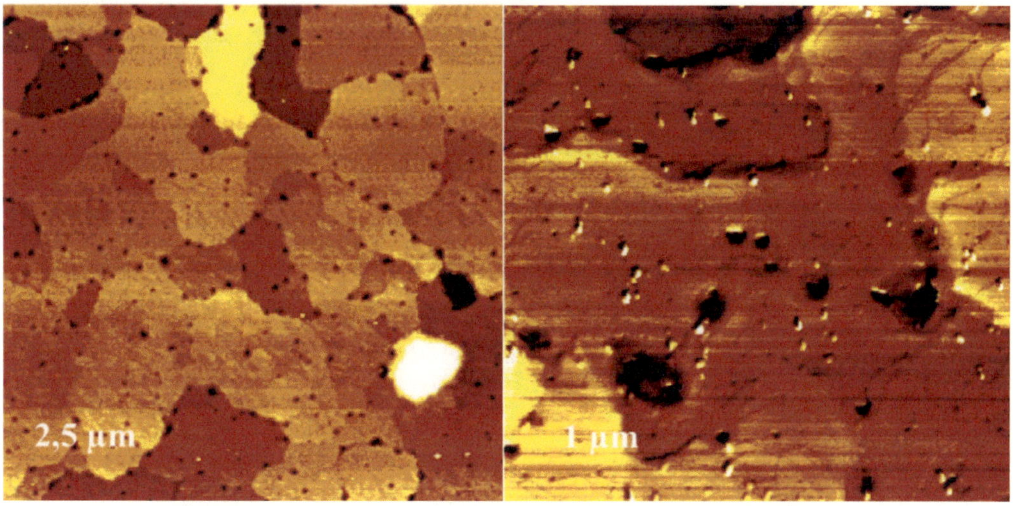

(a) (b)

Fig. 3. AFM images of an Au(111) surface obtained by electron evaporation of gold on mica sheets in a UHV chamber at an evaporation rate of of 1-2 Å s^{-1} for a substrate temperature of 460 °C: 3a) Atomically flat terraces of 500 nm are observed with a size of scanning of 2.5 μm × 2.5 μm; 3b) Atomic steps are distinguished with a size of scanning of 1 μm × 1 μm,.

advantage of AFM imaging in the tapping mode is achieving a direct visualization of surfaces to study the adsorption process without modifying the surface. Therefore, we have performed AFM experiments in an ambient atmosphere, typically 20-25 °C and 30-35 % humidity, using the tapping mode of AFM at a scan frequency of 1-2 Hz. Surface topography has been obtained with uncoated silicon cantilever tips of ~ 15 nm apex diameters. Then our AFM images have been processed with flatten and contrast enhancement processing from Nanoscope III software. Figure 4a shows a 1 μm wide AFM image of a surface exposed for a few seconds to oligonucleotides by immersing in a solution at a concentration of 5 nM in KH_2PO_4 (1 M). This surface exhibits particulates with a height of ~1 nm and a diameter of 15 nm.

How do we attribute these particulates to oligonucleotides? On one hand, oligonucleotides of 25 bases adsorbed on the gold surface through the thiol group and stretched to full length are higher than 16 nm according to SPR measurements (Herne & Tarlov, 1997). On the other hand, if the same oligonucleotide displays segments that are isotopically distributed in space, these authors estimated that the component of the radius of gyration along the direction perpendicular to the surface is on the order of $R_{gz} \approx 1.1 \pm 0.1$ nm (Steel et al., 1998). Thus, it appears that particulates observed by AFM (figure 4a) are oligonucleotides which are curled up in a ball. This globulate conformation of 25-bases oligonucleotides was also described by other authors with AFM (Hansma et al., 1996).

After a longer time of deposition, the surface becomes more covered in particulates, i.e. in oligonucleotides; nevertheless oligonucleotides are still well-distinguishable (figure 4b). In figure 4b, adsorption is inhomogeneous since the molecules are arranged like filaments which seem to follow lines displayed by the surface. Sometimes these lines reproduce the

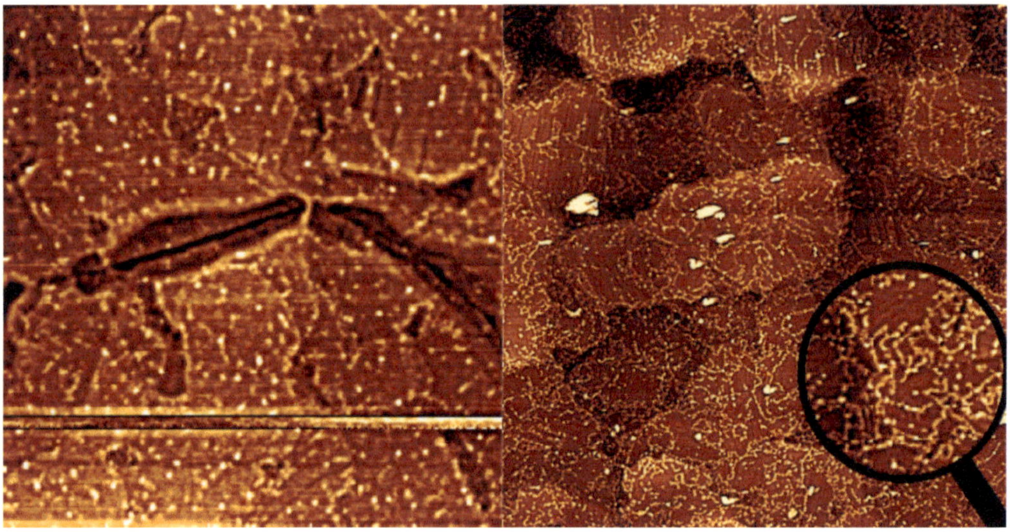

(a) (b)

Fig. 4. AFM images of surfaces exposed to oligonucleotides (5 nM) in a solution of KH2PO4 (1 M): 4a) for a few seconds: the surface exhibits particulates with a height of ~1 nm and a diameter of 15 nm. The size of scanning is 1 μm × 1 μm. 4b) for 10 min: the particulates form a filamentous arrangement following the symmetry of the Au(111) surface (zoom inset). The size of scanning is 2 μm × 2 μm.

symmetry of the Au(111) surface (see the magnified area). Thus, molecules seem to adsorb preferentially at the structure of the surface due to the presence of steps and/or in reconstruction areas. We must emphasize that molecules adsorbed on these lines seem to be connected together because they are close-packed and the lateral resolution of the AFM is limited.

3.3 Physisorption or chemisorption

During contact between the surface and oligonucleotide, molecules are either chemisorbed, i.e. specifically adsorbed via gold-sulfur linkage, or physisorbed, i.e. non-specifically adsorbed via nitrogen interactions of nucleotide side chains. We have studied non-specific adsorption with non-thiolated oligonucleotides. According to Auger Electron Spectroscopy (AES), non-thiolated oligonucleotides are detected whereas AFM images do not display bumps. Thus, bumps observed with thiolated oligonucleotides are due to the linkage through thiol and non-specifically adsorbed molecules are not visible with AFM. This is probably due to the diffusion of non-attached molecules on the surface, which is more rapid than the scanning speed of AFM (Mourougou-Candoni et al., 2003).

How do oligonucleotides adsorb on the surface? As molecules do not have enough time to react with the surface, they are essentially physisorbed, and they reach their equilibrium density in a few seconds. After the surface is removed from the solution, these molecules diffuse and react with the surface becoming chemisorbed. According to our images, this chemisorption is promoted by steps or/and reconstructions of the surface.

3.4 Kinetic of adsorption

The acquisition of AFM images with time of deposition shows clearly that adsorption proceeds in two steps (Mourougou-Candoni et al., 2003):

- In the first step, molecules adsorb instantaneously with a density of 10^{11} molecules cm^{-2} that we are able to count on AFM images (figure 4a). This density cannot be explained by diffusion of oligonucleotides during immersion in solution because their coefficient of diffusion of (6-7) $\times 10^{-7} cm^2 s^{-1}$ (Tinland et al., 1997) is too low. In fact, we explain it by molecules reaching the surface during dipping.
- In the second step, the adsorption increases slowly with a rate of 10^8 molecules $cm^{-2} s^{-1}$ due to diffusion. This rate reflects the chemisorption of oligonucleotides. The kinetic factor of $4\times10^{-4} s^{-1}$ is consistent with the measures for chemisorption of alkanethiol on a gold surface (Lavrich et al., 1998). Considering that this factor is around $(10^{13}\text{-}10^{14}) \times e^{-E/RT} s^{-1}$, we obtain an activation energy, E, around 100 kJ mol^{-1}. This is in the range of the activation energy of surface molecule dissociation. Thus, it corresponds to the reaction activation energy of the thiol group with gold. In addition, the reaction rate can depend on the structure of the surface as displayed by AFM images (figure 4b).

In this two-step mechanism, the density of chemisorbed molecules is proportional to the equilibrium density of physisorbed molecules. Therefore, during incubation in water at ambient temperature, physisorption being limited by electrostatic repulsion between neighboring oligonucleotides due to negative charges of their phosphated backbone, it induces a low chemisorption. Moreover, this chemisorption must be increased by promoting physisorption. Indeed, electrostatic are minimized in our solutions with phosphate KH_2PO_4 (1M) due to high ionic force, which permits to screen oligonucleotides charges. However, we have observed that chemisorption also increases in water at high temperature (60 °C). Thus the electrostatic repulsion described as a limiting factor (Steel et al., 1998) is not sufficient here. In fact, the activation energy that we have calculated gives a kinetic factor for specific reaction 100-fold higher at 60 °C than at room temperature.

Furthermore, the densities of molecules evaluated in these images are drastically different from the values obtained by Huang et al. (Huang E. et al., 2001). With a gold surface similar to ours and with same concentrations, they estimated from their AFM images a density in the 10^9 molecules cm^{-2} range. In fact, they consider some large lumps appearing with a diameter of 26-40 nm as oligonucleotide molecules, which we would attribute to impurities as those visible in figures 4 (or packs of oligonucleotides). However, their AFM images display small features they do not take into account and that we assign to oligonucleotides.

In conclusion, we show that AFM permits to study the adsorption process of isolated molecules such as oligonucleotides on a surface, here gold surface. Indeed AFM in tapping mode provides a direct visualization of oligonucleotide-coupled surfaces with a nanoscopic resolution. In addition AFM coupled with chemical analyses contribute to differentiation between physisorption and chemisorption. Thus, chemisorbed oligonucleotides appear as white bumps of 1 nm height that we can count on the gold surface. In addition, AFM exploration leads to determination of adsorption kinetics in a two-step mechanism. The first instantaneous adsorption concerns essentially molecules, which adsorb non-specifically during dipping of the substrate, reaching their equilibrium density. Then, their reaction with surface is promoted by steps and/or reconstructions of the surface. The increase of density observed in the second step concerns molecules physisorbing from solution and reacting with the surface by diffusion. Finally, AFM allows us to show that this reaction depends on the structure of the surface and to evaluate a kinetic factor increasing with temperature.

4. Imaging self-assembled monolayers

Following the previous work on functionalization of surface with oligonucleotides, we have been interested by using them for hybridization with DNA strands. Therefore, oligonucleotides must be available to hybridization without displaying rapid removal under hybridization or washing conditions. It means that oligonucleotides must be chemically grafted on the surface. Indeed, thiol-metal bonds are on the order of 100 kJ mol^{-1}, making the bond stable in a wide variety of temperature, solvents, and potentials (Vos et al., 2003). Thus for further applications, we have passivated a surface functionalized with a high density of oligonucleotides, using SAMs.

4.1 What is called self-assembled monolayer?

Self-assembled monolayer, or SAM, provides one of the easiest ways to obtain ordered monolayers leading to the preparation of thermodynamically stable monolayers (Nuzzo & Allara, 1986; Ulman, 1991; Dubois & Nuzzo, 1992) as compared to Langmuir–Blodgett (Vos et al., 2003; Madou, 2002) and other techniques, where only physisorbed, thermally unstable mono/multilayer films are obtained. They consist of a monomolecular thick film of organic molecules, which presents a hydrophilic "head-group" and a hydrophobic "tail group". The formation of SAM starts by strong chemisorption of the hydrophilic "head-group", from either vapor or liquid phase (Schwartz, 2001), followed by a slow two-dimensional organization of hydrophobic "tail groups" (Wnek & Bowlin, 2004).

Areas of close-packed molecules nucleate and grow until the surface is covered with a single monolayer. In fact, the monolayer packs tightly due to Van der Waals interactions (Kaifer, 2001; Estroff et al., 2005). Several studies show that long-chain alkane thiols form more well-ordered defect-free monolayers (hydrophobicity increases with the length of alkanethiols) than short-chain alkanethiols, disulphides or sulphides. Aromatic (pi systems like benzene, naphthalene or diphenylene systems) or/and hydrogen-bonded molecules with multiple contacts, containing functional groups like thiols, amines, sulphides, selenides etc. provide improved stability (Bandyopadhyay et al., 1999; Venkataraman et al., 1999; Aslam et al., 2001).

4.2 Passivation with self assembled monolayer

One of the important advantages of SAM is that they can be prepared in the laboratory by simply dipping the desired substrate in the required millimolar solution for a specified time followed by thorough washing with the same solvent and drying, often using a jet of dry argon. In our work, we have investigated the influence of physico-chemical properties of molecules forming the SAM. Therefore, we have carried out passivation of oligonucleotides functionalized gold surface obtained above with SAM. An important property of molecules forming SAM is that they display a hydrophilic "head-group" and a hydrophobic "tail group", but also an "end group" at the end of the tail. This "end group" can be hydrophobic or hydrophilic leading to what we call a "hydrophobic SAM" or a "hydrophilic SAM", respectively. Thus, we are interested by interactions between oligonucleotides and SAM according to properties of this "end group".

4.2.1 Passivation with hydrophobic SAM

One example of molecules which are known to form hydrophobic SAM on gold surface, are alkanethiols (containing ten methyl units), the "end group" being a CH_3. The monolayer formation proceeds in two steps: first physisorption and then diffusion and chemisorption, which lead to an ordered layer due to attractive intermolecular interaction. The balance sheet of these interactions induces a spontaneous and slightly exothermic (ΔE_{ads} 0.2eV) adsorption process of alkanethiols on a gold surface (Dubois & Nuzzo, 1992). We have observed that on surface functionalized with a high density of oligonucleotides (figure 5a), passivation leads to a homogeneous film of alkanethiols, compacting the oligonucleotides along lines (figure 5b). In figure 5b, the trend towards demixing is due to hydrophobic properties of alkanethiols, which push the oligonucleotides on the grain boundaries. Hence oligonucleotides are more or less upright on the surface with a height of several nm. However in this case, we note that passivation with a hydrophobic SAM renders the oligonucleotides not sufficiently available for hybridization, due to steric effects.

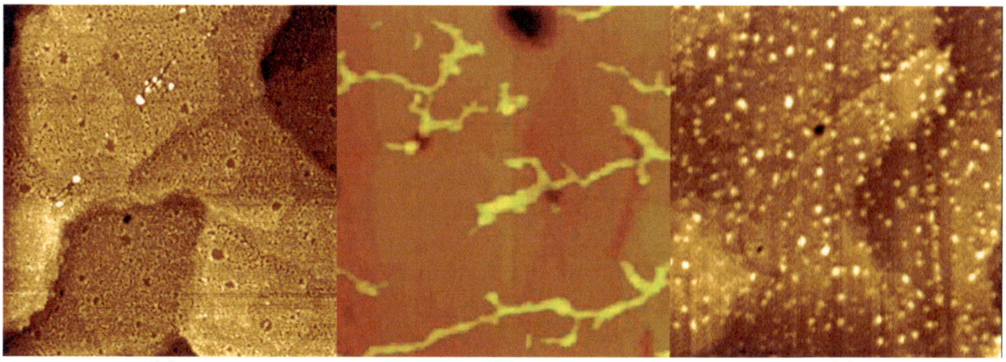

(a) (b) (c)

Fig. 5. Passivation of surface functionalized with oligonucleotides: 5a) AFM image of a surface functionalized with a high density of oligonucleotides: molecules cover the surface with holes of 1 nm depth. The size of scanning is 5 μm × 5 μm and z scale is 3 nm; 5b) AFM image of a surface after immersion in an aqueous solution of alkanethiol: oligonucleotides are grouped together and form compact lines of few nm height, surrounded by a homogeneous film of alkanethiols of 1 nm height. The size of scanning is 3 μm × 3 μm and z scale is 7 nm; 5c) AFM image of surface after immersion in an aqueous solution of mercaptohexanol: oligonucleotides show increased levels of desorption and the remaining molecules are dispersed on the surface. They appear as bumps of 1nm height, which are surrounded by a homogeneous film of mercaptohexanol. The size of scanning is 0.5 μm × 0.5 μm and z scale is 2 nm.

4.2.2 Passivation with hydrophilic SAM

The passivation with hydrophilic SAM has been carried out using mercaptohexanol, an alkylthiol chain containing six methyl units and an OH as "end group". We have observed that this hydrophilic SAM desorbs almost all of the chemisorbed molecules (90%), substituting them by a molecular film (figure 5c). This result notably differs from the one obtained by other authors (Levicky et al., 1998), who measured 20 to 50% of desorption. They attribute these values solely to desorption of physisorbed oligonucleotides. In our case, the strong desorption is probably due to our gold surface with large terraces (figure 3a), where a highly ordered layer of mercaptohexanol can grow. In contrast, their surface of gold evaporated on glass at low temperature shows nanometric crystallites. Hence the organization of their layer of mercaptohexanol is not sufficient to compete with chemisorbed oligonucleotides. In conclusion the passivation with a hydrophilic molecule leads to a surface with only few oligonucleotides, which are well-isolated for further hybridization with a DNA stands.

4.3 Imaging hybridization

The aim of surface functionalized with oligonucleotides and passivated with mercaptohexanol is to be applied as DNA chips. Therefore, oligonucleotides must be available for hybridization with a DNA strand of 1000 bases. In fact, after passivation with mercaptohexanol, oligonucleotides are well-dispersed on the surface. Hence, they acquire a configurational freedom which allows them to form double helix with complementary DNA strands. First, we have obtained two DNA single strands (DNAss) by the retro transcription of a messenger RNA (ARNm) selected for its biological interest. One of these strands being complementary to the oligonucleotide of 25 bases that we have grafted on the gold surface, our aim is to control the selectivity of our oligonucleotide functionalized surface. In order to verify AFM imaging results, we have also radio-labeled with P32 during the retro transcription process.

Once the DNAss is hybridized, the 25 bases of the molecule reacting with the oligonucleotide lead to a double strand which is quite stiff. In comparison, the free part of the DNAss appears like a linear chain of oligonucleotide, which diameter is smaller than the double strand. Hence, this free part is very flexible and can undergo important deformations. That is why it is often represented by a Gaussian polymer (Zhang Y., 2001), meaning that each monomer can be considered as a vector randomly oriented, considering electrostatic repulsion interactions between phosphate groups and pairing between complementary bases. In addition, as hybridization is carried out in a salt buffer, pairing between bases from the same strand can occur, facilitated by presence of counter ions, which neutralize phosphate groups charges (Montanari & Mézard, 2000).

The aim of AFM imaging is to differentiate non-hybridized oligonucleotides to hybridized ones from the different of size. Indeed, we have observed features of 2.5 nm height on hybridized surface (figure 6a), that we attribute to hybridized DNAss. The hybridization is confirmed by radioactivity scanning of a 1 cm^2 surface (figure 6c). In contrast, AFM image of hybridization with a non-complementary DNAss gives a low physisorption (figure 6b), which is confirmed by radioactivity scanning (figure 6d). However, the amount of hybridized molecules counted in AFM images is lower than radioactivity measures. This is probably due to the mobility of certain molecules chains, which renders them hard to observe with AFM.

In addition, some of the features of a "non-hybridized" surface can be attributed to proteins contained in hybridization buffer. Indeed, the mercaptohexanol film makes the surface

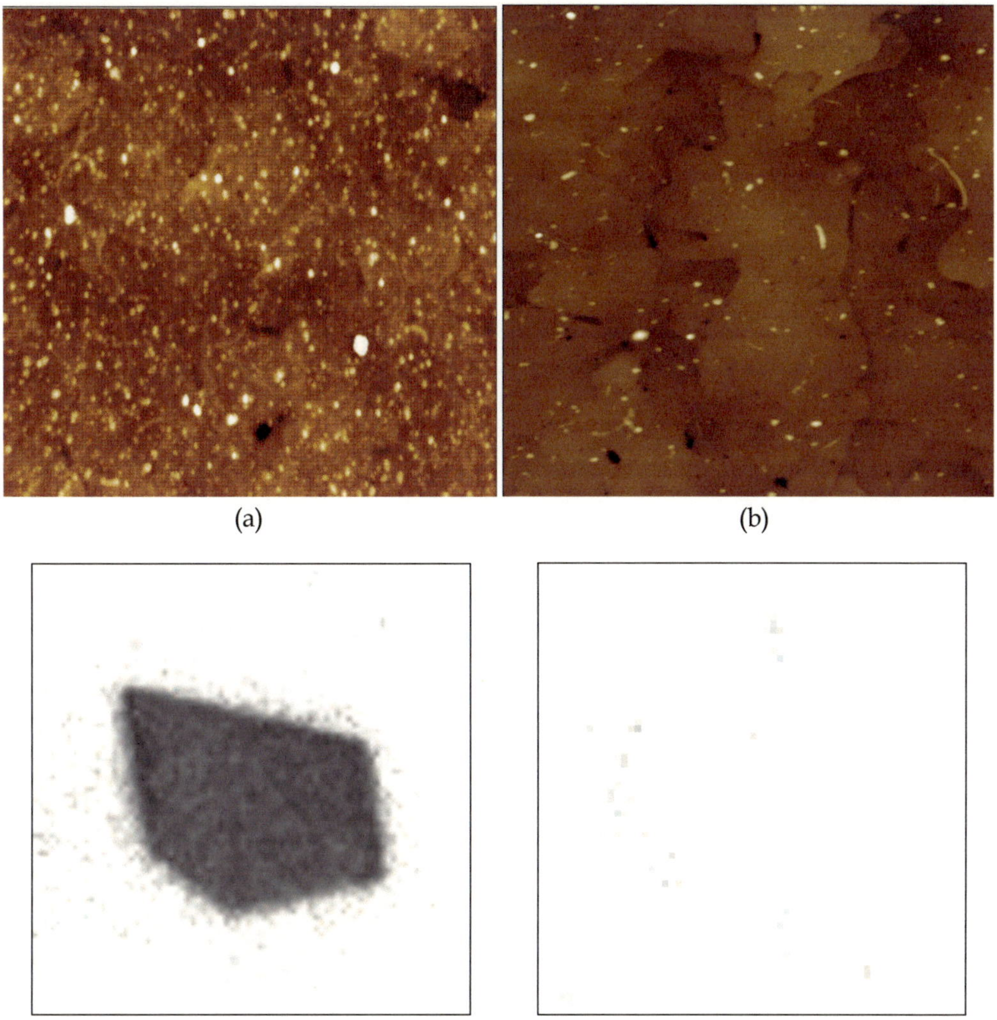

(a) (b) (c) (d)

Fig. 6. Imaging of hybridization on surfaces functionalized with oligonucleotides and passivated with mercaptohexanol: With complementary DNAss : the amount of hybridized molecules evaluated 6a) on AFM image is of 10^3 molecules μm^{-2} and 6c) by radioactivity measurements (surface size of 1 cm^2) is of 5.10^3 molecules μm^{-2}. The size of AFM images is 1 µm × 1 µm and z scale is 7 nm; With non-complementary DNAss : the amount of hybridized molecules evaluated 6b) on AFM image is of 50 molecules μm^{-2} and 6d) by radioactivity measurement (surface size of 1 cm^2) is of 10 molecules μm^{-2}. The size of AFM images is 1 µm × 1 µm and z scale is 7 nm.

hydrophilic due to OH "end groups" present on the surface. Hence, proteins and DNA chains can adsorb on it. Without hybridization, non-complementary DNAss and protein are in competition. Whereas in presence of complementary DNAss, the reaction of hybridization is promoted. Moreover, their chains can be mobile on the surface with low electrostatic interactions with OH, hence becoming less visible to AFM.

In conclusion, AFM tapping mode permits one to image mechanism of passivation with SAM. According to hydrophobity or hydrophilicity properties of the SAM, interactions with molecules present on the surface vary. The hydrophilic SAM appears to let on the surface only the oligonucleotides which are well-chemisorbed and available for reactions. Furthermore, the differentiation between hybridized and non-hybridized oligonucleotides is successfully achieved by tapping mode thanks to size difference. Thus, AFM imaging becomes an alternative way of detecting directly reactions on surface, with the advantage of avoiding the preparation of labeled molecules.

5. Imaging 2D polymerized film

Functionalization with alkylsilane to form 2D polymerized film is of great interest in various fields, such as biosensors (Battistel et al., 1991; Schierbaum, 1994), microelectronics (Kumar et al., 1994; Burtman et al., 1999), catalysis (Juvaste et al., 1999; Yang et al., 2003), etc. For this purpose, alkylsilanes are grafted on glass (Ulman, 1991), silicon (Vandenberg et al., 1991; Kallury et al., 1994; Vrancken et al., 1995; Horr & Arora, 1997; Ek et al., 2003; Zhang & Srinivasan, 2004) or mica (Bezanilla et al., 1995; Lyubchenko et al., 1996; Tätte et al., 2003; Diez-Perez, 2004; Crampton et al., 2005, 2006) surfaces. Generally, it is assumed that molecules adsorb in an ordered film on the surface. Alkyloxy moieties form Si-O covalent bonds between the molecules or with the surface hydroxyl groups to build up a polymeric film anchored on the surface. In the case of bi-functionalized molecules, with a terminal group R such as H_2N^-, HO^-, HS^-, HSO_3^-, Cl^-, and Br^-, the second functionality R is expected to extend from the surface. However, often, more disordered monolayers are observed (Vandenberg et al., 1991; Kallury et al., 1994; Vrancken et al., 1995; Horr & Arora, 1997). Indeed, usually, both terminal groups are able to interact with the surface through hydrogen or electrostatic bonds, resulting in various configurations (Heiney et al., 2000; White & Tripp, 2000). Furthermore, because interactions between the molecules and the surface depend drastically on the substrate properties, a lack of reproducibility in film formation is often observed.

We have been interested by the functionalization of mica for reasons described above. Our molecule of interest for the formation of a 2D polymerized film is an aminosilane: *N*-(2-aminoethyl)-3 aminopropyltrimethoxysilane (AAPS). The adsorption of AAPS was studied on silica, and authors described it as an ordered film anchored on the surface via Si-O covalent bond, the amine functions extending from the surface (Chrisey et al., 1996; Ek et al., 2004). However, no experiment confirming this scheme was reported for AAPS on mica. In general, two ways of immobilizing a film on a surface exist: aqueous and vapor deposition.

5.1 Preparation of the substrate

In contrast to silica, freshly cleaved mica lacks native hydroxyl groups (Crampton et al., 2006), so covalent binding essential for the formation of a well-anchored layer of molecules seems unlikely. This problem is overcome by activating the surface through hydration to open up the silicate bonds (Kim et al., 2002). Two methods of hydration are possible:

- The first method consists of exposing the sample to a jet of steam (Schwartz et al., 1992). Figure 7 shows the evolution of the surface with time of exposition. After 30s of exposure, surface presents 3-5 Å depth holes (figure 7a) and longer exposure, such as 90 s, leads to more or less wide 2D islands with a height of 1 nm (figure 7b). Because this height corresponds to the thickness of one mica leaflet, we attribute these islands to remaining pieces of the outer leaflet of mica, probably after a corrosion of the surface. Because an additional molecule layer also has a height on the order of 1 nm, this kind of surface is obviously not suitable for our study. Unfortunately, steam treatment of mica is not reproducible enough to obtain a surface without such islands.

- The second method of hydration consists of incubating the sample in water at room temperature. After 10 min of incubation, the AFM image shows a flat surface with no islands (figure 7c). In addition, this treatment leads to reproducible hydrated surfaces.

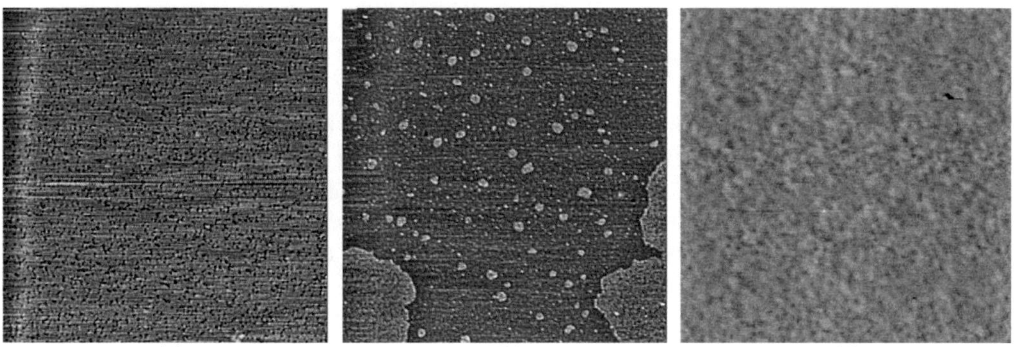

(a) (b) (c)

Fig. 7. AFM images (2 µm × 2 µm size) of the mica surface: 7a) exposed to a jet of steam for 30 s: holes correspond to a depth of 3-5 Å; 7b) exposed to a jet of steam for 90 s: islands correspond to a height of 1 nm; 7c) incubated in water for 10 min: holes correspond to a depth of 3-5 Å.

Finally, the chemical modifications due to both surface treatments are assessed by contact angle measurements. These are done immediately after completion of the treatment. Freshly cleaved mica shows a highly hydrophilic surface with a contact angle smaller than 5° (Seah & Dench, 1979). Incubation in water for 10 min makes it change to 20°. In the case of steam treatment, the contact angle measured on surfaces without islands increases with the time of exposure, also reaching 20°. This small variation in contact angle suggests that the surface is likely to be homogeneous. Thus, both methods similarly modify wetting properties of the surface. Even if we have no indication of the presence or the number of hydroxyl groups on the surface, we observe a lack of AAPS adsorption during the treatment in the vapor phase on a freshly cleaved mica surface.

For the adsorption in the aqueous phase, the molecule film depends neither on the previous hydration nor on the hydration method. This indicates that during the incubation in the solution of AAPS, the surface would be modified just like during incubation in water. Therefore, we have chosen the relevant hydration method depending on whether the subsequent molecule layer is performed through vapor or aqueous deposition. For vapor phase deposition of AAPS, mica is first hydrated by a jet of steam after precautious checking of the quality of the surface by AFM. For aqueous phase deposition, we routinely use the incubation method without checking the surface prior to molecules deposition.

5.2 Deposition in aqueous phase

In aqueous phase, the two amines contained by AAPS molecules can be either protonated or not, according to the solution pH. The mica lattice contains negative binding sites associated with Al and filled with potassium ions, K^+. In fluid, these cations (K^+) can be removed or displaced, as shown by surface force apparatus and XPS, presenting a negative surface potential (Crampton et al., 2005). For instance, protonated AAPS molecules (due to pH) can replace potassium ions, so they can adsorb preferentially on the surface. Therefore, pH must play a decisive role in the adsorption of AAPS on mica. For instance pure water (pH around 6) used to rinse the surface after immersion in AAPS solution, can protonate molecules. However, we have shown with XPS that for low concentrations, the number of molecules left after drying the surface without rinsing can be negligible.

5.2.1 Effect of pH

Experiments carried out by varying pH have allowed us to relate the protonation of AAPS amines to a $pK_{1/2}$ like the one introduced by Holmes-Farley et al. (Holmes-Farley et al, 1988). They defined the $pK_{1/2}$ for a liquid-solid interface as the value of the pH of the solution at which the functional groups at the interface are half-ionized. Thus, we have evaluated a $pK_{1/2}$ of 10-11 for the AAPS-mica interface, explaining the adsorption of AAPS by electrostatic interactions via protonated terminal amines only for pH's under 10 (Mourougou-Candoni & Thibaudau, 2009). In addition, the maximum surface density reached by protonated AAPS molecules is around 40% of the compact monolayer density. In fact, mica displays a large negative surface charge density in solution, which can form electrostatic bonds with protonated amine groups of aminosilane (Trens et al., 1995). Thus, we can relate the density of the protonated AAPS (i.e., 1.7×10^{14} molecules.cm^{-2}) to the density of negative charges on the bare surface, which is on the order of 1.8×10^{14} cm^{-2} (Maslova et al., 2004). Thus, our results clearly indicate that adsorption first proceeds by ionic interaction between the protonated amino groups and the negative charges of the surface until these are neutralized. Then electrostatic repulsion between protonated AAPS prevents their additional adsorption. Subsequently, only neutral molecules (with two free amines) are able to adsorb onto the surface.

5.2.2 Effect of incubation time

Exploring incubation time, we have evaluated that the density of molecule reach rapidly around 50% of the compact monolayer density and saturates at this value obtained by XPS measurements. Therefore, we investigate the configuration of AAPS molecules with AFM imaging in tapping mode (figure 8). We suppose that molecules cover either half of the surface, being upright on it, or the whole surface more or less lying flat on it. For 5 min of exposure, the substrate displays a homogeneous surface with a low roughness in the order of few angstroms (figure 8a); no island or structure of 1 nm height (corresponding to AAPS height) can be seen on the AFM image. Thus, it is clear that these AFM data are more in agreement with molecules lying flat on the surface. For longer exposure, bumps of heterogeneous heights around 0.5-1 nm appear on the layer (figure 8b). These bumps may correspond to small aggregates of upright molecules that are condensed on the surface or that have been already formed in the solution. However, we have not observed the formation of a structured layer of molecules leading to a film of molecules on the surface.

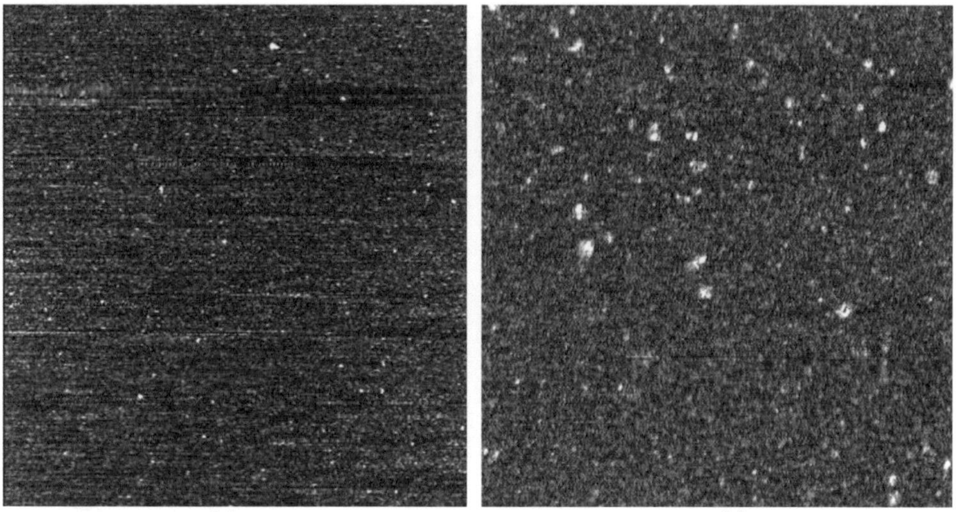
(a) (b)

Fig. 8. AFM images (2 µm × 2 µm size) of hydrated mica surface incubated in a solution of AAPS at 40 µM for (8a) 5 min and (8b) 45 min. The darker to brighter features correspond to 1 nm height.

Although AAPS adsorption in aqueous phase gives interesting results concerning the dependence with pH, we note limitations due to film disordering on the surface and copolymerization of AAPS in the liquid. It must be pointed out that this kind of problems may happen with every alkyloxy molecule because they can polymerize in solution. We insist on the importance of these experiences because they demonstrate clearly that surface analysis techniques must be completed by a direct visualization via AFM in order to study film formation.

5.3 Deposition in vapor phase

5.3.1 Formation of monolayer

To overcome problems of self-polymerization, deposition in the vapor phase can be also proposed because molecular density is lower in the vapor phase. Indeed, self-assembled monolayers have been obtained with silane on silicon (Sugimara et al., 2002). In our experiments, the mica surface is exposed to AAPS vapor under an anhydrous nitrogen atmosphere at room temperature for 15 min to 48 h, and afterward, the surface is imaged by AFM (figures 9). For 15 min of exposure to AAPS, the surface appears rough with few bi-dimensional islands (figure 9a). These islands and the surrounded surface heights are of 0.8 and 0.4-0.5 nm, respectively. This must be compared to the roughness of 0.2 nm of the mica substrate before its exposure to AAPS. After 1 h of exposure, figure 9b shows a quite homogeneous film with holes of 0.8 nm depth (with few bumps).

In addition, the contact angle of a water drop on the surface increases with exposure time, reaching ~50° on the film. This value is in the range of contact angles reported for aminosilanes films (40-63°) (Song et al., 2006). Moreover, because the length of AAPS molecules is on the order of 1 nm, islands are probably formed by condensed upright AAPS

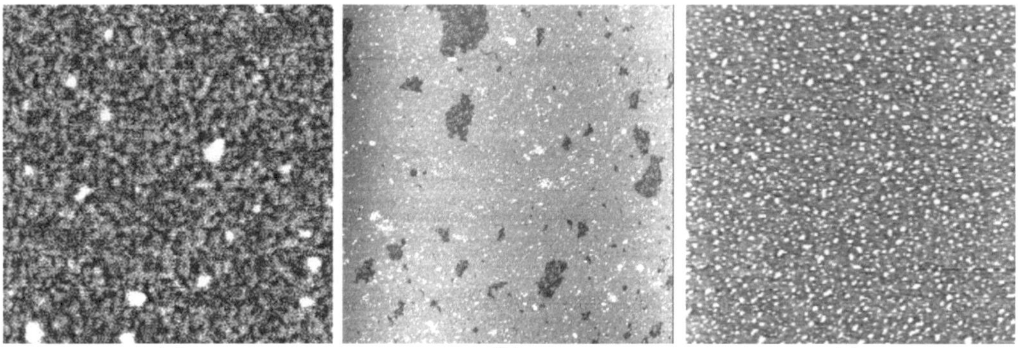

(a) (b) (c)

Fig. 9. AFM images of hydrated mica surfaces exposed to vapor of AAPS under anhydrous nitrogen atmosphere: 9a) For 15 min (1 μm × 1 μm size) the darker to brighter features correspond to 1 nm height; 9b) For 1 h (2 μm × 2 μm size), light gray to dark gray features correspond to 1 nm height; 9c) For 48 h (2 μm × 2 μm size), dark gray to white features correspond to 10 nm height.

molecules (0.8 nm), which are surrounded by prone molecules (0.4-0.5 nm). The film obtained after 1 h of exposure is undoubtedly a monolayer of upright molecules on the surface. According to these results, we infer that molecules first adsorb onto the surface in a disordered phase, and then they condense into islands, which grow and coalesce to form a monolayer.

5.3.2 Restructuration of layers

For a longer treatment (48h), AFM images show that the surface increases in roughness, with bumps of ~2-4 nm height (figure 9c). Hence, after the first monolayer has grown, adsorbed molecules instead form 3D clusters. This phenomenon is similar to the well-known Stransky-Krastanov crystalline growth mode. This mode appears when the interfacial energy between the surface and the first monolayer is lower than the surface energy of the monolayer and when the interfacial energy between the first monolayer and successive layers is higher than the surface energy of successive layers. Actually, this structure is not stable and changes with exposure to ambient atmosphere. Indeed, the surface morphology of the sample presented in figure 9c is obviously modified after 24 h in ambient atmosphere (figure 10a): it is covered with numerous small, bi-dimensional islands of 1.7 nm height and a few larger islands. However, "pinholes" of 0.8 nm depth on the film supporting the islands (figure 10b) indicate that the first monolayer does not drastically change and that the restructuring instead concerns the matter on it. The depletion area surrounding the highest islands (figure 10a) indicates that they grow from the surrounding matter. This is typical of a dewetting phenomenon.

According to this reorganization, it is obvious that molecules are mobile prior to exposure to the ambient atmosphere. The more realistic assumption to explain this mobility is that polymerization is not complete after exposure to AAPS under anhydrous nitrogen atmosphere, certainly due to the lack of water molecules for the hydrolysis of the methoxy ends, whereas when the surface shown in figure 9c is exposed to ambient humidity, hydrolysis

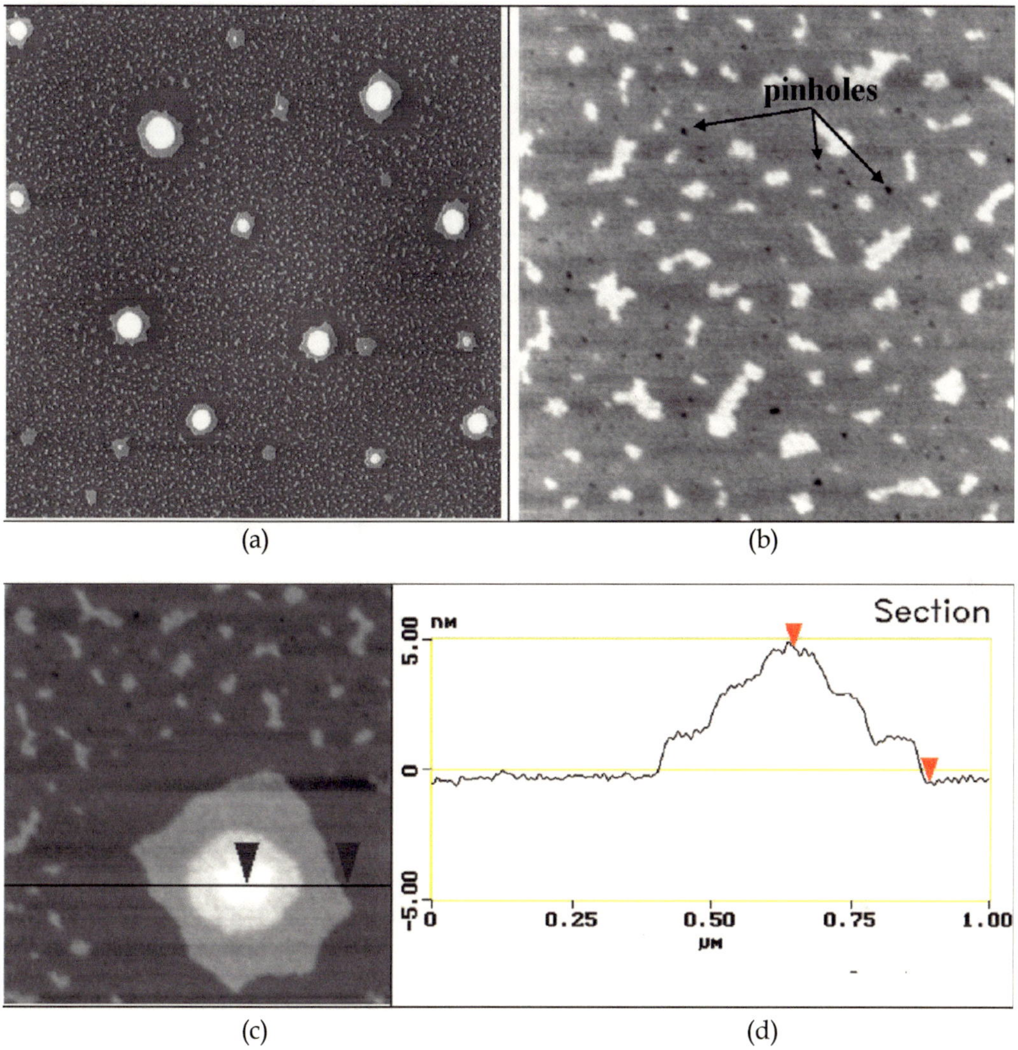

Fig. 10. AFM images of mica surface treated for 48 h to vapor of AAPS and exposed 24 h in ambient atmosphere at room temperature: 10a) The size of the image is of 10 μm × 10 μm, the darker to brighter features correspond to 15 nm height; 10b) Magnified image (2 μm × 2 μm size) of bilayer islands with pinholes of 0.8 nm depth on the film supporting the bilayer islands; 10c) Magnified image (1 μm × 1 μm size) of a high island with superposed bilayers; 10d) Section analysis of the high island of panel 10c.

occurs, which triggers polymerization and film reconstruction. Concerning the larger islands, some of them are of 1.7 nm height, but most display one or more stacked bi-dimensional islands of 1.7 nm height like a set of "Russian dolls". For example, figure 10c shows a large island composed of three stacked bi-dimensional islands of 1.7 nm height (see cross section in figure 10d). Such a stacking indicates an order in the film above the first monolayer, perpendicular to the surface. The quantification of heights measured with AFM (of 0.8 nm for the first monolayer and 1.7 nm for islands) clearly rules out a non-structured film.

5.3.3 Configuration of molecules

This study with AFM imaging and contact angle measurements allows us to deduce a schematic for the formation of AAPS layers on mica. For the first monolayer, a contact angle of ~60° is expected for the 100% amino-terminated monolayer (N. P. Huang et al., 2001). In our case (50°), we clearly obtain a uniform assembly of upright molecules with amine ends oriented mainly outward. In addition, this monolayer does not change from exposure under anhydrous atmosphere to ambient atmosphere (figure 10b). This obviously means that molecules interact among themselves or with the surface when they adsorb under anhydrous atmosphere. However, Si-O covalent bonds must be rare due to the lack of water molecules for the hydrolysis of the methoxy ends. Therefore, molecules are probably self-assembled on the surface via van der Waals interactions.

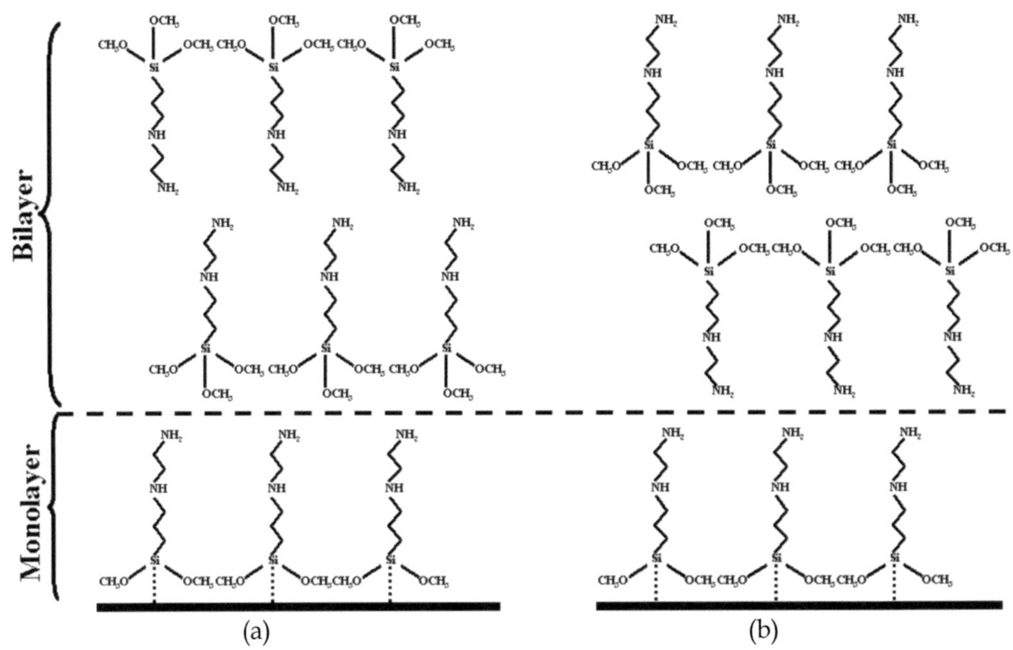

Fig. 11. Possible configurations of the bilayer: molecules in the bilayer are standing either head-to-head or tail-to-tail. (The first monolayer is a self-assembly of upright molecules with amine ends mainly oriented outward.)

For the film above the first monolayer, exposure to ambient atmosphere restructures it in bi-dimensional islands with a perpendicular periodicity of 1.7 nm, which is approximately twice the height of a monolayer. This suggests that islands are formed of one bilayer of upright molecules. If molecules in the bilayer were arranged head to tail, we would also observe a stacking periodicity of 0.8 nm order perpendicular to the surface. Consequently, molecules are standing either head-to-head, or tail-to-tail. According to these remarks, only two (coarse) orientations are possible for AAPS molecules of the film superposed to the first monolayer (figure 11a and b). Moieties displayed at the interface with air are methoxy ends in figure 11a and amine ends in figure 11b. Therefore, contact angle measurements on the bilayer could discriminate between both configurations, but these measurements are quite imprecise, probably due to the mobility of the bilayer. However, if the interaction between a tail and a head is preferential in the interface between the first monolayer and the subsequent film, as in the configuration of figure 9a, then it is also the case inside the bilayer. Therefore configuration 11a is not self-consistent, contrary to configuration 11b.

More precisely, molecules oriented as in figure 11b can display two structures. The first one, hereafter called a double leaflet structure, consists of two superposed leaflets with structure and density similar to the first monolayer, molecules of a leaflet polymerizing with each other (figure 12a). The second structure, hereafter called a single-leaflet structure, consists of only one sheet of 2D polymerized molecules, the tails of these molecules being alternatively localized on each side of the polymerization plan (figure 12b). In this case, the density of tails on each side of the polymerization plan is half of that in the first layer, and we can expect that the tails of molecules are tilted to pack the structure. Of the two structures, the latter seems more realistic to us if we consider their formation. In fact, the double-leaflet structure, figure 12a, implies that molecules of the leaflet close to the monolayer (inner leaflet) must be completely polymerized before the other leaflet (outer leaflet) extends on it. Otherwise a cross-polymerization will occur between both leaflets, and in the limiting case, it will lead to the single-leaflet structure. Therefore, if the double-leaflet structure is valid, we will observe areas with the inner leaflet covered partially by the outer leaflet.

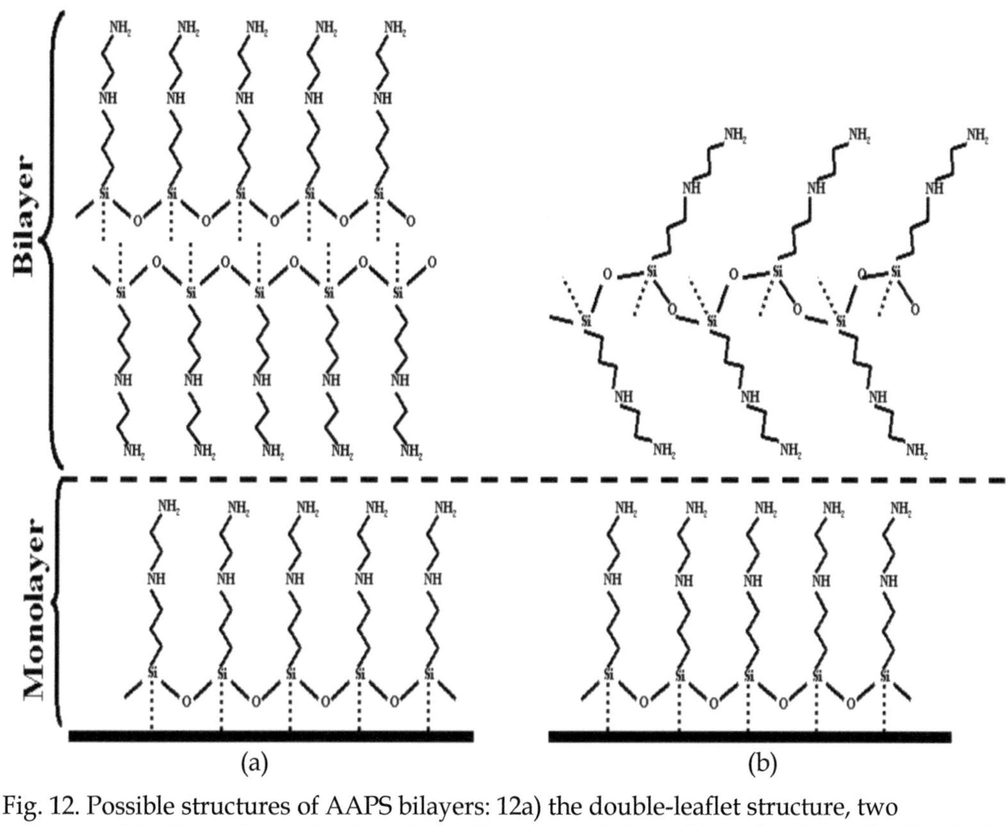

Fig. 12. Possible structures of AAPS bilayers: 12a) the double-leaflet structure, two superposed leaflets with molecules of a leaflet polymerizing with each other; 12b) the single-leaflet structure, one sheet of 2D polymerized molecules.

In addition, the dewetting behavior observed on AFM images in ambient atmosphere is driven by a difference between interfacial energies. In fact, the interfacial energy between the first monolayer and the bilayer must be different from the interfacial energy between bilayers. In the case of the double-leaflet structure, both interfaces are similar, given by the chemistry and the density of tails, which are the same in the monolayer and in the bilayer. In contrast, in the single leaflet structure, the density of tails at interfaces between bilayers is different from the one at the interface between the first monolayer and the bilayer. This undoubtedly leads to different interfacial energies. Thus, the single-leaflet structure correlates with the behavior of bilayers. On the basis of energy considerations or formation mechanisms, configuration 12b seems to be the most realistic structure. In order to determine precisely the organization of the molecules in the bilayer, we have to reach a molecular resolution on these films with AFM.

In conclusion, AFM imaging allows us to study the formation and structure of AAPS on mica thanks to a systematic study of deposition conditions and their effects. It must be pointed out that this kind of exploration must be undertaken to understand functionalization of surface with 2D polymerized films. Thus, in aqueous treatment the interaction of molecules with the surface depends on the pH, as compared to the $pK_{1/2}$ that must be evaluated through AFM imaging and surface analysis techniques. In this work, only for pH's under 10 does the AAPS adsorb on the mica surface by electrostatic interactions via protonated terminal amines and no formation of a structured layer of molecules is observed. Therefore, tapping mode has been used to thoroughly investigate vapor treatment, demonstrating that the film of AAPS is composed of a first monolayer and successive bilayers. We must point out that AFM imaging has lead to the first observation of such an organization in aminosiloxane films, to our knowledge.

6. Development on conventional AFM in tapping mode

We have presented in the parts above various potentialities of conventional AFM in tapping mode for imaging functionalized surfaces. We have based our argumentation on experiments carried out on very different ways of functionalization, such as aqueous or vapor treatments leading to isolated single molecules, SAMs or polymer 2D films. However, parameters such as resolution, environment and speed of imaging must be improved according to the functionalizing process. Therefore, many developments on conventional AFM tapping mode have been carried out contributing to its imaging capacities and its applications.

6.1 Topographic imaging resolution

The first application of AFM in tapping mode is topographical imaging. In this field, the principal requirement is the resolution.

6.1.1 Improvements in tip development

In conventional AFM in tapping mode, we have mentioned that the radius of curvature of the tip and its shape are of great importance for the imaging resolution in air. In addition, the surface chemistry of the tips, usually not well defined, may limit the application of tapping AFM in the investigation of functionalized surfaces. A great breakthrough in terms of resolution comes from carbon nanotubes attached to the end of the tip (figure 13) (Dai et al, 1996; Hafner et al., 2001; Wong et al., 1998a, 1998b). Indeed, carbon nanotube tips possess a high aspect ratio, mechanical robustness, small diameter and a well-defined surface chemistry. The resolution attainable with these tips is comparable with that of other ultimate resolution imaging techniques such as cryogenic electron-microscopy (Koehne, 2011; Kitazawa, 2011). In addition, nanotubes also offer the possibility to be functionalized, exposing, thus, well-defined chemical groups or chemisorbed biomolecules. This opportunity can be exploited to study the spatial distribution of chemical functional groups or complementary biomolecules as for hybridization (Woolley, 2004).

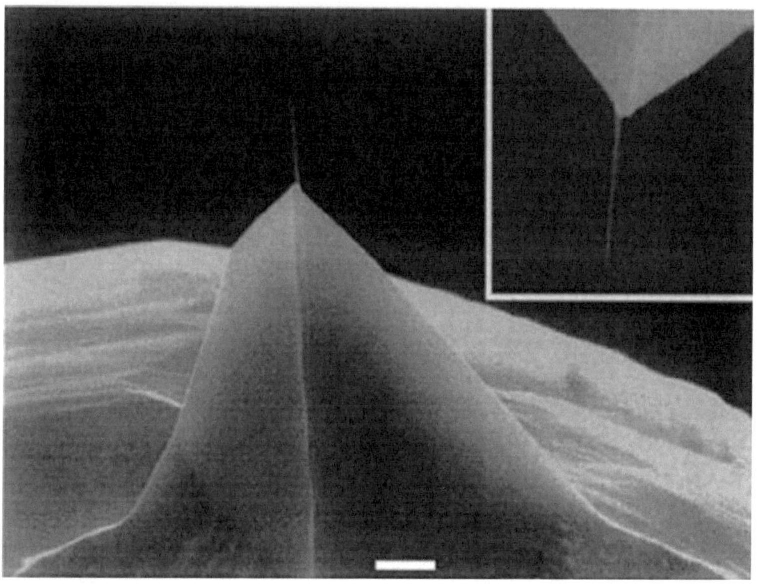

Fig. 13. Carbon nanotube attached to the end of a silicon tip. The inset is a higher magnification view of the same tip rotated 180°◦ relative to the main image (bar = 1 μm) (Alessandrini & Facci, 2005).

6.1.2 Improvement in force control

Resolution can also be improved by accurately controlling the interaction between tip and sample. The variation of the tip-sample force is achieved by changing the amplitude of the freely oscillating tip called driving amplitude, DA, and the set-point amplitude, SP. The effective tip-sample force increases with DA and/or the difference (DA-SP) (Höper et al., 1995) by modifying the set point, which balances the contribution of attractive and repulsive forces. (San Paulo & Garcia, 2000). Thus, an automatically adjusted set-point can produce lower force measurements at higher spatial resolutions (Möller et al., 1999). However, in imaging in air, an attractive force appears due to the layer of water condensation and other contamination which often covers both tip and sample. Indeed, water forms a meniscus pulling the tip and sample together. The resulting strong attractive force is usually of 10 to 100nN, making high-resolution imaging difficult and sometimes causing sample damage. (Dufrêne, 2002). These capillary forces can be eliminated by performing the imaging in aqueous solution, and so maximizing resolution (Alessandrini & Facci, 2005).

6.2 Non-topographical modes of imaging

In contrast to the contact mode, the height images of the tapping mode can show minor, and sometimes, barely detectable variations with changes in the force. In this case, the frequency and phase of the oscillating cantilever are more sensitive to the tip-sample interaction force.

6.2.1 Frequency imaging

The description of the vibrating probe as a harmonic oscillator shows that repulsive tip-sample force interactions cause a shift of the resonant frequency to high frequencies and related phase changes (Dürig et al., 1992). Attractive forces decrease the resonant frequency. The images of frequency shifts provide new information about surface topography and other properties (Babcock et al., 1995). The frequency shift images are not widely used in measurements at ambient conditions because the low Q-factor of the cantilever in air makes it difficult to track the small negative frequency shifts and to use them for the feedback required for imaging in the attractive force regime (Magonov et al.,1997a). Such an operation works well in ultra high vacuum (UHV) where the Q-factor of the oscillating probe is extremely high. Hence, atomic-scale defects of several semiconductor lattices were observed in this mode (Sugawara et al., 1995).

6.2.2 Phase imaging

In tapping AFM, the phase images are often recorded simultaneously with the height images. They show the variations, at different points on the surface, of the phase of the oscillating tip determined at the fundamental resonant frequency of the freely oscillating tip. Therefore, phase of the tip is adjusted to zero before the tip engages the sample. Phase images provide the best contrast of fine morphological and nano-structural features due to their high sensitivity to surface imperfections such as steps, cracks, and the like. On surfaces with local variations of mechanical properties, the phase changes are even more informative (Magonov et al., 1997b). The phase shift being strictly related to the amount of energy dissipated in the tip–sample contact, mapping the phase shift permits to identify regions of different interaction properties (Cleveland et al., 1998, Tamayo & Garcia, 1997). For instance, gold nanoparticles adsorbed on a phospholipidic bilayer functionalizing a surface of mica give topographical images showing gold nanoparticles with blurred outline (figure 14a). In contrast, phase images clearly permits to distinguish gold nanoparticles with well-defined outline (figure 14b). Thus, the stiffness-related contrast of the phase images offers new possibilities for imaging multi-component samples.

6.3 Imaging resolution in liquid

The development of tapping AFM mode in liquid configured an important breakthrough for the application of the AFM in the case of single molecules or films, which are loosely immobilized. Applications of this method concerns also many other objects, like biological materials, which must be observed in their native environment, thereby opening the possibility of analyzing their structural and functional aspects at the sub-molecular level (Kumar et al., 2005). By selecting appropriate buffer conditions, it is generally possible to maintain an applied force in the range of 0.1 to 0.5 nN. Therefore, a preliminary investigation is recommended on pH and ionic strength effects on the image quality in order

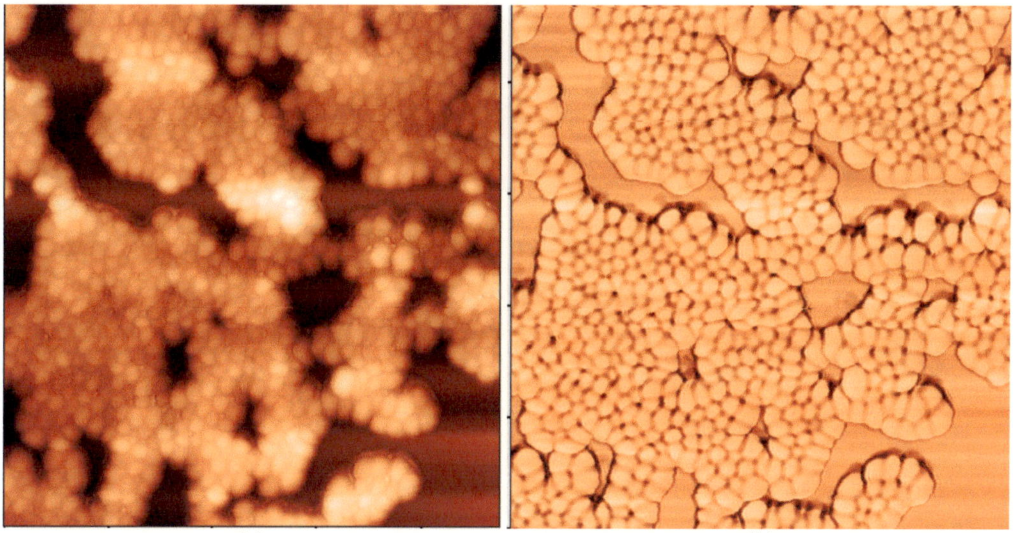

Fig. 14. AFM images of gold nanoparticles adsorbed on a phospholipidic bilayer functionalizing a surface of mica, the size of AFM images is 0.5 μm × 0.5 μm and z scale is 50 nm: 14a) the topographical image shows gold nanoparticles with blurred outline. 14b) the phase image shows nanoparticles with well-defined outline.

to define an optimal imaging environment. Also, because of thermal drift, it is often essential to readjust the applied force between image acquisitions.

For measurements, the sample is immersed in the buffer, in a cell which can be thermostatted, permitting diffusion of molecules and phase transitions of films. An example of the phase transition of a phospholipidic single-bilayer supported on a mica substrate is shown in figure 15 by real time temperature controlled atomic force microscopy. Authors distinguish two-phase transitions in this bilayer arising from the independent melting of each leaflet at different temperatures (Charrier & Thibaudau, 2005). They observe shifts in temperature that they attribute to different leaflet compressions induced by the adsorption of the lipids on the mica substrate. Such studies on fluidity of phospholipid films are a major feature required for technological applications. Indeed because phospholipid bilayers are highly electrically resistant, and ordered, they can be used for biosensor technologies based on electrical and optical detections (Dumas et al., 2011).

However, a fundamental drawback of working in liquid is the reduction of the Q factor of the cantilever. This reduction is caused by the viscosity of the surrounding liquid. The relative high Q value observed in air ensures a high sensitivity since a small shift in the resonance frequency, caused by tip-sample interaction, produces a large drop in the amplitude of the oscillation. In liquids, as the resonance peak is much broader, a small shift in the resonance frequency induces a moderate change in the amplitude of oscillation (Moreno-Herrero et al., 2004). A better way to control the force applied by the tip is an active quality factor control (active-Q). This is a technique which permits to increase the otherwise low quality factor for the oscillating cantilever in liquid and correspondingly to decrease the force applied by the tip on the sample (Alessandrini & Facci, 2005; Tamayo et al., 2000, 2001).

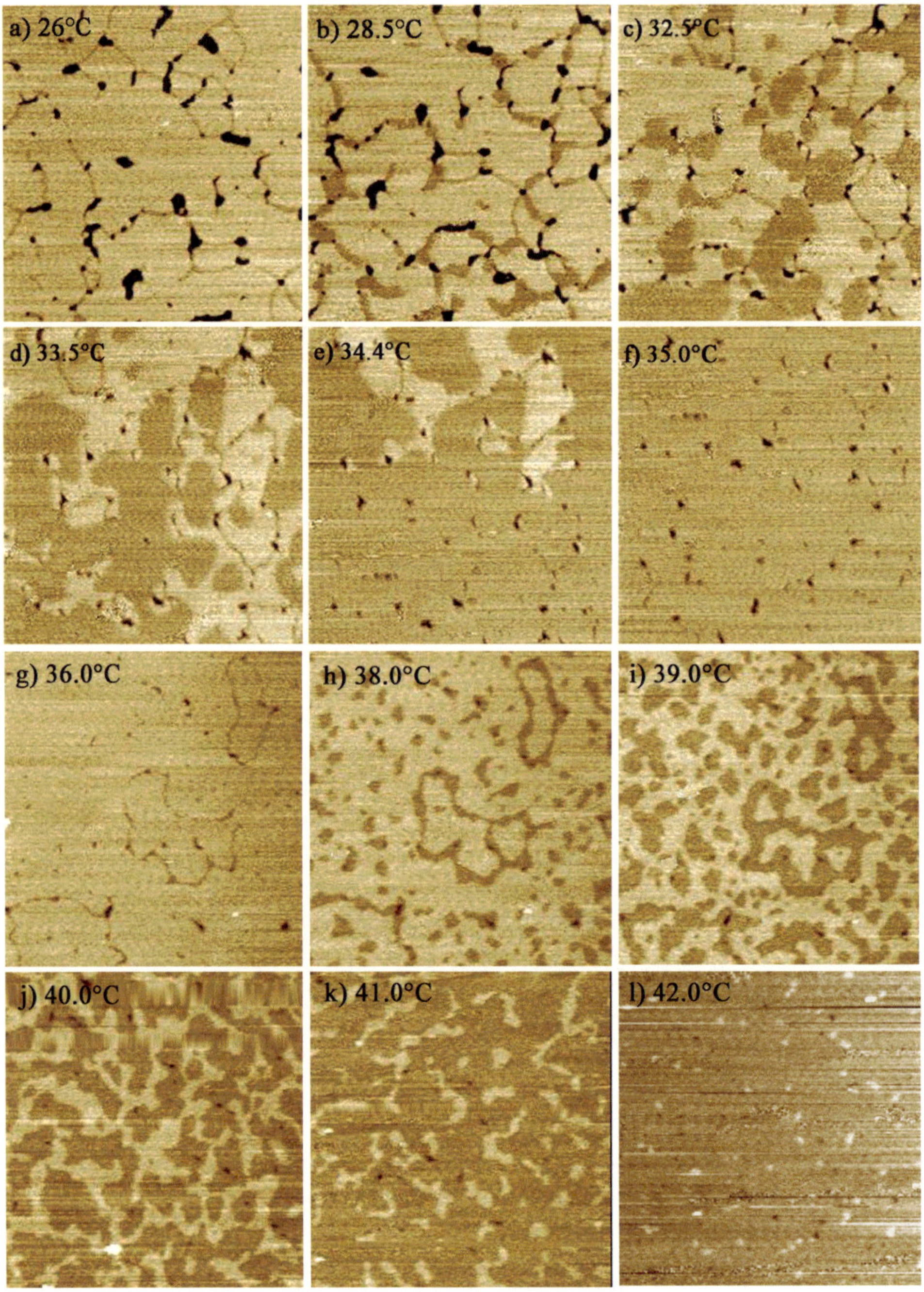

Fig. 15. AFM images (size 3 µm × 3 µm) of the transitions of a supported single-bilayer at different temperatures. The darkest areas are holes in the bilayer. The sample is continuously heated under the AFM tip at a rate of 0.1°C min^{-1}. The temperature indicated on each image corresponds to the temperature in the middle of the image (Charrier & Thibaudau, 2005).

6.4 Improvements on scanning speed

Increasing the scanning speed of AFM in tapping mode permits to follow dynamics of process on functionalized surface, at a nanometer scale. In fact, processes can occur on a millisecond timescale or less, while one image takes generally more than a minute to be captured. The scanning speed is limited by mechanical constraints (Butt et al., 1993). The dynamic of the piezoelectric scanner is a limit for high speed imaging. The dynamic is enhanced by using smaller high-frequency piezo segments to move z-scanner (Mamin et al., 1994; Zhao et al., 2011). Concerning the xy-scanner, an attempt to minimize coupling motions is carried out. Because the scanning speed of each direction may differ, the linear motion stage for a high-speed scanner is designed to have different resonance frequencies for the modes, with one dominant displacement in the desired directions. This unsymmetrical configuration separates the frequencies of two vibration modes with one dominant displacement in each desired direction, and hence suppresses the coupling between motions in two directions (Park & Moon, 2011). Another constraint is to maintain a high signal-to-noise ratio during high speed scanning. Therefore, cantilevers with higher resonant frequencies are needed, while their spring constant should remain constant. For instance, the mass of the cantilevers can be reduced, which permits to combine high resonance frequency with small spring. One way is to reduce the size of cantilevers (9-40 µm) leading to MHz resonance frequency (Walters et al., 1996). Thanks to these cantilevers, authors obtained a sequence of images in liquid at few ms intervals (Ando et al., 2001, Lyubchenko et al., 2011). The last but not the least limiting point is the time taken by the oscillating cantilever to change amplitude (Sulchek et al., 2000). This time can be reduced by implementing an active damping circuit (Sulchek et al., 2002; Fleming et al., 2010).

7. Acknowledgment

I would like to thank Pr. Franck Thibaudau, Dr. Cathy Naud, Dr. Isabelle Meunier and Mr. Jean-Matthieu Barbier for their participation in this work. Dr. Catherine Nguyen and Dr. Béatrice Loriot are thanked for their participation in preparation of biological materials and helpful discussions on DNA hybridization. Dr. Anne Charrier is gratefully thanked for producing comparative height and phase images, figure 14; and images of temperature dependent transitions in liquid AFM, figure 15.

8. References

Ando, T.; Kodera, N.; Takai, E.; Maruyama, D.; Saito, K. & Toda, A. (2001) A high-speed atomic force microscope for studying biological macromolecules, *Proc. Natl Acad. Sci. USA*, Vol. 98, pp. 12468–12472

Alessandrini, A. & Facci, P. (2005) AFM: a versatile tool in biophysics, *Meas. Sci. Technol.*, Vol. 16, pp. R65–R92

Aslam, M.; Bandyopadhyay, K.; Lakshminarayanan, V. & Vijayamohanan, K. (2001) *J. Colloid. Interface Sci.*, Vol. 234, pp. 410

Babcock, K.; Dugas, M.; Manalis, S. & Elings, V. (1995), *MRS Symp. Proc.*, Vol. 355, pp. 311

Bandyopadhyay, K.; Vijayamohanan, K.; Venkataramanan, M. & Pradeep, T. (1999) *Langmuir*, Vol. 15, pp. 5314

Battistel, E.; Bianchi, D. & Rialdi, G. (1991) *Pure Appl. Chem.*, Vol. 63, pp. 1483

Bezanilla, M.; Manne, S.; Laney, D. E.; Lyubchenko, Y. L. & Hansma, H. G. (1995) *Langmuir*, Vol. 11, pp. 655–659

Binnig, G.; Quate, C.F. & Gerber, C. (1986) Atomic Force Microscope. *Phys. Rev. Lett.*, Vol. 56, pp. 930–933

Burtman, V.; Zelichenok, A.; Yakimov, A. & Yitzchaik, S. (1999) In *Semiconducting Polymers: Applications, Properties and Synthesis*; American Chemical Society: Washington, DC, Chap. 25

Butt, H. J. ; Siedle, P. ; Seifert, K. ; Fendler, K. ; Seeger, T. ; Bamberg, E.; Weisenhorn, A. L. ; Goldie, K. & Engel, A. (1993) Scan speed limit in atomic force microscopy, *J. Microsc.*, Vol. 169, pp.75–84

Charrier, A & Thibaudau, F. (2005) Biophys. J., Vol. 89, pp. 1094–1101

Chrisey, L. A.; Lee, G. U. & O'Ferrall, C. E. (1996) *Nucleic Acids Res.*, Vol. 24, pp. 3031-3039

Cleveland, J. P.; Anczykowski, B.; Schmid, A. E. & Elings, V. B. (1998) Energy-dissipation in tapping-mode atomic-force microscopy, *Appl. Phys. Lett.*, Vol. 72, pp. 2613–2615

Cloarec, J. P.; Martin, J. R.; Polychronakos, C.; Lawrence, I.; Lawrence, M. F.; Souteyrand, E. (1999) *Sens. Actuators B*, Vol.58, pp. 394-398

Crampton, N.; Bonass, W. A.; Kirkham, J. & Thomson, N. (2005) *Langmuir*, Vol. 21, pp. 7884–7891

Crampton, N.; Bonass, W. A.; Kirkham, J. & Thomson, N. (2006) *Ultrmicroscopy*, Vol. *106*, pp. 765–770

Dai, H.; Hafner, J. H. & Lieber, C. M. (1996) Nanotubes as nanoprobes in scanning probe microscopy, *Nature*, Vol. 384, pp. 147–51

Diez-Perez, I.; Luna, M.; Teheran, F.; Ogletree, D. F.; Sanz, F. & Salmeron, M. (2004) *Langmuir*, Vol. 20, pp. 1284

Dubois, L. H. & Nuzzo, R. G. (1992) Synthesis, structure and properties of model organic surfaces, *Annu. Rev. Phys. Chem.*, Vol. 43, pp. 437–463

Dufêne, Y. F. (2002) Atomic Force Microscopy, a Powerful Tool in Microbiology, *Journal of bacteriology*, Vol. 184, No. 19, pp. 5205–5213

Dumas, C.; El Zein, R.; Dallaporta, H.; & Charrier, A. (2011), Autonomic Self-Healing Lipid Monolayer: A New Class of Ultra-Thin Dielectric, *Langmuir*, DOI. 10.1021/la202333n

Dürig, U.; Zuger, O. & Stadler, A. (1992) *J. Appl. Phys.*, Vol. 72, pp. 1778

Ek, S.; Iiskola, E. I.; Niinistï, L.; Vaittinen, J.; Pakkanen, T. T.; Keränen, J. & Auroux, A. (2003) *Langmuir*, Vol. *19*, pp. 10601-10609

Ek, S.; Iiskola, E. I. & Niinistö, L. (2004) *J. Phys. Chem. B*, Vol. 108, pp. 9650–9655

Estroff, L. A.; Kriebel, J. K.; Nuzzo, R. G. & Whitesides, G. M. (2005) Self-Assembled Monolayers of Thiolates on Metals as a Form of Nanotechnology, *Chem. Rev.*, Vol. 105, n°4, pp. 1103–1170

Fleming, A.J.; Aphale, S.S.; Moheimani, S.O.R. (2010) A New Method for Robust Damping and Tracking Control of Scanning Probe Microscope Positioning Stages, *IEEE Transactions on nanotechnology*, Vol. 9, N°4, pp. 438-448

Hafner, J. H.; Cheung, C-L.; Woolley, A. T.& Lieber, C. M. (2001) Structural and functional imaging with carbon nanotube AFM probes, *Prog. Biophys. Mol. Biol.*, Vol. 77, pp. 73–110

Hansma, H. G.; Revenko, I.; Kerry, K. & Laney, D. E. (1996) *Nucleic Acids Res.*, Vol. 24, No. 4, 713-720
Heiney, P. A.; Grüneberg, K.; Fang, J.; Dulcey, C. & Shashidhar, R. (2000) *Langmuir*, Vol. 6, pp. 2651
Herne, T. M. & Tarlov, M. J. (1997) *J. Am. Chem. Soc.*, Vol. 119, pp. 8916- 8920
Holmes-Farley, S. R.; Bain, C. D. & Whitesides, G. M. (1988) *Langmuir*, Vol. 4, pp. 921–937
Höper, R.; Gesang, T.; Possart, W.; Hennemann, O-D. & Boseck, S. (1995) *Ultramicroscopy*, Vol. 60, pp. 17
Horr, T. J. & Arora, P. S. (1997) *Colloid Surf., A*, Vol. 126, pp. 113
Huang, N. P.; Michel, R.; Voros, J.; Textor, M.; Hofer, R.; Rossi, A.; Elbert, D. L.; Hubbel, J. A. & Spencer, N. D. (2001) *Langmuir*, Vol. 17, pp. 489
Huang, E.; Satjapipat, M.; Han, S. & Zhou, F. (2001) *Langmuir* , Vol. 17, pp. 1215-1224
Jalili, N. & Laxminarayana, K. (2004) Mechatronics, Vol. 14, pp. 907–945
Juvaste, H.; Iiskola, E. I. & Pakkanen, T. T. (1999) *J. Organomet. Chem.*,Vol. 587, pp. 38
Kaifer, A. (2001) *Supramolecular Electrochemistry*, Coral Gables. Wiley VCH. pp. 191–193
Kallury, K. M. R.; Macdonald, P. M. & Thompson, M. (1994) *Langmuir , 10*, 492.
Kelley, S. O.; Barton, J. K.; Jackson, N. M.; McPherson, L. D.; Potter, A. B.; Spain, E. M.; Allen, M. J. and Hill, M. G. (1998) *Langmuir*, Vol. 14, No. 24, 6781-6784
Kim, S.; Christenson, H. K. & Curry, J. E. (2002) *Langmuir*, Vol. 18, pp. 2125–2129
Kitazawa, M. ; Ito, S.; Yagi, A.; Sakai, N.; Uekusa, Y.; Ohta, R.; Inaba, K.; Hayashi, A.; Hayashi, Y.; Tanemura, M. (2011) High-Resolution Imaging of Plasmid DNA in Liquids in Dynamic Mode Atomic Force Microscopy Using a Carbon Nanofiber Tip, *Japaneses journal of applied physics*, Vol. 50, N°8, special issue
Klein, H.; Blanc, W.; Pierrisnard, R. ; Fauquet, C. & Dumas, Ph. (2000) *Eur. Phys. J. B*, Vol. 14, pp. 371-376
Koehne, J. E.; Stevens, R. M.; Zink, T.; Deng, Z.; Chen, H.; Weng, I. C.; Liu, F. T. & Liu, G. Y. (2011) Using carbon nanotube probes for high-resolution three-dimensional imaging of cells, *Ultramicroscopy*, Vol. 111, N°8, pp.1155-62
Kumar, A.; Biebuyck, H. A. & Whitesides, G. M. (1994) *Langmuir*, Vol. 10, pp. 1498
Kumar, S.; Chaudhury, K.; Sen, P. & Guhal, S. K. (2005) Atomic force microscopy: a powerful tool for high-resolution imaging of spermatozoa, *Journal of Nanobiotechnology*, Vol. 3, N°9, pp. 1-6
Lavrich, D. J.; Wetterer, S. M.;. Bernasek, S. L. & Scoles, G. (1998) *J. Phys. Chem. B*, Vol. 102, pp. 3456-3465
Levicky, R.; Herne, T. M.; Tarlov, M. J. & Satija S. K. (1998) Using self assembly to control the structure of DNA monolayers on gold : a neutron reflectivity study, *J. Am. Chem. Soc.*, Vol. 120, pp. 9787
Lisdat, F.; Ge, B. & Scheller, F. W. (1999) *Electrochem. Commun.*, Vol. 1, pp. 65-68
Lyubchenko, Y. L.; Blankenship, R. E.; Gall, A. A.; Lindsay, S. M.; Thiemann, O.; Simpson, L. & Shlyakhtenko, L. S. (1996) *Scanning Microsc. Suppl.*, Vol. 10, pp. 97
Lyubchenko, Y.L.; Shlyakhtenko, L.S. & Ando, T. (2011) Imaging of nucleic acids with atomic force microscopy, Methods, Vol. 54, N°2, pp. 274-283.
Madou, M. (2002) *Fundamentals of Microfabrication: The Science of Miniaturization*, CRC, pp. 62–63
Magonov, S. N. & Reneker, D. H.. (1997a) Characterization of polymer surfaces with atomic force microscopy, *Annu. Rev. Mater. Sci.*, Vol. 27, pp. 175–222

Magonov, S. N.; Elings, V. & Whangbo, M-H. (1997b) Phase imaging and stiffness in tapping mode AFM, *Surf. Sci.*, Vol. 375, pp. 385–391

Mamin, H. J.; Birk, H.; Wimmer, P. & Rugar, D. (1994) High-speed scanning-tunneling-microscopy—principles and applications, *J. Appl. Phys.*, Vol. 75, pp. 161–168

Maslova, M. V.; Gerasimova, L. G. & Forsling, W. (2004) *Colloid J., Vol. 6*, pp. 322–328

Möller, C.; Allen, M.; Elings, V.; Engel, A. & Müller, D.J. (1999) Tapping-Mode Atomic Force Microscopy Produces Faithful High-Resolution Images of Protein Surfaces, *Biophys. J.*, Vol. 77, pp. 1150–1158

Montanari, A. & Mézard, M. (2000) Hairpin Formation and Elongation of Biomolecules, *Phys. Rev. Lett.*, Vol. 86, pp. 2178

Moreno-Herrero, F.; Colchero, J. ; Gomez-Herrero, J.; & Baro, A. M. (2004) Atomic force microscopy contact, tapping, and jumping modes for imaging biological samples in liquids, *Physical Review E*, Vol. 69, pp.031915

Mourougou-Candoni, N.; Naud, C. & Thibaudau, F. (2003) Adsorption of thiolated oligonucleotides on gold surfaces: An atomic force microscopy study, *Langmuir*, Vol. 19, pp. 682-686

Mourougou-Candoni, N. & Thibaudau, F. (2009) Formation of aminosilane film on Mica, *J. Phys. Chem. B*,Vol. 113, pp. 13026–13034

Müller, D. J.; Fotiadis, D.; Scheuring, S.; Muller, S. A. & Engel, A. (1999) Electrostatically balanced subnanometer imaging of biological specimens by atomic force microscope, *Biophys J.*, Vol. 76, pp. 1101–11

Nuzzo, R. G. & Allara, D. L. (1986) *J. Am. Chem. Soc,*. Vol. 105, pp. 4481

Ohnesorge, F. & Binnig, G. (1993) True atomic resolution by atomic force microscopy through repulsive and attractive forces, *Science,* Vol. 260, pp. 1451–1456

Park, J.K. & Moon, W. K. (2011) Development of XY scanner with minimized coupling motions for high-speed atomic force microscope, *Journal of central south inversity of technology*, Vol.18, N°3, pp. 697-703

Peterlinz, A.; Georgiadis, M.; Herne, T. M.; Tarlov, M. J. (1997) *J. Am. Chem. Soc.*, Vol. 119, pp. 3401-3402

San Paulo, A. & Garcia, R. (2000) High-resolution imaging of antibodies by tapping-mode atomic force microscopy: attractive and repulsive tip–sample interaction regimes , *Biophys. J.*, Vol. 78, pp. 1599–605

Schierbaum, K.; Weiss, T.; Van Velzen, E. T.; Engbersen, J.; Reinhoudt, D. & Cöpel, W. (1994) *Science*, Vol. 265, pp. 1413

Schwartz, D. K.; Steinberg, S.; Israelachvili, J. & Zasadzinski, J. A. N. (1992) *Phys. Rev. Lett.*, Vol. 69, pp. 3354

Schwartz, D.K. (2001) Mechanisms and Kinetics of Self-Assembled Monolayer Formation, *Annu. Rev. Phys. Chem.*, Vol. 52, pp. 107–137

Seah, M. P. & Dench, W. A. (1979) *Surf. Interface Anal., Vol. 1*, pp. 2

Shlyakhtenko, L. S.; Gall, A. A.; Weimer, J. J.; Hawn D. D. & Lyubchenko, Y. L. (1999) *Biophys. J.*, Vol. 77, pp. 568-576

Song, X.; Zhai, J.; Wang, Y. & Jiang, L. (2006) *J. Colloid Interface Sci.*, Vol. 298, pp. 267

Sugawara, Y.; Ohta, M.; Ueyama, H. and Morita, S. (1995) *Science,* Vol. 270, pp. 1646

Steel, A. B.; Herne, T. M. & Tarlov, M. J. (1998) *Anal. Chem.*, Vol. 70, pp. 4670-4677

Sugimara, H.; Hozumi, A.; Kayemana, T. & Takai, O. (2002) *Surf. Interface Anal.*, Vol. 24, pp. 550

Sulchek, T.; Yaralioglu, G. G.; Quate, C. F.; & Minne, S. C. (2002) Characterization and optimisation of scan speed for tapping-mode atomic force microscopy, *Rev. Sci. Instrum.*, Vol. 73, pp. 2928–2936

Sulchek, T.; Hsieh, R.; Adams, J. D.; Yaralioglu, G. G.; Minne, S. C.; Quate, C. F.; Cleveland, J. P.; Atalar, A. & Adderton, D. M. (2000) High-speed tapping mode imaging with active Q control for atomic force microscopy, *Appl. Phys. Lett., Vol.* 76, pp. 1473–1475

Tamayo, J. & Garcia, R. (1996) Deformation, contact time, and phase-contrast in tapping mode scanning force microscopy, *Langmuir* , Vol. 2, pp. 4430–4435

Tamayo, J. & Garcia, R. (1997) Effects of elastic and inelastic interactions on phase-contrast images in tapping-mode scanning force microscopy, *Appl. Phys. Lett.*, Vol. 7, pp. 1 2394–12396

Tamayo, J.; Humphris, A. D. L. & Miles, M. J.; (2000) Piconewton regime dynamic force microscopy in liquid, *Appl. Phys. Lett.*, Vol. 77, pp. 582–584

Tamayo, J.; Humphris, A. D. L.; Owen, R. J.; & Miles, M. J. (2001) High-Q dynamic force microscopy in liquid and its application to living cells, *Biophys. J.*, Vol. 81, pp. 526–37

Tätte, T.; Saal, K.; Kink, I.; Kurg, A.; Lohmus, R.; Mäeorg, U.; Rahi, M.; Rinken, A. & Lohmus, A. (2003) *Surf. Sci.*, Vol. 532, pp. 1085–1091

Tinland, B.; Pluen, A.; Sturm, J. & Weill, G. (1997) *Macromolecules* , Vol. 30, pp. 5763-5765

Trens, P.; Denoyel, R. & Rouquerol, J. (1995) *Langmuir* 1995, Vol. 11, pp. 551–554

Ulman, A. (1991) *An Introduction to Ultrathin Organic Films: From Langmuir–Blodgett to self-assembly;* Academic Press: Boston, MA

Vandenberg, E. T.; Bertilson, L.; Liedberg, B.; Uvdal, K.; Erlandsson, R.; Elwing, H. & Lundstrom, I. (1991) *J. Colloid Interface Sci.*, Vol. 17, pp. 103

Venkataramanan, M.; Skanh, G.; Bandyopadhyay, K.; Vijayamohanan, K. & Pradeep, T. (1999) *J. Colloid. Interface Sci.*, Vol. 212, pp. 553

Vos, J. G.; Forster, R. J. & Keyes T. A. (2003) *Interfacial Supramolecular Assemblies.* Wiley, pp. 88–94.

Vrancken, K. C.; Possemiers, K.; Van der Voort, P. & Vansant, E. F. (1995) *Colloid Surf., A* , Vol. *98*, pp. 235

Walters, D. A.; Cleveland, J. P.; Thomson, N. H.; Hansma, P. K.; Wendman, M. A.; Gurley, G. & Elings, V (1996) Short cantilevers for atomic force microscopy, *Rev. Sci. Instrum.*, Vol. 67, pp. 3583–3590

White, L. D. and Tripp, C. P. (2000) *J. Colloid Interface Sci.*, Vol. 232, pp. 400–407

Wnek, G. & Bowlin, G. L. (2004) *Encyclopedia of Biomaterials and Biomedical Engineering.* Informa Healthcare. pp. 1331-1333.

Wong, S. S.; Harper, J. D.; Lansbury, P. T. & Lieber, C. M. (1998a) Carbon nanotube tips: high-resolution probes for imaging biological systems, *J. Am. Chem. Soc.*, Vol. 120, pp. 603–604

Wong, S. S.; Joselevich, E.; Woolley, A. T.; Cheung, C-L. & Lieber C. M. (1998b) Covalently functionalized nanotubes asnanometer-sized probes in chemistry and biology, *Nature,* Vol. 394, pp. 52–5

Woolley, A.T. (2004) Biofunctionalization of carbon nanotubes for atomic force microscopy imaging, *Methods in molecular biology*, Vol. 283, pp. 305-319

Yang, Y.; Zhou, R.; Zhao, S.; Li, Q. & Zheng, X. (2003) *J. Mol. Catal. A: Chem.*,Vol. 192, pp. 303

Zhang, Y.; Zhou, H. & Ou-Yang, Z. C. (2001) Stretching Single-Stranded DNA: Interplay of Electrostatic, Base-Pairing, and Base-Pair Stacking Interactions, *Biophys. J.*, Vol. 81, pp. 1133

Zhang, F. & Srinivasan, M. P. (2004) *Langmuir,* Vol. 20, pp. 2309

Zhao, J.; Guo, T.; Ma, L.; Fu, X. & Hu, X.T. (2011) Metrological atomic force microscope with self-sensing measuring head, *Sensors and actuators A-physical*, Vol.167, N°2, pp. 267-272

Part 2

Biological Molecules, Proteins and Polymers

4

AFM Measurements to Investigate Particulates and Their Interactions with Biological Macromolecules

L. Latterini and L. Tarpani
Department of Chemistry, Center of Excellence for Nanostructured and Innovative Materials, University of Perugia
Italy

1. Introduction

In recent years much attention has been paid to the development of metrology methods to investigate particulate matter and its interaction with bio-molecules. This interest is triggered by the potential applications of nanoparticle-biomolecule hybrid systems in different areas such as bio-sensing, catalysis, target delivery, selective recognition, etc. (Amelia et al., 2010; Bellezza et al., 2009; Latterini & Amelia, 2009; Joralemon et al., 2005; Nehilla et al., 2005; Rosi & Mirkin, 2005). Furthermore, a better understanding of the interactions between particles and biomolecules could help to optimize the ability to reduce the exposure to particulate matter in working environments.

In the last decade AFM methods based on a vibrating tip to explore a surface topography experienced a significant transformation which allowed them to reach nm-resolution imaging and become sensitive tools to investigate tip-sample interactions down to sub-nm resolution (García & Pérez, 2002). Hence the chance is to develop quantitative procedures to study material properties with high spatial resolution even without affecting the softest samples. These achievements have shown that AFM methods can be used as a valid alternative to other well established techniques (such as electron microscopies) in the study of nanostructured materials. The good spatial resolution of AFM measurements can be achieved without any sample pre-treatments thus overcoming the limitations in the sample preparation involved in electron microscopies. AFM imaging appears particularly attractive to characterize particulate matter based on organic materials with high spatial resolution without any concerns about scattering cross sections and sample treatment procedures. Extremely interesting in this context is the possibility to use AFM to characterize particles conjugated to biological macromolecules. Indeed, AFM scanning showed a good accuracy to obtain size distributions for colloidal particle samples comparable to dynamic light scattering techniques or even better if the samples were polydispersed (Hoo et al., 2008)

In the present contribution, particulate matter, either intentionally prepared with designed dimensional, morphological and chemical properties or produced in working environments during the phases of metal processing or combustion processes, were dimensionally characterized and information on their surface morphology were obtained.

The characterization of particulates or colloidal nanoparticles in the presence of protein was used to obtain valuable information on the nanoparticle-protein interactions and eventually on the disposition of the macromolecules with respect to the particles. The presented results will be discussed in terms of experimental conditions to enhance or to quench the particulate-biomolecule interaction in order to control the stability of hybrid materials.

2. Results

Wet chemical synthesis for colloidal nanoparticle preparation have recently attracted much attention with the aim to optimize the procedures to work in mild conditions (atmospheric pressure, temperature below 100°C); in these conditions, the colloidal samples can be easily characterized by polydisperse size distributions and non-homogeneous shapes. AFM imaging can provide a fast investigation tool to characterize nanoparticle preparations without a prior knowledge of the size distributions and shape. Furthermore, the acquisition of AFM data can give valuable information on the thickness of the stabilizer shell, which has to be necessarily used to control the nanoparticle growth in solution and it is worth to be taken into account as particle constituent. For nanomaterials, the size distribution, surface area, shape, aggregation state and composition strongly affect their biological activity since these properties have an influence on their interactions with biomolecules. AFM in tapping mode has been used to study nanoparticles deposited on mica and to investigate their interactions with proteins and DNA.

2.1 Dimensional characterization of colloidal nanoparticles and particulates

AFM topography imaging was helpful to obtain information on the growth mechanism of CdS nanocrystals prepared in water by thermolysis of a single precursor ((2,2′-bpy)Cd(SC{O}Ph_2)) and the thioglycerol at a constant molar ratio of 1:2.5 and at different refluxing times (from 30′ to 5 hours). In particular, the size distribution in the different samples was monitored by AFM measurements. In Figure 1, AFM images recorded on the samples with shortest and longest reaction times, respectively, are reported together with the related size distribution analysis, based on gaussian functions. For the sample refluxed for 30′, an average size of 2.2±0.1 nm was determined. On the other hand, for the sample obtained with longer refluxing times, the size distribution appears more complex and two populations can be found: the first with the average size centered at 3.1±0.1 nm and the second (although with lower frequency) having the mean diameter at 4.8±0.3 nm. The size distribution analysis confirmed that the nanocrystal dimensions increased with the refluxing time and underlined that different populations are formed during the nanocrystal growth. In fact, the size histograms showed that, during the growth, the mean diameter increased together with an impressive change in the distribution width. The sample obtained after 30′ refluxing presented a broad size distribution (width 2.2 nm), while in the sample obtained with longer refluxing times the most frequent distribution becomes much narrower (width 1.2 nm) and a very broad nanocrystal population (width 6.3 nm) appeared. Since the samples were obtained from the same preparation procedure and contained the same capping agent concentration, the dimension change cannot be attributed to a stabilizer effect. This behaviour can be explained considering that the nanocrystal growth is controlled by surface processes. Most likely the growth is because

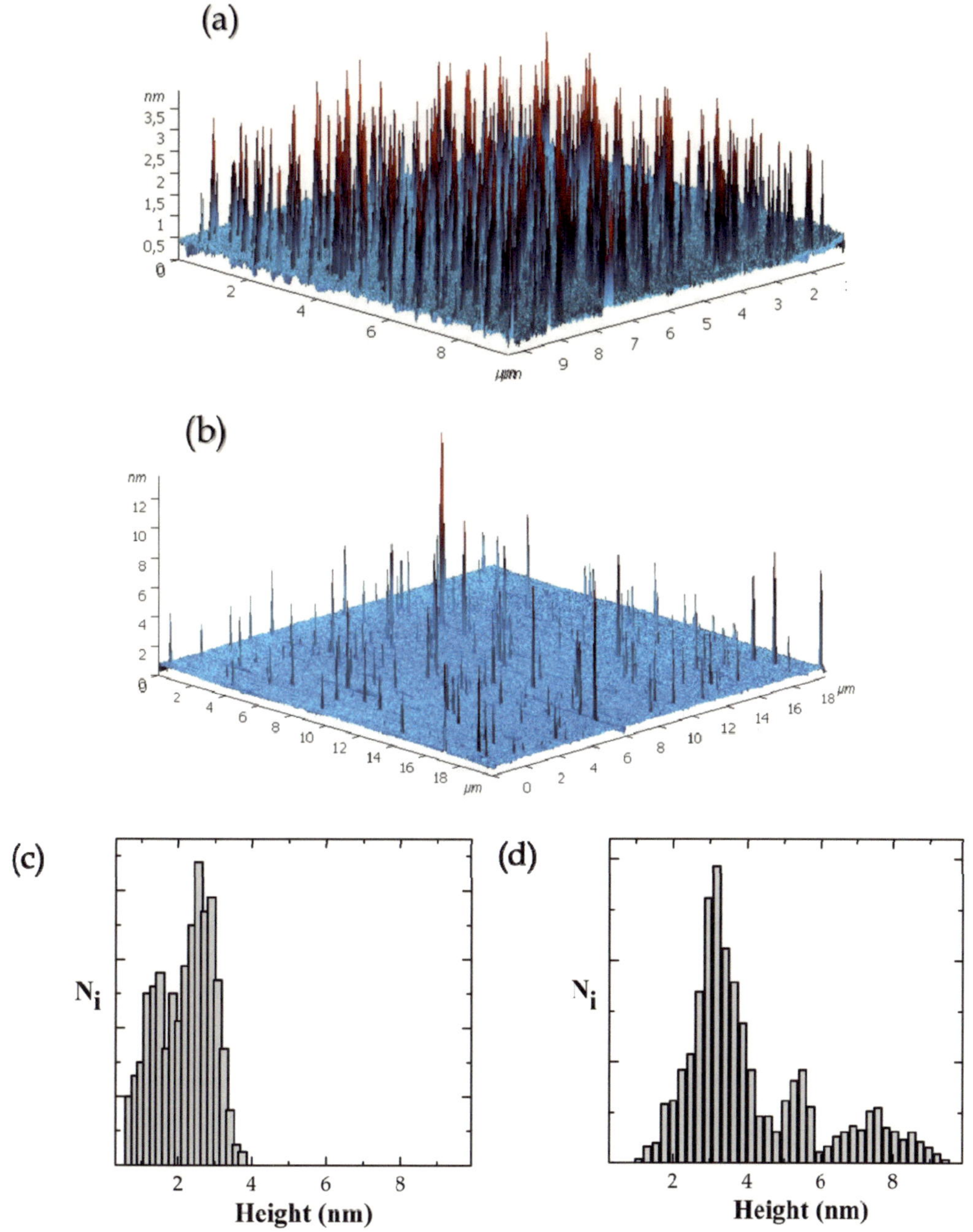

Fig. 1. 3-D topography images of CdS nanocrystal refluxed with thioglycerol for 30′ (a) and 5 hours (b) together with their relative height distributions (c, d respectively)

the diffusion of the seeds on the nuclei surface is quite rapid, and therefore it leads to a very broad size. Furthermore, the difficulties to control the growth lead to the development of defects in the crystal structures as confirmed by luminescence studies which show trap states emission (Latterini & Amelia, 2009).

In the case of metal nanoparticles suspensions, the comparison between topography and phase images allowed us to make the hypothesis that the stabilizer shell dimensions cannot be neglected. Gold nanoparticles were prepared in water upon in-situ reduction of Au(III) by citrate anions, which play the double role of reduction agent and stabilizer. AFM images showed isolated nanoparticles with a spherical shape (Figure 2a). The phase images (Figure 2b), recorded simultaneously with the topography images, have shown different contrast for every single grain; indeed a brighter spot corresponding to a higher oscillation phase was observed inside every grain in the phase imaging mode. Similar differences in contrast were not observed in the topography images, suggesting that the grain is actually a nanocomposite material having components which interact differently with the AFM tip. Thus a hypothesis was made that in the chemical composition of colloidal nanoparticles an important component is the organic stabilizer. This hypothesis was further supported by TEM images and from the comparison between AFM and TEM size distribution, an estimate of the stabilizer shell thickness of few nm, depending on the experimental conditions during the synthesis, can be obtained.

In order to explore the effect of citrate ion concentration on the properties of particles, preparations were carried out keeping constant the Au(III) amount and reducing to one half the citrate concentration. AFM images indicated that with lower citrate concentrations the average particles size was smaller (12 ± 0.3 nm compared to 20 ± 0.2 nm obtained by doubling the citrate content) and the distribution of the dimensions was narrower. These observations indicated that the increase of citrate concentration induced a faster and more efficient nucleation process and allowed better control of the particle growth through a diffusion controlled process, although a thickening of the stabilizer shell cannot be excluded.

Silica nanoparticles prepared via the Stöber method could be easily visualized and characterized through AFM scanning, once the suspension was spin-coated on a mica support (Figure 3a). AFM acquisitions show the spherical shape of the nanoparticles with an averaged diameter of 70 nm as a result of a quite narrow distribution. Additionally, the nanoparticle surface appeared regular and without roughness (Figure 3b). The lack of observing pores on the nanoparticle surface by AFM scanning was most likely because the cavities are smaller than the AFM tips (about 1 nm). Generally the void particles appear well separated on mica, indicating that the surface charges act as efficient capping agents. When the silica particle surface is covalently functionalized with organic dyes, such as fluorescein or 9-aminoacridine, the particle height resulted increased by a factor of two or three (Figure 3c) and the grains do not appear isolated any more, as already observed for similar systems (Latterini & Amelia, 2009). These morphology changes were attributed to the presence of the aromatic dye molecules on the particle surface which reduce the net charge and are able to form aggregate species stabilized by π-π stacking. The occurrence of these aggregate species might strongly be reduced in suspension samples for the presence of solvation interactions, but they are predominant in solid state and can strongly affect the chemical-physical behaviour of the samples. Thus attention should be paid in the detection of these aggregated species when devices are prepared from suspensions. AFM is one of the few methods which allows one to visualize the formation of these assemblies.

The particulates produced in working environments during material processing were collected through a standard device which was designed to collect and separate aerosol through dimensional properties. Briefly, a Sioutas Cascade Impactor provides a five step

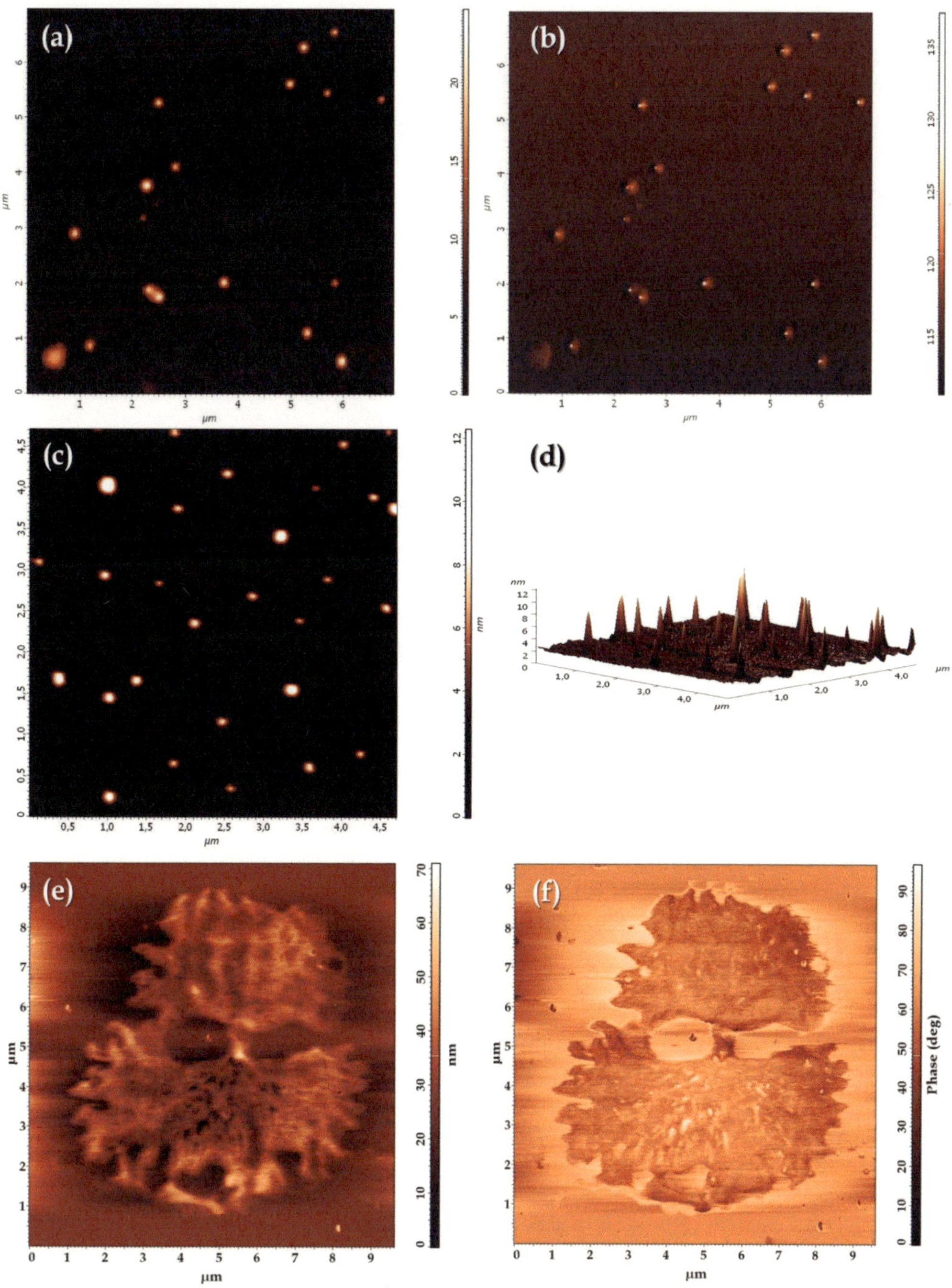

Fig. 2. (upper panel) AFM images in topography (a) and phase (b) mode of gold nanoparticles stabilized by citrate cations prepared with [Au(III)]/[citrate] of 1:14; (middle panel) 2-D (c) and 3-D (d) topography images of gold nanoparticles prepared with [Au(III)]/[citrate] of 1:7; (lower panel) AFM images in topography (e) and phase (f) of gold nanoparticles upon interaction with bacterial DNA.

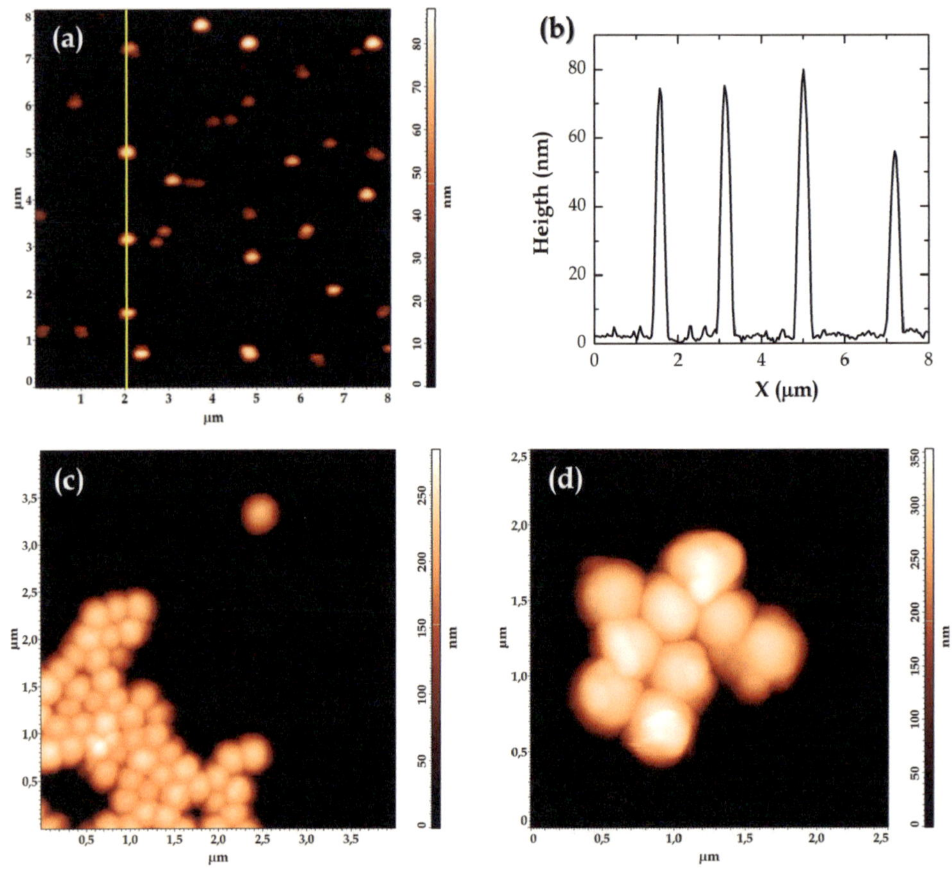

Fig. 3. (upper panel) AFM images in topography (a) and x-scan line (b) of void silica nanoparticles; (lower panel) AFM images in topography of fluorescein-functionalized silica nanoparticles (c) and void silica nanoparticles (d) in the presence of BSA.

collection which corresponds to the following 50% cut-point of 2.5 μm, 1.0 μm, 0.5 μm, 0.25 μm (filters A, B, C and D, respectively) on a 25 mm PTFE filter. The Impactor has a final step to collect the particles below the < 0.25 μm cut - point on a 37 mm PTFE filter (filter AF) equipped with a sample pump capable of maintaining a constant flow rate (about 9 l/min). For the morphological/dimensional characterization of the particulate through AFM imaging, the collected particulate was desorbed from the collection filters, since the latter presented a very rough surface which did not allow to have enough resolution. Each filter was transferred in 10 mL vials; in each vial 5 mL of water were added. The vials were then sealed and the desorption was carried out by ultrasonication for 20 minutes at room temperature. The morphological analysis was carried out upon deposition of the obtained suspensions on mica. The AFM images were collected in tapping mode in order to avoid sample degradation or removal. The AFM images show that the shape of the particulates formed is influenced by the nature of the working processes taking place during the sample collection, as well as the environmental conditions (temperature, pressure, material concentration). In particular, spherical objects were observed from the samples collected in places where digging process were carried out or where metals were treated at high temperatures, while the samples collected in environments where blade are used (such as for wood processing) presented particles with quite sharp edges. Since the recent literature evidenced that the particle shape and size can affect their delivery and toxicity (Lewinski et al., 2008), the creation of a database containing the characterization of particulates produced in industrial working locations is particularly important to reduce the negative effects to personnel from exposure to these particulates within the working environment. Furthermore, the dimensional characterization has to be investigated in deeper details and AFM imaging provides a fast investigation tool which can give high resolution information. AFM topography images showed that the micron-size particulates collected in places where digging operations are carried out, or during metal processing, are constituted by smaller particles with dimensions between 15 and 100 nm. Even the samples desorbed from the collection filters with higher dimensional cut (Figure 4a, b and d) are constituted by smaller nanoparticles which form agglomerates with bigger dimensions. However, within the agglomerates, the nanostructure is maintained, as shown by the jagged linescan (Figure 4c) which presents steps about 25 nm height and can be attributed to the single nanoparticles composing the agglomerate.

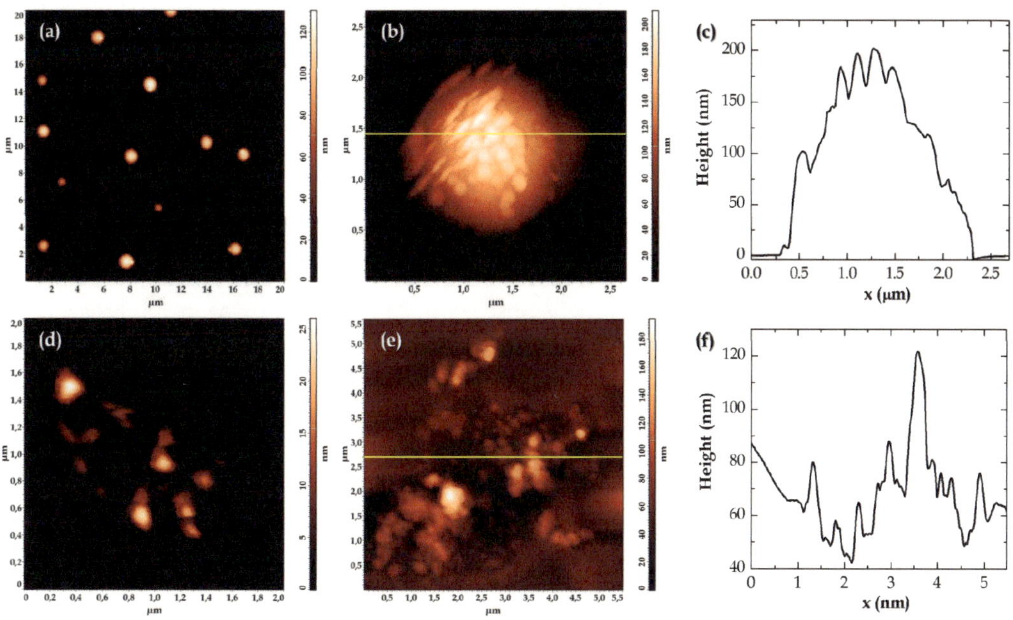

Fig. 4. (upper panel) AFM images representing the topography (a,b) and x-scan line (c) of nanoparticulate collected during digging operations (cut-off filter = 0.25 μm); (lower panel) AFM images representing the topography of nanoparticulate collected during metal welding operations (cut-off filter = 0.25 μm) in the absence (d) and in the presence of bacterial DNA (e) together with x-scan line graph (f) taken from the image (e).

2.2 Investigations of the interactions between nanoparticles and biomolecules

The interactions between colloidal nanoparticles and biomolecules were investigated by AFM through an analysis of the grain dimensions and morphology and the data in the absence of the biomolecules compared to those obtained in the presence of biomolecules.

Generally for all the colloidal nanoparticles under investigation, a marked increase in grain dimensions was observed upon interaction with protein or bacterial DNA. In particular gold nanoparticles bearing citrate ions on the surface interact efficiently with bacterial DNA. The interaction is so strong to be optically visualized by colour changes of the gold suspensions; the well know, intense red colour of gold suspensions turns to an intense blue upon addition of DNA (about 10^{-4} M in base pair). This behaviour is obviously due to modifications of the Surface Plasmon Resonance (SPR) of the gold colloids, which is a deeply investigated phenomenon due to the potential application for sensing and labelling (Latterini & Tarpani, 2011). However, a much weaker effect can be observed when the single DNA base or mixtures of bases are added to gold colloids, thus the effect has to be related to DNA structure. AFM images recorded on gold-DNA complex deposited on mica (Figure 2e-f) show that the colloids are no longer detectable as individuals, but the samples are instead characterized by supramolecular architectures whose dimensions can reach the μm scale. This observation, together with the SPR shift to longer wavelength, suggested that DNA strands tend to accumulate around the metal particles likely replacing, at least in part, the citrate anions leading to micron-size aggregates formation. Inside these aggregates, gold colloids come into closer contact, as highlighted by the SPR shift, which is in agreement with literature data (Ghosh & Pal, 2007). The lack of clearly detecting the metal nanostructure even in phase mode is probably due to the fact that they are buried inside the biological layer which is estimated to be tens of nm thick if the average diameter of the pristine gold nanoparticles (12±0.3 nm) is taken into account.

A similar aggregation phenomenon was observed also when bacterial or calf thymus DNA solutions were added to the suspensions of particulates collected from metal welding operations. In this case the metal nanoparticles are not intentionally prepared and stabilized thus interactions with DNA strands are enhanced to reach a better stabilization in the water media. As a results, particles with dimensions below 25 nm (Figure 4d) in the presence of DNA form aggregate structures with an overall dimension in the order of hundreds of nm.

A clustering effect was observed for silica nanoparticles when they were topographically imaged in the presence of Bovine Serum Albumine (BSA). In particular, the grain dimensions increased when the void silica nanoparticles were deposited in the presence of BSA; for 80 nm diameter particle, an increase by a factor of 4 was observed in the height and a larger effect was observed in the width (Figure 3d). These effects have been attributed to the adsorption of the protein on the surface of the silica nanoparticles, as previously observed for similar systems (Bellezza et al., 2009; Latterini & Amelia, 2009). Indeed, the net negative charge present on the void silica nanoparticles in aqueous neutral media can have an important role in controlling the adsorption of the protein which presents a positive net surface charge in the same pH conditions. This adsorption process resulted in a shielding effect from the negative charges which stabilized the naked particle and maintained isolation; thus the silica nanoparticles with BSA adsorbed on the surface tend to form clustered structures. However, no clear evidence was obtained by AFM to determine the conformation of the protein on the surface of the particles.

AFM can be also a valid means to study and comprehend the mechanism behind the interaction between organic nanomaterials and biomolecules. The protein Bovine Serum Albumin (BSA) is used as model biomolecule to investigate its interaction with polystyrene nanoparticles (PS NPs) synthesized in our group.

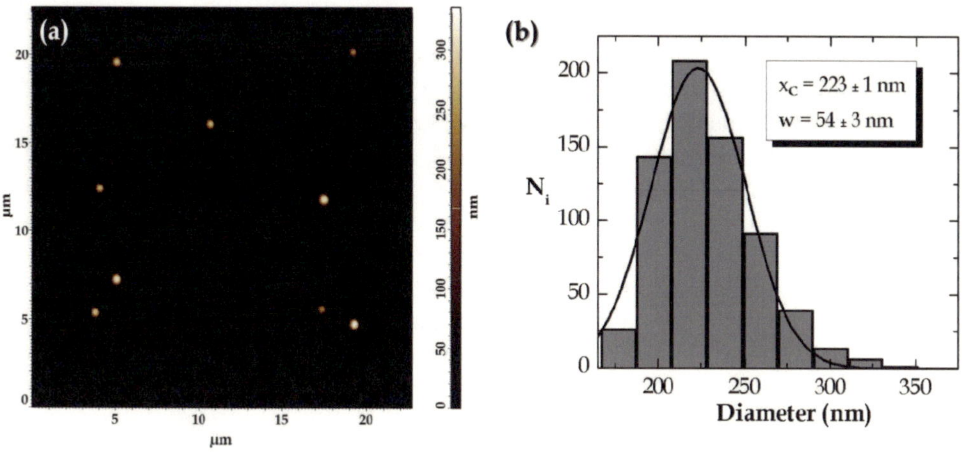

Fig. 5. AFM images representing the topography (a) of polystyrene NPs deposited on mica and relative size distribution built up from AFM images in (b).

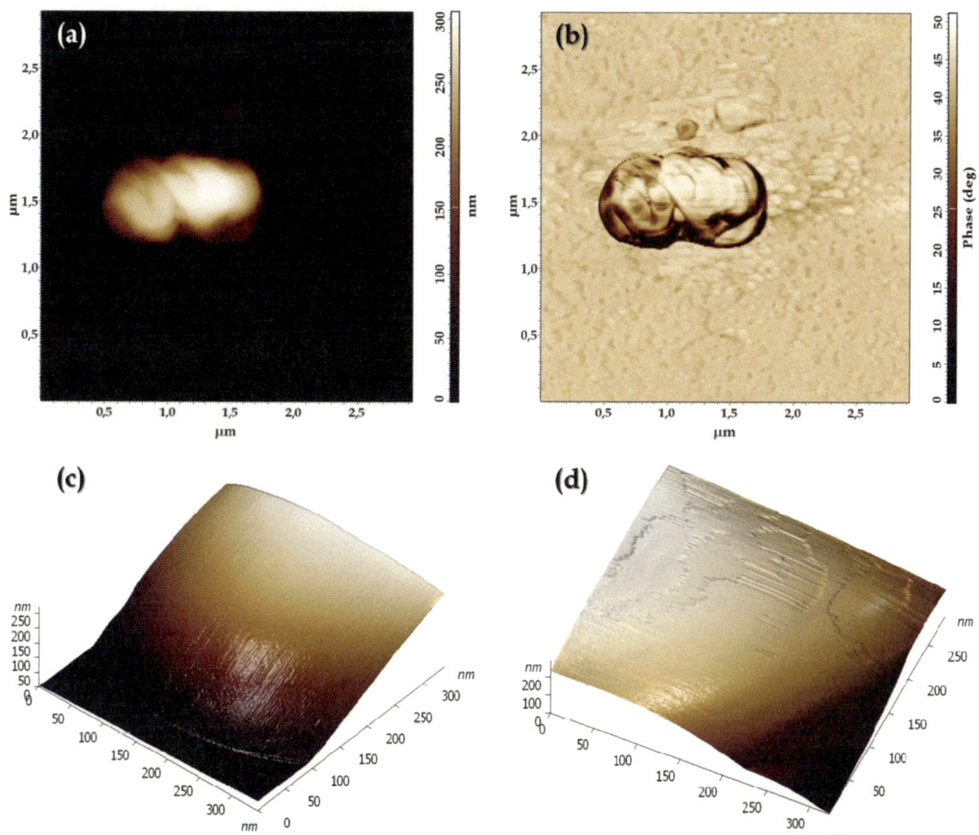

Fig. 6. (upper panel) AFM images representing the topography (a) and phase (b) of polystyrene NPs deposited on mica after BSA adsorption; (lower panel) 3-D AFM image of a polystyrene NP surface before (c) and after (d) BSA adsorption.

AFM topography images of a PS NPs sample deposited on mica by spin-coating demonstrate the presence of spherical particles with a smooth surface (Figure 5a). The height histogram built up from the AFM images (taking into account at least 500 particles) indicates that the nanoparticles are quite polydisperse with a mean diameter of about 230 nm (Figure 5b). A 10^{-3} M aqueous solution of BSA was then added to the synthesized PS NPs and AFM topography images were collected after deposition on mica. Upon interaction with the protein, the images clearly show the formation of aggregates with an elongated shape but the same Z-height of the single nanoparticles (Figure 6a-b). The data seem to indicate that the adsorbed protein acts as a linker between the nanostructures binding them together in groups of three or four. It is known in literature (Yoon et al., 1996) that BSA can be adsorbed on a surface according to two different orientations: side-on, in which the longer side (14 nm) adheres to the surface or end-on, in which the shorter side (4 nm) is involved in the adsorption. A schematic representation of these two types of interaction is shown in Figure 7b. In this particular case, topography images in high resolution of the PS NPs surface were taken after BSA adsorption. The resulting 3-D topographic images demonstrate that upon interaction with BSA (Figure 6d) there is an increase of the surface roughness and the formation of a single protein layer adsorbed on the polystyrene nanoparticles. As shown by the x-scan profile (Figure 7a), this layer has a height of about 4 nm, thus confirming that BSA is adsorbed onto the polymeric NPs in the side-on orientation.

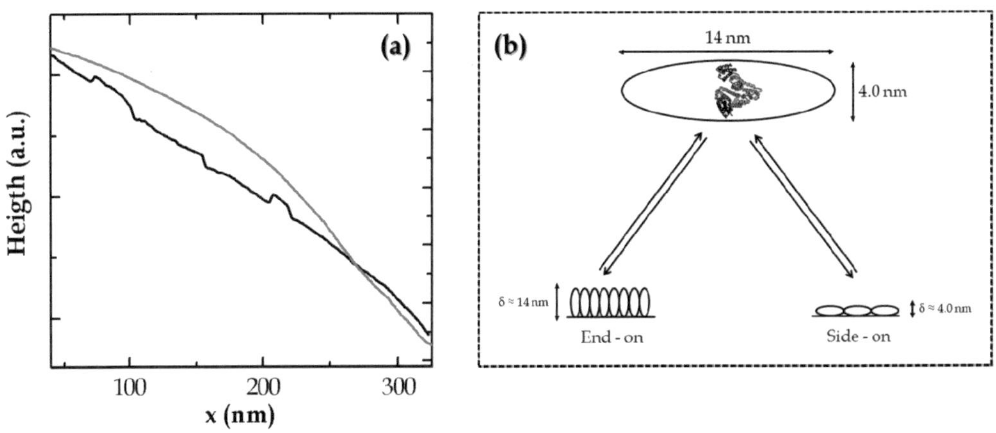

Fig. 7. (a) X-scan line graph of polystyrene NPs surface before (gray line) and after (black line) BSA adsorption; (b) Scheme of the possible orientations of BSA adsorbed on a solid surface

3. Conclusions

AFM scanning has been used to characterize, from a dimensional and morphological point of view, colloidal nanoparticles prepared intentionally with designed properties and particulates collected in working environments. The data obtained from AFM topography imaging, once statistically analyzed, were helpful to obtain information on the growth mechanism of CdS nanocrystals and gold nanoparticles. Indeed, a broadening of size distribution of CdS colloids suggested that the growth was mainly controlled by surface processes; on the other hand, the narrowing of dimensional populations for gold nanoparticles indicated that the growth could occur through a diffusion controlled process. Interestingly, the comparison between topography and phase images allowed us to make the hypothesis that the stabilizer shell around the particles has a dimension of few nm thus colloidal nanoparticles can be better regarded as nanocomposites. Silica nanoparticles prepared through a sol-gel method were successfully imaged in topography mode and appeared well dispersed, with a narrow size distribution and a smooth surface.

AFM appears to be a valid tool also for a fast and high resolution analysis of particulates collected in working environments. Thus AFM imaging can be useful for the creation of a database on dimension and morphology of particulates produced in different working environments in order to evaluate their toxicity in relation to the tools and the conditions used. AFM topography images showed that the micron-size particulates collected in places where digging or welding operation are carried out are actually constituted by smaller particles with dimensions between 15 and 100 nm.

AFM is a valid mean to study and comprehend the interactions between nanomaterials and biomolecules. Generally for all the investigated nanoparticles, a marked increase in grain dimensions was observed upon interaction with protein or DNA. AFM images recorded on nanoparticle-biomolecule conjugates demonstrated that the effect is due to the formation of supramolecular architectures whose dimensions can reach the μm scale, in which electrostatic interactions might have an important role. Only in the case of polystyrene particles with 220 nm diameter, the BSA molecules adsorbed on their surface are arranged in an ordered conformation. The line-scan analysis through topographic images allowed us to establish the BSA orientation.

4. Acknowledgment

This work is supported both by the University of Perugia and the Department of the University for the Scientific and Technological Research (MIUR-Rome). Authors are grateful to INAIL for financial support through a research agreement (May 2010-2012) and for providing the samples collected in working environments.

5. References

Amelia, M.; Flamini, R.; Latterini L. (2010). Recovery of CdS nanocrystal defects through conjugation with proteins. *Langmuir*, Vol. *26*, pp 10129–10134, ISSN 0743-7463

Bellezza, F.; Cipiciani, A.; Latterini, L.; Posati, T.; Sassi,P. (2009). Structure and Catalytic Behaviour of Myoglobin adsorbed onto Nanosized Hydrotalcites. *Langmuir*, Vol. *25*, pp 10918–10924, ISSN 0743-7463

Dedecker, P.; Hotta, J.I.; Flors, C.; Sliwa, M.; Uji-I, H.; Roeffaers, M.B.J.; Ando, R.; Mizuno, H.; Miyawaki, A. & Hofkens, J. (2007). Subdiffraction imaging through the selective donut-mode depletion of thermally stable photoswitchable fluorophores: numerical analysis and application to the fluorescent protein Dronpa. *J. Am. Chem. Soc.*, Vol.129, No.51, (December 2007), pp. 16132-16141, ISSN 0002-7863

García, R. & Pérez, R. (2002). Dynamic atomic force microscopy methods. *Surface Science Reports*, Vol.47, No.6-8, (April 2002), pp. 197-301, ISSN 0167-5729

Ghosh, S.K. & Pal T., (2007). Interparticle coupling effect on the surface plasmon resonance of gold nanoparticles: from theory to applications. *Chem. Rev.*, Vol.107, No.11, , pp. 4797-4862, ISSN 0009-2665

Hoo, C.M.; Starostin, N.; West, P.; Mecartney, M.L. (2008). A comparison of atomic force (AFM) and dynamic light scattering (DLS) methods to characterize nanoparticle size distributions, J. Nanopart.Res. Vol. 10, pp. 89-96.

Irrgang, J.; Ksienczyk J.; Lapiene V. & Niemeyer C.M. (2009). Analysis of Non-Covalent Bioconjugation of Colloidal Nanoparticles by Means of Atomic Force Microscopy and Data Clustering. *ChemPhysChem,* Vol.10, No.9-10, (July 2009), pp. 1483-1491, ISSN 1439-4235

Joralemon, M.J.; Smith, N.L.; Holowka, D.; Baird, B. & Wooley, K.L. (2005). Antigen-decorated shell cross-linked nanoparticles: Synthesis, characterization, and antibody interactions. *Bioconj. Chem.,* Vol.16, No.5, (September-October 2005), pp. 1246-1256, ISSN 1043-1802

Knemeyer, J.P.; Marme, N. & Sauer, M. (2000). Probes for detection of specific DNA sequences at the single-molecule level. *Anal. Chem.,* Vol.72, No.16, (August 2000), pp. 3717-3724, ISSN 0003-2700

Latterini, L.; Amelia, M., (2009). Sensing proteins with luminescent silica particles. *Langmuir,* Vol. *25,* pp 4767–4773, ISSN 0743-7463

Latterini, L. & Tarpani L. (2011). Hierarchical assembly of nanostructures to decouple fluorescence and photothermal effect. *J.Phys.Chem.C,* DOI: 10.1021/jp208124x, ISSN 1932-7455

Lewinski, N. ; Colvin, V. & Drezek, R. (2008). Cytotoxicity of Nanoparticles, *Small,* Vol.4, No. 1, 26 – 49, ISSN 1613-6829

Nehilla, B.J.; Vu, T.Q. & Desai, T.A. (2005). Stoichiometry-dependent formation of quantum dot-antibody bioconjugates: A complementary atomic force microscopy and agarose gel electrophoresis study. *J. Phys. Chem. B,* Vol.109, No.44, (November 2005), pp. 20724-20730, ISSN 1520-6106

Passeri, R.; Aloisi, G.G.; Elisei, F.; Latterini, L.; Caronna, T.; Fontana, F. & Sora, I.N. (2009). Photophysical properties of N-alkylated azahelicene derivatives as DNA intercalators: counterion effects. *Photochem. Photobiol. Sci.,* Vol.8, No.11, (August 2009), pp. 1574-1582, ISSN 1474-905X

Rosi, N.L. & Mirkin, C.A. (2005). Nanostructures in biodiagnostics. *Chem. Rev.,* Vol.105, No.4, (April 2005), pp. 1547-1562, ISSN 0009-2665

Yoon, J.-Y.; Park, H.-Y.; Kim, J.-H.; Kim, W.-S. (1996), Adsorption of BSA on highly carboxylated microspheres-quantitative effects of surface functional groups and interaction forces *J. Colloid Interface Sci.,* Vol.*177,* 613-620, ISSN 0021-9797

5

AFM Imaging of Biological Supramolecules by a Molecular Imprinting-Based Immobilization Process on a Photopolymer

Taiji Ikawa
Toyota Central Research and Development Laboratories, Inc.
Japan

1. Introduction

Biologically derived molecules (biomolecules) are extremely diverse in their physical sizes, chemical and structural properties. They form supramolecular assemblies *in vivo/vitro* through noncovalent interactions (e.g., hydrogen bonding, hydrophobic interactions, π-π interactions, and/or electrostatic). The structures of the supramolecular assemblies change with the concentrations of salts and the biomolecules itself. Efficient immobilization of various biomolecules and their assemblies is a key aspect of many applications including microarray technologies, (Kambhampati (Ed.), 2003; Schena (Ed.), 2004) biotechnology in general (Mayers, 2002; Whitesides, 2001) and structural analysis based on AFM.

Structures and functions of the biomolecules and their assemblies are susceptible to physical and chemical surface properties and nanotopography of the substrate, and such interfacial forces effect a nanoscale change in molecular shape and structure. (Ostuni, et al., 2001; Ramsden, 1993; Wahlgren & Arnebrant, 1993) The first problem to be overcome is the tendency for biomolecules to denature on contact with the substrate surfaces. Extensive approaches have been developed, using either covalent attachment or noncovalent affinity binding (Mayers, 2002). The covalent coupling process can achieve stable coupling, but it needs complexity and cost of derivation steps, and limited sites for attachment leads to shorter lifetime. The process has a possibility of denaturation by the chemical treatment. On the other hand, the noncovalent affinity binding process is the simplest approach to the immobilization but it tends not to be stable, and activity of biomolecule is often lost in time-dependent structural changes (Ramsden, 1993). For example, mica surface provides an atomically flat surface, but the surface repels most of the biomolecules due to its negative charge. Multivalent cation or chemical modification process are used to avoid repulsion (Bezanilla et al.,1995; Hansma, 2001; Lamture et al., 1994), however, the structures of the supramolecular assemblies changed with the concentrations of salts (Wong et al., 2003).

A recent study for the noncovalent affinity binding process has been directed toward the selective adsorption of biomolecules using nanopatterned surfaces (Cunin et al., 2001; Curtis & Eilkinson, 2001; Shi et al.,1999) and/or molecularly imprinted polymers (Alexander et al., 2003; Haupt, 2003) so as to hold the 3-dimensional structure of the biomolecules. However, these approaches have met with limited success due to their complicated chemical processes and the often expensive facilities required for nanofabrication.

In this chapter, a new technique for the noncovalent immobilization of the biomolecules using a polymer containing azobenzene moiety (azopolymer) is presented (Ikawa et al. 2006, 2007, 2010). The principle of the technique is simple; the azopolymer surface deforms along contours of nano-scale macromolecules during photoirradiation, effectively immobilizing the macromolecules without chemical modification (Fig. 1). That means the molecular shape is imprinted on the azopolymer surface by the photo-irradiation.

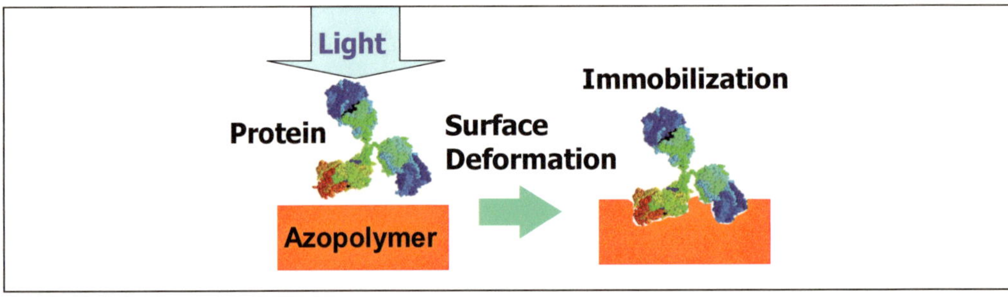

Fig. 1. Principle of the immobilization of protein.

The technique is well suited for imaging biomolecules, especially for AFM, providing a non-reactive, non-ionic, and flat surface (the surface roughness can be < 0.3 nm) on which the complex supramolecular assemblies can be immobilized with little conformational change in the native aqueous environment. The immobilization process dramatically reduces the thermal motion of biomolecules, leading to higher imaging resolution allowing individual biomolecules to be resolved.

The nano-scale biomolecules such as deoxyribonucleic acid (DNA), immunoglobulin G (IgG), and tobacco mosaic viruses (TMV) are demonstrated to be immobilized on such an azopolymer surface by photoirradiation because of a topographic change in the azopolymer surface with the biomolecules after photoirradiation. The imaging technique is also shown to investigate the phase behaviour of cytoskeletal muscle protein aggregates as a function of concentration of the multivalent cation. The data provided direct experimental evidence of a coil-on-coil (braided) structure and the two dimensional nematic rafts discovered by recent x-ray studies (Wong, 2003) and theoretical treatments (Borukhov,1997).

2. Principle of the immobilization of biomolecules on the azopolymer

2.1 Photoinduced motions in azopolymer

2.1.1 Photoisomerization of azobenzenes

Azobenzene and its derivatives can exist in two forms that differ in the isomerization state of the azo group (-N=N-) (Fig. 2) (Rau, 1990). One is the trans-form, which has the stable rod-like form in shape. The other is the cis-form, which has the relatively unstable bent form. The stable trans-form isomerizes into the unstable cis-form when the azobenezenes absorb light. Cis to trans back isomerization can take place thermally and/or photochemically.

Azobenzenes have been classified into three groups by spectroscopic analysis: azobenzene-type molecules, aminoazobenzene-type molecules and pseudo-stilbene-type molecules (Fig. 2)

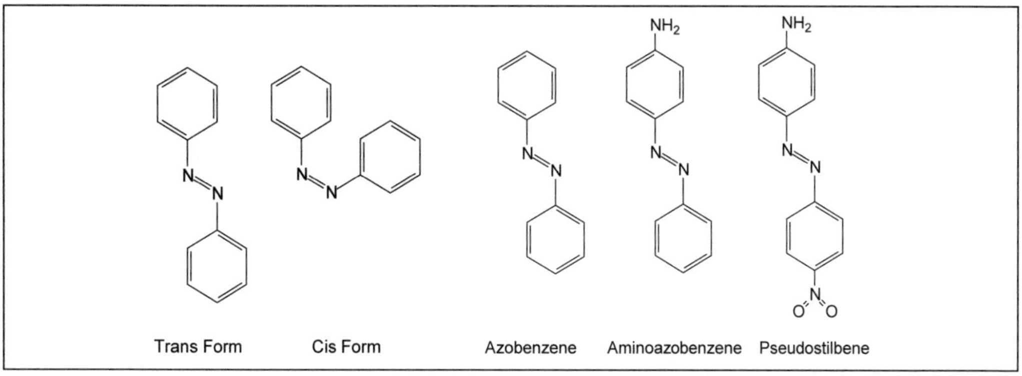

Fig. 2. Isomers of azobenzene and three groups of azobenzene derivatives.

(Natansohn & Rochon, 2002; Rau, 1990). Azobenzene-type molecules have two absorption bands due to π-π^* and n-π^* transition with relatively poor overlap between the two bands. The lifetime of the cis isomer is relatively long up to hours and more. Aminoazobenzene-type molecules show significant overlap of the two absorption bands and the lifetime of the cis isomer is shorter. Pseudo-stilbene-type molecules, where 4- and 4'-positions of the two azobenzene rings are substituted with electron-donating and electron-withdrawing groups, has the two bands overlapped on around the same energy level and the lifetime of the cis isomer is shortest up to second range. Since the π-π^* and n-π^* bands are practically superimposed, light for photoactivation of the trans-cis isomerization will also photoactivate the cis-trans isomerization, which will significantly speed up the whole process. The process can be repeated under illumination, and thus, pseudo-stilbene-type molecules are the best molecules for inducing drastic changes to their surrounding matrix.

2.1.2 Photoisomerization-induced motions in azopolymer

Azobenzenes undergo repeated photoisomerization during photoirradiation even in a glassy-state polymer. Nonbound azobenzenes can affect their environment if they are dissolved in a polymer matrix. The molecular motions of azobenzenes induce the multi level motions in the polymer. The motions can be roughly classified into the following three types (Natansohn & Rochon, 2002).

The first type of motion is the photo-induced orientation of chromophores in a polymer matrix. With linearly polarized light, the photoisomerization is only activated when the chromophore's transition dipolemoment axis has a component parallel to the light polarization. The direction perpendicular to the light polarization is excluded from optical activation and become enriched in chromophores. The concentration of the chromophores aligned perpendicular to the light polarization steadily increases under illumination with polarized light, until a saturation level is attained. This motion produces dichroism and birefringence in polymers (Todorov et al., 1984). Pseudo-stilbene-type azobenzenes is the best molecule for inducing photo-induced orientation because of their fast isomerization process. Aminoazobenzenes are good candidates for the motion, but azobenzenes shows little photoinduced orientation due to their slow back isomerization process.

The second type is domain level motions in conjunction with chromophore motions. To induce this type of motion, the azobenzenes should be part of ordered and/or constrained matrix, for example, liquid crystalline, semi crystalline, Langmuir-Brodgett or monolayer films. Any type of azobenzenes are useful for inducing this kind of motion. In case the azobenzenes undergo photo-isomerization and alignment in the constrained matrix, liquid crystals domains reorient to a direction perpendicular to the light polarization(Ichimura, 2000). Also, the photoisomerization can act as a trigger to disrupt an ordered phase of liquid crystals, which is the most common case found in the literature. The difference in shape between the E (trans) azobenzene isomer and the Z (cis) provides a powerful mesogen (E) and an effective liquid crystalline phase disruptor (Z, with some exceptions).

The third type is massive macroscopic motion at an even larger scale. The photo-illumination with interference pattern of the laser beams produces relief patterns on the polymer surface (Fig. 3) (Kim et al., 1995; Rochon et al., 1995). Direct exposure to the laser beam also forms a dent structure on the polymer surface. To induce this kind of motion, pseudo-stilbene-type azobenzenes is the best molecule and it requires that the azobenzenes should be connected to polymers. This motion has been considered to be a photo-driven mass transport effect because total volume of the polymer is almost the same after photo-illumination, which is quiet different from other conventional microscopic surface processing. Various driving forces behind it have been proposed such as internal pressure (Rochon et al., 1995), light intensity gradient (Kim et al., 195), and intermolecular interaction (Pedersen et al., 1997). However, neither the mass transport effect itself nor the nature of the driving force has been directly confirmed. Recently, Karageorgiev et al. reported the observation of light-induced isothermal transition of the polymer film from a solid phase to a fluid phase by atomic force microscopy (Karageorgiev et al., 2005). In their report, the polymer behaves like a viscoelatic fluid during photo-illumination, whereas the fluidity is affected by the light field vector. The result suggests that the photoisomerization motion of the azobenzene plasticizes the polymer matrix during photo-illumination, which is considered to be the first step of the massive macroscopic motion of the polymer.

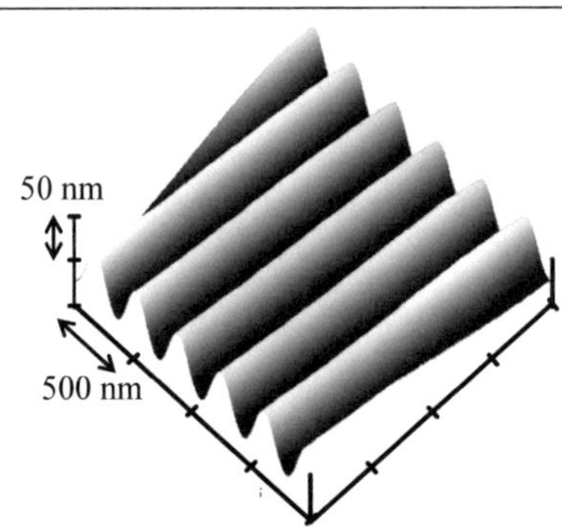

Fig. 3. A relief pattern formed on an azopolymer surface by exposure to an interference pattern of light, imaged by atomic force microscopy.

2.1.3 Surface deformation of azopolymers by sub-micron sized dielectric particle

The author's research group found that a topographical change could be induced on the surface of azobenzene-containing polymers by means of photo-illumination with a monolayer of polystyrene (PS) particles of submicron diameter (Hasegawa, 2001; Ikawa et al. 2000; Kawata et al., 1999). The experimental technique to display this phenomenon is very simple: (1) a monolayer of PS particles was formed on the surface of the azopolymer film; (2) the polymer film was exposed to a laser beam; (3) after removing the particles, hexagonally arrayed dents, of which diameter were nearly the same as the PS particles, were formed on the surface (Fig. 4). The dents structure with a diameter from 1000 nm to 20 nm could be achieved. The author explored the mechanism of the nanoscale deformation of the azopolymer based on (1) size effects of the small particles on the nanostructure formation, (2) the electric field calculated by Mie scattering theory, and (3) the visco-elasticity analyzed by scanning probe microscopy (Ikawa, 2001). The result implies that "the optical near field" of the PS particles that are smaller than the wavelength of the incident light can cause the nano-scale surface deformation of the azopolymer. This technique itself was considered to be an entirely new nano-structure fabrication technique, and showed the potential of the azopolymer for the application to near-field imaging (Kawata, 1999) and optical data storage (Hasegawa, 2001).

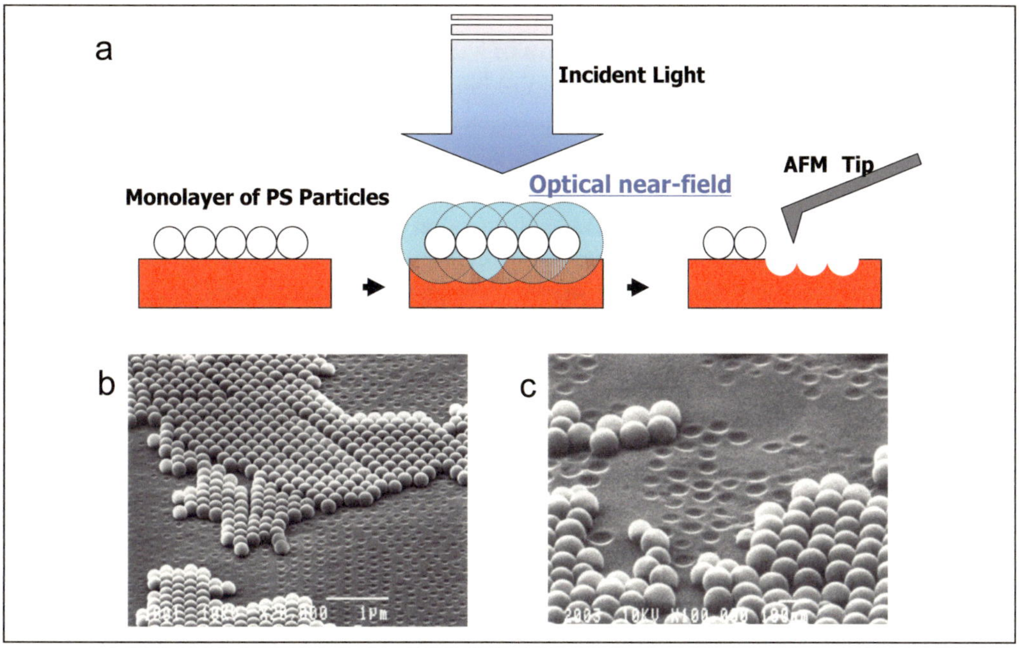

Fig. 4. (a) Schematic representation of the nanostructure patterning by spherical particles. (b) and (c) SEM images of the azopolymer surfaces treated by (b) the particles of 241 nm in diameter and (c) the particles of 98 nm in diameter. The particles were partially removed from the surface by sonication.

2.2 Immobilization of small particles on the azopolymer surface and AFM imaging

In the course of these studies, the author found that the small particles on the azopolymer can be immobilized by photo-illumination (Ikawa, 2006). As shown in Fig. 4, the deformed surface is considered to effectively sustain the particles. Of particular interest is that not only PS particles but biomolecules including globular proteins, filamentous proteins and deoxyribonucleic acids (DNA) can be immobilized on the azo polymer.

The author confirmed that the azopolymer surface deform along the shapes of the small particles, suggesting that the small particles are physically immobilized on the surface because of the increase in the contact area between the small particles and the polymer. The immunological and enzymatic studies showed that the immobilized proteins keep their vital activities (Ikawa, 2006). This new concept for the immobilization of the biological macromolecules has the distinct potential for biological applications including protein chip application (Mouri, 2010) and biological imaging (Ikawa, 2007). Moreover, it provides a new concept of the fabrication of two-dimensional array of spherical particles (Watanabe, 2010).

Following section, nano-scale particles including both deoxyribonucleic acid (DNA) and proteins are shown to be immobilized on the surface of the azopolymer only by photoirradiation. Atomic force microscopy (AFM) reveals that the polymer surface deforms along the contour of the nano-scale particles and physically holds them upon photo-irradiation. Immunological and enzymatic studies presents that proteins immobilized on the polymer surface retained their original functionality.

2.2.1 Experimental technique: Preparation of azopolymer films and photoimmobilization of biomolecules on the films

Two kinds of azopolymers were used in the experiment. **Polymer 1:** A urethane-urea copolymer containing disperse red 19 was synthesized (Ikawa et al., 2001; Kawata et al., 1999). The polymer had a molecular weight of 170,000 (relative to polystyrene), a glass transition temperature (Tg) of 145°C and an absorption maximum of 475 nm. Contact angles of water and ethylene glycol to the polymer were 83° and 58°, respectively. Changes in the absorption spectrum and the contact angles cannot be detected before and after 1-hour photoirradiation with 25 mW/cm^2 of light from a 5x10 arrays of blue light emitting diodes (LEDs, Toyoda Gosei). The absorbance at a wavelength of 470 nm for the film was 5% lower than the absorbance at the wavelength of 475 nm (λ_{max}). UV−vis absorption spectra of the film before and after photoirradiation were obtained by a Shimadzu UV-2000 spectrophotometer. **Polymer 2:** Poly{4'-[[[2-(methacryloyloxy) ethyl]ethyl] amino]-4-cyanoazobenzene-co-methyl methacrylate} (15 mol% azobenzene moiety) was obtained by free-radical polymerization (Ikawa, 2006 and 2010). The polymer had a molecular weight of 25,000, a Tg of 102°C and an absorption maximum of 447 nm. Contact angle of water and ethylene glycol to the polymer were 75° and 53°, respectively. Changes in the absorption spectrum and the contact angles cannot be detected before and after 1-hour photoirradiation with 25 mW/cm^2 of light from LEDs. The absorbance at a wavelength of 470 nm for the film was 10% lower than the absorbance at the wavelength of 450 nm (λ_{max}). The 50 nm-thick azopolymer films were prepared on amino-conjugated glass slides by spin coating from a pyridine solution. Mean roughnesses (Ra) of the bare azopolymers surfaces were around 0.6 nm, being about the same before and after photoirradiation without those biomolecules.

Changes in the azopolymer surface topography with λ-DNA, Immunoglobulin G (IgG), and Tobacco mosaic virus (TMV) before and after photoirradiation were probed by atomic force microscopy (AFM). **λ-DNA**: An aqueous solution of 1 mg/mL λ-DNA was spin-coated onto the azopolymer (polymer 1) surface and then the surface was irradiated with laser light of 488 nm in wavelength and 10 mW/cm^2 in optical power densities for 10 min. The surface was observed by contact-mode AFM (Digital Instruments Nanoscope E) and a silicon nitrite cantilever (the typical tip radius of curvature is 15 nm, Nanoworld). **IgG:** 1 μL of a phosphate buffered saline solution (PBS) containing fluorophore (Cy5)-linked IgG (Funakoshi) was spotted on the azopolymer (polymer 2) surface. After evaporating the solution, the surface was irradiated with light from the 5x10 arrays of blue LEDs for 30 min; optical power density at the polymer surface was measured by an Ophir optical power meter and was around 25 mW/cm^2. Then, the surface was washed for 30 min with PBS containing 0.01 wt% Tween20 as a nonionic surfactant. The amount of the immobilized IgG was confirmed by the fluorescence intensity of the spot. The fluorescence intensity increased linearly with the concentration of IgG in the spotting solution and saturated around 2 μg/mL. Under this condition, the area density of IgG on the spot was about 2.5 ng/mm^2, corresponding to the amount calculated for a close-packed monolayer of IgG. For the AFM experiments, the spotting solution containing 0.5 μg/mL IgG was selected, so as to avoid the formation of the multilayer. The surface image was obtained by tapping-mode AFM (Digital Instruments, Dimension 3100) and a sharp silicon cantilever (the tip radius of curvature is under 5 nm. Nanoworld). The azobenzene-containing polymer surface was then washed with PBS containing 2 wt% of sodium dodecyl sulfate (SDS) to remove IgG. After confirming that the fluorescence from the spot had disappeared, a further AFM image was obtained. **TMV:** TMV was purchased from BIOREBA AG. Purification of TMV was performed by a Beckman XL-90 ultracentrifuge system. Stock solution of TMV was desalted and diluted by buffer exchange using Milipore Micocon YM-10 filter units. The final concentration of the TMV solution was 5.5 μg/mL of TMV and 10 μM of PBS. 2 μL of working solution was spotted on the azopolymer film, and then the solution was dried naturally. The film was then irradiated with light at a wavelength of 470 nm from an array of blue LEDs (25 mW/cm^2). The film surface was observed by a contact-mode AFM (Nanoscope E, Digital Instruments) with a silicon nitrite cantilever (ORC8, the typical tip radius of curvature was 15 nm; the spring constant was 0.05 N/m, Veeco). After AFM imaging, the film was rinsed overnight in an aqueous solution of 1 wt % sodium dodecyl sulfate to remove TMV from the film surface and was observed by AFM again.

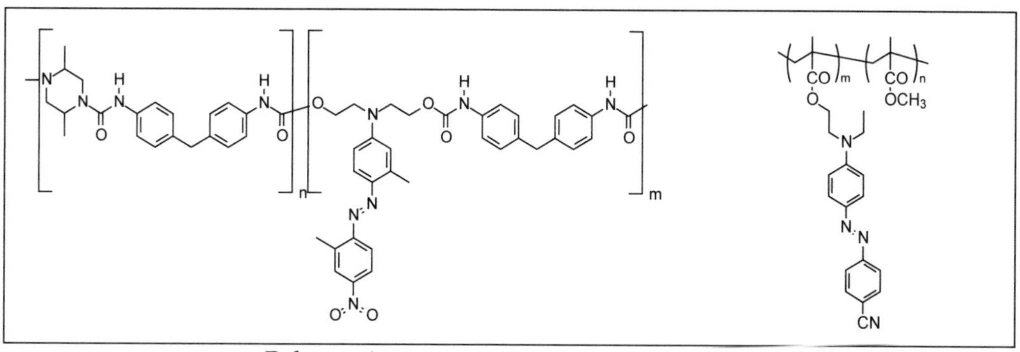

Polymer 1 Polymer 2

Fig. 5. Chemical structures of azopolymers in this study.

2.2.2 λ-DNA

λ-DNA as fibrous biomolecules is demonstrated to be immobilized on the azopolymer surface. The fibrous object in Fig. 6a is considered to be a bundle of λ-DNA (the diameter of the bundle is about 50 nm), which has been immobilized on the azopolymer surface by

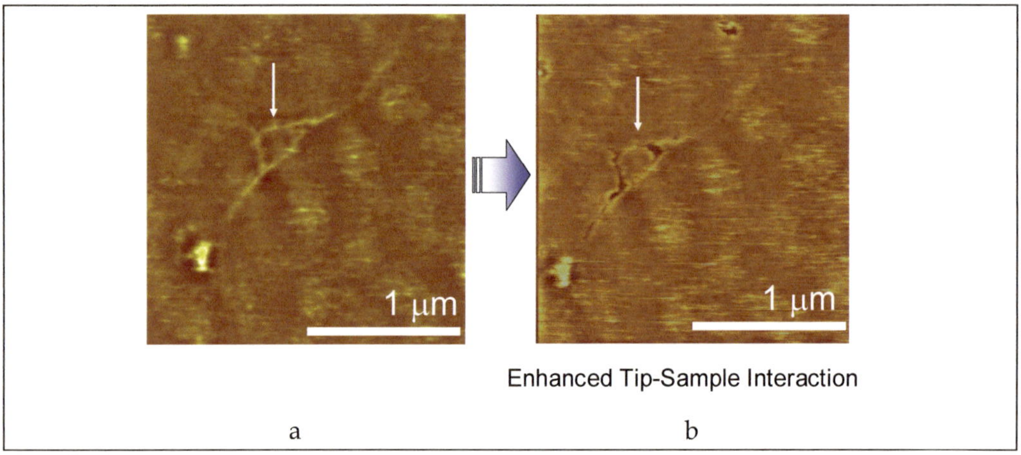

Fig. 6. The surface deformation on the azopolymer with DNA. a and b are contact-mode AFM images of the polymer surface covered with λ-DNA (The image height is from 0 to 20 nm). a, First scan of the surface covered with λ-DNA. b, the same image taken with a higher contact force after the first scan.

spin-casting from the DNA aqueous solutions and subsequent photoirradiation with laser light. By increasing the applied force of the AFM tip (Fig. 6b), the fibrous object is wiped away by the tip and it can be seen that the shape of the fibrous object is clearly imprinted as a fibrous valley on the azopolymer.

2.2.3 Immunoblobulin G

The globular biomolecules also can be immobilized on the azopolymer. Fig. 7 is AFM images of the IgG immobilized on the azopolymer surface. In Fig.7 a the azopolymer surface is covered with a layer of small granulated particles with 10 to 30 nm in diameter and around 8 nm in height (The height was estimated from the defects and the edge of the layer. Red markers in Fig. 7a.). The sizes of the particles are nearly equivalent to one subunit of IgG (about 10 nm, Fig. 1), considering the image includes the AFM tip-convolution artifact. The layer is so flat that the IgG monolayer is believed to be formed on the azopolymer surface. Fig. 7b shows an AFM image of the same area after washing the surface with PBS containing 2 wt% of SDS to remove the IgG layer. The dents of about 20 nm in diameter and 2 nm in depth are observed on the surface (a typical example is indicated by green markers in Fig. 7b, cross-section. Larger dents are also observed (red markers)). In contrast, as shown in Fig. 7c, no dents are formed on the azopolymer surface where no IgG was deposited. Comparing these images and cross sections, the dents formed on the azopolymer surface in Fig. 7b is considered to be mirroring the surface shape of the IgG layer shown in Fig. 7a.

Next, the retention of IgG on the azopolymer surface was investigated. Fig. 8a shows how the retention of fluorophore (Cy5)-linked IgG on the azobenzene-containing polymer surface changes with the photoirradiation time. The residual amount of IgG increases with the photoirradiation time and saturates over 30 min of photoirradiation. This time-dependent behavior is analogous to the polymer surface deformation; the deformation is increased with the photoirradiation time but is inclined to saturate. To investigate this

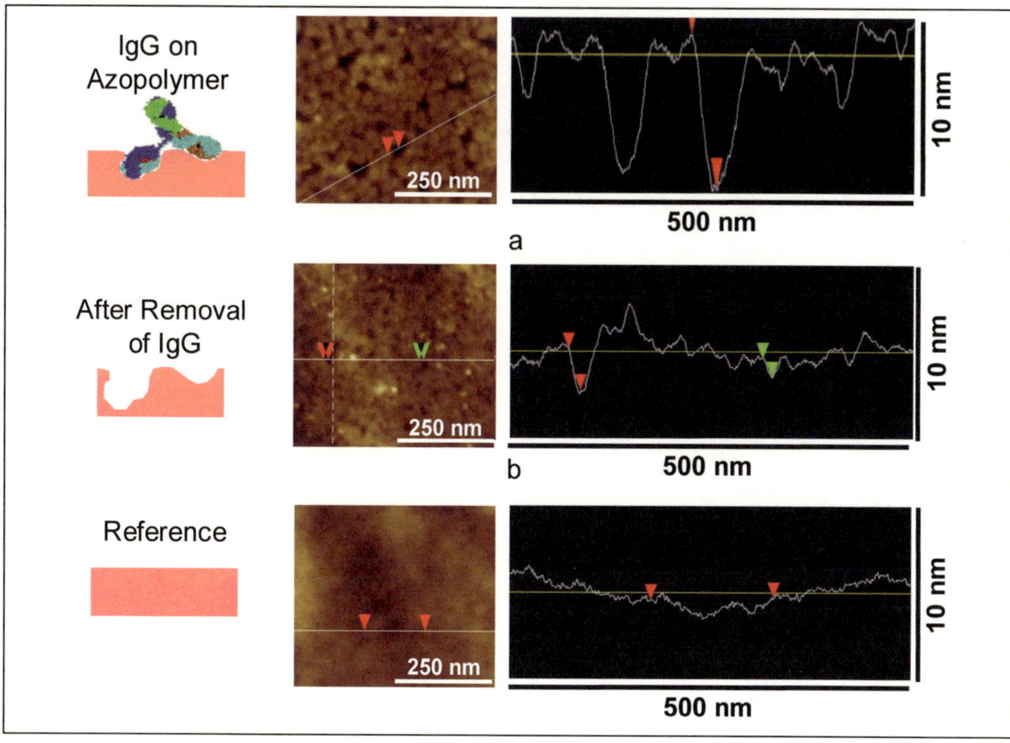

Fig. 7. The surface deformation on the azopolymer with IgG. a, A tapping-mode AFM image of the polymer surface covered with IgG. b, The same image taken after removal of the IgG by washing with PBS containing 2 wt% SDS. c, A control showing the bare azopolymerr surface after photoirradiation. This image was taken at the outside of the above IgG spot.

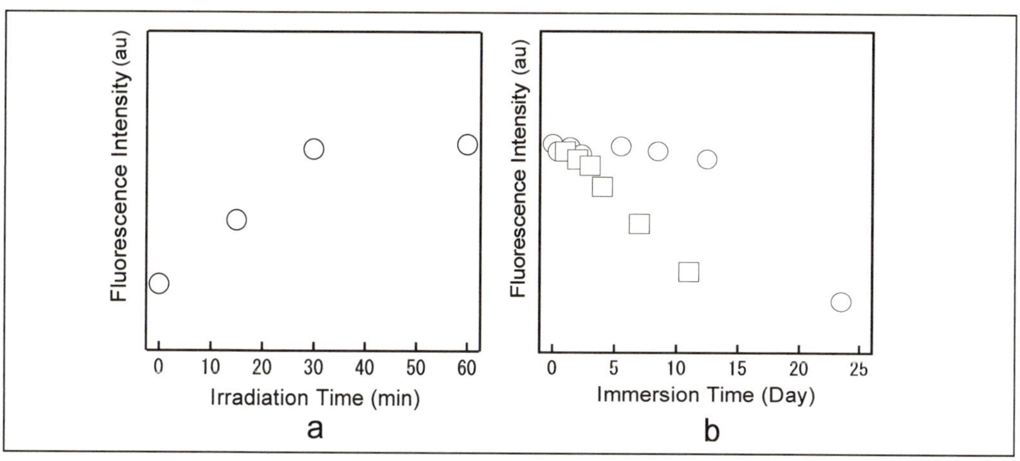

Fig. 8. The retention of fluorophore (Cy5)-linked IgG on the azopolymer surface after the photoirradiation. a, Photoirradiation time dependence of residual amounts of Cy5-linked IgG on the polymer. b, Desorption of IgG from the polymer surface in PBS after 30 min photoirradiation. Circles and squares denote results for 4 °C and room temperature, respectively.

desorption behavior further, the IgG-modified polymer surface which was photoirradiated for 30 min was soaked in PBS at room temperature and 4 °C (Fig. 8b). The IgG molecules immobilized on the polymer surface desorb very slowly on a time scale of several days, in contrast to a time scale of tens of minutes for the IgG molecules with the shorter photoirradiation time. Note that IgG molecules can be removed by just soaking in water. This suggests that the IgG molecules are physically, not chemically, immobilized on the polymer surface.

Activities of immobilized proteins, IgG on the azopolymer were investigated as follows. The temporal stability of the IgG activity was shown in Fig. 9. In Fig. 9a, the fluorescent IgG is immobilized on the lines of the spots A and B as controls, and the non-fluorescent IgG is immobilized on the lines of the spots C and D, and the spots has been reacted to the fluorescent antigenic IgG. The fluorescence intensity of the spots C and D are about 40 % of the intensity of the spots A and B. This means that 40% of the immobilized IgG is capable of capturing the antigens in solutions. Considering the steric hindrance between the IgG molecules, the activity of the immobilized IgG is very high. The immobilized IgG has been kept functioning very well for at least 6 months by the storage at 4 °C (Fig. 9). In the same way dozens of antibodies has been confirmed to continue to exhibit reactivity to specific antigens after immobilization on azopolymer.

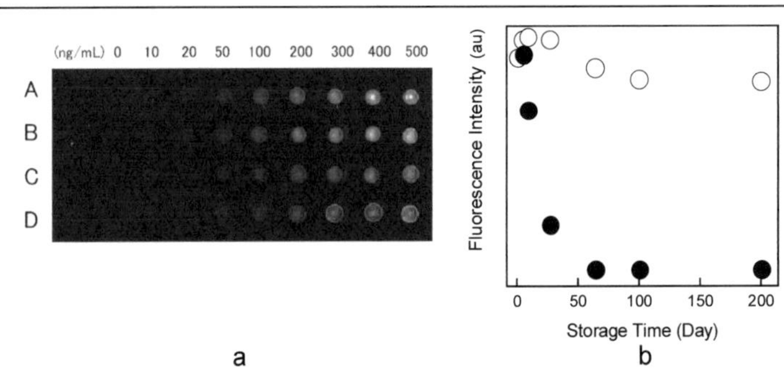

Fig. 9. The immunological activity of IgG immobilized on the azobenzene-containing polymer surface. a, A fluorescence image of the IgG spots (Cy5-linked Rabbit IgG was immobilized on A and B as controls, and Goat IgG to Rabbit IgG(H+L) was on C and D. The spot C and D had been reacted to Cy5-linked Rabbit IgG in the aqueous solution. b, The temporal stability of the IgG activity. Hollow and solid circles denote results for storage at 4 °C and at room temperature on dry condition, respectively.

2.2.4 Tobacco mosaic viruses

Fig. 10 shows contact-mode AFM images of the azopolymer surface treated with TMV. Shown in Fig. 10 a–c are the images of the sample in the presence of TMV for different photoirradiation times of 0, 10, and 20 min, respectively. All images show rod-shaped particles with a typical length of around 300 nm; however, the rods are not of uniform length. Some rods are shorter than 300 nm, and some are connected at each end. Several aggregations of granular particles are also observed in Fig. 10c. The granular particles on Fig. 10c were also observed on the samples of which preparation conditions were the same with Fig. 10a,b. Frequency of the appearance of the granular particles depended on the

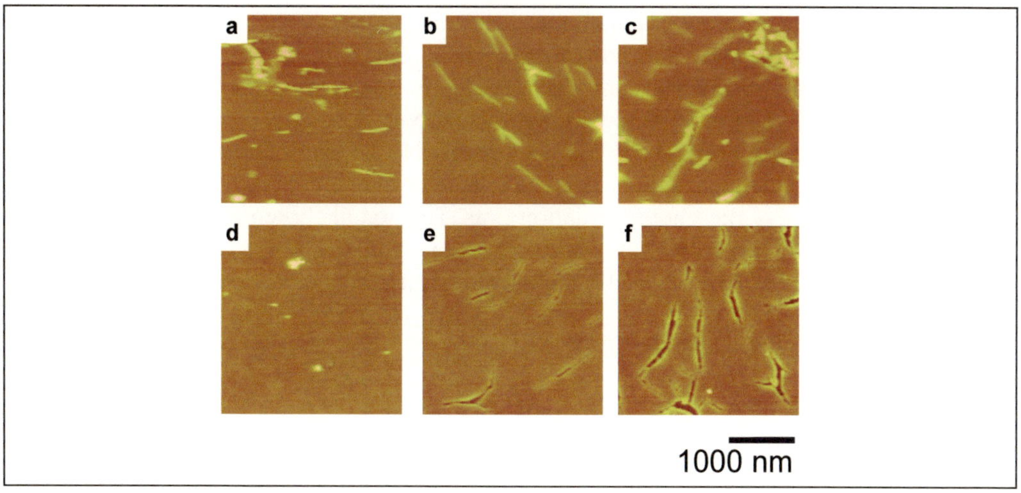

Fig. 10. AFM images of the azopolymer surface: (a–c) azopolymer surface in the presence of TMV; (d–f) azopolymer surface after washing the surface by detergent. (a, d) Without photoirradiation, (b, e) 10 min photoirradiation, and (c, f) 20 min photoirradiation.

sample preservation time; the frequency increased with increasing the preservation time after purification of the TMV stock solution. The granular particles were, therefore, not formed by the photoirradiation but formed during the preservation. These structures coincide with the structure seen by electron microscopy; the rods and the granular particles are attributed to TMV and decomposed materials from TMV (Casper, 1963; Shenton, 1999; Schramm, 1951).

Comparing Fig. 10a with Fig. 10b and Fig. 10c, strong image noises appear, and most of the rod-shaped particles are aligned parallel to the horizontal scanning direction in Fig. 10a. This strongly suggests that the rod-shaped particles on the surface are moved and aligned by the probe tip during scanning due to the unstable adsorption of TMV on the azopolymer surface. On the other hand, clear images of the rod-shaped particle are obtained in Fig. 10b,c. The heights of the rod-shaped particles gradually decrease with the photoirradiation time (Fig. 11a). This suggests that the rod-shaped particles are embedded into the azopolymer surface during the photoirradiation; therefore, the rods are immobilized firmly against the scanning of the probe tip. It must be noted that most of the rod-shaped particles are located in diagonal directions in Figure 10b. This is not due to the scanning of the probe tip, but rather to the flow of the buffer solution during the sample preparation, because the direction of the particles is different at each position even on the same sample. The TMV particles might be aligned along the convection flow during evaporating the solvent; for example, the convection flow was along the diagonal direction during the sample preparation in Fig. 10b.

Shown in Fig. 10d–f are contact-mode AFM images of the azopolymer surface after removal of TMV by washing with detergents; the samples were fabricated for different photoirradiation times of 0, 10, and 20 min, respectively. The flat surface with some small debris is observed in Fig. 10d. No deformation is caused on the azopolymer surface without photoirradiation. On the other hand, the observed structure of the grooves in Fig. 10e,f complements that of the rodlike particles shown in Fig. 10b,c, indicating that TMV shape is imprinted on the azopolymer surface by the photoirradiation.

Fig. 11 represents a detailed AFM analysis of the rod-shaped particles and the grooves on the azopolymer. The lateral and longitudinal cross sections of the typical rod-shaped particles on the azopolymer surface are shown in Figure 11a,b. From these cross sections, the rod-shaped particles are found to lay flat on the azopolymer surface, and the particles are gradually embedded while keeping their sides parallel to the azopolymer surface during the photoirradiation. Figure 11c shows a change in the average height of the rod-shaped particles as a function of the photoirradiation time. The height shown in the inset in Fig. 11c is averaged from 100 particles in several AFM images of the same sample. The average height decreases from 12 to 5 nm as the photoirradiation time increases from 0 to 30 min.

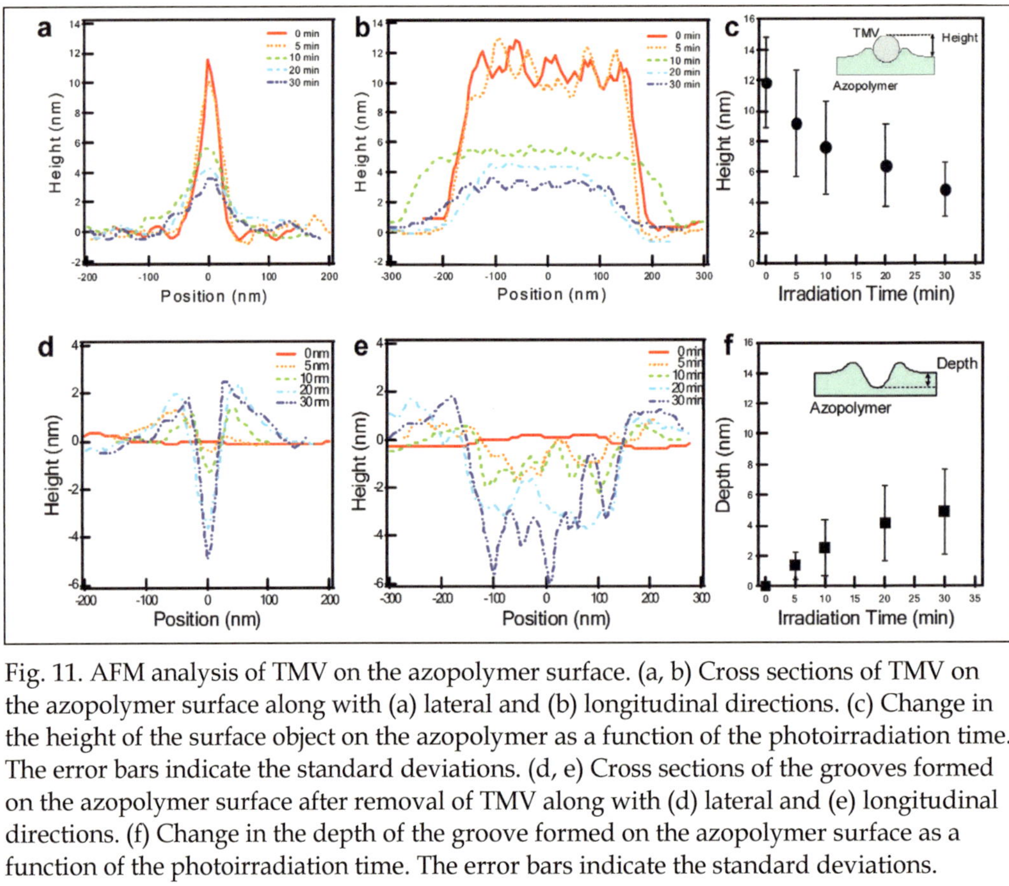

Fig. 11. AFM analysis of TMV on the azopolymer surface. (a, b) Cross sections of TMV on the azopolymer surface along with (a) lateral and (b) longitudinal directions. (c) Change in the height of the surface object on the azopolymer as a function of the photoirradiation time. The error bars indicate the standard deviations. (d, e) Cross sections of the grooves formed on the azopolymer surface after removal of TMV along with (d) lateral and (e) longitudinal directions. (f) Change in the depth of the groove formed on the azopolymer surface as a function of the photoirradiation time. The error bars indicate the standard deviations.

In the lateral cross sections in Fig. 11a, the full width at half-maxima (fwhm) of the peaks are around 30 nm, which is twice as large as the 18 nm diameter of TMV. This is due to the common imaging artifacts from a convolution of the probe geometry and the samples. Likewise, the average height at 0 min photoirradiation is 12 nm in Fig. 11c, which is smaller than the TMV diameter of 18 nm. This must be due to the strong interaction between the probe tip and TMV by the contact mode AFM operation, together with the unstable adsorption of TMV during the scanning in the AFM operation as shown in Fig. 10a. Although the cross sections contain these artifacts, it is evident that the height of the particles gradually decreases on a time scale of minutes during the photoirradiation.

The lateral and longitudinal cross sections of the typical grooves on the azopolymer surface after removal of the rod-shaped particles are shown in Fig. 11d,e. The lateral cross sections in Figure 11d show that the depth of the groove increases with the photoirradiation time accompanied by an uplift of the rim of the groove. The distance between the peaks of the rim is around 50 nm, which is 3 times larger than the diameter of TMV. The observed distance between the rims is accurate because the geometry of the sample surface, rather than of the probe, establishes the line profile of the peaks of the groove. On the other hand, the depth of the groove possibly appears small due to the probe tip not reaching the bottom of the groove. A change in the average depth of the grooves formed on the azopolymer surface as a function of the photoirradiation time is shown in Fig. 11f. The depth, defined in the inset in Fig. 11f, is averaged from 100 grooves in several AFM images of the same sample. By increasing the photoirradiation time to 30 min, the average depth of the grooves was increased to 5 nm. Sums of the average height in Figure 11c and the average depth in Figure 11f at the same photoirradiation time are kept constant at around 10 nm, which is smaller than the 18 nm diameter of TMV. The groove depth might be slightly underestimated due to the probe tip not reaching the bottom of the groove.

Based on the AFM analysis, the behavior of the azopolymer surface with TMV during the photoirradiation is summarized. As the photoirradiation time increases, TMV gradually embeds into the azopolymer surface because of the formation of the complement groove just beneath TMV. The groove depth increases with the uplift of the groove rim during the photoirradiation, but the distance between the groove rims stays constant at around 50 nm, 3 times larger than the diameter of TMV. To be precise, the geometry of the grooves on the azopolymer surface is slightly different from that of TMV. Finally, over half of the TMV body embeds into the groove after 30 min of photoirradiation. Overall, these results indicate that both the azopolymer surface deform along the shape of TMV during the photoirradiation. As a result, the contact-mode scanning of the probe tip in the AFM operations supports TMV in the groove formed on the azopolymer surface.

3. AFM imaging of supramolecular assmblieds on the azopolymer

3.1 Supramolecular assemblies of actin filament

In this section, a structural study of supramolecular assemblies of cytoskeletal filamentous (F-) actin in the presence of divalent cation is presented (Ikawa et al., 2007). F-actin is a double-stranded helical filament made of the protein G-actin, can be considered as a semi-flexible and highly charged polyelectrolyte, with diameter $D_A \sim 80Å$, persistence length $\xi_A \sim 10$ μm and anionic liner charge density $\lambda_A \sim -e/2.5$ Å. (Egelman, 2004; Wong et al., 2003) *In vitro*, F-actin in the presence of divalent cations assembles into gel-like networks and bundles that resemble their cellular counterparts formed with linker proteins. The F-actin/divalent cation aggregation has been used as a good model system, both experimentally and theoretically, for studying biological polyelectrolyte association. Recent experiments using high resolution sall-angle X-ray scattering (SAXS) showed that with high concentration of divalent cations, F-actin forms bundles consisting of filaments that are closely packed in a distorted hexagonal arrangement. (Egelman, 2004; Wong et al., 2003) Within a small range in the low cation concentration regime, a unique layered structure consisting of stacks of nematic F-actin rafts was observed. The detailed structural phase behaviour of the F-actin supramolecular assembly challenges present theoretical model in many aspects. (Borukhov and Bruinsma 2001; Ha &

Liu, 1997; Lee et al., 2004) Clearly, in addition to the average structures revealed by XRD, to have a detailed view of the individual structural elements (filaments, bundles and networks) at the molecular level would provide much insight into the interactions that drive the self-assembly process of biological polyelectrolytes.

The AFM imaging technique based on the azopolymer was used to investigate the phase behaviour of F-actin aggregates as a function of concentration of the divalent cation Mg^{2+}. The data provided direct experimental evidence of a coil-on-coil (braided) structure of F-actin bundles formed at high Mg^{2+} concentrations. At intermediate Mg^{2+} concentrations, the data showed the first images of the two dimensional nematic rafts discovered by recent x-ray studies (Wong et al., 2003) and theoretical treatments. (Borukhov & Bruinsma, 2001)

3.1.1 Experimental procedure

F-actin was polymerized from lyophilized monomeric Globular (G-) actin (2mg/ml) from rabbit skeletal muscle. (Wong et al., 2003) F-actin length was controlled by the addition of an appropriate amount of 1 mg/mL gelsolin. The photoimmobilization process used to prepare the F-actin/Mg^{2+} samples is as follows. F-actin and magnesium chloride solutions are spotted (each spot contains 1 μL of $MgCl_2$ and 1 μL of F-actin) and mixed on the surface of a spin-coated azopolymer film (polymer 2), on a glass substrate. Each sample (substrate) contains an array of spots (typically 6-8) with different concentrations of F-actin and Mg^{2+}. The film was then sealed inside a humidity chamber to prevent evaporation and irradiated for 60 minutes with light (470 nm) from a 6x10 array of blue light emitting diodes (LED) with an optical power density of 10 mW/cm^2. After washing the surface to remove excess sample, the substrate was probed by using a Digital Instruments Dimension 30000 scanning probe microscope in tapping-mode with a standard silicon cantilever (tip radius of curvature ~ 20 nm).

3.1.2 AFM image of F-actin filament and its assembly

An AFM image and an axial height trace of a single F-actin filament immobilized on the azo polymer surface is shown in Fig. 12. The height trace shows periodic variation with a typical repeating distance of 35 nm matching the pitch of the F-actin. The observed pitch varies from 30 nm to 40 nm, which is consistent with previous electron microscopy observations that F-actin is a helix with a random variable twist (Egelman, 2004; Egelman et al., 1982). The observed height (3 nm - 4 nm from valley to peak) of the filament is about half of the actual F-actin diameter (6-8 nm), suggesting that the filament is about halfway embedded into the azopolymer film after photoirradiation. The typical observed width of a single filament measured perpendicular to the filament is around 20 nm, about 3 times greater than the actual diameter of F-actin, which can be attributed to a tip-sample convolution effect. Even though it is difficult to remove this tip-sample convolution effect, it is not difficult to differentiate between single filaments and bundles based on their apparent diameter.

Fig. 13a-c demonstrates the progressive association of long actin filaments (up to ~10 μm in length, no gelsolin) with increasing Mg^{2+} concentration (0 mM, 10 mM, 80 mM, respectively) on the azo polymer surface. The F-actin solution with 0 mM Mg^{2+} exhibits an uncondensed isotropic phase (Fig. 13a), with filaments maintaining large distances and intersecting angles (~90 degrees) between them to minimize electrostatic repulsion. With 10 mM Mg^{2+}

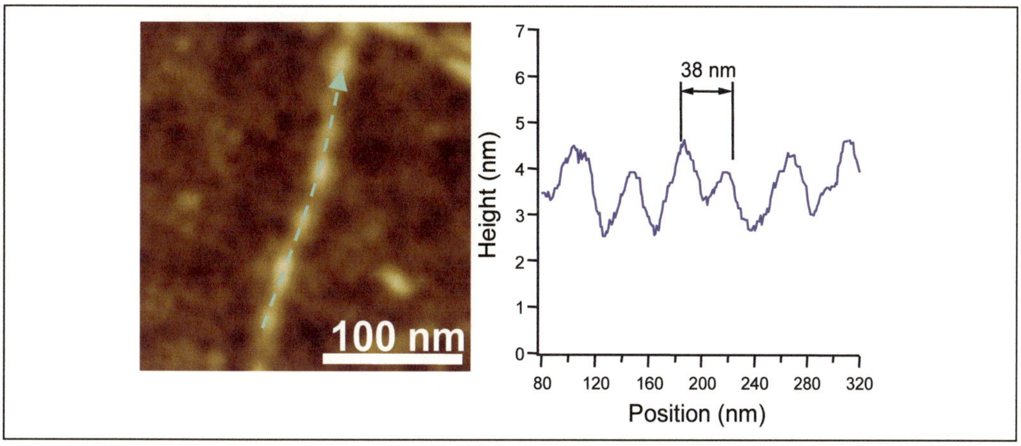

Fig. 12. An AFM image of a single F-actin filament and a height trace along the single filament showing periodic variations corresponding to F-actin twists.

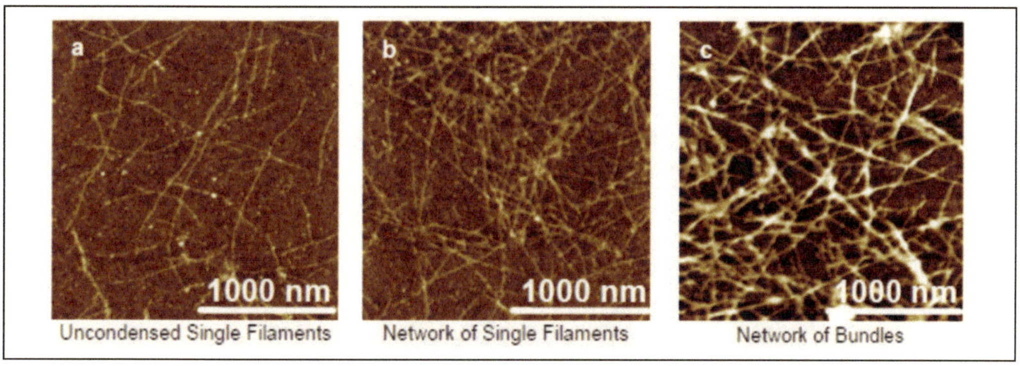

Fig. 13. AFM images showing the progressive association of long (no gelsolin) actin filaments as a function of Mg^{2+} concentration. (a) Isotropic phase of F-actin (0 mM Mg^{2+}). (b) Network of F-actin (10 mM Mg^{2+}). (c) Network of F-actin bundles (80 mM Mg^{2+}). The phase map was obtained from one azo-polymer sample containing multiple spots of F-actin/ Mg^{2+} mixed at different ratios.

(Fig.13b), the distances between filaments become smaller and the filaments form a network structure with smaller intersecting angles between filaments. The network consists of predominantly single filaments of F-actin. At 80 mM Mg^{2+} (Fig.13c), however, a different network structure composed of mostly thick filaments (F-actin bundles), is observed. The single filaments and bundles are entangled and oriented randomly in the network, suggesting little excluded volume interaction which drives liquid crystalline ordering in the more concentrated solution. Interestingly, the bundles observed in the networks appear to be fairly uniform in diameter and large bundles were rarely seen under this condition. This suggests that there might be a growth limit of the bundle size, which has been predicted theoretically. Overall, the phase behaviour observed in the AFM images is consistent with the previous results obtained using x-ray diffraction and optical microscopy. However, the high resolution data allowed us to examine the structures at a single filament or bundle level, which led to observations relevant to several important unanswered questions about F-actin assemblies.

There has been much discussion about the structure of bundles that are formed by charged biopolymers at high counter-ion concentrations. One of the intriguing possibilities is whether the F-actin could form helical coil within a bundle.(Shao et al., 2000) Analogous structures have been theoretically predicted, but never experimentally verified. Using the current technique, direct evidence of the coil-on-coil (braided) bundle structure at higher cation concentrations has been found(>20 mM Mg^{2+}). In Fig. 14a,b, two examples of the braided bundles formed with short F-actin (average length = 680 nm controlled with gelsolin) and 80 mM Mg^{2+} are shown. Under this condition, co-existence of both single filaments and bundles were observed, which can be easily differentiated in the magnified images by their apparent diameter. Following the trace lines, it can be seen that the bundles unravel at their ends into three or more single filaments. The braided configuration of the bundle is especially obvious in Fig. 14b. The braided structure is found to exist in a wide range of Mg^{2+} concentrations (5 mM to 160 mM), from the uncondensed phase to the bundled phase. In comparison, such spiral structures were not readily discernible in the bundles that are formed by longer filaments (Fig. 14c). One could argue that the longer filaments are more prone to kinetic hindrance to forming braided structures due to increased difficulty in rotational movements.

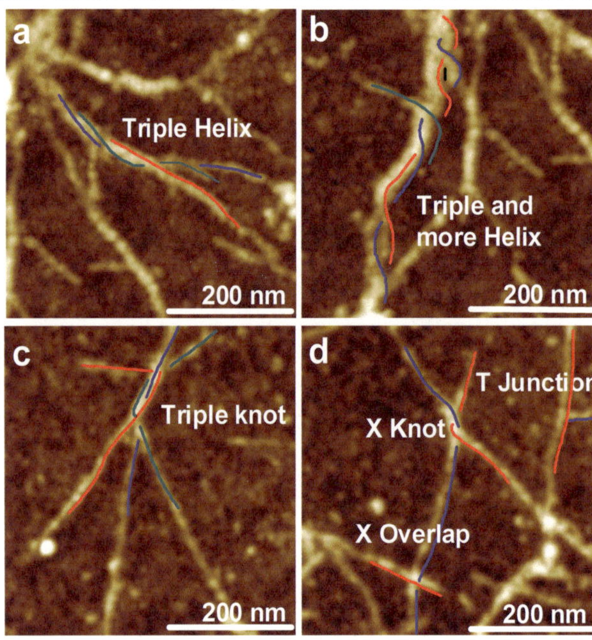

Fig. 14. Braided structures of short F-actin (average length 680 nm) bundles and precursor junctions. (a, b) Braided bundles at high concentration of Mg^{2+} (80 mM). The bundle in image (a) consists of three filaments and the bundle in (b) consists possibly of more than three filaments. (c, d) Junction-type precursor structures formed in the uncondensed phase of F-actin with 5 mM Mg^{2+}. All the images are 0-10 nm in height.

AFM images of F-actin at lower Mg^{2+} concentrations offered some clues as to how the helical bundles may be formed. Fig. 14c,d show several distinct F-actin junctions (points where single filaments are joined or crossed) observed at 5 mM Mg^{2+} concentration. In Fig. 14c, three filaments form a knot structure of about 100 nm in length, and the knot unravels at both ends into three single filaments with fairly large angular separation. Also, entangled points formed by two filaments are observed in Fig. 14d. In the same image, two other types of joints could be seen: an X overlap in which the two filaments simply cross each other and a T junction where the end of one filament is seemingly attached to another filament at a near 90 degree angle. All these junctions can be considered as precursor sites of the more extensive helical bundle structure shown in Fig. 14a,b at higher Mg^{2+} concentrations.

The braided bundle structure may have been present in previous images of F-actin bundles obtained using electron microscopy, AFM, and confocal optical microscopy, but was not recognized as such. For example, high resolution cryo-AFM images of F-actin clearly showed the existence of braided bundles. (Shao et al., 2000) Synchrotron x-ray diffraction data showed that the close packing pattern of the bundle deviates from an exact hexagonal arrangement ($q10=0.089Å^{-1}$ and $q11 = 0.139$ $Å^{-1}$, respectively), which may be partially attributed to the braided arrangement of some F-actin inside the bundle. (Angelini, et al., 2003, Wong, et al. 2003) The observed axial repeat distance of the braided bundles is around 100 nm (Fig. 14b,c), comparable to the pitch of a single F-actin twisted structure. This strongly suggests that the F-actin filament follows the topology of the twist of F-actin in order to achieve tighter packing.

It is important to note that the existence of braided F-actin bundles does not necessarily contradict the earlier conclusion of hexagonal packing of filaments inside the bundles. Because of the limited statistical sampling of AFM imaging and the large F-actin length distribution, it is likely that the actual samples contain both structures, with hexagonal bundles being the prevalent structure giving rise to the x-ray diffraction peaks.

The structures formed in the intermediate range of concentration are of particular interests, as previous x-ray studies revealed in this regime an unique phase composed of lamellar stacks of crossed rafts (L_{XR} phase; Wong, et al. 2003). Such a structure, formed with 20 mM of Mg^{2+}, is shown in Fig. 15a. The filaments form a 2D nematic-like rafts with a lateral repeat distance of about 12 nm, slightly larger than the F-actin diameter. The rafts are stacked at a large angle from each other, as was deduced from x-ray data, which showed a series of strong (00L) harmonic peaks due to stacking. The raft-like structures can be observed in a wide range of Mg^{2+} concentration (5-40 mM) with short F-actin and were much less dominant with longer filaments. This is consistent with the phase diagram compiled with x-ray data. (Wong et al., 2003) Similar structure has been observed in the system consisting of microtubules and divalent cations, suggesting a certain degree of universality of phase behaviour of rod-like biological filaments with divalent cations.

The 2D nemtic-like rafts were found to coexist with aggregated perpendicular filaments at slightly lower Mg^{2+} concentrations (5-10 mM), as shown in Fig. 15b, which is consistent with recent molecular dynamic simulation predictions that isolated stiff polyelectrolyte filaments in general evolve from aggregated perpendicular filaments to aggregated parallel rods.16 The theoretical treatment also describes that the aggregated perpendicular filaments can form two-dimensional rafts. (Borukhov et al., 2001) This image clearly shows the coexistence of the parallel filaments and the perpendicular one.

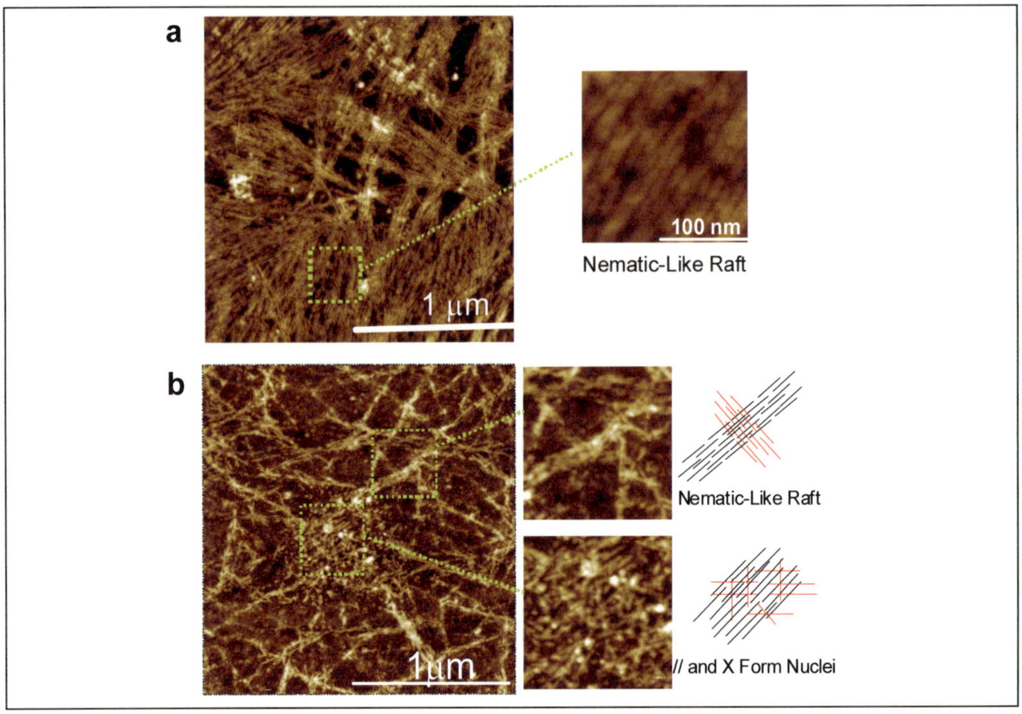

Fig. 15. AFM images of intermediate phases of short F-actin (average length 170 nm) Mg^{2+}. (a) A phase consists of the nematic-like rafts with 20 mM Mg^{2+}. In part, the rafts are stacked. (b) A phase consists of both the nematic-like rafts and the perpendicular aggregates with 10 mM Mg^{2+}.

Based on the above AFM images, the phase diagram of the supramolecular assembly of F-actin was summarized in Fig. 16. The structures of the assemblies changes with concentration of Mg^{2+} and length of the filaments, which is consistent with the previous X-ray study and the theoretical predictions. (Borukhov et al., 2001; Wong et al, 2003) The AFM study clearly shows the first-time-seen images of the following structures: (1) the cross stacking of the 2D nematic-like rafts of short F-actin at intermediate concentration of Mg^{2+} (5 - 10 mM) and (2) the braided bundle structure at high concentration of Mg^{2+} (more than 20 mM).

3.2 AFM image of myosin filaments

Cytoskeletal motorproteins myosin associated with actin filament tracks through a head region, called motor domain, that binds and hydrolyzes ATP. The Myosin from muscle protein called Myosin II, which generates the force for muscle contraction. Myosin II is an elongated protein that is formed from two heavy chains and two copies of each of two light chains. Each of the heavy chains has a globular head chains at its N-terminus that contains the force-generating domain, followed by a very long amino acid sequence that forms an extended coiled-coil that mediates heavy chain dimerization. The two light chain bind close to the N-terminal head domain, while the long coiled-coile tail bundles itself with the tails of other myosin molecules. These tail-tail interaction *in vivo* results in the formation of larger bipolar thick filaments (Alberts et al., 2002).

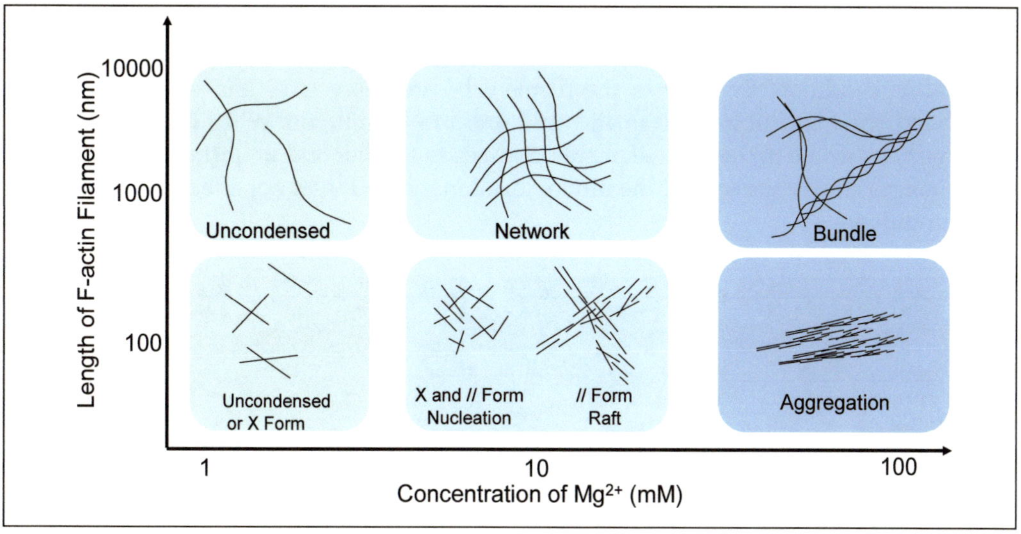

Fig. 16. A phase diagram of the supramolecular assembly of F-actin as a function of Mg^{2+} concentration.

The assembly of the myosin *in vitro* can be regulated by ionic strength and preparation condition (Offer, 1987). When the salt concentration of solution of myosin is reduced, either by dilution or by dialysis, the myosin molecules polymerize into filaments; the tendency for filament formation increases as either the salt concentration or pH is reduced. The structure of the synthetic filaments formed is not fixed but varies grossly with the final ionic condition and the rate at which the salt concentration is reduced.

The structure of the myosin filaments is analysed by AFM imaging using the azopolymer. Myosin from rabbit skeletal muscle (22 mg/ml containing 20 mM TES, pH7.0, 0.6 M NaCl, 50 % of glycerole, Prozyme) was diluted or dialyzed by aqueous buffer solution containing imidazole, potassium chloride, magnesium chloride. Final concentration of the buffer was summarized in Table 1. The photoimmobilization process used to prepare the myosin filament samples is as follows. The myosin filament solutions are spotted (each spot contains 1 μL) on the surface of a spin-coated azopolymer film (polymer 2), on a glass substrate. The film was then sealed inside a humidity chamber to prevent evaporation and irradiated for 60 minutes with light (470 nm) from a 6x10 array of blue light emitting diodes (LED) with an optical power density of 25 mW/cm^2. After washing the surface to remove excess sample, the substrate was probed by using a Digital Instruments Nanoscope E scanning probe microscope in contact-mode with a standard silicon cantilever (tip radius of curvature ~ 20 nm).

sample	Concentration of Myosin (mg/mL)	pH	Buffer Imidazole (mM)	KCl (mM)	$MgCl_2$ (mM)	Preparaton Method	Filament Size Lentgh(nm)	Diameter(nm)
a	0.25	7.4	20	25	4	Dialysis	>10000	5 - 20
b	0.2	7.4	20	25	4	Dilution	>2000	5 - 10
c	0.77	7.4	20	25	160	Dilution	500	2 - 5
d	0.71	7.4	20	500	4	Dilution	200	2

Table 1. Preparation condition for AFM imaging of the myosin filament in Fig. 17.

Fig. 17 shows the AFM images of the myosin filaments immobilized on the azopolymer surface. Comparing Fig. 17a and b, the size of the filament is shown to be affected by the preparation condition. By dialysis, the filament became very large and entangled, on the other hand, the filament became smaller and uniform by dilution. When the ionic strength of the buffer became higher, the filaments changes to smaller and uniform size (Fig. 17b,c). These images clearly shows that the immobilization method does not affected by the buffer ionic condition.

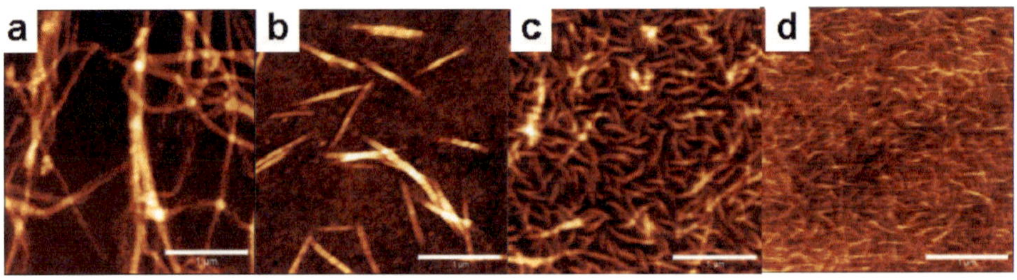

Fig. 17. AFM Images of Myosin Filaments immobilized on the Azopolymer surface. Scale bar 1000 nm. a, b, c and d corresponds in Table 1

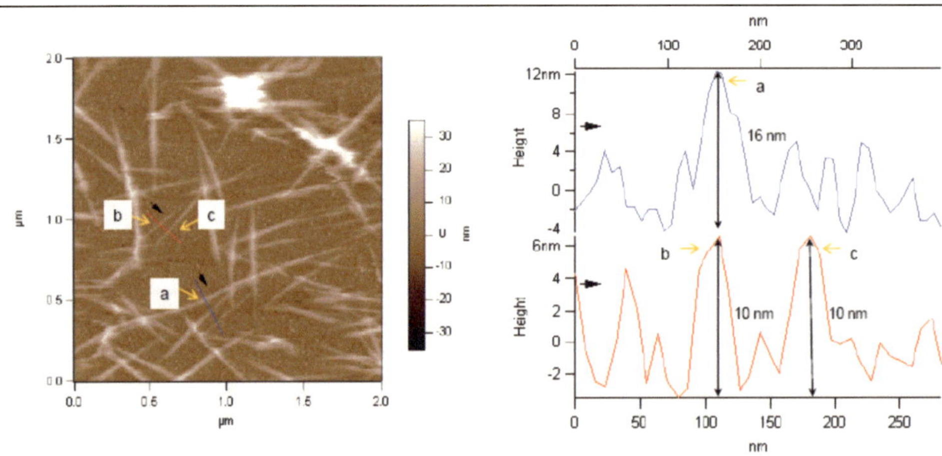

a b

Fig. 18. AFM image of myosin filament obtained in fluid condition. 2-dimensional image (a) and the cross section (b).

The AFM imaging of myosin is also performed in fluid conditon. After immobilizing the myosin in the buffer on the azopolymer by photoirradiation, the solution is rinsed by the same buffer. Immediately, the fluid imaging is performed by Asylum Research MFP-3D-BIO Atomic Force Microscope in tapping-mode.

Fig. 18 shows the AFM image of Myosin filament, the buffer conditon is same as the sample b in Table 1 and Fig 18b. This image clearly shows that the myosin filaments are immobilzed on the azopolymer surface even in the fluid condition and the filament size is almost the same as the one obtained even in air conditon by contact-mode AFM, which is higher sample-tip interaction. The experiments shows that the ionic strength is not affected by the immobilization on the azopolymer, and that the AFM images obtained both in fluid and air conditon are the essentially the same.

4. Conclusion

The immobilization technique using the azopolymer is well-suited for AFM imaging of biomolecules and their assembly because it can provide a non-reactive, non-ionic, and flat surface on which the complex supramolecular assemblies can be immobilized in the native aqueous environment, reducing the possibility of chemical denaturation of the immobilization objects. The immobilization process dramatically reduces the thermal motion of biomolecules, leading to higher imaging resolution allowing individual biomolecules to be resolved without interference from the substrate. Clear biomolecule images appeared on the azopolymer surface after the photoirradiation, even by using contact-mode AFM where interaction between the probe tip and the sample is relatively strong.

There is an important disadvantage when compared with atomically flat mica surface as a substrate for AFM imaging; the information about the height of the object is spoiled by its embedding into the azopolymer surface. However, comparing the observed height of the object with the groove formed on the azopolymer surface, the true height can be estimated. Another disadvantage is that the azopolymer used in this experiment is inadequate for the immobilization of highly charged objects like TMV in the aqueous condition. (Note that general hydrophilic proteins, for example IgG, green fluorescent protein, and F-actin, could be immobilized on the same azopolymer surface in aqueous media.). To immobilize highly charged objects like TMV in the aqueous condition, introduction of a counter charged functional group to the azopolymer is essential.

In summary the technique is of greater advantage than the conventional methods in points of versatility and simplicity for AFM imaging biomolecules and their assembly.

5. Acknowledgment

Author thanks C.R. Safinya, Youli Li, Kai Ewert, L.S. Hirst, N. Bouxsein, M.C. Choi and R. Beck for useful discussions. Author thanks Y. Kato, T. Yamada, M. Shiozawa, M. Narita, M. Mouri, F. Hoshino, T. Mitsuoka, T. Matsuyama, H. Takahashi, O. Watanabe and S. Ito for their kind support for this work. Author thanks H. Takami and H. Sugasawa of Asyrum Technology Co. Ltd for fluid imaging of myosin.

6. References

Alberts, B.; Johnson, A.; Lewis, J., Rall, M.; Roberts, K. & Walter, P. (2002) Chapter 16, Molecular motors, In *Molecular Biology of the Cell 4th Ed.*, pp.949-952 Garland Science, New York, USA

Alexander, C.; Davidson, L. & Hayes, W., (2003), Imprinted polymers: artificial molecular recognition materials with applications in synthesis and catalysis. *Tetrahedron, Vol.*59, pp.2025-2057

Angelini, T.E.; Liang, H.; Wriggers, W. & Wong, G.C.L., (2003) Like-charge attraction between polyelectrolytes induced by counterion charge density waves, *Proc. Natl. Acad. Sci. USA*, Vol. 100, pp.8634-8637

Bezanilla, M.; Manne, S.; Laney, D.E.; Lyubchenko, Y.L. & Hansma, H.G. (1995), Adsorption of DNA to mica, silylated mica and minerals: characterization by atomic force microscopy. *Langmuir*, vol. 11, pp.655-659

Borukhov, I. & Bruinsma, R.F., (1997), Counterion-mediated attraction between two like-charged rods. *Phys. Rev. Lett.* vol.79, 1289-1292

Borukhov, I. & Bruinsma, R. F., (2001) Raft instability of biopolymer gels. *Phys. Rev. Lett.* Vol.87, 158101

Casper, D.L.D., Assembly and stability of the tobacco mosaic virus particle. *Adv. Protein Chem.* Vol.18, pp.37-121

Curtis, A. & Wilkinson, C., (2001), Nantotechniques and approaches in biotechnology. *Trends in biotechnology, Vol.* 19, pp.97-101

Cunin, F.; Schmedake, T.A.; Link, J.R.; Li, Y.Y.; Koh, J.; Bhatia, S. N. & Sailor, M. J. (2002) Biomolecular screening with encoded porous silicon photonic crystals. *Nature Materials, Vol.* 1, pp.39-41

Egelman, E.H. (2004) Acrosomal actin: twists and turns of a versatile filament. *Curr. Biol.* Vol.14, R959

Egelman, E. H., Francis, N., DeRosier, D. J., (1982), F-actin is a helix with a random variable twist. *Nature*, Vol. 298, pp. 131-135

Ha, B.-Y. & Liu, J. A., (1997), Counterion-mediated attraction between two like-charged rods. *Phys. Rev. Lett.*, Vol.79, pp.1289-1292

Hansma, H.G., (2001) Surface biology of DNA by atomic force microscopy. *Annual Rev. Phys. Chem.*, Vol.52, pp.71-92

Hasegawa, M.; Ikawa, T.; Tsuchmori, M.; Watanabe, O.; Kawata, Y., (2001) Topographical nanostructure patterning on the surface of a thin film of polyurethane containing azobezene moiety using the optical near field around polystyrene spheres. *Macromolecules*, Vol.34, pp7471-7476

Haupt, K.,(2003) Imprinted polymers - Taylor-made mimics of antibodies and receptors. *Chem. Comm.* pp.171-178.

Ichimura, K., (2000) Photoalignment of liquid-crystal systems. *Chem. Rev.*, Vol.100, 1847

Ikawa, T.; Hoshino, F.; Matsuyama, T.; Takahashi, H. & Watanabe, O., (2006), Molecular-shape imprinting and immobilization of biomolecules on a polymer containing azo dye, *Langmuir*, Vol.22, No.6, pp.2747-2753

Ikawa, T.; Hoshino, F.; Watanabe, O.; Li, Y.; Pincus, P. & Safinya, C.R., (2007), Molecular-scale imaging of F-actin assemblies immobilized on a photopolymer surface, *Phys. Rev. Lett.*, Vol.98, 018101

Ikawa, T.; Kato, Y.; Yamada, T.; Shiozawa, M.; Narita, M.; Mouri, M.; Hoshino, F.; Osamu, W.; Tawata, M. & Shimoyama, H., (2010),Virus-templated photoimprint on the surface of an azobenzene-containing polymer, *Langmuir*, Vol.26, No.15, pp.12673-12679

Ikawa, T.; Mitsuoka, T.; Hasegawa, M.; Tsuchimori, M.; Watanabe, O.; Kawata, Y.; Egami, C.; Sugihara, O.; Okamoto, N. (2000) Optical near field induced change in viscoelasticity on an azobenzene-containing polymer surface. *J. Phys. Chem., B.* Vol.104, pp 9055-9058

Ikawa, T.; Mitsuoka, T.; Hasegawa, M.; Tsuchimori, M.; Watanabe, O. & Kawata, Y., (2001) Azobenzene polymer surface deformation due to the gradient force of the optical near field of monodispersed polystyrene spheres. *Phys. Rev. B.*, Vol. 64, 195408

Kambhampati, D., (Ed.) , (2003), In: *Protein Microarray Technology*, Wiley-VCH, Weinheim, Germany

Karageogiev, P.; Neher, D.; Schulz, B.; Stiller, B.; Pietsch, U.; Giersig, M. & Brehmer, L. (2005) From anisotropic photo-fluidity towards nanomanipulation in the optical near-field, *Nature Mater.* Vol.4, pp.699-703

Kawata, Y.; Egami, O.; Nakamura, O.; Sugihara, M.; Okamoto, M.; Tsuchimori, M. & Watanabe, O., (1999) Non-optically probing near-field microscopy, *Opt. Commun.* Vol.161, pp.6

Kim, D.Y.; Li, L.;Kumar, J. & Tripathy, S.K.,(1995) Laser-induced holographic surface relief gratings on nonlinear optical polymer films, *Appl. Phys. Lett.* Vol.66, pp.1166-1168

Lamture, J.B.; Beattie, K.L.; Burke, B.E.; Eggers, M.D.; Ehrlich, D.J.; Fowler, R.; Hollies, M.A.; Kosicki, B.B.; Reich, R.K.; Smith, S.R.; Varma, R.S. & Hogan, M.E., (1994) Direct detection of nucleic acid hybridization on the surface of a charge coupled device, *Nucleic Acids Res.*, Vol. 22, pp. 2121

Lee, K-C.; Borukhov, I.; Gelbart, W. M.; Liu, A.J.; Stevens, M. J. ,(2004), Effect of mono- and multivalent salts on angle-dependent attractions between charged rods. *Phys. Rev. Lett. Vol.* 93, 128101

Mayers, A. G., (2002), In: *Biomolecular Sensors*, Gizeli, E., Lowe, R. C., (Eds), Taylor and Francis, London, England

Mouri, M.; Ikawa, T.; Narita, M.; Hoshino, F. & Watanabe, O., (2010) Orientation Control of Photo-Immobilized Antibodies on the Surface of Azobenzene-Containing Polymers by the Introduction of Functional Groups, *Macromol, Biosci.*, Vol. 10, pp.612

Natanshon, A. & Rochon, P., (2002) Photoinduced motions in azo-containing polymers, *Chem. Rev.*, Vol.102, pp. 4139

Offer, G. (1987), Chapter 12 Myosin filaments, In *Fibrous Protein Structure*, PP.307-356, Academic Press, N

Ostuni, E.; Chapman, R. G.; Holmlin, R. E.; Takayama, S. & G. M. Whitesides, (2001) A survey of structure-property relationships of surfaces that resist the adsorption of protein, *Langmuir*, Vol.17, pp.5605-5620

Ramsden, J. J., (1993) Experimental methods for investigating protein adsorption kinetics at surfaces, *Quarterly Reviews of Biophysics*, Vol.27, pp.41-105

Rau, H.; (1990), In *Photochemistry and Photophysics*, J. K. Rabek, (Ed.), CRC Press: Boca Raton, Flance, Vol. 2, pp.119-121.

Rochon, P.; Batalla, E. & Natansohn, A., (1995) Optically induced surface gratings on azoaromatic polymer films, *Appl. Phys. Lett.* Vol.66, pp.136-138

Schena, M., (Ed.), (2004), In: *Protein Microarray*, Jones and Bartlett Publishers, Sudbury, USA.

Schramm, G. & Wiedeman, M.,(1951) , *Z. Naturforsch. B*, Vol. 6, 379

Shao, Z.; Shi, D. & Somlyo A.V. (2000), Cryoatomic force microscopy of filamentous actin, *Biophys. J.*, Vol. 78, pp. 950-958

Shenton, W.; Douglass, T.; Young, M.; Stubbs, G.; Mann, S. (1999) Inorganic–organic nanotube composites from template mineralization of tobacco mosaic virus, *Adv. Mater.*, Vol.11, pp.253-256

Shi, H.; Tsai, W-B.; Garrison, M.D.; Ferrari, S. & Ratner, B. D., (1999) Template-imprinted nanostructured surfaces for protein recognition, *Nature, Vol.*398, pp.593-597

Todorov,T.; Nikolova, L., Tomova, N., (1984) Polarization holography. 1: A new high-efficiency organic material with reversible photoinduced birefringence, *Appl. Opt.* Vol. 23, pp. 4309-4312

Wahlgren, M. & Arnebrant, T., (1991) Protein adsorption to solid surfaces., *TIBTECH, Vol.*9, pp.201-208.

Watanabe, O.; Ikawa, T.; Kato, T.; Tawata, M. & Shimoyama, H. (2006) Area-selective photoimmobilization of a two-dimensional array of colloidal spheres on a photodeformed template formed in photoresponsive azopolymer film, *Applied Physics Letters, Vol.* 88, 204107-204109

Wong, G.C.L.; Lin, A.; Tang, J.X.; Li, Y.; Janmey, P.A. & Safinya, C.R., (2003) Structure of actin cross-linked with alpha-actinin: A network of bundles, *Phys. Rev. Lett.*,Vol.91, 08103.

Whitesides, G. M.; Ostuni, E.; Takayama, S.; Jiang, X. & Ingber, D. E. (2001) Soft Lithography In Biology And Biochemistry, *Annu. Rev. Biomed. Eng.Vol.* 3, pp. 335-373.

6

Protein Interactions on Phospholipid Bilayer, Studied by AFM Under Physiological Conditions

Špela Irman[1,2], Miha Škarabot[3,4], Igor Muševič[3,4] and Borut Božič[1,2]
[1]*University Medical Centre, Division of Internal Medicine, Department of Rheumatology*
[2]*University in Ljubljana, Faculty of Pharmacy, Chair for Clinical Biochemistry*
[3]*Jožef Stefan Institute, Department of Condensed Matter Physics*
[4]*University in Ljubljana, Faculty of Mathematics and Physics*
Slovenia

1. Introduction

In this Chapter we would like to share our experience using the atomic force microscope (AFM) within the field of biochemistry. We present the preparation, observation and study of solid supported phospholipid bilayers with AFM. Because phospholipid surfaces are one of the most important places for the interaction between different molecules in the living beings, the knowledge of their preparation and study is essential. Second, we present three examples of protein molecules interacting on the aforementioned phospholipid surfaces: annexin A5, β_2-glycoprotein I, and antibodies. Each section of the Chapter contains all the details that allow the reproduction of: solid supported phospholipid bilayers; annexin A5 crystallization on solid supported phospholipid bilayers; β_2- glycoprotein I agglomeration on solid supported phospholipid bilayers; binding of antibodies to mica; and study of effects and interaction of specific antigen-antibody pairs. Practical instructions at the end of each section present some very useful suggestions when performing the same or similar experiments.

2. Introduction to use of atomic force microscopy in biochemistry

Since the invention of AFM in the year 1986 (Binning et al., 1986), the AFM has become very important tool in the field of biochemistry (Bippes & Müller, 2011). AFM has been used for 3D imaging of molecules (DNA, proteins, polysaccharides), structures (membranes, phospholipid structures, bacteria, cells) and their interaction (Shao et al., 1996; Gadegaard, 2006). Beside imaging, force spectroscopy has been used to reveal biochemistry processes on a molecular level (Rief et al., 1997; Oesterhelt et al., 2000). AFM has also been used for manipulation of biological material (Fotiadis et al., 2002; Thalhammer et al., 1997). High nanometer resolution, simple sample preparation (no need for vacuum), the ability to measure forces between 10^{-4} N and 10^{-12} N and possibility of the »in situ« study in dry or in liquid environment are the most straightforward advantages of AFM.

2.1 Basic principles

Figure 1 presents basic working principle and key elements of the AFM: sensitive cantilever with the sharp tip (AFM probe), piezoelectric scanner which moves the sample in all directions and an optical detection system which is measuring the cantilever bending. AFM can operate in different imaging modes, where the tip is scanning the sample surface to obtain the surface topography, or in force mode where the tip is approaching and retracting the sample to measure the force between the tip and the sample. The key element of the AFM is the probe, since the sharp tip of the probe is interacting with the sample and it measures and controls forces with the surface. Different probes have tips with different chemical and physical properties, which govern the adsorption of the sample components on the tip, what could have big impact on the imaging (modification of the tip apex) and measuring forces. The tips can also be functionalized in order to achieve different chemical activity of the tip (silanization) or particular biological specificities (functionalization with the antigen, antibody, etc.). Big advantage of the AFM comparing to other imaging techniques is in the fact, that samples could be studied in the ambient conditions or in different buffer solutions, which can mimic natural conditions for biological samples. Biological samples are usually studied on a particular platform also called a substrate (more details on the substrates further in the text). The right choice of a substrate is very important, since the substrate can governs the samples properties.

2.2 Modes of operation

AFM can be operated in different imaging modes, where the most common are contact and oscillation mode, or in force mode. Decision about which mode to use is dependent on the sample characteristic and the properties of the sample we want to study.

2.2.1 Contact mode imaging

Contact mode is the original and the most accurate imaging AFM mode, where the tip is brought into the hard contact with the sample surface and it is scanned across the surface. The cantilever deflection, and thus the contact force, are kept constant during the scanning by using a feedback loop. Images are generated by mapping the vertical position of the sample (or cantilever) as it moves up and down to maintain the constant force between the tip and the surface. The deviation of the cantilever deflection from its constant value is recorded as well and provides the error signal, or deflection image, which represents the slope. In contact mode the tip is dragged with relatively high velocity across the studied surface. This results in a friction force between the moving tip and the surface of the sample, which exerts shearing force on the sample. The result is a shear deformation of the sample surface. Therefore, the contact mode is more appropriate when examining the samples with relatively rigid surfaces (crystalline samples) or samples with high self-healing characteristics (phospholipid bilayers). For soft biological samples the contact force should be maintained as low as possible.

2.2.2 Oscillation mode imaging

In the oscillation, or dynamic, mode the cantilever is oscillated with very high frequency, close to the resonant frequency of the cantilever. The most popular oscillation mode is the

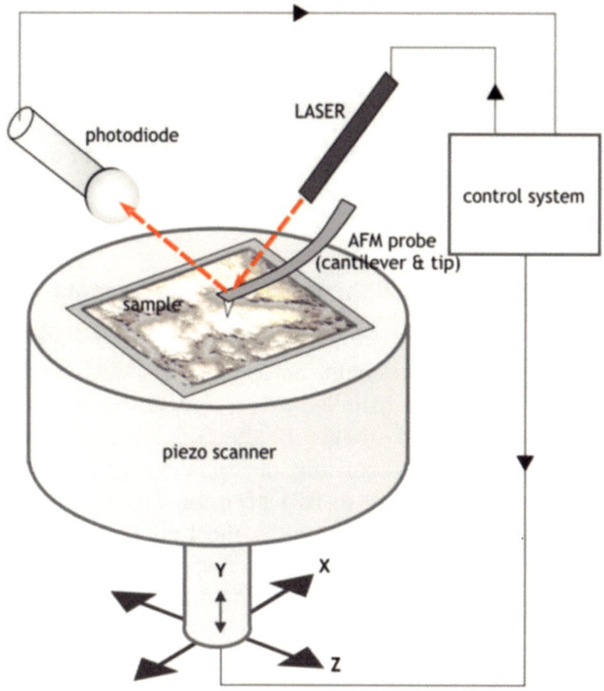

Fig. 1. Basic components and work principle of the atomic force microscope. The basic component of the microscope is a very sharp tip, which is mounted to cantilever. When measurement takes place, the forces between the sample and the tip cause deformation of the cantilever that bends according to the scanned surface. The bending of the cantilever is the most frequently detected optically by a reflected laser beam. The laser beam is directed to the upper side of the cantilever and reflected to the photo-detector (photodiode). The signal from photo-detector is then directed to the computer controlled hardware unit where the feedback electronics moves the sample, which lies on the piezoelectric scanner. In contact mode the laser beam is directed all the time to the same position on the photodiode, so the tip is following the sample surface. The computer transforms the information of scanner movement to the image shown on the monitor.

intermittent contact, or "tapping", mode, where the tip touches the sample surface only once during the oscillation cycle. When the tip is in the contact with the surface, the amplitude of the oscillation is slightly decreased and it is usually used as a feedback parameter. Images are generated by mapping the vertical distances that scanner moves to maintain the constant amplitude during scanning. This mode was developed in order to eliminate the lateral forces, which can damage samples, especially the biological ones.

For even more delicate samples one can use the non-contact mode. Here the tip during oscillation does not touch the sample surface. It oscillates above the sample surface with small amplitude and the distance between tip and sample is controlled by cantilever's resonance frequency which is maintained by the feedback loop. However, this mode does not reach the resolution of contact and tapping mode due to the relatively big separation between tip and sample.

2.2.3 Force spectroscopy mode

In force mode the tip is approaching and retracting from the sample above the same point and it measures the interaction between the tip and the sample. The result of this measurement is distance dependent force curve and not the 3D topographical image of the surface. High resolution of this measurement (piconewton range at nanometer distances) can provide accurate information about intra- and intermolecular interactions and mechanical sample properties.

2.3 Atomic force microscope used in the presented experiments

All our AFM measurements were performed in a liquid environment using a Nanoscope IIIa-MultiMode AFM (Digital Instruments, Santa Barbara, CA) equipped with E (15μm range) scanner. Mica substrates were installed into a contact mode fluid cell. Using AFM we have measured forces and acquired images in the contact mode using oxide-sharpened silicon nitride tips (MSCT-AUNM silicon nitride tip, Veeco, Camarillo, CA) mounted on cantilevers with nominal force constant of 0.01 N/m or 0.03 N/m, with typical curvature radius of 15 nm. We used different scanning rates, most often 5 Hz. The scanning force was kept at the lowest possible value by continuously adjusting the set point during imaging. All experiments were performed at 25°C (Irman et al., 2009, 2010, 2011; Žager et al., 2011).

3. Preparation and study of solid-supported phospholipid bilayers by atomic force microscope

During the past decade a large number of different membrane system have been described, including solid-supported phospholipid bilayers (SPBs), polymer-cushioned lipid bilayers, hybrid bilayers, tethered lipid bilayers, suspended lipid bilayers or supported vesicular layers, all of them having a potential bio-technological applications (reviewed in Richter et al., 2006). However, for our experimental purposes we chosen the *in vitro* model of SPBs because: a.) SPBs are easy to prepare and b.) together with atomic force microscopy this *in vitro* model offers measurements in real time in liquid environment, and therefore *in situ* observation and evaluation of interactions of particular molecules on phospholipid surfaces. SPBs are well suited to analyze lipid domain formation, intermembrane interactions, or membrane processes such as protein adsorption, protein self-assembly, protein localization at lipid phase boundaries and protein function.

3.1 Formation of solid-supported phospholipid bilayers

The mechanism of SPBs formation from large unilamellar vesicles was pioneered by Brian and McConell (Brian & McConnell, 1984): adsorbed vesicles fuse among themselves until critical size is reached, and then rupture to form bilayer disks (Brian & McConnell, 1984; Lipowsky & Seifert, 1991; Seifert, 1997; Reviakine & Brisson, 2000). The one-step procedure allows creating SLBs of different lipid mixtures. Such SLBs form a fluid two dimensional space allowing free diffusion in translation and rotation of lipid molecules and lipid-associated proteins. It was recognized that several factors govern SPB formation: lipid vesicles used for their construction (their composition, charge, size and physical state); aqueous environment (its composition, pH and ionic strength); and nature of support (its surface charge, chemical composition and roughness) on which SPB is formed. A number of reports have revealed difficulties to form

SPBs on surfaces such as gold, $SrTiO_2$, TiO_2 or platinum, leaving mica and silicon-based materials, such as glass, Si_3N_4 or silica as the most common surfaces used for preparation of SPBs. It was recognized that the interactions between lipids and solid support strongly affect the properties (inter-leaflet distribution of lipids in the SPBs) and the quality (integrity) of the final SPB (reviewed in Richter et al., 2006).

3.2 Mica as a solid support

In our study mica was chosen as solid support. Mica is molecularly smooth and hydrophilic and consists of negatively charged layers bound together by positively charged interlayer of K^+. In aqueous solutions, a mica cleavage surface becomes negatively charged due to the dissociation of K^+. It was reported that mica causes asymmetrical inter-leaflet distribution of phosphatidylcholine and phosphatidylserine (PS) containing mixtures of phospholipids, with more PS on mica-facing leaflet of SPB. The asymmetry on mica was suggested to originate from a specific calcium-mediated interaction between the support and PS (Richter & Brisson, 2005). In general it was found that calcium promotes the adsorption and rupture of vesicles and subsequent SPB formation. Effects are particularly strong on mica, since only mmol/l concentration of the ion is sufficient to generate significant effect.

3.3 Mica-supported phospholipid bilayers simulate the physiological conditions of the cell surface

3.3.1 Recipe for preparation of mica-supported phospholipid bilayers

Planar, mica-SPBs are formed from 0.5 g/l suspension of large unilamellar sonicated phospholipid vesicles in HEPES buffered saline (HBS; 10 mM HEPES, 150 mM NaCl), pH 7.5, with 1.5 or 2 mmol/l of $CaCl_2$. For preparation of HBS Water for injections from Braun (Melsungen, Germany) is used. Large unilamellar sonicated phospholipid vesicles are prepared as follows: Appropriate amounts of lipids either synthetic (30 % dioleil-phosphatidyserine in the mixture with dioleil-phosphatidylcholine (Avanti Polar Lipids, Alabaster, AL, USA)), or naturally derived phospholipids (30 % L-α-phosphatidylserine in the mixture with L-α-phosphatidylcholine (Sigma- Aldrich, St. Luis, MO, USA)), are dissolved in chloroform. The solvent is evaporated under low pressure in the presence of N_2 for at least 30 min. HBS with calcium is added to the newly generated lipid film, yielding a 0.5 mg/ml multilamellar vesicle suspension. Unilamellar vesicles are obtained using a bath sonicator (UZ 4R, Iskra, Kranj, Slovenia). Prepared vesicles could be studied by light scattering (Zeta Sizer 3000, Malvern Instruments, England, UK) and/or direct observation with AFM.

SPB is formed by deposition of 120 μl of freshly sonicated vesicles onto a cleaved mica surface (Provac AG, Balzers, Liechtenstein) followed by incubation for 60 min at room temperature. Further treatment of the sample to form the SPBs on mica is however dependent on the phospholipid mixture that is used for preparation of vesicles and the properties of vesicles themselves. If the vesicles are prepared from phospholipids, and the average Tm (Tm is a gel to liquid crystal transition temperature) of the phospholipid mixture is over the room temperature, then sample should be further heated to the Tm or above (in our experimental model the Tm for mixture from naturally derived phospholipids was designated 41°C) for 10 min. When using the phospholipid mixture with the Tm that is below the room temperature, no further heating of the sample is necessary (as was in our case with the vesicles from synthetic phospholipids). The excess lipids are removed by exchanging the solution covering mica with buffer, and the sample is then installed in the contact mode fluid cell in the AFM. The microscope is allowed to thermally equilibrate for a minimum of 15 min before imaging.

3.3.2 Our comments to mica-supported phospholipid bilayers

The developed *in vitro* model of mica-SPBs starts by preparation and characterization of phospholipid vesicles, we found that by slightly changing only two conditions when preparing the vesicles, the strength of the vacuum and pressure under which N_2 was blown in the system, we were able to measure vesicles of different sizes, from 60 nm to 300 nm. An increase in vacuum coupled with a decrease N_2 pressure decreased the sizes of vesicles. An increase of the sonification time decreased the sizes of vesicles. Polydispersity of the vesicles was strongly dependent on the quality of chemicals used for preparation of vesicles and the time of sonification. In general, the longer the time of sonification, the less polydisperse were the vesicles. But after certain time of sonification, poydispersity began to grow. For production of unilamellar vesicles we have also used the extrusion method, where multilamellar vesicles dispersion were extruded through polycarbonate membranes with an average pore size of 50 nm, 100 nm and 200 nm. The vesicles made by extrusion method were around 20-30 nm larger than the sizes of the pores used and more homogeneous in comparison with vesicles made by sonification. Nevertheless, for our formation of SPBs on mica, vesicles made with sonification were used, and sizes around 200 nm proved to be the most useful. When studying vesicles with AFM, contact and tapping mode were used for imaging (Figure 2A).

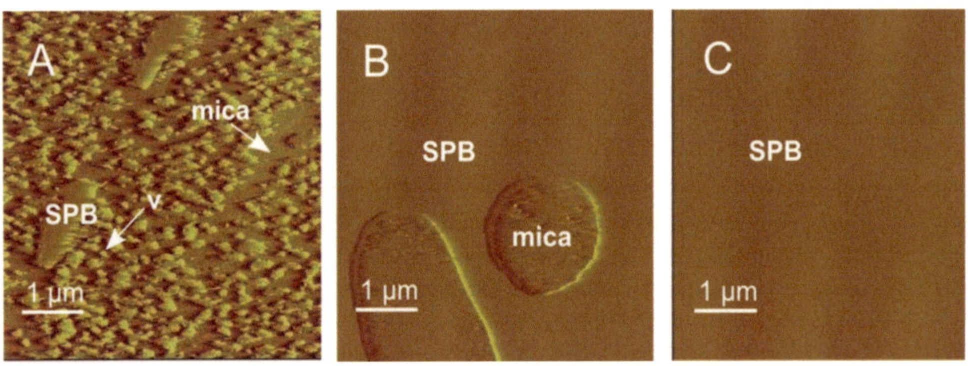

Fig. 2. Deflection images of vesicles, discontinuous and continuous SPBs, made in AFM contact mode. A.) 0.5 mg/ml sonicated unilamellar vesicles solution (30 % dioleil-PS in the mixture with dioleil-phosphatidylcholine in HBS with 1.5mmol/l of calcium) after 15 min incubation in AFM fluid cell. Phospholipid vesicles (v) with sizes from 60 nm to 250 nm can be observed. Some vesicles have already started to fuse among themselves to form SPB patches. B.) A discontinuous SPB. C.) A continuous SPB, where a completely flat surface can be observed.

The next step was preparation and characterization of SPBs. We found that formation of SPBs from naturally derived phospholipids was influenced by slightly different fatty acid compositions of both L-α-PS and L-α-phosphatidylcholine between the batches used. Several combinations of conditions (incubation time at room temperature, temperature and duration of heating) have to be experimentally tested to generate reproducible formation of phospholipid bilayers. Phase transition temperature for the mixture of naturally derived phospholipids used in our experimental model was determined experimentally to be approximately 41°C. The work with synthetic dioleil-PS and dioleil-phosphatidylcholine was much more straightforward due to the fixed composition of synthetic phospholipids: we did not have to change anything, once the protocol for formation of SPBs was established. Thicknesses of phospholipid bilayers from naturally derived and synthetical phospholipids on mica measured by imaging with AFM in the contact mode were approximately 3.6 nm. The thicknesses were therefore lower than expected (around 6 nm). In AFM contact mode the tip is dragged with relatively high velocity across the surface of the SPB. This results in a friction force between the moving tip and the upper surface of the SPB, which exerts shearing force on the SPB. The consequence is a shear deformation of SPB, tilting of the molecules in the bilayer and a smaller apparent thickness of the SPB. Using force measurements we have determined the average force required for penetration into the phospholipid bilayers, which was approximately 0.4 nN. We also measured the thicknesses of the bilayers being penetrated and determined them to be approximately 5.3 nm (Irman et al., 2009). The presence of SPB was confirmed by imaging and force measurements as presented in Figure 2 and Figure 3. Figure 3 further supports the existence of phospholipid bilayer since two monolayers that together form phospholipid bilayer are clearly visible.

With the use of naturally derived phospholipids, we can mimic the conditions in the human body much better than with synthetic ones (Irman et al., 2009).

3.3.3 Practical instructions

1. AFM offers nanoscale observation. Therefore, selection of chemically, microbiologically and physically extra pure reagents (water, buffers and phospholipids) for preparation of SPBs is essential.
2. Since phospholipids are prone to oxidation and microbiological contamination one should make sure that phospholipids used are fresh and properly handled. When preparing the vesicles avoid: a.) overheating the phospholipid mixture during the sonification, b.) the contact of phospholipid mixture with air oxygen (use inert atmosphere: nitrogen, argon).
3. The amount of the phospholipids to form the bilayer should be sufficient. When using the 0.5 mg/ml phospholipid vesicles solution in particular buffer system (presence of mmol/l calcium is advisory), approximately 120 µl of the vesicles solution should be deposited onto a freshly cleaved mica surface.
4. In order to achieve the sufficient concentration of the vesicles on mica surface for their further fusion, the vesicles should be incubated on mica at room temperature for 60 minutes.
5. If the Tm of the used phospholipid mixture is higher than the room temperature, the sample has to be heated at the defined Tm for about 10 to 15 minutes. If the Tm of the mixture is at or below the room temperature no heating is necessary to achieve the fusion of the vesicles.
6. The removal of excess lipids is achieved by exchanging the solution covering mica with buffer.
7. The sample is then installed in the fluid cell (contact mode or tapping mode fluid cell) in the AFM. The SPBs in the fluid cell should be covered with the buffer all the time.

However, avoid flushing the SPBs sample with the buffer before the microscope thermally equilibrates which usually takes a minimum of 15 min.

8. Perform AFM measurements: imaging, force measurements.

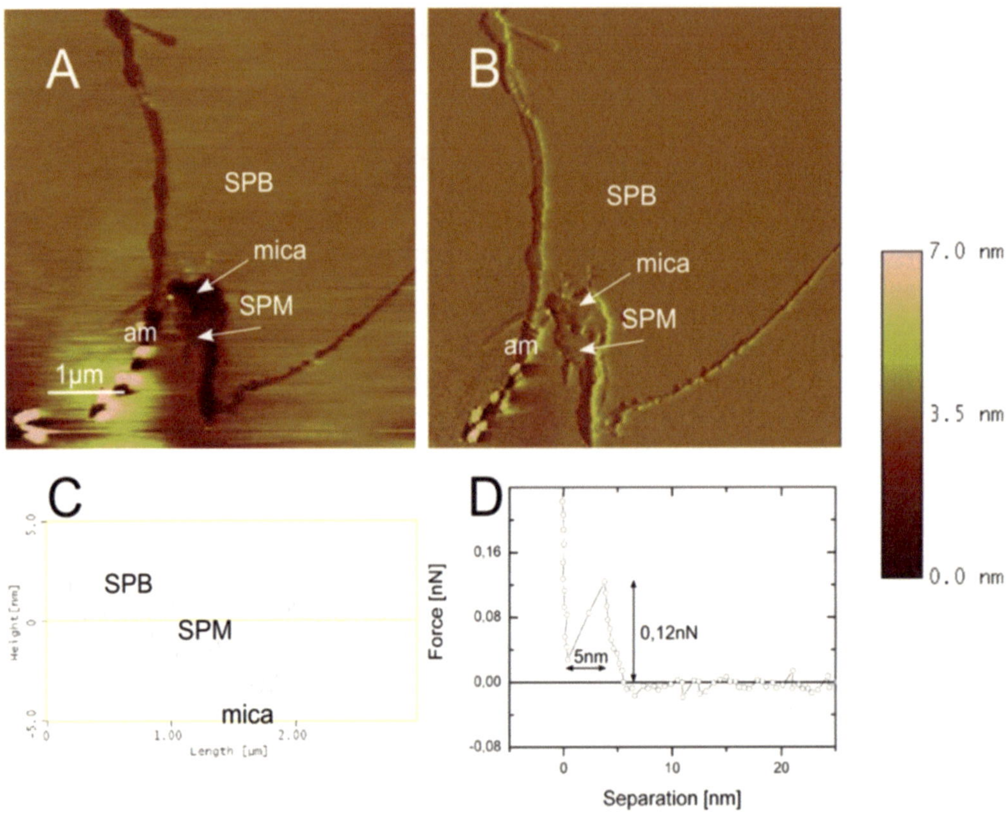

Fig. 3. AFM height and deflection images, height cross section and force measurement of SPB, disrupted with the AFM tip and measured in the contact mode AFM fluid cell. As a buffer above SPB, HBS with 2 mmol/l of calcium was used. This figure presents evidence that the phospholipid vesicles form phospholipid bilayer and not monolayer on mica. (A) AFM height image, where three layers: mica, first phospholipid monolayer (SPM) and second monolayer, which together form the SPB, are measured. Some accumulated material (am) can also be deduced. (B) AFM deflection image of the same surface as in image A, where all three layers are more clearly visible. (C) Height cross section of image A, indicating first phospholipid monolayer is 2 nm higher and the phospholipid bilayer is 4 nm higher than mica. (D) Force measurement showing that the tip is penetrating through SPB about 5 nm thick, with the required force for penetration of 0.12 nN.

4. Models of basic protein interaction - AFM study of annexin A5, β_2-glycoprotein I and antibodies

In this section we give three examples of the proteins that are physiologically present in human body. We present their interaction with phospholipid surfaces, mica, as well as their interactions with each other.

4.1 Crystallization of annexin A5 on phospholipid membranes

4.1.1 Annexin A5's characteristics

Annexin A5 (ANX A5) is an example of protein that forms crystalline lattice over the exposed phospholipid surfaces. ANX A5 is a 35.7 kDa member of the annexin family, which consists of water-soluble, structurally related and calcium-dependent phospholipid binding proteins (Benz & Hofmann, 1997; Gerke et al., 2005; van Genderen et al., 2008). ANX A5 is formed of four domains solely made of α-helices, and is shaped like concave disk with calcium and phospholipid-binding domains present on the convex side (Huber et al., 1990). ANX A5 molecules are monomeric in solution, however, after binding to phospholipid membrane, they spontaneously form tightly bound trimers. The membrane bound trimers self-organize into two types of 2D crystals, with p3 or p6 symmetry (Oling et al., 1998). The mechanism of ANX A5 crystallization on negatively charged phospholipid membranes in the presence of calcium has been thoroughly described (Reviakine et al., 1998, 2000, 2001; Richter et al., 2005; Irman et al., 2009) and it is here schematically shown in Figure 4.

To date, many physiological roles of ANX A5 have been proposed. It is generally accepted that its physiological significance is closely connected to the ability to bind in a calcium-dependent and reversible manner to negatively charged phospholipids, PS in particular. The anticoagulant properties of the protein are a consequence of ANX A5 crystallization on phospholipid membranes, resulting in a lattice of protein over phospholipid surfaces. This blocks the availability of phospholipid surfaces for coagulation reactions. The anticoagulant activity was connected also to more specific properties of ANX A5, such as down-regulation of surface-expressed tissue factor (Ravassa et al., 2005). Several other biological characteristics of ANX A5 have been described, including calcium-channel activities (Rojas et al., 1990; Berendes et al., 1993; Liemann et al., 1996), regulation of phospholipase A2 (van Heerde et al., 1995; Russo-Marie, 1990), cytosolic protein kinase C (van Heerde et al., 1995; Russo-Marie, 1990), inhibition of phagocytosis of apoptotic cells by both activated and inactivated macrophages (Callahan et al., 2000), inhibition of microparticle generation and induction of a novel endocytic pathway (Kenis et al., 2004).

4.1.2 Recipe for preparation and study of crystalline annexin A5 on mica-supported phospholipid bilayers

In order to study ANX A5 crystallization on SPBs, an appropriate amount of 10-40 mg/l ANX A5 (we used ANX A5 isolated from human placenta (Sigma- Aldrich, St. Luis, MO, USA)) in HBS with 1.5-20 mmol/l of calcium is injected into the fluid cell of the AFM with prepared SPB. HBS-Ca^{2+} is prepared in Water for injections (Braun, Melsungen, Germany). The SPBs could be formed of naturally derived: L-α-PS (Sigma- Aldrich, St. Luis, MO, USA) and L-α-phosphatidylcholine, (Sigma- Aldrich, St. Luis, MO, USA) or synthetic: dioleil-PS and dioleil-phosphatidylcholine, (Avanti Polar Lipids, Alabaster, AL, USA). The presence of ANX A5 crystalline shield is studied by imaging and force measurements (Irman et al., 2009, 2011).

4.1.3 Our comments on annexin A5 crystallization on mica supported phospholipid bilayers

We found that ANX A5 is able to self-assemble on planar phospholipid bilayers on mica, from synthetic or naturally derived phospholipids. It was found that 2D crystallization of

ANX A5 on phospholipid bilayers depends on concentration of calcium, PS and ANX A5 (Reviakine et al., 1998, 2000, 2001; Richter et al., 2005; Irman et al., 2009). By fixed weight share of the PS in the phospholipid mixture with the phosphatidylcholine, 30 %, and 21 mg/l of ANX A5 in HBS with 2 mmol/l of calcium, the p6 crystal form of ANX A5 was documented (unit cell: a = b = 20 nm, γ = 60°). Under identical conditions and 10 times higher concentration of calcium, ANX A5 self-assembled in two different crystallization forms, signed p6 and p3 (unit cell: a = b = 7 nm, γ = 60°). Figure 4 represents insight into gradual crystallization of ANX A5 on SPBs, as detected by AFM in the contact mode. In Figure 4 both, p3 and p6, crystal forms of ANX A5 are presented.

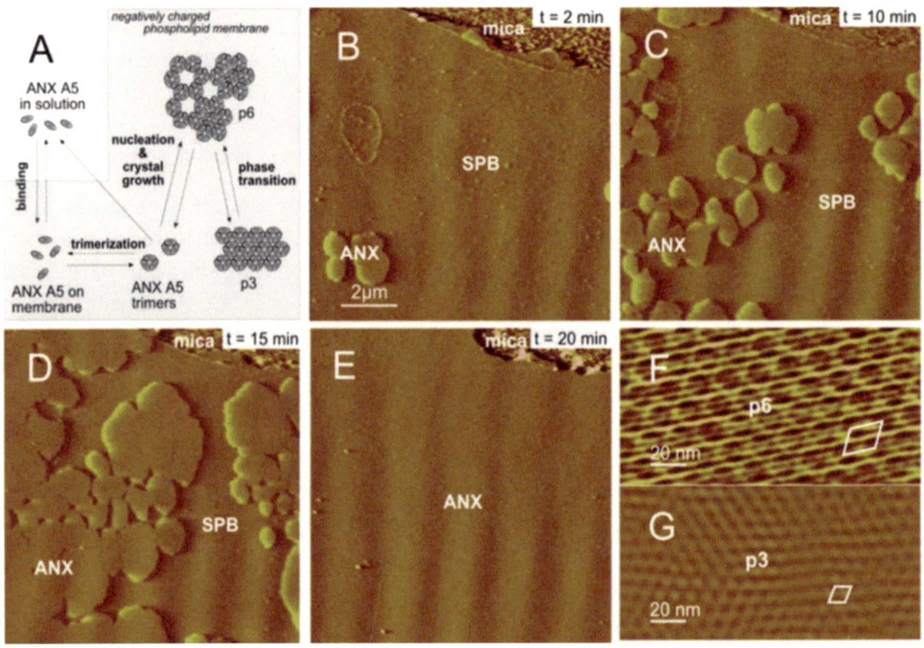

Fig. 4. Scheme and a time sequence of AFM deflection images of ANX A5 crystallization on SPB, measured in the contact mode. (A) Scheme of ANX A5 crystallization on negatively charged phospholipid surfaces in the presence of calcium ions (Govorukhina et al., 2003): Monomeric ANX A5 binds to membrane in a calcium-dependent manner where it forms trimers. The trimers crystallize in two dimensions. The holes in the honeycomb-like lattice of p6 symmetry can be filled with additional non-crystalline trimers, also called central trimers. At high protein coverage, a phase transition of the first order into a more densely packed crystal form with p3 symmetry can occur. When reducing the concentration of ANX A5 or calcium or both, the process is reversed and desorption takes place; (B) 10 mg/l ANX A5 in HBS with 1.5 mmol/l of calcium was used for observation of its crystallization on SPB. SPB contained 30% α-L-PS and 70% α-L- phosphatidylcholine. Image was measured 5 minutes, (C) 10 minutes, (D) 15 minutes and (E) 20 minutes after ANX A5 was administrated into the fluid cell of AFM. Growth of ANX A5 crystalline domains can be deduced. In image E the whole SPB is covered with crystalline ANX A5. ANX A5 crystalline domains are around 2.9 nm higher than SPB on which they grow. (F) p6 crystal form of ANX A5 (unit cell: a=b=20 nm and γ = 60°) and (G) p3 crystal form of ANX A5 (unit cell: a=b=7 nm and γ = 60°). Fourier transformation filtering (NanoScope Reference Manual, 1996) is applied in images F and G.

When studying crystallization using more physiological like conditions (10 mg/l of ANX A5 in HBS with 1.5 mmol/l calcium on phospholipid bilayers containing 30 % of L-α-PS), the p6 crystal form was predominantly found. The thickness of ANX A5 crystalline layer over phospholipids was determined to be around 2.9 nm. By performing force measurements we found that the crystallized ANX A5 layer on phospholipid bilayers could be elastically deformed, but could not be ruptured with forces up to 1nN. Demonstration that native ANX A5 is able to spontaneously crystallize on naturally derived phospholipids is supporting the putative role of ANX A5 crystal structures as a possible antithrombotic shield (in detail in Irman et al., 2009, 2011).

The process of ANX A5 desorption from crystalline ANX A5 on SPBs was also studied. Desorption can be achieved by reducing the concentration of ANX A5 above the studied surfaces. For observation of desorption of ANX A5 from the crystalline ANX A5 on SPBs we used pure buffer, HBS with 1.5 mmol/l of calcium. We started our observation with ANX A5 p3 crystal form and by allowing the degradation process to continue due to time, p3 gradually transformed into less dense p6 crystal form of crystalline ANX A5, and crystalline p6 domains then began to break under the minimum force of the AFM tip (Figure 5). Force measurement studies showed that during the process of desorption, the ANX A5 crystalline layer which was in p6 crystal form, with the holes (desorbed hexamers-signed as h in the Figure 5) could be penetrated. The AFM tip penetrated through a 5 nm thick layer, most probably representing the SPB. The desorption process made previously stable ANX A5 crystal structure on SPB mechanically very unstable (it could be ruptured by imaging the surface with minimum scanning force).

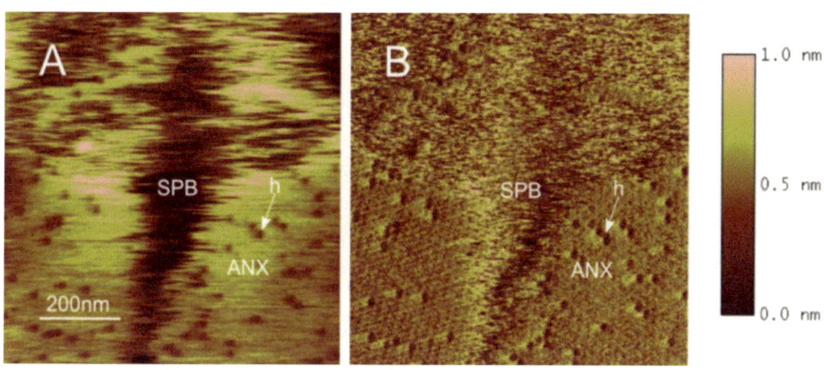

Fig. 5. AFM height and deflection images of breaking ANX A5 (10 mg/l in HBS with 1.5 mmol/l of calcium) p6 crystalline domains with the AFM tip when observing and studying the process of annexin desorption from SPB. Images were measured in contact mode at a minimum scanning force. (A) AFM height image presenting the p6 crystalline domains of ANX A5 on SPB, which are missing the hexamers (h) in the structure, due to the process of desorption. The AFM tip is breaking the crystalline domains during the scanning the studied surface, indicating the mechanical instability of the observed surface. (B) AFM deflection image of image A, where the topography of the surface can be more clearly deduced.

4.1.4 Practical instructions

1. ANX crystallization will occur with reagents (water, buffers, phospholipids, proteins) that are chemically, microbiologically and physically extra pure.

2. Different proteins need different composition of phospholipid surface in order to crystallize successfully. Make sure that phospholipid components that govern the crystallization are present and intact (phospholipids are prone to oxidation, microbiological contamination).
3. Make sure that other reagents (ions) that govern the crystallization process are present and in adequate concentration (in the buffer system).
4. For crystallization studies use the protein that is as highly purified and as fresh as possible. Impurities and degradation products may disturb the protein crystallization as well as observation of the crystallization by AFM (impurities may accumulate on the tip of the AFM cantilever and therefore cause worse resolution).
5. Prepare a phospholipid surface. Inspect it in the appropriate AFM fluid cell.
6. Inject the appropriate amount of the protein in the appropriate buffer into the AFM fluid cell.
7. Before measuring, the AFM should be thermally stabilized (approximately 15 minutes). When observing the crystallization of proteins, the AFM contact mode is appropriate.

4.2 Agglomeration of β_2-glycoprotein I on phospholipid membranes

4.2.1 β_2-glycoprotein I's characteristics

β_2-glycoprotein I (β_2-GPI) is an example of the protein that agglomerates on phospholipid surfaces. β_2-GPI is a glycoprotein of 54 kDa, with plasma concentration of about 150 mg/l. The crystal structure of the protein is composed of five domains that form a circular conformation or an elongated J-shaped conformation with overall dimensions of 13.2 x 7.2 x 2.0 nm^3 (Bouma et al., 1999; Scwarzenbacher et al., 1999; Agar et al., 2010). Each domain consists of 60 amino acids, except for domain V. Domain V consists of 82 amino acids due to C-terminal extension of 19 amino acids and an insertion of 6 amino acids, forming a hydrophobic loop. In addition, domain V carries a definite positive charge arising from 14 lysine residues. These specific structures of domain V are responsible for the binding properties of β_2-GPI to anionic phospholipids (Hamdan et al., 2007; Frank et al., 2009; Miyakis et al., 2004; Sodin-Šemrl & Rozman, 2007). Upon binding to negatively charged phospholipid surfaces, conformation of β_2-GPI changes and oligomerization (clustering) of the protein molecules on the phospholipid surface occurs (Gamsjaeger et al., 2005). Physiologically, β_2-GPI has been shown to be involved in the mechanisms such as inhibition of the coagulation pathway, platelet prothrombinase activity and platelet aggregation (reviewed in Lutters et al., 2003).

4.2.2 Recipe for study of agglomeration of β_2-glycoprotein I on mica-supported phospholipid surfaces

In order to study β_2-GPI agglomeration on prepared SPBs, an appropriate amount of the protein (in our experimental model we used 0.15 g/l of β_2-GPI purified from pooled human plasma (Čučnik et al., 2004) and dissolved in HBS with 1.5 mmol/l of calcium) is injected into the fluid cell of the AFM with preformed SPB. HBS is prepared in Water for injections (Braun, Melsungen, Germany). In our experimental model SPBs are prepared of 30% w/w L-α-PS (Sigma- Aldrich, St. Luis, MO, USA) in the mixture with L-α-phosphatidylcholine (Sigma- Aldrich, St. Luis, MO, USA). The agglomeration of β_2-GPI on SPBs is studied by imaging and force measurements (Irman et al., 2010; Žager et al., 2011).

4.2.3 Our comments on agglomeration of β_2-glycoprotein I on mica-supported phospholipid surfaces

β_2-GPI I clusters (0.15 g/l of β_2-GPI I in HBS containing 1.5 mmol/l of calcium) were detected approximately 3.1 nm higher than the phospholipid surface on which they were formed, measured in the contact mode. The measured heights of β_2-GPI clusters are lower than expected from the dimensions of the β_2-GPI molecule (13.2 x 7.2 x 2.0 nm^3) and confirm the horizontal-like orientation of the molecule on phospholipid bilayers (Hamdan et al., 2007). However, the specific nature of AFM measurements in contact mode should also be considered. The observed agglomeration of β_2-GPI on SPBs, as confirmed by our AFM experiments, was suggested as a reaction mechanism comprising two steps: i.) initial binding of the protein to the lipids, ii.) subsequent formation of protein clusters. Binding of the protein on the phospholipids was recognized to be mainly of electrostatic and also hydrophobic nature (Frank et al., 2009; Gamsjaeger et al., 2005). Greater binding of β_2-GPI to SPBs has been detected in the presence of more negatively charged net surface of SPBs within a reduced calcium environment (Gamsjaeger et al., 2005; Willems et al.,1996). When using discontinuous SPBs, β_2-GPI bound to mica patches when these are exposed. Because the mica surface is hydrophilic and slightly negatively charged, the interactions between protein and the support are likely to be mainly of electrostatic nature. Measured heights of the protein clusters on mica are approximately 8 nm. Since no insertion of the glycoprotein domains into mica is possible, vertical orientation of the β_2-glycoprotein I molecules on mica is expected (in detail in Irman et al., 2010; Žager et al., 2011).

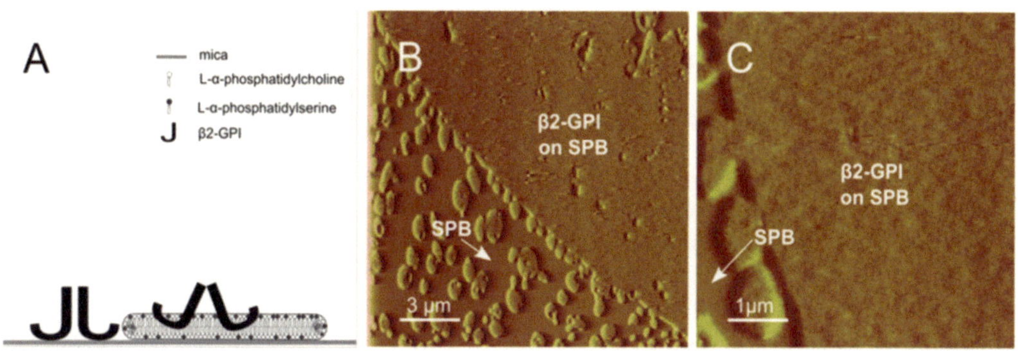

Fig. 6. Scheme and AFM deflection images of β_2GPI binding to SPBs and mica. A.) Scheme of β_2GPI binding to SPBs and mica. Notice a horizontal-like orientation on SPBs and vertical orientation of the molecule on mica. (B) AFM deflection images of binding β2-GPI (0.15 g/l in HBS with 1.5 mmol/l of calcium) to continuous SPB (no mica exposed). (C.) Magnified deflection image of the protein clusters on SPB.

4.2.4 Practical instructions

1. Select chemically, microbiologically and physically extra pure reagents (water, buffers, phospholipids, proteins).
2. Different proteins need different composition of phospholipid surface in order to agglomerate successfully. Make sure that phospholipid components that govern the agglomeration are present and intact (phospholipids are prone to oxidation, microbiological contamination).

3. Make sure that other reagents (ions) that govern the agglomeration process are present and in adequate concentration.
4. For agglomeration studies use the protein that is as highly purified and as fresh as possible. Impurities and degradation products may disturb the protein crystallization as well as observation of the agglomeration by AFM (impurities may accumulate on the tip of the AFM cantilever and therefore cause worse resolution).
5. Prepare appropriate phospholipid surface. Inspect the phospholipid surface in the contact or tapping AFM fluid cell.
6. Inject appropriate amount of the protein in the appropriate buffer system in the AFM fluid cell.
7. Allow to thermally stabilize (approximately 15 minutes). Measure.

4.3 AFM study of antibodies

4.3.1 The use of AFM in studies of antibodies and their interaction with antigens

Antibodies are a part of the specific humoral immune response, which target and neutralize the foreign objects (bacteria, viruses, tumors) in vertebrate body. Antibodies are glycoproteins belonging to the immunoglobulin superfamily. Immunoglobulins G (IgG) which are more thoroughly considered in this section of the Chapter are just one of possible antibodies isotypes. IgG is a 150 kDa globular molecule, 14.2 x 8.5 x 3.8 nm^3 (Silverton et al., 1977; Marquart et al., 1980; Deisenhofen, 1981), consisting of four polypeptide chains. These four segments are held together by disulphide bonds and noncovalent hydrophobic interactions, making the native state of the protein in aqueous solution relatively robust. Therefore, it is expected that the protein molecule on the surface should be largely a globular assembly, although some local deformations might occur because of protein-surface and protein-protein interactions (Xu et al., 2006).

AFM offers the study of antibodies on a molecular level and in an aqueous environment. Therefore, the possibilities regarding the use of AFM for the study of antibody-antigen interaction are numerous. AFM has been used: a.) to study the structure and binding characteristics of antibodies or antigens on a particular platform. In this section, the results of the study of binding characteristics of IgG molecules on SPBs and mica in aqueous medium (HBS with 1.5 mmol/l of calcium) are presented; b.) to directly study specific interactions between antibodies and antigens employed. Results are achieved by using the AFM probes functionalized with antigen or antibody molecules (Hinterdorfer et al., 1996; Allen et al., 1997); c.) to measure the effects of antibody-antigen interactions. AFM played very important role in visually presenting the possible pathophysiology in autoimmune diseases called antiphospholipid syndrome (Rand et al., 2008; Irman et al., 2010, 2011; Žager et al., 2011), as presented in the next section (Section 5) of the Chapter. As such, AFM could also be used in the evaluation of the biological drugs activity.

4.3.2 Recipe for studying the antibodies interaction on mica

In our experimental model IgG are purified from a sera of healthy blood donor with MAbTrapTM Kit (Amersham, GE Healthcare, Little Chalfont, UK), according to manufacturer's instructions. After purification, the preparations are dialyzed against HBS containing 1.5 mM of calcium, pH 7.5. HBS is prepared in Water for injections (Braun,

Melsungen, Germany). Concentrations of purified proteins are determined spectrophotometrically (Camspec M501 Single Beam Scanning UV/Visible Spectrophotometer, Camspec Ltd., Cambridge, UK), using the extinction coefficient of 14.0 for the 1% IgG solution. The binding of IgG in HBS with 1.5 mM $CaCl_2$ to mica substrates is measured in the AFM contact mode fluid cell: Mica substrates are installed into the fluid cell and sealed with the O-ring. Then the solution of antibodies (0.001 g/l or 10 g/l IgG in HBS containing 1.5 mM calcium) is administrated into the system. The results are obtained by imaging with continuously adjusting the set point to the minimum value of the scanning force. The binding of antibodies to mica and SPBs is studied also on discontinuous SPBs (SPBs that are not covering the whole mica surface).

4.3.3 Our comments on molecular and technical aspects

When imaging binding of 0.001 g/l IgG in HBS containing 1.5 mmol/l of calcium on mica, we found that IgG bind weakly and gradually to mica surface, as shown in Figure 7. The assemblies could be carried away by the AFM tip, with scanning force set just above the minimum (Figure 7 C).

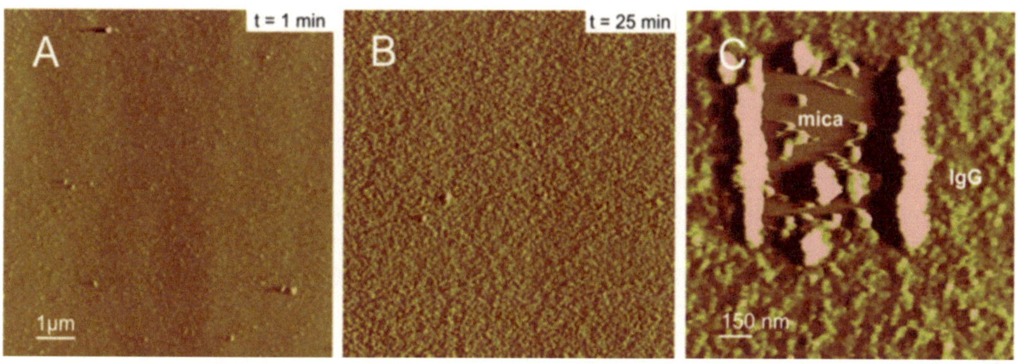

Fig. 7. Time sequence of AFM deflection images of IgG (1 mg/l in HBS containing 1.5 mmol/l of calcium) binding to mica, measured in the contact mode. IgG started binding to mica immediately after applying the solution into the AFM fluid cell. Image (A) was measured 1 minute and (B) 25 minutes after applying IgG to mica. More adsorbed or maybe even accumulated material can be deduced in image B. (C) When increasing the scanning force above minimum, the AFM tip carried away the IgG molecules. Globular assemblies can be deduced from image C.

IgG molecules had shapes of globular assemblies with diameters ranging from 30 to 50 nm and heights from 2 to 5 nm. In Figure 8 one such assembly is magnified. Dimensions of globular assemblies measured on mica led us to the assumption that we are observing most probably single antibodies or even clusters of IgG molecules together. In addition, the orientation of IgG on mica is most probably random: "flat on" (antibody lying flat on the surface), "side on" (Fab and Fc closer to the surface), "end on" (Fc closer to the surface) and "head on" (Fab closer to the surface). Great discrepancy in dimensions (overestimation of object size) of observed single molecules of IgG could be explained by the nature of AFM measurements with the tip (Ramirez-Aguilar 1998, Howald 1994). The sharper and more flexible the tip of AFM cantilever is used, the more precisely the surface can be described.

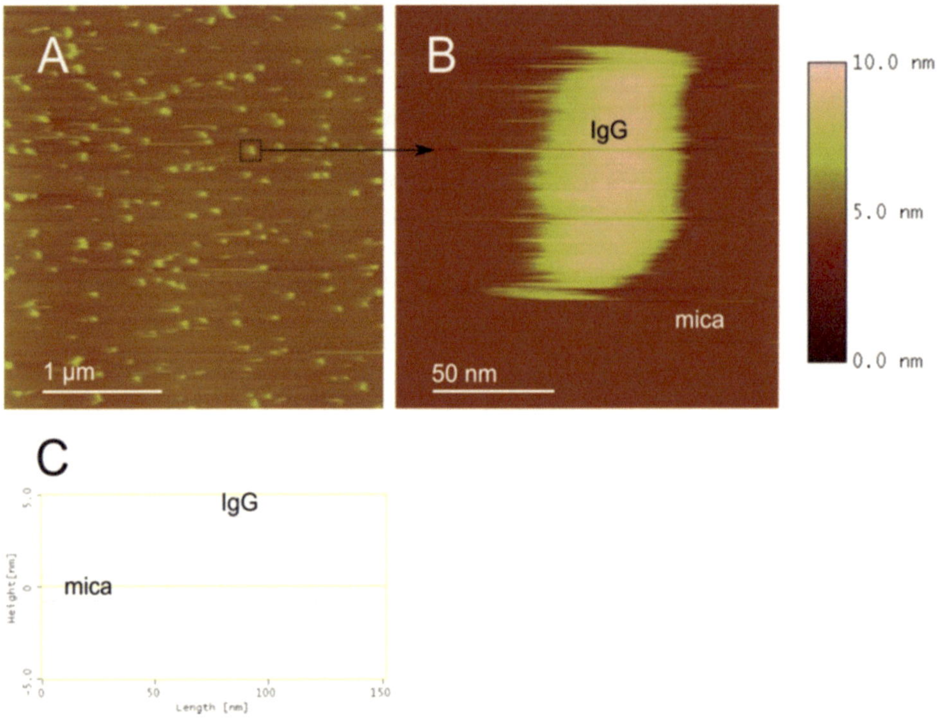

Fig. 8. AFM height images and height cross section of the IgG (1 mg/l in HBS with 1.5 mmol/l of calcium) assembly, measured in the contact mode. (A) Image of IgG assemblies on mica, with diameters ranging from 30 to 50 nm and heights from 2 to 5 nm. (B) Image represents single assembly with dimensions 40 x 80 x 5 nm^3. (C) From cross section profile of image B one can measure height of studied assembly of about 4.5 nm.

Because the mica surface is hydrophilic and slightly negatively charged, the interactions between IgG and the support are likely to be mainly of electrostatic nature.

When using the physiological concentration of IgG in HBS containing 1.5 mM of calcium, the observed globular assemblies randomly interconnected with each other, leading to the formation of loose antibody patches on mica, and they were measured to be 4.9 ± 1 nm higher than SPBs (Figure 9).

To conclude, we found that antibodies bound weakly, randomly and most probably electrostatically to the exposed mica surface. They further agglomerated into loose protein patches. No binding of studied IgG antibodies (from a healthy blood donor) directly to phospholipid bilayers could be detected.

4.3.4 Practical instructions

1. Study of antibodies structure and binding by AFM requires the use of at least microbiologically and physically extra pure antibodies. Chemical and biological purity is mandatory when studying the specific interactions. Impurities could make the observations far less specific. Microbiological, physical and chemical extra purity for all other reagents that are present in the experimental model is mandatory as well.

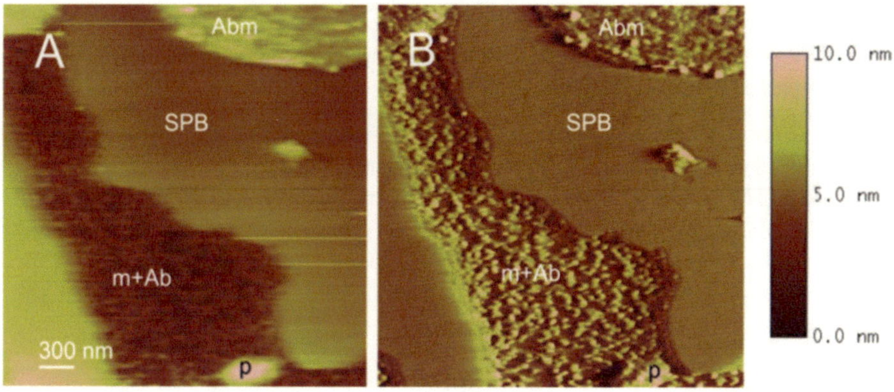

Fig. 9. AFM height and deflection images of IgG adsorption (10 g/l in HBS containing 1.5 mM of calcium) to mica patches of discontinuous SPB, measured in the contact mode fluid cell. (A) On the image, three surfaces can be observed: loose antibody layer on mica (Abm) that can be measured around 5 nm above SPB; the SPB layer (SPB), about 4 nm above mica; and mica with some antibodies that only started to adsorb or accumulate (m+Ab). One can deduce that assemblies on m+Ab, representing IgG, started randomly interconnect with each other to form the loose antibody patch on mica (p). On the Abm, the antibody patch is already formed. No binding of antibodies to the SPB was measured. (B) The deflection image of the same surface as in image A. All three surfaces can be more clearly observed. Globular assemblies can be deduced.

2. When studying the structure of antibodies one should consider the change in specificities and possibly the structure of antibodies as well, when using the antibodies that are being subjected to different isolation procedures (Omersel et al., 2010).
3. When focusing the study of the antibodies on their structure, one should use AFM imaging modes with less friction force interaction- oscillation modes.

5. Models of increased complexity – AFM study of specific antibody-antigen interactions on the *in vitro* model of phospholipid bilayer

AFM is a very useful method to study a variety of molecules, structures and the interactions between them, including an antigen-antibody and protein-membrane interactions. In the field of autoimmunity, knowledge about interactions among antiphospholipid antibodies and ANX A5 are of crucial importance to understand etiopathogenesis of antiphospholipid syndrome and to find new therapeutic targets. Antiphospholipid syndrome is an autoimmune disease which is characterized by the core clinical manifestation of thrombosis, venous or arterial, and recurrent foetal loss (Miyakis et al., 2006; Wilson et al., 1999; Ashersone et al., 2002). The family of antiphospholipid antibodies, when found in persistently high levels, present the laboratory criteria for the diagnosis of antiphospholipid syndrome. Antiphospholipid antibodies are very heterogeneous and combine antibodies directed toward: i.) phospholipids (cardiolipin, phosphatidylserine), ii.) different protein cofactors (β_2-GPI, prothrombin, ANX A5, protein S, protein C, low and high molecular weight kininogens and others), and iii.) complexes of protein cofactor-phospholipid (Meroni & Shoenfeld, 2008; Arnout & Vermylen, 2002; Shoenfeld, 2002). Many pathologic mechanisms of antiphospholipid antibodies associated with the antiphospholipid syndrome have been suggested so far. One of the possible mechanisms was 1998 presented by Rand et al.: antiphospholipid antibodies interfere with a formation of ANX A5 crystalline shield over blood vessels and therefore diminish the proteins anticoagulant protective role (Rand et al., 1998, 2008).

In this Section we present the results of our study of ANX A5 and antiphospholipid antibodies (anti- β_2- glycoprotein I antibodies, anti-annexin A5 antibodies) interaction on a molecular level. The missing knowledge was acquired by the use of SPBs, simulating the activated cell phospholipid surface, and the use of AFM. Visualization of antigen-antibody interactions in their native aqueous environment with a nanometer resolution and the use of native reagents (phospholipids, ANX A5, β_2-GPI and antibodies) present the main advantages of our experimental model.

5.1 Study of interaction of annexin A5 and anti-annexin A5 antibodies on mica-supported phospholipid bilayer

5.1.1 Anti-annexin A5 autoantibodies

Anti-annexin A5 antibodies (anti-ANX A5) were first detected 17 years ago and were recognized as a subgroup of antiphospholipid autoantibodies (Matsuda et al., 1994). Since then, anti-ANX A5 have been associated with the occurrence of recurrent pregnancy losses, pre-eclampsia, *in vitro* fertilization failures and/or thrombotic events in patients with pregnancy complications and systemic autoimmune diseases such as systemic lupus erythematosus, antiphospholipid syndrome and rheumatoid arthritis (Matsuda et al., 1994; Rodriguez-Garcia et al., 1996; Kaburaki et al., 1997; Satoh et al., 1999; Nojima et al., 2001; Matsubayashi et al., 2001; Gris et al., 2003; Bizzaro et al., 2005; Zammiti et al., 2006, Božič et al., 2005). However, mechanisms through which these antibodies affect the mentioned pathological processes have not yet been elucidated. We have focused our study on the direct effect of anti-ANX A5 on ANX A5, a potent anticoagulant protein.

5.1.2 Recipe for study of anti-annexin antibodies and annexin A5 interaction on the mica-supported phospholipid bilayers

In brief, SPBs are prepared on mica, simulating the physiological conditions of the cell surface. On SPBs, ANX A5 is completely or/and incompletely crystallized. Effects of IgG are studied by imaging using AFM in the contact mode (in detail in Irman et al., 2011).

For the study of interaction of anti-ANX A5 and crystalline ANX A5 on SPBs, sera are acquired and selected from the sera bank of the Department of Rheumatology (University Medical Centre Ljubljana, Ljubljana, Slovenia). Hundred samples of sera are pre-tested by an *in-house* or commercial enzyme-linked immunosorbent assay for the presence of different subtypes of antiphospholipid antibodies. The antiphospholipid antibodies tested are: anti-cardiolipin antibodies (Božič et al., 1997); anti-β_2-glycoprotein I antibodies (anti-β_2-GPI) (Čučnik et al., 2004a); anti-prothrombin antibodies (Ambrožič et al., 2002); and anti-ANX A5 (Orgentec Diagnostica, Mainz, Germany). 6 sera are selected according to clinical features of the patient, immunologic tests and availability (adequate volume stored). The obtained samples are grouped into the group A (autoimmune venous thrombosis), B (autoimmune obstetric complications) and C (controls). Total IgG from our selected sera are purified with MAbTrap™ Kit (Amersham, GE Healthcare, Little Chalfont, UK), according to the manufacturer's instructions. After purification, the preparations are dialysed against HBS containing 1.5 mM calcium (HBS-Ca^{2+}), pH 7.5. HBS-Ca^{2+} is prepared in Water for injections

(Braun, Melsungen, Germany). Concentrations of purified proteins are determined spectrophotometrically (Camspec M501 Single Beam Scanning UV/Visible Spectrophotometer, Camspec Ltd., Cambridge, UK), using the extinction coefficient of 14.0 for the 1% IgG solution. Concentrations of IgG samples used in further AFM study are 10 g/l in HBS-Ca^{2+}.

The effects of particular IgG (patients' and healthy blood donor's) are studied on incompletely and completely crystallized ANX A5 on SPBs: SPBs are prepared of 30 % w/w L-α-PS (Sigma- Aldrich, St. Luis, MO, USA) in the mixture with L-α-phosphatidylcholine (Sigma- Aldrich, St. Luis, MO, USA). After the presence of SPB is confirmed, 10 mg/l ANX A5 isolated from human placenta (Sigma- Aldrich, St. Luis, MO, USA) in HBS-Ca^{2+} is injected into the fluid cell of the AFM. When the presence of ANX A5 crystalline shield, incompletely or completely covering the SPB is detected, IgG are added to the ANX A5 solution covering the SPB. ANX A5 concentration is kept at 10 mg/l. The effects of IgG on crystalline ANX A5 are measured by AFM for another 60 minutes. Results from the experiment where applying antibodies before the ANX A5 to SPBs, are also resolved.

Effects of the isolated IgG on the velocity of ANX A5 crystallization on SPBs are studied as well: ANX A5 (10 mg/l in HBS-Ca^{2+}) is injected into the fluid cell of AFM on the SPB, and the time needed for ANX A5 to cover all the SPB's surface is measured. The HBS-Ca^{2+} is then used in order to remove the bound ANX A5 of the phospholipid surface (desorption). After ANX A5 desorbed completely from SPB, a mixture of particular IgG and 10 mg/l ANX A5 in HBS-Ca^{2+} is added and the time needed for complete coverage of SPB's surface with crystalline ANX A5 in the presence of particular IgG is measured.

5.1.3 Our comments on technical and clinical aspects

Our study revealed two different effects of anti-ANX A5 IgGs (Irman et al., 2011): i.) a disruption of incompletely crystallized ANX A5 shield as presented in Figure 10 (IgG samples from patients with autoimmune venous thrombosis), and ii.) a decrease in velocity of ANX A5 crystallization (IgG samples from patients with autoimmune recurrent pregnancy losses). Therefore, our study confirms the heterogeneous effects of anti-ANX A5 on crystalline ANX A5 over planar mica-supported SPBs. This supports their distinct roles in pathogenic mechanism and also offers an explanation for different clinical conditions, such as autoimmune thrombosis or obstetric complications in the antiphospholipid syndrome. The observed different effects of anti-ANX A5 containing IgG samples on incompletely crystallized ANX A5 are due to the heterogeneity in epitope specificity and in avidity of anti-ANX A5. No disruptive effects of the studied IgG on the intact ANX A5 crystal shield (completely covering the SPB) suggests that anti-ANX A5 cannot be the primary cause but more likely potentiate the effect of other pathological factors. Pathological potential of anti-ANX A5 should therefore be considered as a "*second hit*", but for pathologies in human body to develop the "*first hit*" (genetic and environmental pathological factors influencing the expression, translation or structure of ANX A5 and therefore its binding to phospholipid surfaces and its 2-D crystallization) should also be present (Arnout & Vermylen, 2002).

To conclude, new approaches are necessary in laboratory diagnostics, based on the knowledge obtained by AFM studies, since the detection of anti-ANX A5 in the plasma by the routinely used methods is not able to identify their fine specificity and to differentiate between patients concerning their risk for annexinopathies.

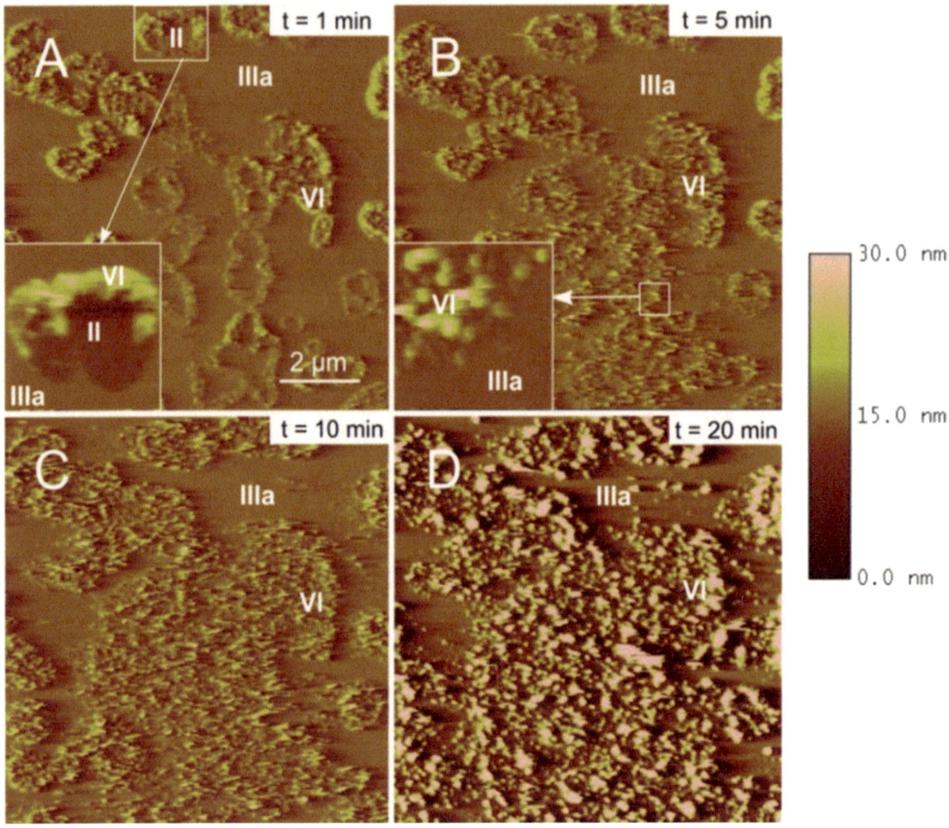

Fig. 10. Time sequence of AFM height and deflection images of the effect of sample IgG-A1(patient with autoimmune venous thrombosis) on ANX A5, not completely covering the SPB. After application of IgG-A1 to ANX A5 incomplete crystalline layer that is 64% covering the continuous SPB, antibodies start to bind to the lateral epitopes of crystalline ANX A5 and cause the disruption of ANX A5 protective shield. Image (A) is measured immediately, (B) 5 min (50% of SPB covered with crystalline ANX A5), (C) 10 min (33% of SPB covered with crystalline ANX A5) and (D) 20 min (28% of SPB covered with crystalline ANX A5) after IgG-A1 were applied. On the left lower corner of image (A), there is a magnified part of that image presented as 1.2 X 1.2 mm^2 height image. We detected that IgG-A1 bind to the lateral epitopes of crystalline ANX A5 (IIIa), which is around 2.6 nm higher that SPB (II). Antibody patches are around 3 nm higher than crystalline ANX A5. In the left lower corner of the image (B) there is magnified, 1.4 X 1.4 mm2, height image of ANX A5 crystalline (IIIa) and antibody patches (VI). It was measured, that antibody patches are in some parts approximately 1 nm lower and in some parts up to 12 nm higher, than crystalline ANX A5, suggesting that antibodies indeed disrupt the ANX A5 protective shield. (D) This height image shows the second layer of IgG-A1, most probably anti-ANX A5, 8-12 nm higher than the layer of antibodies that disrupted the crystalline ANX A5 (latticing of immune complexes of ANX A5 and anti-ANX A5). Reprinted and modified from Irman Š., Škarabot M., Muševič I., Rozman B., Božič B.. Effects of anti-annexin antibodies on annexin A5 anticoagulant shield, as observed by atomic force microscopy. Journal of Autoimmunity 2011;36:98-105, with permission from Elsevier.

5.2 Study of interaction between annexin A5 and β_2-glycoprotein I and anti- β_2-glycoprotein I antibodies pair on mica-supported phospholipid bilayers

5.2.1 Anti- β_2-glycoprotein I autoantibodies

Among the most studied antiphospholipid antibodies are anti-β_2-glycoprotein I antibodies (anti-β_2-GPI). Anti-β_2-GPI of different isotypes, directed toward different epitopes of the antigen molecule and of different avidity, have been associated with various clinical manifestations (Shoenfeld 2003): thrombosis and pregnancy complications in patients with antiphospholipid syndrome (de Laat et al., 2006a, 2006b, 2007; Rand et al., 2008; Čučnik et al., 2004b; Ioanou et al., 2007) described in patients with systemic lupus erythematosus (Čučnik et al., 2004b), in infectious diseases (Arvieux et al., 2002) and childhood atopic dermatitis (Ambrožič et al., 2002), in patients with stroke and acute coronary syndrome (Bizzaro et al., 2010). Disruption of ANX A5 protective crystalline structure by complexes of β_2-GPI and anti-β_2-GPI on phospholipid surfaces presents one of their possible pathological mechanisms of action.

5.2.2 Recipe for the study of the effects of β_2-glycoprotein I and anti- β_2-glycoprotein I antibodies pair on crystalline annexin A5 on mica-supported phospholipid bilayers

In brief, SPBs are prepared on mica, simulating the physiological conditions of the cell surface. On SPBs, ANX A5 is completely or/and incompletely crystallized. Effects of β_2-GPI and/or isolated IgG are studied by imaging using AFM in the contact mode (in detail in Irman et al., 2010; Žager et al., 2011).

For the purposes of the study, sera were selected from the sera bank of the Department of Rheumatology (University Medical Centre, Ljubljana, Slovenia). Sera are pre-tested by an *in-house* or commercial enzyme-linked immunosorbent assay for the presence of different subtypes of antiphospholipid antibodies: anti-cardiolipin antibodies (Božič et al., 1997), anti-β_2-GPI antibodies (Čučnik et al., 2004a), anti-prothrombin antibodies (Ambrožič et al., 2002) and anti-ANX A5 antibodies (Orgentec Diagnostica, Mainz, Germany). In the present study, sera were selected according to clinical features of the patient, immunologic tests and availability (adequate volume stored). Total IgG from selected sera are purified with MAbTrap™ Kit (Amersham, GE Healthcare, Little Chalfont, UK), according to manufacturer's instructions. After purification, the preparations are dialyzed against HBS-Ca^{2+}, pH 7.5. HBS-Ca^{2+} is prepared in Water for injections (Braun, Melsungen, Germany). Part of isolated IgG, after affinity purification with MAbTrap™ Kit, are dialyzed against phosphate buffered saline (PBS) and then further subjected to isolation of anti-β_2-GPI by an in-house affinity column (Čučnik et al., 2004b). Isolated anti-β_2-GPI are dialyzed against HBS-Ca^{2+}. Concentrations of purified proteins are determined spectrophotometrically (Camspec M501 Single Beam Scanning UV/Visible Spectrophotometer, Camspec Ltd., Cambridge, UK), using the extinction coefficient of 14.0 for the 1% IgG solution. Obtained samples are designated: i.) sample IgGA, 10 g/l, IgG fraction from a patient A with primary antiphospholipid syndrome who suffered from venous thrombosis and is positive for IgG anti-cardiolipin antibodies and anti-β_2-GPI; ii.) sample anti-β_2-GPIA, 0.4 g/l, isolated anti-β_2-GPI from a patient A, IgG isotype; and iii.) sample IgGB, 10 g/l, IgG fraction from a healthy blood donor without antiphospholipid antibodies.

The effects of particular IgG (patients' and healthy blood donor's) are studied on incompletely and completely crystallized ANX A5 on SPBs. SPBs are prepared of 30 % w/w L-α-PS (Sigma-Aldrich, St. Luis, MO, USA) in the mixture with L-α-phosphatidylcholine (Sigma- Aldrich, St. Luis, MO, USA). After the presence of SPB is confirmed, 10 mg/l ANX A5 isolated from human placenta (Sigma- Aldrich, St. Luis, MO, USA) in HBS-Ca^{2+} is injected into the fluid cell of the AFM. When the presence of ANX A5 crystalline shield, incompletely or completely covering the SPB is detected, IgG and/or 0.15 g/l β_2-GPI (purified from pooled human plasma (Čučnik et al., 2004a), in HBS-Ca^{2+}) are added to the ANX A5 solution covering the SPB. ANX A5 concentration is kept at 10 mg/l. The effects of IgG and/or β_2-GPI on crystalline ANX A5 are measured by AFM for another 60 minutes. Results from the experiment where applying antigen-antibody pair before the ANX A5 to SPBs, are also resolved.

5.2.3 Our comments on technical and clinical aspects

When experimenting with isolated anti-β_2-GPI (sample anti-β_2-GPIA), the β_2-GPI-anti-β_2-GPI pair grew on SPBs, but only in the presence of incompletely crystallized ANX A5 (Figure 11). No effect on crystalline ANX A5 was observed, when using the IgG fraction (which contained also anti-β_2-GPI) from the same patient. The observed *in vitro* effect only by isolated anti-β_2-GPI could be explained by different titers of anti-β_2-GPI. Anti-β_2-GPI in sample anti-β_2-GPIA were 10 x more concentrated than in sample IgGA (100 x above the cut off, determined by an *in-house* anti-β_2-GPI enzyme-linked immunosorbent assay (Čučnik et al., 2004b)). Avidity and epitope specificity of anti-β_2-GPI for β_2-GPI in the samples IgGA and anti-β_2-GPIA were identical as a result of using the same polyclonal antibody fraction. However, patient A has determined (by an *in-house* kaotrophic anti-β_2-GPI enzyme-linked immunosorbent assay) high avidity anti-β_2-GPI profile, which should not be neglected, when considering the reasons for ability for growth of β_2-GPI-anti-β_2-GPI pair in the presence of incomplete crystalline ANX A5 on SPBs (Božič et al., 2007; Žager et al., 2011). Since the antigen-antibody complex was unable to bind to SPB when the phospholipid surface was completely covered with ANX A5, we can deduce that the presence of pathological anti-β_2-GPI alone is not sufficient to cause disruption of ANX A5 crystalline shield, and therefore thrombosis. Our results correlate to clinical observations by which not all patients with positive antiphospholipid antibodies develop clinical manifestations and, in the ones that do, the thrombotic events occur only occasionally in spite of the persistent presence of antiphospholipid antibodies. Taken together, our results indicate that the hypothesis of antiphospholipid antibodies (more specifically, anti-β_2-GPI) mediated disruption of the ANX A5 protective shield is possible. However, the pathological potential of anti-β_2-GPI should be considered only as a necessary *"second hit"*, as is also the case with before disguised anti-ANX A5 (Arnout & Vermylen, 2002).

To conclude, we confirmed the proposed thrombomodulatory effect of β_2-GPI- anti-β_2-GPI pair to ANX A5 by *in vitro* model with higher physiological similarity to circumstances in human body, and AFM ability to visualize the interaction in real time and at a nanomolecular scale. Knowledge about molecular interactions between ANX A5 and antiphospholipid antibodies is prerequisite for the improvement of laboratory diagnostics of patients with anti-ANX A5 and a basis for possible new target therapy. AFM confirmed its role as very powerful tool for evaluation of pathological events "in situ", in aqueous environment and on a molecular level.

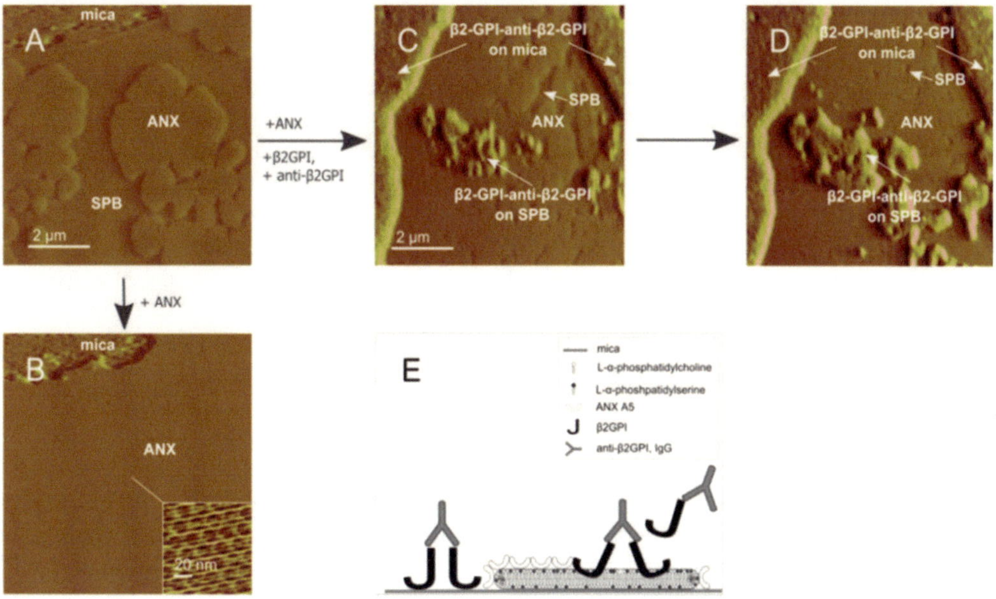

Fig. 11. AFM deflection images and a scheme of the effect of β_2-GPI and isolated anti-β_2-GPI (from patient A, suffering from primary phospholipid syndrome) on crystalline ANX A5 on SPBs. (A) Image of mica and crystalline ANX A5 (10 mg/l in HBS-Ca^{2+}) not completely covering the SPB; (B) after 15 min of incubating the ANX A5 solution (10 mg/l in HBS-Ca^{2+}) over the SPB crystalline ANX A5 completely covered the SPB. The right lower corner shows 100 X 100 nm^2 ANX A5 crystalline structure where p6 crystal form can be observed; (C) however, if β_2-GPI (0.15 g/l in HBS-Ca^{2+}) and anti-β_2-GPI isolated from sample A (0.4 g/l in HBS-Ca^{2+}) were added to the ANX A5 (10 mg/l in HBS-Ca^{2+}) solution covering the incomplete crystalline ANX A5 layer over the SPB, the complexes of β_2-GPI and isolated anti-β_2-GPI on SPB were measured as well. Antibodies and antigen formed complexes with apparently sufficient affinity to bind to SPB in the presence of crystalline ANX A5. The complexes of β_2-GPI and isolated anti-β_2-GPI bound to exposed mica surface as well; (D) image of further lateral growth of β_2-GPI-isolated anti-β_2-GPI patches on SPB in the presence of incompletely crystallized ANX A5 on SPB is shown; (E) scheme of binding complexes of β_2-GPI and isolated anti-β_2-GPI on mica and to SPB in the presence of incompletely crystallized ANX A5. Reprinted and modified from Žager U., Irman Š., Lunder M., Škarabot M., Muševič I., Hodnik V., Anderluh G., Čučnik S., Kveder T., Rozman B., Božič B.. Immunochemical properties and pathological relevance of anti-b2-glycoprotein I antibodies of different avidity. International Immunology 2011;23(8):511-8, with permission from The Japanese Society for Immunology and the Oxford University Press.

5.2.4 Practical instructions

1. In order to study the antibodies, their interaction with antigens, or the consequences of that interaction, antibodies should be microbiologically and physically extra pure. Chemical and biological purity is mandatory when studying the specific interactions. Impurities could make the observations far less specific. Microbiological, physical and chemical extra purity for all other reagents that are present in the experimental model is mandatory as well.

2. In order to ensure physiological relevance of the studied *in vitro* model, naturally derived reagents (phospholipids, proteins) should be used. However, one should consider the change in specificities of antibodies that are being subjected to different isolation procedures (Omersel et al., 2010).
3. When studying the specific interaction between the particular antibody-antigen pair one could use the force mode and different imaging AFM modes (contact, tapping, non-contact, ect.)
4. Monoclonality or polyclonality of specific antibodies should be considered for each experiment separately. Fine paratope heterogeneity and affinity heterogeneity may greatly influence results (in plus or in minus).
5. When studying the structure of antibodies or specific interaction between specific antibody-antigen pairs, concentrations of the reagents should be low.

6. Conclusion

In this Chapter we have described our experiences by AFM, studying protein-protein interactions on the phospholipid membranes in the *in vitro* simulated physiological conditions. Practical suggestions for preparation of SPBs are presented and upgraded with observations of single protein interactions - spontaneous crystallization of ANX A5, agglomeration of β_2-GPI, and antibody interactions. Some interpretation of AFM usefulness for research work with systems of increased complexity are shown - AFM study of specific antibody-antigen interactions on the *in vitro* model of phospholipid bilayer, supported by own experimental data and suggestions for successful work. Biological systems are hardly simulated in the *in vitro* conditions, due to their high level of complexity. However, AFM appears very usable tool in biochemistry which makes multimolecular interactions and micro environmental characteristics of the used models visible and therefore closer to our understanding.

7. References

Agar, C., van Os, G. M., Morgelin, M., Sprenger, R. R., Marquart, J. A., Urbanus, R.T., Derksen, R. H. W. M., Meijers, J. C. M. & de Groot, P. G. (2010). Beta2- glycoprotein I can exist in 2 conformations: implications for our understanding of the antiphospholipid syndrome. *Blood* 116:1336-43

Allen, S., Chen, X., Davies, J., Davies, M. C., Dawkes, A. C., Edwards, J. C., Roberts, C. J., Sefton, J., Tendler, S. J. & Williams, P. M. (1997). Detection of antigen-antibody binding events with the atomic force microscope. *Biochemistry* 36:7457–63.

Ambrožič, A., Avčin, T., Ichikawa, K., Kveder, T., Matsuura, E., Hojnik, M., Atsumi, T., Rozman, B. & Koike, T. (2002). Anti-beta2-glycoprotein I antibodies in children with atopic dermatitis. *Int Immunol* 14:823-30.

Ambrožič, A., Kveder, T., Žigon, P. & Božič, B. (2002). A modified ELISA for the detection of phosphatidylserine dependent anti-prothrombin antibodies with increased sensitivity and specificity. *Ann Rheum Dis* 61:218-9.

Arnout, J. & Vermylen, J. (2002). Current status and implications of autoimmune antiphospholipid antibodies in relation to thrombotic disease. *J Throm Haemost* 1:931-42.

Arvieux, J., Renaudineaeu, Y., Mane, I., Perraut, R., Krilis, S. A. & Youinou, P. (2002). Distinguishing features of anti-beta 2 glycoprotein I antibodies between patients with leprosy and the antiphosholipid sydrome. *Throm Haemost* 87:599-605.

Asherson, R. A., Cervera, R., Piette, J.C. & Shoenfeld, Y. (2002). *The antiphospholipid syndrome II. Autoimmune thrombosis.* Elsevier Science B V, Amsterdam, 145-360

Binning, G., Quoate, CF. & Gerber, CH. (1986). Atomic force microscope. *Phys Rev Lett* 56: 930-3.

Bippes, CA. & Müller, DJ. (2011). High-resolution atomic force microscopy and spectroscopy of native membrane proteins. *Rep Prog Phys* 74: doi:10.1088/0034-4885/74/8/086601.

Bizzaro, N., Tonutti, E., Villalta, D., Tampoia, M. & Tozzoli, R. (2005). Prevalence and clinical correlation of anti-phospholipid binding protein antibodies in anticardiolipin-negative patients with systemic lupus erythematosus and women with unexplained recurrent miscarriages. *Arch Pathol Lab Med* 129:61-8.

Benz, J. & Hofmann, A. (1997). Annexins: From structure to function. *Biol Chem* 378:177-83.

Berendes, R., Voges, D., Demange, D, Huber, P. & Burger, A. (1993). Structure-functon analysis of the ion channel selectivity filter in human annexin V. *Science* 262:427-30.

Bizzaro, N., Chinellato, M., Villalta, D., Antico, A., Tonutti, E., Tozzoli, R. (2010). Antibodies to the β_2-GPI domains IV/V in patients with stroke and acute coronary syndrome: results of a prospective case-control study. Abstract on *7th international congress on Autoimmunity*, Ljubljana.

Bouma, B., de Groot, P. G., van den Elsen, A. M. H., Ravelli, R. B. G., Schouten, A., Simmelink, M. J. A., Derksen, R. H. W. M., Kroon, J. & Gros, P. (1999). Adhesion mechanism of human β_2-glycoprotein I to phospholipids based on its crystal structure. *The EMBO Journal* 18:5166-74.

Brian, A. A. & McConnell, H. M. (1984). Allogeneic stimulation of cytotoxic T cells by supported planar membranes.*Proc Natl Acad Sci U.S.A.* 81:6159-63.

Božič, B., Kveder, T., Stegnar, M., Marosini-Berus, E., Kos-Golja, M., Peternel, P. & Rozman, B. (1997). Influence of degraded phosphatidylserine on binding of antiphospholipid antibodies. *Int Arch Allerg Immunol* 112:19-26.

Božič, B., Irman, Š., Gašperšič, N., Kveder, T. & Rozman, B. (2005). Antibodies against annexin A5: detection pitfalls and clinical associations. *Autoimmunity* 38: 425-430.

Božič, B., Čučnik, S., Kveder, T. & Rozman, B. (2007). Affinity and avidity of autoantibodies. *In* Shoenfeld, Y., Gershwin, M. E., Meroni, P. L.. *Autoantibodies.* Elsevier B. V., Boston, 21-8.

Callahan, M. K., Williamson, P. & Schleger, R. A. (2000). Surface expression of phosphatidylserine on macrophages is required for phagocytosis of apoptotic tymocytes. *Cell Death Differ* 6:645-53.

Čučnik, S., Križaj, I., Rozman, B., Kveder, T. & Božič, B. (2004). Concomitant isolation of protein C inhibitor and unnicked beta2-glycoprotein I. *Clin Chem Lab Med* 42:171-4.

Čučnik, S., Kveder, T., Križaj, I., Rozman, B. & Božič, B. (2004). High-avidity β2-glycoprotein I antibodies in patients with antiphospholipid syndrome. *Ann Rheum Dis* 63:1478-82.

Deisenhofer, J. (1981). The secondary structure of Protein G', a robust molecule. *Biochemistry* 20:2361-70.

de Laat, B., Dersken, R. H. W. M. & de Groot, P. G. (2006). High-avidity anti-β_2-glycoprotein I antobodies highly correlate with thrombosis in contrast to low-avidity anti-β_2-glycoprotein I antibodies. *J Throm Haemost* 4:1619-21.

de Laat, B., Derksen, R. H. W. M., van Lummel, M., Pennings, M. T. T. & de Groot, P. G. (2006). Pathogenic anti- β_2-glycoprotein I antibodies recognize domain I of β_2-glycoprotein I only after a conformational change. *Blood* 107:1916-24.

de Laat, B., Wu, X. X., van Lummel, M., Derksen, R. H. W. M., de Groot, P. G. & Rand, J. H. (2007). Correlation between antiphospholipid antibodies that recognize domain I of β_2-glycoprotein I and a reduction in the anticoagulant activity of annexin A5. *Blood* 109:1490-4.

Fotiadis, D., Scheuring, S., Muller, S. A, Engel, A. & Müller, D. J.(2002). Imaging and manipulation of biological structures with the AFM. *Micron* 33:385-97.

Frank, M., Sodin-Šemrl, S., Irman, Š., Božič, B. & Rozman, B. (2009). β_2-glycoprotein I and annexin A5 phospholipid interactions: Artificial and cell membranes. *Autoimmun Rev* 9:5-10.

Gadegaard, N. (2006). Atomic force microscopy in biology: technology and techniques. *Biotech Histochem* 81:87-97.

Gamsjaeger, R., Johs, A., Gries, A., Gruber, H. J., Romanin, C., Prassl, R. & Hinterdorfer, P. (2005). Membrane binding of β_2-glycoprotein I can be described by a two-state reaction model: an atomic force microscopy and surface plasmon resonance study. *Biochem J* 389:665–73.

Gerke, V., Creutz, C. E. & Moss, S. E. (2005). Annexins:linking Ca^{2+} signalling to membrane dynamics. *Nat Rev Mol Cell Biol* 6:449-61.

Govorukhina, N., Bergsma-Schutter, A., Mazeres-Dubut, C., Mazeres, S., Drakopoulou, E., Bystrykh, L., Oling, F., Mukhopadhyay, A., Reviakine, I., Laikee Him, J. & Brisson, A. (2003). *In* Bondorowicz- Pikula, J., editor. *Annexins: Biological importance and annexin-related pathologies.* Landes Bioscience, Georgetown, 37-55.

Gris, J. C., Perneger, T. V., Quere, I., Mercier, E., Fabbro-Peray, P., Lavigne-Lissalde, G., Hoffet, M., Dechaud, H., Boyer, J.-C., Ripart-Neveu , S., Tailland, M.-L., Daures, J.-P., Mares, P. & Dauzat, M. (2003). Antiphospholipid / antiprotein antibodies, hemostasis-related autoantibodies, and plasma homocystein as risk factor for first pregnancy loss: A matched case-control study. *Blood* 102:3504–13.

Hamdan, R., Maiti, S. N. & Schroit, A. J. (2007). Interaction of β_2-glycoprotein I with phosphatidylserine-containing membranes: Ligand-dependent conformational alterations initiate bivalent binding. *Biochem* 46:10612-20.

Hinterdorfer, P., Baumgartner, W., Gruber, H. J., Schilcher, K., & Schindler H. (1996). Detection and localization of individual antibody-antigen recognition events by atomic force microscopy. *Proc Natl Acad Sci U S A* 93:3477–81.

Howald, L., Haefke, H., Luthi, R., Meyer, E., Gerth, G., Rudin, H. & Guntherodt H.-J. (1994). Ultrahigh-vacuum scanning force microscopy: atomic-scale resolution at monatomic cleavage steps. *Phys Rev B:Condens Matter* 49:5651-6.

Huber, R., Romisch, J. & Paques, E. (1990). The crystal and molecular structure of human annexin V, an anticoagulant protein that binds calcium and membranes. *EMBO J* 9:3867-74.

Ioannou, Y., Pericleous, C., Giles, I., Latchman, D. S., Isenberg, D. A. & Rahman, A. (2007). Binding of antiphospholipid antibodies to discontinuous epitopes on domain I of human β_2-glycoprotein I. *Arthritis & Rheumatism* 56:280-90.

Irman, Š., Škarabot, M., Muševič, I., Rozman, B. & Božič, B. (2009). *In vitro* model of annexin A5 crystallization on natural phospholipid bilayers observed by atomic force microscopy. *Autoimmunity* 42:414-23.

Irman, Š., Škarabot, M., Muševič, I., Rozman, B. & Božič, B. (2010). Thrombomodulatory effect of anti-b2-glycoprotein I antibodies on crystalline annexin A5 on phospholipid bilayers, as observed by atomic force microscopy. *eJIFCC* 21.

Irman, Š., Škarabot, M., Muševič, I., Rozman, B. & Božič, B. (2011). Effects of anti-annexin antibodies on annexin A5 anticoagulant shield, as observed by atomic force microscopy. *J Autoimmun* 36:98-105.

Kaburaki, J., Kuwana, M., Yamamoto, M., Kawai, S. & Ikeda, Y. (1997). Clinical significance of anti-annexin antibodies in patients with systemic lupus erythematosus. *Am J Hematol* 54:209-13.

Kenis, H., van Genderen, H., Bennaghmouch, A., Rinia, H. A., Frederik, P., Narula, J., Hofstra, L. & Reutelingsperger, C. P. (2004). Cell surface-expressed phosphatidylserine and annexin A5 open a novel portal of cell entry. *J Biol Chem* 279:52623-9.

Leonenko, Z. V., Carnini, A. & Cramb, D.T. (2000). Supported planar bilayer formation by vesicle fusion: the interaction of phospholipid vesicles with surfaces and the effect of gramicidin on bilayer properties using atomic force microscopy. *Biochim Biophys Acta* 1509:131-47.

Liemann, S., Benz, J., Burger, A., Voges, D., Hofmann, A. & Huber, R. (1996). Structural and functional characterization of the voltage sensor in the ion channel human annexin V. *J Mol Biol* 258:555-61.

Lipowsky, R. & Seifert, U. (1991). Adhesion of vesicles and membranes. *Mol Cryst Liq Cryst* 202:17–25.

Lutters, B. C., Derksen, R. H., Tekelenburg, W. L., Lenting, P. J., Arnout, J. & de Groot, P. G. (2003). Dimers of β2-glycoprotein I increase platelet deposition to collagen via interaction with phospholipids and the apolipoprotein E receptor 2'. *J Biol Chem* 278:33831–8.

Marti, O., Drake, B. & Hansma, P. K. (1987). Atomic force microscopy of liquid-covered surfaces: atomic resolution images. *Appl. Phys. Lett.*51:484–6.

Marquart, M., Deisenhofer, J., Huber, R. & Palm, J. (1980). The three-dimensional structure of an intact monoclonal antibody for canine lymphom. *J Mol Biol* 141:369-91.

Matsubayashi, H., Arai, T., Izumi, S., Sugi, T., McIntyre, J. A. & Makino, T. (2001). Anti-annexin V antibodies in patients with early pregnancy loss or implantation failures. *Fertil Steril* 76:694-9.

Matsuda, J., Saitoh, N., Gohchi, K., Gotoh, M., Tsukamoto, M. (1994). Anti-annexin V antibody in systemic lupus erythematosus patients with lupus anticoagulant and/or anticardiolipin antibody. *Am J Hemathol* 47:56-8.

Meroni, P. L. & Shoenfeld, Y. (2008). Predictive, protective, orphan autoantibodies: The example of anti-phospholipid antibodies. *Autoimmun Rev* 7:585-7.

Miyakis, S., Ginnakopoulos, B. & Krilis, S. A. (2004). Beta 2 glycoprotein I- function in health and disease. *Thrombosis Research* 114:335-46.

Miyakis, S., Lockshin, M. D., Atsumi, T., Branch, D. W., Brey, R. L., Cervera, R., Derksen, R. H., de Groot, P. G., Koike, T., Meroni, P. L., Reber, G., Shoenfeld, Y., Tincani, A., Vlachoyiannopoulos, P. G. & Krilis, S. A. (2006). International consensus statement on an update of the classification criteria for definite antiphospholipid syndrome (APS).*J Throm Haemost* 4:295-306.

Nojima, J., Kuratsune, H., Suehisa, E., Futsukichi, Y., Yamanishi, H., Machii, T., Iwatani, Y. & Kanakura Y. (2001). Association between the prevalence of antibodies to beta(2)-glycoprotein I, prothrombin, protein C, protein S, and annexin V in patients with systemic lupus erythematosus and thrombotic and thrombocytopenic complications. *Clin Chem* 47:1008-15.

Oesterhelt, F., Oestrehelt, D., Pfeiffer M., Engel, A., Gaub, H. E. Müller, D. J. (2000). Unfolding Pathways of Individual Bacteriorhodopsins. *Science* 288:143-6.

Oling, F., Bergsma-Schutter, W. & Brisson, A. (1998). Trimers, dimers of trimers, trimers of trimers are common building blocks of annexin A5 two-dimensional crystals. *J Struct Biol* 133:55-63.

Omersel, J., Žager, U., Kveder, T. & Božič, B. (2010). Alteration of antibody specificity during isolation and storage. *J Immunoassay Immunochem* 31:45-59.

Ramirez-Aguilar, K. A. & Rowlen, K. L. (1998). Tip characterization from AFM images of nanometric spherical particles. *Langmuir* 14:2562-6.

Rand, J. H., Wu, X. X., Andree, H. A. M., Ross, A. J. B., Rusinova, E., Gascon-Lema, M. G., Calandri, C. & Harpel, P. C. (1998). Antiphospholipid antibodies accelerate plasma coagulation by inhibiting annexin V binding to phospholipids: A "Lupus Procoagulant" phenomenom. *Blood* 92:1652-60.

Rand, J. H., Wu, X. X., Quinn, A. S., Chen, P. P., McCrae, K. R., Bovill, E. G. & Taatjes, D. J. (2003). Human monoclonal antiphospholipid antibodies disrupt the annexin A5 anticoagulant crystal shield on phospholipid bilayers: evidence from atomic force microscopy. *Am J of Pathol* 163:1193-1200.

Rand, J. H., Wu, X. X., Quinn, A. S. & Taatjes, D. J. (2008). Resistance to annexin A5 anticoagulant activity: a thrombogenic mechanism for the antiphospholipid syndrome. *Lupus* 17:922-30.

Ravassa, S., Bennaghmouch, A., Kenis, H., Lindhout, T., Hackeng, T., Narula, J., Hofstra, L. & Reutelingsperger, C. (2005). Annexin A5 down-regulates surface expression of tissue factor: a novel mechanism of regulating the membrane receptor repertoire. *J Biol Chem* 280:6028-35.

Reviakine, I., Bergsma-Schutter, W. & Brisson, A. (1998). Growth of protein 2D crystals on supported planar lipid bilayers imaged in situ by AFM. *J Struct Biol* 121:356-61.

Reviakine, I., Bergsma-Schutter, W., Marezes-Dubut, C., Govorukhina, N. & Brisson, A. (2000). Surface topography of the p3 and p6 annexin v crystal forms determined by atomic force microscopy. *J Struct Biol* 131:234-9.

Reviakine, I. & Brisson, A. (2000). Formation of supported phosholipid bilayers from unilamellar vesicles investigated by atomic force microscopy. *Langmuir* 16:1806-15.

Reviakine, I., Bergsma-Schutter, W., Mozorov, A. N. & Brisson, A. (2001). Two-dimensional crystallization of annexin A5 on phospholipid bilayers and monolayers: a solid-solid phase transition between crystal forms. *Langmuir* 17:1680-6.

Rief, M., Oesterhelt, F., Heymann, B. & Gaub, H. E. (1997). Single Molecule Force Spectroscopy on Polysaccharides by Atomic Force Microscopy. *Science* 275:1295-97.

Richter, R. P. & Brisson, A. (2005). Following the formation of supported lipid bilayers on mica: A study combining AFM, QCM-D, and ellipsometry. *Biophys J* 88:3422–33.

Richter, R. P., Lai Kee Him, J., Tessier, B., Tessier, C. & Brisson, A. (2005). On the kinetics of adsorption and two dimensional self-assembly of annexin A5 on supported lipid bilayers. *Biophys J* 89: 3372-85.

Richter, R. P., Berat, R. & Brisson A. (2006). Formation of solid-supported lipid bilayers: an integarted view. *Langmuir* 22:3497-505.

Rodriguez-Garcia, M. I., Fernandez, J. A., Rodrigez, A., Fernandez, M. P., Gutierrez, C. & Torre-Alonso, J. C. (1996). Annexin V autoantibodies in rheumatoid arthritis. *Ann Rheum Dis* 55:895–900.

Rojas, E., Pollard, H. B., Haigler, H. T., Parra, C. & Burns, A. L. (1990). Calcium-activated endonexin II forms calcium channels across acidic phospholipid bilayer membranes. *J Biol Chem* 265:21207-15.

Russo-Marie, F. (1990). Annexin V and phospholipid metabolism. *Clin Chem Lab Med* 37:2287-91.

Satoh, A., Suzuki, K., Takayama, E., Kojima, K., Hidaka, T., Kawakami, M., Matsumoto, I. & Ohsuzu, F. (1999). Detection of anti-annexin IV and V antibodies in patients with antiphospholipid syndrome and systemic lupus erythematosus. *J Rheumatol* 26:1715-20.

Schwarzenbacher, R., Zeth, K., Diederichs, K., Gries, A., Kostner, G. M., Laggner, P. & Prassl, R. (1999). Crystal structure of human β_2-glycoprotein I: implications for phospholipid binding and the antiphospholipid syndrome. *The EMBO Journal* 18:6228-39.

Seifert, U. (1997). Configurations of fluid membranes and vesicles. *Adv Phys* 46:13–137.

Shao, Z., Mou, J., Czajkowsky, D. M., Yang, J. & Yuan, J.Y. (1996). Biological atomic force microscopy:what is achieved and what is needed. *Advances in physics* 45:1-86.

Shoenfeld, Y. (2002). Immunology and pathophysiology of the antiphospholipid syndrome. *In* Asherson, R. A.,Cervera, R., Piette, J.-C., Shoenfeld, Y. *The antiphospholipid syndrome II.* Elsevier, Amsterdam, 23-144.

Shoenfeld, Y., Krause, I., Kvapil, F., Sulkes, J., Lev, S., von Landenberg, P., Font, J., Zaech, J., Cervera, R., Piette, J. C., Boffa, M. C., Kamashta, M. A., Bertolaccini, M. L., Hughes, G. R. V., Youinou, P., Meroni, P. L., Pengo, V., Alves, J. D., Tincani, A., Szegedi, G., Lakos, G., Sturfelt, G., Jonsen, A., Koike, T., Sanmarco, M., Ruffatti, A., Ulcova-Gallova, Z., Praprotnik, S., Rozman, B., Lorber, M., Vriezman, V. B. & Blank, M. (2003). Prevalence and clinical correlation of antibodies against six β_2-glycoprotein I-related peptides in the antiphospholipid syndrome. *J Clin Immunol* 23:377-83.

Silverton, E. W., Navia, M. A. & Davies, D. R. (1977). Three-dimensional structure of an intact immunoglobulin. *Proc Natl Acad Sci U S A* 74:5140-4.

Sodin-Šemrl, S. & Rozman, B. (2007). β_2-glycoprotein I and its clinical significance: From gene sequence to protein levels. *Autoimmun Rev* 6:547-52.

Thalhammer, S., Stark, R. W., Müller, S., Wienberg, J. & Heckl, W. M. (1997). The atomic force microscope as a new microdissecting tool for the generation of genetic probes. *J Struct Biol* 119:232-7.

van Genderen, H. O., Kenis, H., Hofstra, L., Narula, J. & Reutelingsperger, C. P. M. (2008). Extracellular annexin A5: Functions of phosphatidylserine-binding and two-dimensional crystallization. *Biochim Biophys Acta* 1783:953-63.

van Heerde, W. L., de Groot, P. G. & Reutelingsperger, C. P. M. (1995). The Complexity of the phospholipid binding protein annexin V. *Thromb Haemostas* 73:172-9.

Zammiti, W., Mtiraoui, N., Hidar, S., Fekih, M., Almawi, W. Y. & Mahjoub, T. (2006). Antibodies to β_2-glycoprotein I and annexin V in women with early and late idiopathic recurrent spontaneous abortions. *Gynecol Obstet* 274:261-5.

Žager, U., Irman, Š., Lunder, M., Škarabot, M., Muševič, I., Hodnik, V., Anderluh, G., Čučnik, S., Kveder, T., Rozman, B. & Božič, B. (2011). Immunochemical properties and pathological relevance of anti-b2-glycoprotein I antibodies of different avidity. *Int Immunol* 23:511-8.

Willems, G. M., Janssen, M. P., Pelsers, M. M. A. L., Comfurius, P., Galli, M., Zwaal, R. F. A. & Bevers, E. M. (1996). Role of divalency in the high-affinity binding of anticardiolipin antibody-β_2-glycoprotein I complexes to lipid membranes. *Biochem* 35:13833-42.

Wilson, W. A., Gharavi, A. E., Koike, T., Lockshin, M. D., Branch, D. W., Piette, J. C., Brey, R., Derksen, R., Harris, E. N., Hughes, G. R., Triplett, D. A. & Khamashta, M. A. (1999). International consensus statement on preliminary classification criteria for definite antiphosholipid syndrome:report of interational workshop. *Arthritis Rheum* 42:1309-11.

Xu, H., Zhao, X., Grant, C. & Lu, J. R. (2006). Orientation of monoclonal antibody adsorbed at the solid/solution interface: a combined study using atomic force microscopy and neutron reflectivity. *Langmuir* 22:6313-20.

7

Nanomechanics of Amyloid Materials Studied by Atomic Force Microscopy

Guanghong Zeng, Yusheng Duan,
Flemming Besenbacher and Mingdong Dong
Interdisciplinary Nanoscience Center (iNANO), Aarhus University
Denmark

1. Introduction

1.1 Amyloid materials and their mechanical properties

Amyloids are usually used to refer to a wide range of fibrous nanostructures formed from natural and synthetic proteins and peptides. The self-propagating protein aggregates are rich in β-sheets, which stack in hundreds to thousands units perpendicular to the fibrous axis, forming fibrils 5-15 nm in width and several micrometers in length (Dobson, 1999; Jaroniec et al., 2004; Luhrs et al., 2005; Sawaya et al., 2007; Wasmer et al., 2008). The structural trait gives amyloids the so called "cross-β" diffraction pattern under X-ray crystallography as well as some tinctorial properties which they share in common, such as Congo red and thioflavin-T binding ability (Westermark et al., 1999) and the characteristic apple-green birefringence under polarized light when stained with Congo red.

While the study of amyloids was initiated a long time ago, the interest in exploring their structures and understanding the structural basis of their formation has been mainly stimulated by their association with neurodegenerative disorders such as Alzheimer's, and Parkinson's diseases (Selkoe, 2001; Tan & Pepys, 1994). Amyloidosis, the process in which soluble protein are deposited pathologically to form amyloid plaques, is believed to be the central step which initiates a series of events which eventually lead to neuron degeneration (Bucciantini et al., 2002; Paravastu et al., 2008). As more diseases such as type II diabetes, Creutzfeldt-Jakob disease (CJD or "Mad Cow" disease), and rheumatoid arthritis are found to be related to amyloidosis (Chiti & Dobson, 2006), amyloids have gained notorious reputation for a long time. However, during the past 10 years, it has been found that many living organisms take advantage of specific proteins' ability to form fibrous amyloids to perform their ordinary functions (Fowler et al., 2007). Bacteria form an extracellular amyloid matrix for their surface adhesion and colony formation (Chapman et al., 2002); in mammal cells, amyloids facilitate and regulate the synthesis of melanin (Fowler et al., 2005); they also serves as a regulatory motif in human hemostasis (Shibayama et al., 1999). These discoveries make amyloids very interesting because of their dual identities as pathogenic factors and functional components.

From the aspect of nanoengineering, amyloids are unique materials because of their highly ordered structure. The cooperative hydrogen-bonds between the well-stacked β-sheets allows amyloid fibrils to grow into microns in length, reaching maximum strength in supermolecular assemblies (Fowler, et al., 2005) that can hardly be achieved by artificial materials. Similar structures are found in silk, one of the natural materials with the highest strength. With their unique well-ordered fibrous structure, amyloid fibrils have found applications in template synthesis for metal nanowires (Carny et al., 2006; Reches & Gazit, 2003; Scheibel et al., 2003), solar cells (Barrau et al., 2008; Channon et al., 2009; Liang et al., 2008), tissue engineering (Ellis-Behnke et al., 2006; Holmes et al., 2000), and drug delivery (Maji et al., 2008).

Understanding the mechanical properties are crucial to biological materials, as the mechanical information reveals their structural origin as well as how the materials contribute to the biological system by interacting with other components. This is especially challenging for amyloids, not only because of their micrometer length and nanometer width which makes them inaccessible for traditional mechanical tests, but also because they have hierarchical structures. Several thin fibrils, or protofilaments, are assembled in a twisted way to form an amyloid fibril. To make it even worse, more and more evidence suggests that amyloids are structurally diverse (Toyama & Weissman, 2011). Therefore it is necessary to measure the mechanical properties at a single fibril level, which falls in the range of nanometers.

1.2 AFM as a unique tool for nanomechanics of amyloid materials

Because the width of the amyloid fibril is usually several nanometers, we have to turn to single-molecular force techniques to explore their nanomechanics. Although new techniques are emerging constantly, the most commonly used ones for single-molecule manipulation and force spectroscopy are atomic force microscopy (AFM), optical tweezers, and magnetic tweezers (Neuman & Nagy, 2008). Optical tweezers and magnetic tweezers share a common mechanism, where objects are trapped either in an optical field (Ashkin et al., 1986) or in a magnetic field (Strick et al., 2000). In both methods, the interaction forces are determined by displacement from the trapped location when no external forces are present. The stiffness of the trapping is linearly determined by the strength of optical trapping or magnetic field, which is tuned by the setup of the laser system or magnets. Thus both methods are able to detect very low force, down to 10^{-1} pN for optical tweezers and 10^{-3} pN for magnetic tweezers. However, the upper limit of the detection is determined by the strength of the trapping force as well as the linear range, which is up to 100 pN for both methods (Neuman & Nagy, 2008). Unfortunately, in many cases of nanomechanical measurement beyond the molecular level, the forces go right out of this limit.

Atomic force microscopy (AFM) (Binnig et al., 1986), operating with a completely different mechanism, is a solution to these cases. Among the three techniques discussed, AFM is perhaps the most popular one. AFM works with a simple mechanism (Figure 1). Basically, it works with a force probe, which is a microfabricated cantilever with a sharp tip mounted on one end. As a piezo system controls the scanning of the tip on the sample surface in the horizontal (x and y) and vertical (z) direction, the deflection of the cantilever as a result of the interactions between the tip and sample is translated by a laser beam reflected on the back of the cantilever. Displacement of the laser beam on the photodiode is recorded as an amplified signal of the cantilever deflection. AFM allows the mapping of the surface down to sub-nanometer range, and works on all types of surfaces, regardless of whether they are

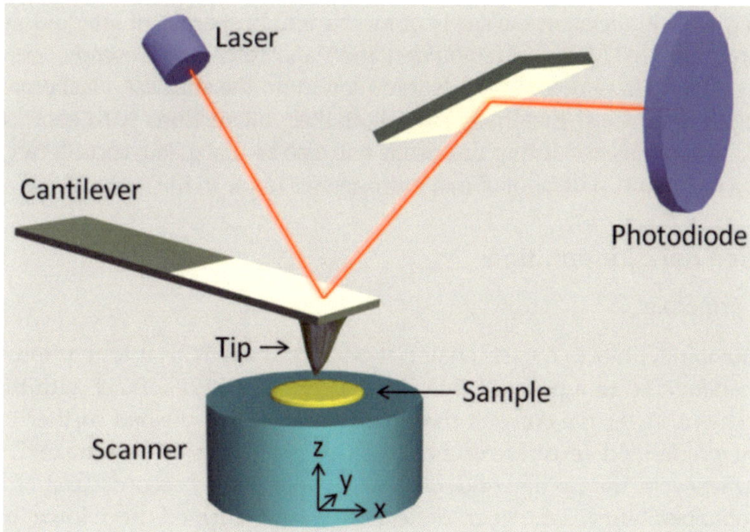

Fig. 1. Schematic illustration of the principles of AFM. The scanner is composed of three piezo components, which control the horizontal (x and y) and vertical (z) movement of the sample.

conductive or not. Another major advantage is that AFM works in liquid environment, which makes it superior to other imaging techniques for the measurement of biological samples under physiological conditions. Besides, sample preparation is simple and fast, compared to other imaging techniques such as electron microscopy.

Although AFM was initially developed for imaging, it is also a powerful tool for the measurement of forces with piconewton resolution. In the force spectroscopy mode (Weisenhorn et al., 1989), instead of scanning across the sample surface, the AFM probe moves vertically at a specified point on the sample, recording a deflection-displacement curve, which is subsequently converted to a force-extension curve by suitable calibrations. Within the operation range, the cantilever behaves as a linear spring. Therefore, the force detected by AFM is determined by the spring constant of the cantilevers used. Due to the large size and relatively high stiffness of the cantilevers, AFM operates at a much higher force range compared to that of the optical and magnetic tweezers, typically from 10 pN to 10^4 pN. The broad detection range is enabled by the extensive choices of cantilevers for a specific measurement.

Another advantage for AFM is the combination of high resolution imaging and force spectroscopy, which makes it possible to locate the region of interest in nanometer precision, especially when the objects have heterogeneous features, such as the case in amyloid materials. Also, it is a major advantage for AFM to operate at physiological conditions, which allows the investigation of amyloid fibrils under conditions similar to their native environment. For these reasons, although AFM is a new tool for amyloid research with the first paper published in 1995 (Oda et al., 1995), it has become a major tool for the characterization of amyloid materials, providing complementary and unique possibilities for amyloid research compared to the electron microscopy, which had been the major imaging tool for bio-samples such as amyloid materials before AFM was invented.

In this chapter, we will focus on the study of mechanical properties of amyloid materials with AFM. By introducing AFM based nanoindentation and force spectroscopy, we are going to illustrate how AFM as a nanotool reveals information on the stiffness, elastic properties, and rupture strength of amyloid materials, as well as their interactions with each other and the environment. Limitations and future directions will also be discussed, considering that AFM is a fast evolving technique, with a lot of major progresses made in the recent years.

2. AFM based nanoindentation

2.1 General principle

In a typical nanoindentation measurement, it usually starts with a topography image. The tip is then maneuvered to a point of interest, and brought into contact with the sample by vertical movement. After the contact, the tip and sample are pushed further towards each other, until a predefined force is reached. At this point the tip is retracted. During this approach-retract cycle, the cantilever deflection is continuously recorded, and force-distance curves are obtained after cantilever deflection is transformed into force by cantilever calibration. The curves are then fitted with suitable model to give the mechanical properties of the sample.

During the force experiment, the instrument records the deflection of the cantilever (d) (which is defined by the change of reflection angle (θ) of the laser beam) versus the displacement of the z piezo (Z). In order to convert the deflection vs. displacement curve to force vs. indentation curve, which is a premise for the fitting of the results, several treatment and calibration steps have to be taken. First, the indentation δ is calculated by subtracting cantilever deflection d with z piezo displacement Z:

$$\delta = Z - d \tag{1}$$

as illustrated in Figure 2. It is noteworthy to mention that the tip-sample contact point has to be determined before the calculation, as the z piezo has already traveled some distance before reaching the sample surface, and the previous displacement before tip-sample contact has to be excluded in order to calculate indention depth. The tip-sample contact point is marked by the onset of cantilever deflection, which is small from the beginning. As a result, the tip-sample contact point has to be estimated from the whole deflection-displacement curve.

The second step is to determine the relationship between cantilever deflection and force, which requires the calibration of cantilever sensitivity and spring constant. Cantilever sensitivity defines the relationship between cantilever deflection and detector voltage change. It is determined by pressing the tip on a hard surface, whose deformation is negligible during the measurement. By recording the z displacement ΔZ and detector voltage change ΔV, the sensitivity is given by:

$$S = \frac{\Delta V}{\Delta Z} \tag{2}$$

As the surface is assumed to be intact, the z displacement equals to the cantilever deflection. Thus in further measurements, cantilever deflection is calculated as:

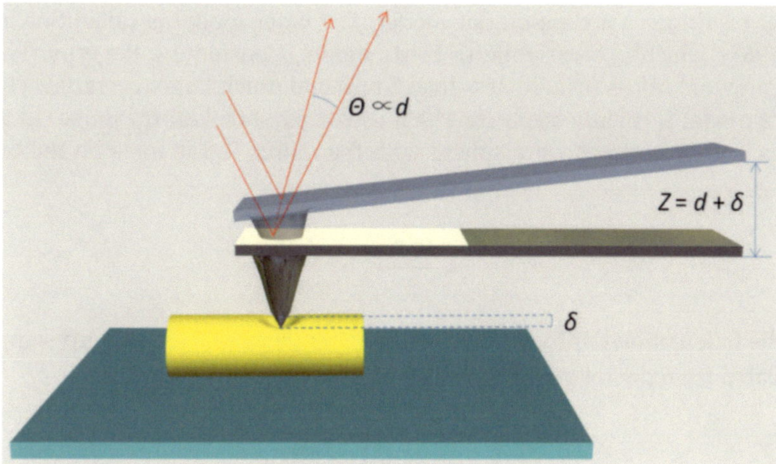

Fig. 2. The relationship of z piezo displacement (Z), cantilever deflection (d) and indentation (δ).

$$d = \frac{\Delta V}{S} \tag{3}$$

A cantilever is regarded as a spring, which means the force on the tip is determined by the deflection and cantilever spring constant according to Hooke's law:

$$F = k \times d \tag{4}$$

Every batch of AFM probe comes with a nominal value of cantilever spring constant. However, due to the systematic error generated during probe fabrication, cantilever properties vary among one batch. Therefore, it is necessary to calibrate the spring constant for each probe used. There are several methods to determine the spring constant of the cantilever with similar uncertainties (Cook, et al., 2006; Gibson et al., 2005; Ohler, 2007). The most commonly used calibration method is the thermal noise method, which has an uncertainty of 5% (Ohler, 2007).

After obtaining the force vs. indentation curve, the curve is submitted to mechanical modeling. Hertz model is a classic model of contact mechanics, which deals with two perfect elastic, homogeneous, and smooth objects pressing against each other (Johnson, 1985). The Hertzian model does not consider adhesion between the two surfaces. If adhesion forces are significant and cannot be omitted, non-Hertzian models such as the Johnson-Kendall-Roberts (JKR) model (Johnson et al., 1971) and the Derjaguin-Muller-Toporov (DMT) model (Derjaguin et al., 1975; Muller et al., 1983) should be used. The JKR and DMT model assumes the presence of short-range adhesion forces within the contact area and long-range adhesion forces outside the contact area, respectively. In most cases of amyloid indentation study, there is only insignificant adhesion between tip and sample, so the Hertz model is mainly used.

In a typical Hertz model, the AFM tip is modeled as having a paraboloidal shape. This is valid when the indentation is small compared to the tip radius, resulting in a sphere-on-flat model. If the indentation is much larger than the tip radius, then the tip can be considered as a rigid cone, resulting in a cone-on-flat model. The latter model is called Sneddon model (Sneddon, 1965), which is a variation of Hertz model. Considering the typical indentation available in amyloid fibrils (usually less than 5 nm) and much larger tip radius (10 - 30 nm), classic Hertz model is mainly applied, which uses a paraboloidal tip shape. In this case, if the AFM tip is approximated by a sphere with the radius R, the force on the cantilever is given by:

$$F = \frac{4\sqrt{R}}{3} E^{*} \delta^{3/2} \tag{5}$$

where δ is the indentation depth, and E^{*} is the effective modulus of the tip-sample system. E^{*} is calculated from the following equation:

$$\frac{1}{E^{*}} = \frac{1-\upsilon_{tip}^{2}}{E_{tip}} + \frac{1-\upsilon_{sample}^{2}}{E_{sample}} \tag{6}$$

where E_{tip} , υ_{tip} and E_{sample} , υ_{sample} are the Young's moduli and the Poisson's ratios for the tip and sample, respectively. Usually the AFM tip is much harder than the sample, so the effective modulus is given by:

$$E^{*} = \frac{E_{sample}}{1-\upsilon_{sample}^{2}} \tag{7}$$

Therefore the force on the cantilever is calculated as:

$$F = \frac{4E\sqrt{R}}{3\,(1-\upsilon^{2})} \delta^{3/2} \tag{8}$$

where E, υ, R, δ. refer to the Young's modulus, Poisson's ratio, tip radius, indention depth, respectively. Poisson's ratio for amyloid is often guessed to be around 0.3.

The tip radius can be determined by two different methods. The preferred method is using electron microscopy to image the tip after the measurements (Guo & Akhremitchev, 2006). The resulting image might have a low contrast due to the low electron density of silicon nitride, which can be improved by sputtering a layer of metal on the tip. An alternative method is using the tip to scan a test sample with sharp morphology (sharper than the tip), and the resulting image can be analyzed by convolution models to get the estimated tip radius (Zenhausern et al., 1992). Previous study showed that the systematic error for the tip sample convolution method is about 30% (VanLandingham et al., 2005), which means that electron microscopy is, in principal, a more precise method to determine the tip radius. However, electron microscopy requires considerable time and effort to obtain quantifiable results.

Another concern is the finite sample thickness. When the indention depth is significant compared to the sample thickness, the sample cannot be regarded as infinitely thick. In this situation, the substrate also contributes to the mechanical response of the tip-sample system, resulting in a deviated Young's modulus. This effect can be corrected by calculating correction factors using the uncorrected Young's modulus and normalized force (Akhremitchev & Walker, 1999; Guo & Akhremitchev, 2006). After all the calibration and approximation, the force can be linearly fitted against indentation by equation 8 and the Young's modulus is obtained.

2.2 Applications

An early AFM indentation measurement was conducted on insulin amyloid fibrils adsorbed on mica surface (Guo & Akhremitchev, 2006). The obtained force curves showed no adhesion between the tip and fibril, by which it was rationalized that the Hertz model could be used to fit the force curve. Besides, no significant indentation hysteresis was observed, suggesting a purely elastic response of the fibril to the compressive load. Considering that some fibrils were thin compared to indentation depth (height distribution ranges from 2.5 to 14 nm), correction for finite sample thickness was conducted. Variation of modulus values along the same fibril is low, suggesting similar supramolecular structure along the fibril. However, the modulus distribution among different fibrils is pretty broad, ranging from 10 to 30 MPa. The broad distribution of the Young's modulus among fibrils suggests variation in the internal packing density, and therefore different supramolecular structures (Guo & Akhremitchev, 2006), confirming the structure heterogeneity of amyloid fibrils. The result also agrees well with the observed broad distribution of the morphology, with fibril heights range from 2.5 to 14 nm. The measured Young's modulus value is significantly lower than that of the globular protein crystals (from 200 MPa to 1 GPa) (Alonso & Goldmann, 2003; Morozov & Morozova, 1993), which suggests that amyloid fibrils are relatively loosely packed, as the protofilaments are usually separated by water (Perutz et al., 2002).

It is important to note that the above method only measures the mechanical response of amyloid fibrils perpendicular to the fibril axis. It is not surprising that measured Young's modulus is low, as the fibrils are packed from protofilaments by non-specific intermolecular interactions, resulting in loose packing. However, along the fibril axis, the fibrils are constructed by β strands stacking together by intermolecular multivalent hydrogen-bonding. Thus a much higher stiffness is expected along the axis direction.

The measurement of the elastic and shear moduli along the axis are enabled by miniaturization of the standard three-point bending test with AFM (Kis et al., 2002; Salvetat et al., 1999), as illustrated in Figure 3 (Dobson, et al., 2006). Insulin amyloid fibrils are suspended over a microfabricated groove. The AFM tip was pressed against the fibril until it broke and the tip touched the bottom of the groove. The recorded force curve can be divided into four regions: region 1, the tip didn't touch the fibril; region 2, linear region, the tip contacted and deformed the fibril; region 3, nonlinear region, the tip continued to deform the fibril until it broke; region 4, linear region, the tip was pressed against the substrate, so the mechanical response corresponds to the cantilever spring constant. By considering a simple geometric model, the rupture strength of the amyloid fibril was determined to be 0.6 ± 0.4 GPa, comparable to that of spider silk (1-1.5 GPa) (Vollrath & Knight, 2001) and steel (0.6-1.8 GPa) (Shackelford et al., 1995). By measuring the mechanical response along the fibril at different fraction of the total suspended length, the results were fitted to a model and the elastic and shear moduli were determined to be $E = 3.3 \pm 0.4$ GPa and $G = 0.28 \pm 0.2$ GPa. This result confirms the previous argument that the stiffness amyloid fibril along the axis is much higher than that perpendicular to the axis.

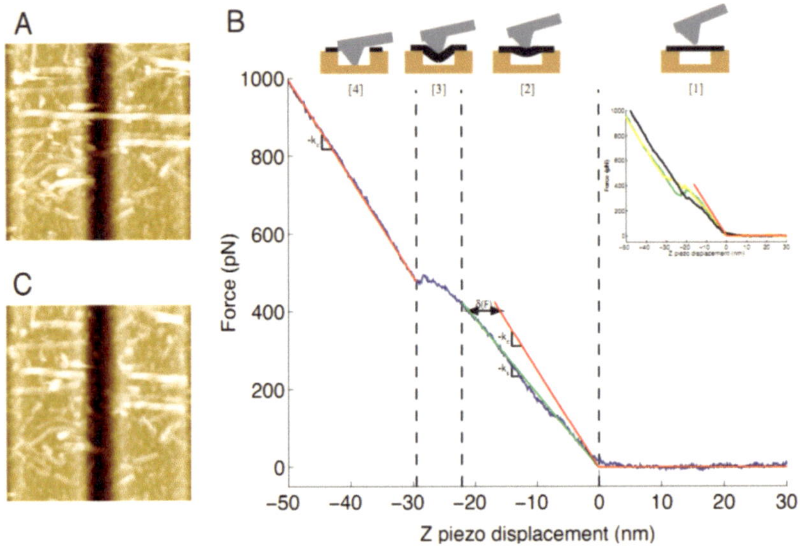

Fig. 3. Three-point bending test of amyloid fibrils with AFM (Dobson et al., 2006).

In the same paper, the authors invented a novel way to estimate the bending rigidity of the amyloid fibril. Fibrils were deposited onto mica surface, and their topographic data were acquired by tapping mode AFM and then submitted to statistical analysis based on thermal fluctuation. The resulting persistence length and bending rigidity agrees pretty well with those from force spectroscopy.

The huge difference between the axial and radial moduli is confirmed by analysis of the comparison of nanoindentation results on different location along the poly (ValGlyGlyLeuGly) amyloid fibrils (Flamia et al., 2008). As shown in Figure 4, AFM indentation was performed on three kinds of locations: fibril on silicon substrate, fibril on another fibril, and fibril suspended between two fibrils. The result is that the force versus distance curves showed identical mechanical response on different points. This result indicates that the fibril buckles instead of bends (pattern c versus pattern b in Figure 4 down part), which is the consequence of much higher axial stiffness compared to radial stiffness.

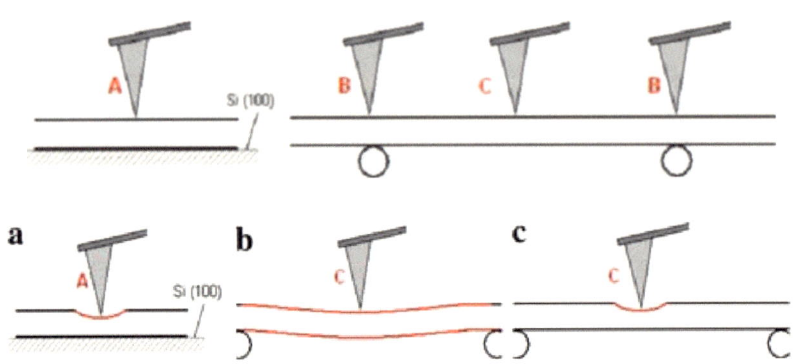

Fig. 4. Illustration of the different indentation locations along amyloid fibrils (up) and the expected deformation patterns (down) (Flamia, et al., 2008).

AFM based nanoindentation has also been applied to measure the stiffness of artificially self-assembled peptide nanotubes (Kol et al., 2005). A linear response was observed when the peptide nanotube on mica surface was pressed with AFM tip. The apparent point stiffness was obtained as the effective spring constant. The effective spring constant is the sum of the cantilever and nanotube spring constants, which gives the following relationship:

$$\frac{1}{k_{eff}} = \frac{1}{k_{cant}} + \frac{1}{k_{nano}} \tag{9}$$

By fitting the spring constant and the geometric configuration of the nanotube with a mechanical model, it was estimated that the Young's modulus reaches as high as 19 GPa, much higher than most biological structures such as microtubules (about 1 GPa) (de Pablo et al., 2003). The implication of the result is that artificial peptide nanotubes are even more efficiently packed than amyloid fibrils, making them promising for novel nanostructured materials.

3. AFM based force spectroscopy

3.1 General principle

The operation process of AFM based force spectroscopy is similar to that of indentation, but the purpose is quite different. A typical force spectroscopy cycle composes of four steps: (1) tip approaches the sample by vertical movement; (2) tip touches the sample with desired force and time and begins to retract; (3) tip adsorbs a molecule and stretches the molecule while retracting; (4) The molecule detaches from the surface. During the process, z piezo displacement is recorded. The extension of the molecule is calculated by subtracting cantilever deflection from z piezo displacement and adjusted according to how long the piezo has travelled before reaching the sample (maximum tip-sample separation). The resulted curve is usually called force-extension curve in force spectroscopy.

The mechanical response when a polymer molecule is stretched can be fitted by theoretical models (dash line in Figure 5 (4)). The most commonly used models are freely-jointed chain (FJC) and worm-like chain (WLC) models. Freely-jointed chain is the simplest ideal model for polymer. It assumes the polymer is composed of freely jointed rigid rods which move independently from each other. In contrast, WLC model describes the polymer chain as an isotropic, continuously flexible chain. WLC model is more suitable for stiffer polymers, with constrains between the movements of adjacent segments. As amyloid fibrils have high bending rigidity, they are modeled with WLC theory in nearly all related publications. The equation for WLC model is given as:

$$\frac{1}{\gamma} = \frac{1}{k_c \upsilon}\left(1 + \frac{k_c L_C}{4}\sqrt{\frac{F_p}{F^3}}\right) \tag{10}$$

Where k_c is the spring constant, υ is tip velocity, L_c and L_p are two parameters obtained from the WLC fitting, representing contour length and persistence length, respectively, F is rupture force (pN), γ is the loading rate, and

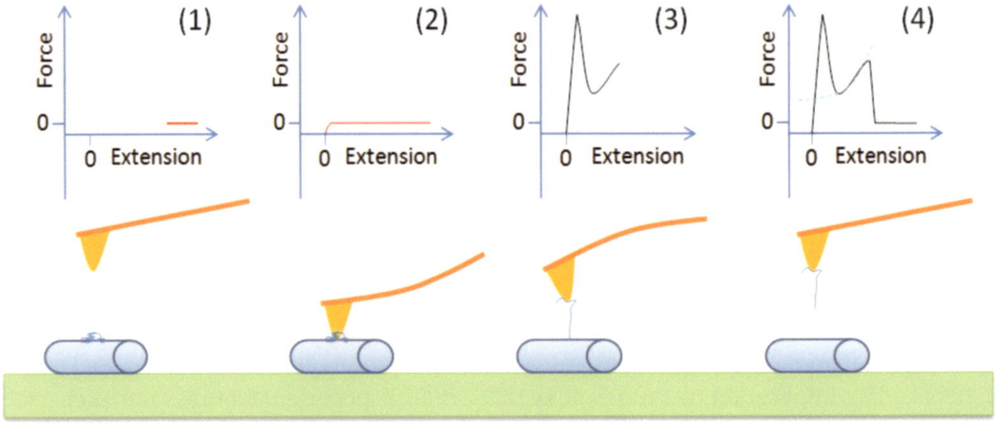

Fig. 5. General principle of AFM based force spectroscopy.

$$F_p = \frac{k_B T}{L_p} \tag{11}$$

3.2 Applications

As amyloid fibrils are usually heterogeneous assemblies, their force spectroscopy is often complicated and sometimes challenging to understand. In the AFM manipulation of the Aβ1-40 and Aβ25-35 fibrils (Kellermayer et al., 2005), the resulting force curves exhibited two distinct mechanical responses: (1) fully reversible, non-linear elasticity with WLC fitted contour length often exceeding 100 nm (Figure 6A); (2) force platform characterized with long distance constant force stretching followed by abrupt force drop (Figure 6B). In most cases, the two patterns are superposed onto each other (Figure 6C, 6D).

The force plateau indicates that a molecule or fibril was being desorbed, peeled off, or unzipped from the mother fibril. During the manipulation of amyloid fibrils with AFM tip, there are three possible candidates: the whole fibril, the protofilaments, or individual β-sheets. A piece of key evidence comes from the AFM imaging of the point before and after manipulation. It was observed that the helical morphology of the fibrils was identical before and after manipulation, which indicates that the fibril and protofilaments were probably intact, otherwise the morphology of the fibril would have been disturbed. Therefore, it is only possible that individual β-sheets were desorbed from the fibrils, which was not visible under normal AFM imaging. Furthermore, the non-linear elastic force response was fitted to WLC model, and the resulted persistent length of 0.38 ± 0.06 nm is comparable with that of a fully unfolded protein chain (titin, 0.4 nm) (Rief et al., 1997; Tskhovrebova et al., 1997). The β-sheet (s) can withstand force as high as 600 pN (Figure 6A), which can be explained by the parallel cooperative hydrogen-bonds along the axial direction.

It is surprising that the both the force plateaus and force steps are highly reversible and repeatable, with no loading-rate dependency. This implies that the associated state of the β-sheets is highly favored and stabilized within the amyloid fibrils (Kellermayer, et al., 2005), which partly explains the high stability of amyloid fibrils.

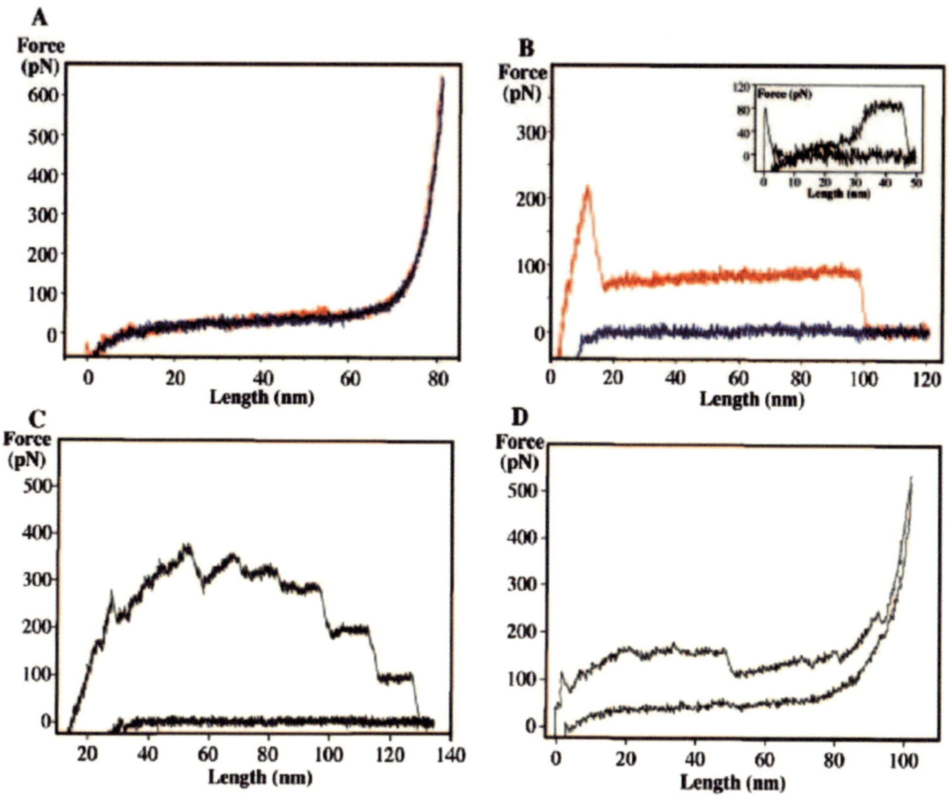

Fig. 6. Force curves of Aβ amyloid fibrils manipulated by AFM (Kellermayer, et al., 2005).

Once the force curve pattern has been recognized and related with specific interactions within the amyloid fibrils, quantitative information of the interactions can be revealed, thanks to the high sensitivity of AFM force measurement. In a following work, the unzipping force of β-sheets from the Aβ1-42 (full-length neurotoxic peptide associated with Alzheimer's disease) amyloid fibrils is compared with that of Aβ1-40 mentioned above. With two extra amino acid residues added to the C-terminus, the unzipping force falls from about 33 pN to about 23 pN, which suggests that the amyloid fibrils are destabilized by the additional two residues.

In principle, if the tip contacts the β-sheets on the amyloid fibril in the right place, a single molecular stretch should be observed. This was achieved in the AFM manipulation of amyloid fibrils formed from an 11 amino acid peptide segments of transthyratin, TTR (Fukuma et al., 2006; Mostaert & Jarvis, 2007). When the force spectroscopy was conducted on TTR fibrils, similar plateaus were observed, corresponding to the peeling off of β-sheets from the fibrils; in addition, force curves with sawtooth pattern were also captured (Figure 7), which were attributed to the successive unraveling of the peptide molecules from the fibril bulk.

The sawtooth pattern of the force spectroscopy of amyloid structures has helped identify amyloid fibrils as functional components in natural adhesive (Mostaert et al., 2006). Extracellular polymeric substances (EPS) are responsible for the adhesive properties of algae. The presence of amyloid structures were revealed by the characteristic green-gold

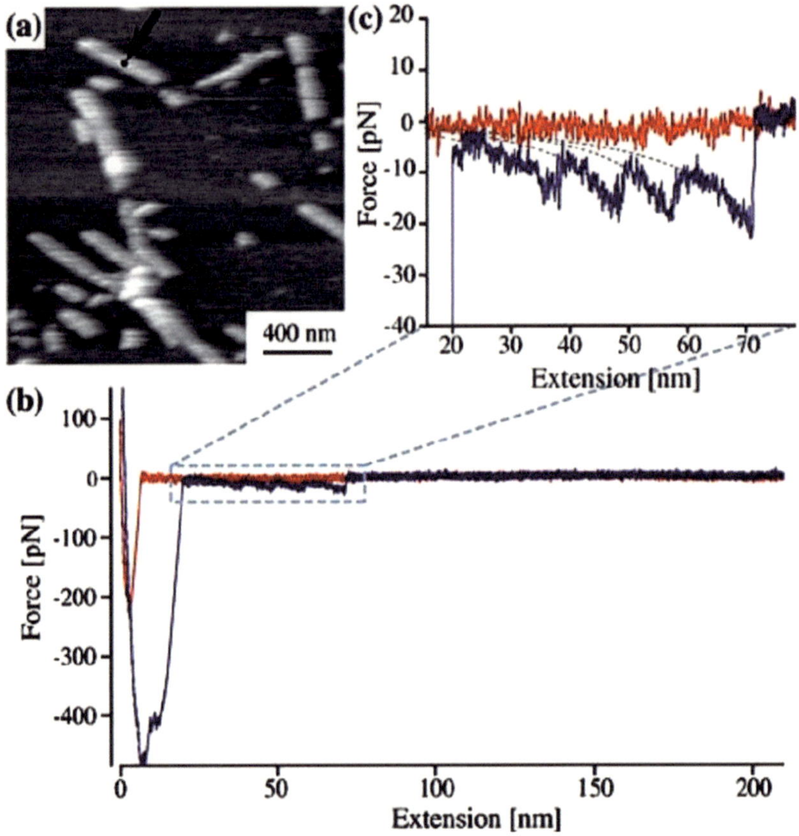

Fig. 7. Sawtooth like force curve obtained by the AFM manipulation of TTR amyloid fibrils (Fukuma, et al., 2006).

birefringence observed with cross-polarized light after Congo red dye staining. However, either direct imaging by AFM or separation from the EPS matrix is very difficult because of the complex structure and composition of EPS. However, under AFM force spectroscopy, uniform and reproducible sawtooth patterns were observed in high abundance, appearing in 20% to 50% of all the obtained force curves, depending on different regions. By fitting with WLC model, a mean persistence length of 0.34 ± 0.18 nm was obtained, which is similar to that of the titin protein (0.4 nm) (Rief, et al., 1997; Tskhovrebova, et al., 1997) or tenascin (0.42 nm) (Oberhauser et al., 1998). The mean value of the force peaks was also found to be typical for systems containing hydrogen-bonded β-sheets (Brockwell et al., 2005). Therefore, it is reasonable to propose the possible presence of highly ordered amyloid structures in EPS.

More recently, the role of amyloid fibrils in natural adhesives was confirmed by an extensive study on barnacle cement (Sullan, et al., 2009). The versatility of the AFM technique was well illustrated in this work. First, an AFM imaging was conducted to reveal the diverse morphologies of the sample, as shown in Figure 8. Then, AFM indentation tests were performed at three points in images C, D, and E. The corresponding structures were large regular rods, unstructured aggregates, and the matrix, having elastic moduli of 20-90 MPa, 0.2-2 MPa, and 1-10 MPa, respectively. Furthermore, force spectroscopy was

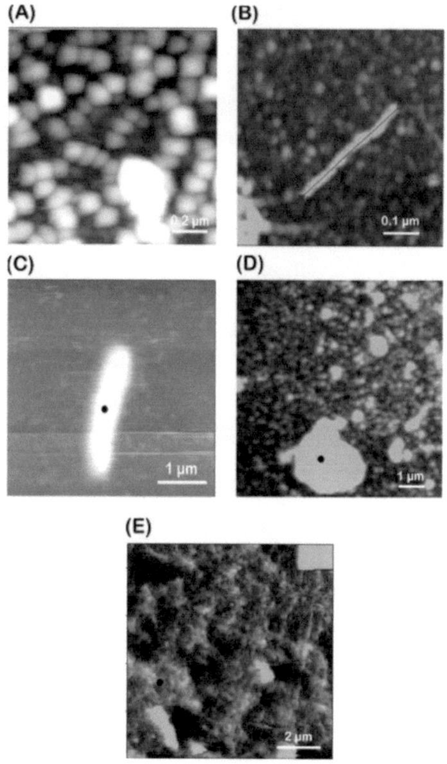

Fig. 8. A-E: Different morphologies in the barnacle cement sample. Black dots in C, D, E indicates the AFM indentation points (Sullan et al., 2009).

performed. The sawtooth pattern was observed when the tip was indented into the matrix and pulled out. However, even more periodic sawtooth pattern was obtained when the "fly-fishing" method (Rief, et al., 1997) was used. This method avoids indentation into the matrix, thus reduces the possibility of picking up multiple molecules in a single pull. Fitting the force curve with WLC model gave a persistence length of 0.35 ± 0.05 nm, which agrees pretty well with previous results on amyloid fibrils (Kellermayer, et al., 2005; Mostaert, et al., 2006). In addition, FT-IR spectroscopy and dye (Congo red and thioflavin T) staining confirmed the presence of β-sheet and amyloid structures in the sample.

The force curve patterns of amyloid fibrils under AFM manipulation are closely related to the structure and mechanical stability of the fibrils. AFM force spectroscopy on mature amyloid fibrils formed by glucagon peptides, which has uniform twisted fibrillar structures, revealed a simple force curve pattern (M. D. Dong, et al., 2008). All of the force curves exhibited non-linear elastic mechanical response followed by one or several rupture events. The absence of force plateau, which is a characteristic pattern of the unzipping of β-sheets from the fibril, implies that the high packing density in mature glucagon amyloid fibrils allows a stable confinement of the peptide molecules in the twisted fibrillar structure, in contrast to Aβ amyloid fibrils (Karsai et al., 2006; Kellermayer, et al., 2005). The stable structure is further confirmed by repeatedly stretching a single fibril for 1000 times. The resultant force curves showed surprisingly reversible and reproducible non-linear elasticity, with a narrow distribution of both the rupture length and rupture force (Figure 9 (a)). The remarkable clean and well-defined force curves are explained by the binding of the tip to a single amyloid fibril and subsequent successive stretching between the tip and substrate, with each stretch ending with the fibril being detached from the substrate (Figure 9 (b), vi2).

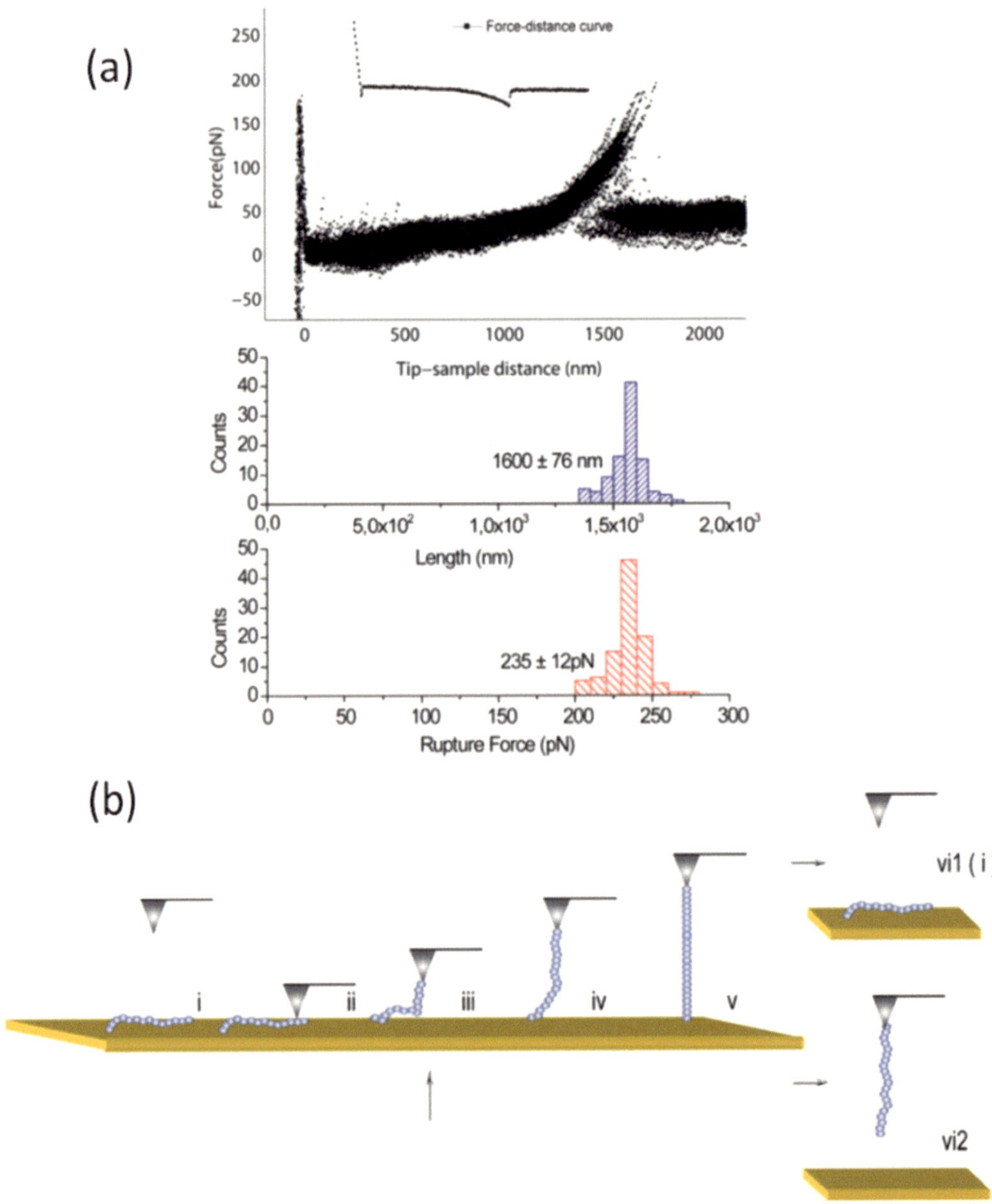

Fig. 9. Nonlinear elastic response recorded in a successive stretching (a) and schematic illustration of the possible stretching models (b) (M. D. Dong et al., 2008).

By varying the preparation conditions, the effect of disturbing factors on the mechanical stability of amyloid fibril formation can be explored. Recently, the effect of shear on the formation of β-lactoglobulin (β-Lg) amyloid fibrils is investigated with AFM imaging and force spectroscopy (Dunstan et al., 2009). Three conditions were investigated: nature environment, variable shear, and controlled shear. Force plateau, which was attributed to the peeling off of β-sheets from the amyloid fibrils, was used as an indicator of the mechanical strength of the assembled fibrils. Amyloid fibrils formed from controlled shear have significantly lower mechanical strength (force magnitude ~20 pN) than those formed from variable shear (~100 pN). This result indicates that variant shear induced fibrils are densely packed and well-ordered. The conclusion is further supported by AFM imaging. For variable shear induced fibrils, twisted morphology, which is of higher order, was observed. The presence of thick fibrils (5~8 nm) was the result of the assembly of protofibrils. In contrast, the controlled shear induced fibrils have lower height (~4 nm) and "string-of-beads" morphology, which is believed to be formed from partially unfolded monomers. Therefore, the variable shear induced fibrils are in a more mature state and those formed from controlled shear are less mature.

In most AFM based force spectroscopy measurements, the sample is attached to the tip by non-specific, intermolecular interactions. The method is straightforward and easy to perform. However, if more precise binding of the molecule is required, covalent bonding provide much more control on the binding position as well as guaranteed binding stability. In a force spectroscopy study of amyloid formed from human prion protein (PrP90-231), protein was attached by linking the engineered Cys residue to gold-covered AFM tip by gold-thiol bonding (Ganchev et al., 2008). In contrast to the irregular and poorly reproducible curves observed for the wild-type protein or Cys-variant (at position 103) probed with silicon nitride tip, similar elastic stretching was observed for each force curve of the covalently linked system. The contour length histogram from the WLC modeling of the force curves is well-defined, with 24-25 nm as the maximum, suggesting that ~63-66 residues can be stretched entropically before the whole protein is fully pulled out from the amyloid fibrils (assuming 0.38 nm per residue in a fully extended conformation), as illustrated in Figure 10. It is reasonable to assume that the ~63-66 residues are located out of the hydrogen-bonded core and the residues involved in the fibril core start at residue ~166-169. Further evidence was provided by moving the engineered Cys residue to position 90, which resulted similar starting point at residue ~164-166. Thus the results are reliable and provide important information for the structure of PrP amyloid fibrils.

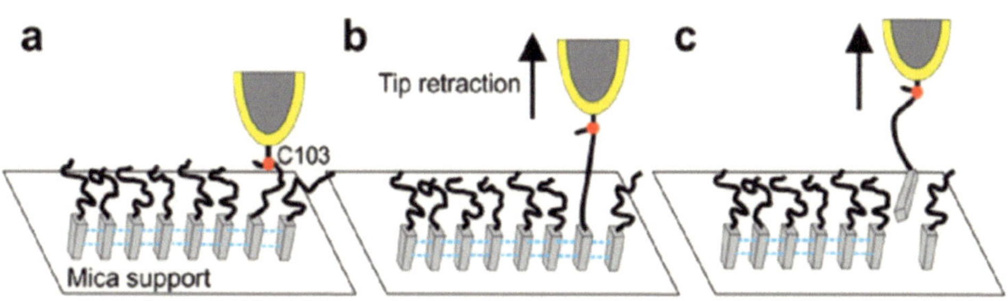

Fig. 10. Illustration of the stretching of a protein and final pull out from the core of amyloid fibrils (Ganchev, et al., 2008).

In another recent example, α-synuclein proteins (which forms amyloid associated with Parkinson's disease) were covalently attached to the tip and substrate surface separately, and their interaction was probed by AFM force spectroscopy. The testing pH was varied to investigate pH dependency. It has long been recognized that amyloid fibril formation is facilitated in acidic pH (Stine et al., 2003). The rupture force between the two proteins increases with decreasing pH, suggesting that lower pH increases the protein intermolecular interactions, facilitating protein aggregation to form amyloid fibrils, which is consistent with previous results (Lyubchenko et al., 2005). By pulling the molecules at different pulling rates, the dynamics of protein interactions can be revealed. The so-called dynamic force spectroscopy was again performed at different pH. At all pH, the rupture force increases dramatically with loading rate (pulling rate), which is defined as high loading rate dependency. By fitting with appropriate model, the lifetime of the molecular complex (dimer) was determined to be seconds, which is significantly longer than nanosecond lifetime from a recent report on structure dynamics of the α-synuclein monomer (Tsigelny et al., 2007). As a result, the formation of protein dimer significantly increases the stability of the protein molecules, which might serve as a critical nucleation step towards the aggregation of proteins to form amyloid fibrils.

4. Conclusion and perspectives

In this chapter, we have learnt from works published in the past 6 years that AFM is a powerful tool for studying the nanomechanics of amyloid materials. Typical working modes such as nanoindentation, force spectroscopy with stretching of the amyloid fibrils, or unzipping of β-sheets from the fibrils can be performed on a single platform (Figure 11 (a), (b), (c)). Combined with AFM imaging, AFM based nanoindentation makes it possible to identify a specific amyloid fibril and measure its mechanical response. The method has also revealed the huge different between the axial and radial Young's moduli of the amyloid fibrils, which is closely related to their molecular structures. AFM based force spectroscopy has showed several response pattern of amyloid fibrils under AFM manipulation. Depending on their composition and structural stability, unzipping of β-sheets, stretching of peptide molecules, stretching of an amyloid fibril have been observed. The force curve patterns, either non-linear elastic response or plateau or the superposing of the two, have been related to the morphology, packing density, stage of maturation, as well as the interactions with the environment.

The field of amyloid nanomechanics is still quite young, and what has been done has only utilized a fraction of the powerfulness of AFM. For example, covalent attachment of amyloid fibrils on the AFM tip for force spectroscopy, which will provide high accuracy and efficiency of binding, has rarely been used (Ganchev, et al., 2008; Yu et al., 2008). We expect more sophisticated AFM technique like tip modification, dynamic force spectroscopy, etc., would push AFM based research on amyloid mechanical properties to more fundamental level, single molecule force spectroscopy (SMFS), for example (Figure 11 (d)). If the tip is modified with a peptide chain or protein molecule, the interaction between single peptide or protein molecule and amyloid fibril can be probed by AFM based SMFS. The proposed method would help to identify amyloid proteins interacting with important cell surface receptors, as these proteins may be directly involved in toxicity. In addition we expect this method will also reveal more information about the surface properties, chemical composition of amyloid materials, and modulating the activity between amyloid proteins and cells.

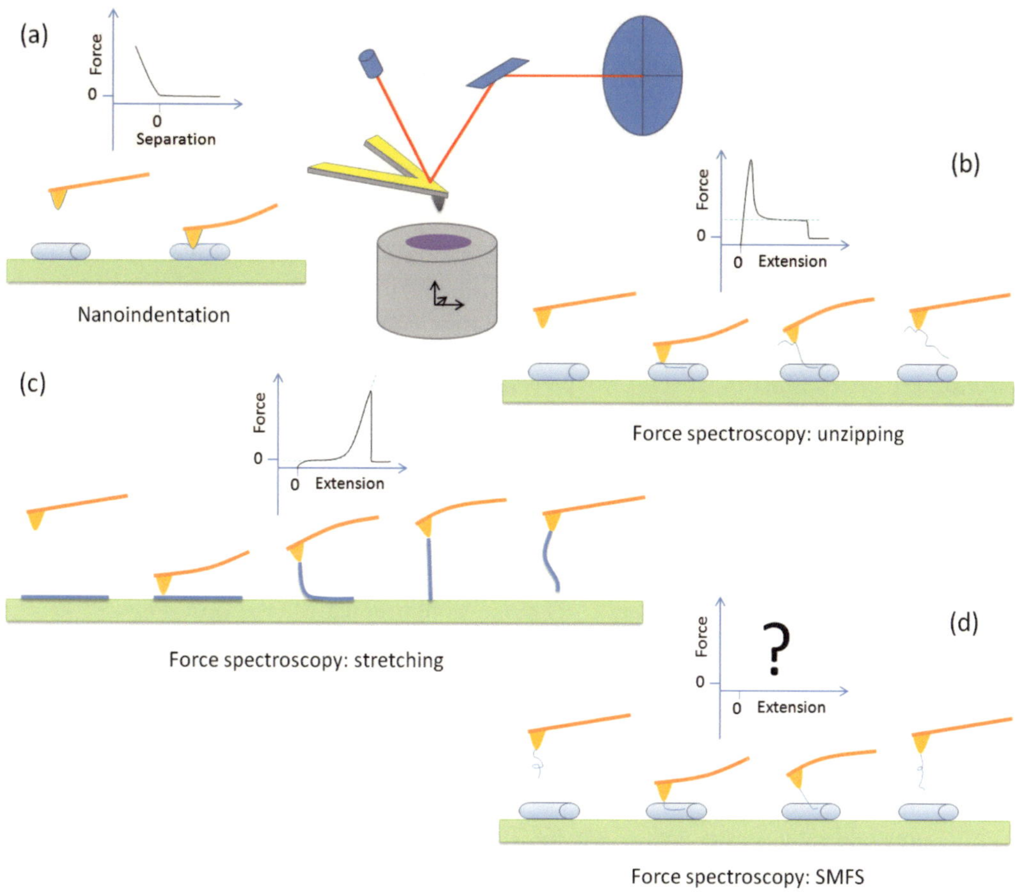

Fig. 11. Summary of AFM based study on the nanomechanics of amyloid materials and future possibility.

On the other hand, AFM is a fast-developing technique, with new progresses being made every year. Among them, quantitative nanomechanical mapping (QNM) (M. Dong & Sahin, 2011; M. D. Dong et al., 2009) is noteworthy, as it has already been applied to measurement mechanical properties of amyloid fibrils (Adamcik et al., 2011; Sweers et al., 2011). QNM records a force curve at every point on the sample and uses peak force value of the force curve as imaging feedback. The advantage is that mechanical properties such as Young's modulus, adhesion, deformation, and dissipation can be calculated and exported simultaneously in real time. QNM makes the measurement of surface mechanical properties quite straightforward (Adamcik, et al., 2011).

The ability of mapping surface mechanical properties without compromising the resolution is attractive, as it will be helpful to study the heterogeneity of amyloid fibrils, identifying different stages of amyloid growth.

However, potential problems may exist in the convenient measurement technique. Because normally data analysis is automatically processed, users have limited control, which makes it hard to correct errors from finite sample thickness, deviation from standard model, etc., according to the specific system investigated (Sweers, et al., 2011). Thus it is still very important to understand the data analysis process and evaluate potential system errors it may bring about.

5. References

Adamcik, J., Berquand, A., & Mezzenga, R. (2011). Single-step direct measurement of amyloid fibrils stiffness by peak force quantitative nanomechanical atomic force microscopy. *Applied Physics Letters, 98* (19), 193701.

Akhremitchev, B. B., & Walker, G. C. (1999). Finite sample thickness effects on elasticity determination using atomic force microscopy. *Langmuir, 15* (17), 5630-5634.

Alonso, J. L., & Goldmann, W. H. (2003). Feeling the forces: atomic force microscopy in cell biology. *Life Sciences, 72* (23), 2553-2560.

Ashkin, A., Dziedzic, J. M., Bjorkholm, J. E., & Chu, S. (1986). Observation of a Single-Beam Gradient Force Optical Trap for Dielectric Particles. *Optics Letters, 11* (5), 288-290.

Barrau, S., Zhang, F., Herland, A., Mammo, W., Andersson, M. R., & Inganas, O. (2008). Integration of amyloid nanowires in organic solar cells. *Applied Physics Letters, 93* (2), 023307.

Binnig, G., Quate, C. F., & Gerber, C. (1986). Atomic Force Microscope. *Physical Review Letters, 56* (9), 930-933.

Brockwell, D. J., Beddard, G. S., Paci, E., West, D. K., Olmsted, P. D., Smith, D. A., et al. (2005). Mechanically unfolding the small, topologically simple protein L. *Biophysical Journal, 89* (1), 506-519.

Bucciantini, M., Giannoni, E., Chiti, F., Baroni, F., Formigli, L., Zurdo, J. S., et al. (2002). Inherent toxicity of aggregates implies a common mechanism for protein misfolding diseases. *Nature, 416* (6880), 507-511.

Carny, O., Shalev, D. E., & Gazit, E. (2006). Fabrication of coaxial metal nanocables using a self-assembled peptide nanotube scaffold. *Nano Letters, 6* (8), 1594-1597.

Channon, K. J., Devlin, G. L., & MacPhee, C. E. (2009). Efficient Energy Transfer within Self-Assembling Peptide Fibers: A Route to Light-Harvesting Nanomaterials. *Journal of the American Chemical Society, 131* (35), 12520-12521.

Chapman, M. R., Robinson, L. S., Pinkner, J. S., Roth, R., Heuser, J., Hammar, M., et al. (2002). Role of Escherichia coli curli operons in directing amyloid fiber formation. *Science, 295* (5556), 851-855.

Chiti, F., & Dobson, C. M. (2006). Protein misfolding, functional amyloid, and human disease. *Annual Review of Biochemistry, 75*, 333-366.

Cook, S., Schaffer, T. E., Chynoweth, K. M., Wigton, M., Simmonds, R. W., & Lang, K. M. (2006). Practical implementation of dynamic methods for measuring atomic force microscope cantilever spring constants. *Nanotechnology, 17* (9), 2135-2145.

de Pablo, P. J., Schaap, I. A. T., MacKintosh, F. C., & Schmidt, C. F. (2003). Deformation and collapse of microtubules on the nanometer scale. *Physical Review Letters, 91* (9), 098101.

Derjaguin, B. V., Muller, V. M., & Toporov, Y. P. (1975). Effect of contact deformations on the adhesion of particles. *Journal of Colloid and Interface Science, 53* (2), 314-326.

Dobson, C. M. (1999). Protein misfolding, evolution and disease. *Trends in Biochemical Sciences, 24* (9), 329-332.

Dobson, C. M., Smith, J. F., Knowles, T. P. J., MacPhee, C. E., & Welland, M. E. (2006). Characterization of the nanoscale properties of individual amyloid fibrils. *Proceedings of the National Academy of Sciences of the United States of America, 103* (43), 15806-15811.

Dong, M., & Sahin, O. (2011). A nanomechanical interface to rapid single-molecule interactions. [10.1038/ncomms1246]. *Nature Communications, 2*, 247.

Dong, M. D., Hovgaard, M. B., Mamdouh, W., Xu, S. L., Otzen, D. E., & Besenbacher, F. (2008). AFM-based force spectroscopy measurements of mature amyloid fibrils of the peptide glucagon. *Nanotechnology, 19* (38), 384013.

Dong, M. D., Husale, S., & Sahin, O. (2009). Determination of protein structural flexibility by microsecond force spectroscopy. *Nature Nanotechnology, 4* (8), 514-517.

Dunstan, D. E., Hamilton-Brown, P., Asimakis, P., Ducker, W., & Bertolini, J. (2009). Shear-induced structure and mechanics of beta-lactoglobulin amyloid fibrils. *Soft Matter, 5* (24), 5020-5028.

Ellis-Behnke, R. G., Liang, Y. X., You, S. W., Tay, D. K. C., Zhang, S. G., So, K. F., et al. (2006). Nano neuro knitting: Peptide nanofiber scaffold for brain repair and axon regeneration with functional return of vision (vol 103, pg 5054, 2006). *Proceedings of the National Academy of Sciences of the United States of America, 103* (19), 7530-7530.

Flamia, R., Zhdan, P. A., Castle, J. E., & Tamburro, A. M. (2008). Comment on the mechanical properties of the amyloid fibre, poly (ValGlyGlyLeuGly), obtained by a novel AFM methodology. *Journal of Materials Science, 43* (1), 395-397.

Fowler, D. M., Koulov, A. V., Alory-Jost, C., Marks, M. S., Balch, W. E., & Kelly, J. W. (2005). Functional Amyloid Formation within Mammalian Tissue. *PLoS Biol, 4* (1), e6.

Fowler, D. M., Koulov, A. V., Balch, W. E., & Kelly, J. W. (2007). Functional amyloid - from bacteria to humans. *Trends in Biochemical Sciences, 32* (5), 217-224.

Fukuma, T., Mostaert, A. S., & Jarvis, S. P. (2006). Explanation for the mechanical strength of amyloid fibrils. *Tribology Letters, 22* (3), 233-237.

Ganchev, D. N., Cobb, N. J., Surewicz, K., & Surewicz, W. K. (2008). Nanomechanical properties of human prion protein amyloid as probed by force spectroscopy. *Biophysical Journal, 95* (6), 2909-2915.

Gibson, C. T., Smith, D. A., & Roberts, C. J. (2005). Calibration of silicon atomic force microscope cantilevers. *Nanotechnology, 16* (2), 234-238.

Guo, S., & Akhremitchev, B. B. (2006). Packing Density and Structural Heterogeneity of Insulin Amyloid Fibrils Measured by AFM Nanoindentation. *Biomacromolecules, 7* (5), 1630-1636.

Holmes, T. C., de Lacalle, S., Su, X., Liu, G. S., Rich, A., & Zhang, S. G. (2000). Extensive neurite outgrowth and active synapse formation on self-assembling peptide scaffolds. *Proceedings of the National Academy of Sciences of the United States of America, 97* (12), 6728-6733.

Jaroniec, C. P., MacPhee, C. E., Bajaj, V. S., McMahon, M. T., Dobson, C. M., & Griffin, R. G. (2004). High-resolution molecular structure of a peptide in an amyloid fibril determined by magic angle spinning NMR spectroscopy. *Proceedings of the National Academy of Sciences of the United States of America, 101* (3), 711-716.

Johnson, K. L. (1985). Contact mechanics. Cambridge, U.K.: Cambridge University Press.

Johnson, K. L., Kendall, K., & Roberts, A. D. (1971). Surface Energy and the Contact of Elastic Solids. *Proceedings of the Royal Society of London. A. Mathematical and Physical Sciences, 324* (1558), 301-313.

Karsai, Á., Mártonfalvi, Z., Nagy, A., Grama, L., Penke, B., & Kellermayer, M. S. Z. (2006). Mechanical manipulation of Alzheimer's amyloid β1–42 fibrils. *Journal of Structural Biology, 155* (2), 316-326.

Kellermayer, M. S. Z., Grama, L., Karsai, A., Nagy, A., Kahn, A., Datki, Z. L., et al. (2005). Reversible mechanical unzipping of amyloid beta-fibrils. *Journal of Biological Chemistry, 280* (9), 8464-8470.

Kis, A., Kasas, S., Babic, B., Kulik, A. J., Benoit, W., Briggs, G. A. D., et al. (2002). Nanomechanics of microtubules. *Physical Review Letters, 89* (24), 248101.

Kol, N., Adler-Abramovich, L., Barlam, D., Shneck, R. Z., Gazit, E., & Rousso, I. (2005). Self-assembled peptide nanotubes are uniquely rigid bioinspired supramolecular structures. *Nano Letters, 5* (7), 1343-1346.

Liang, Y., Guo, P., Pingali, S. V., Pabit, S., Thiyagarajan, P., Berland, K. M., et al. (2008). Light harvesting antenna on an amyloid scaffold. *Chemical Communications* (48), 6522-6524.

Luhrs, T., Ritter, C., Adrian, M., Riek-Loher, D., Bohrmann, B., Doeli, H., et al. (2005). 3D structure of Alzheimer's amyloid-beta (1-42) fibrils. *Proceedings of the National Academy of Sciences of the United States of America, 102* (48), 17342-17347.

Lyubchenko, Y. L., McAllister, C., Karymov, M. A., Kawano, Y., Lushnikov, A. Y., Mikheikin, A., et al. (2005). Protein interactions and misfolding analyzed by AFM force spectroscopy. *Journal of Molecular Biology, 354* (5), 1028-1042.

Maji, S. K., Schubert, D., Rivier, C., Lee, S., Rivier, J. E., & Riek, R. (2008). Amyloid as a depot for the formulation of long-acting drugs. *Plos Biology, 6* (2), 240-252.

Morozov, V. N., & Morozova, T. Y. (1993). Elasticity of Globular-Proteins - the Relation between Mechanics, Thermodynamics and Mobility. *Journal of Biomolecular Structure & Dynamics, 11* (3), 459-481.

Mostaert, A. S., Higgins, M. J., Fukuma, T., Rindi, F., & Jarvis, S. P. (2006). Nanoscale mechanical characterisation of amyloid fibrils discovered in a natural adhesive. *Journal of Biological Physics, 32* (5), 393-401.

Mostaert, A. S., & Jarvis, S. P. (2007). Beneficial characteristics of mechanically functional amyloid fibrils evolutionarily preserved in natural adhesives. *Nanotechnology, 18* (4).

Muller, V. M., Derjaguin, B. V., & Toporov, Y. P. (1983). On two methods of calculation of the force of sticking of an elastic sphere to a rigid plane. *Colloids and Surfaces, 7* (3), 251-259.

Neuman, K. C., & Nagy, A. (2008). Single-molecule force spectroscopy: optical tweezers, magnetic tweezers and atomic force microscopy. [10.1038/nmeth.1218]. *Nature Methods, 5* (6), 491-505.

Oberhauser, A. F., Marszalek, P. E., Erickson, H. P., & Fernandez, J. M. (1998). The molecular elasticity of the extracellular matrix protein tenascin. *Nature, 393* (6681), 181-185.

Oda, T., Wals, P., Osterburg, H. H., Johnson, S. A., Pasinetti, G. M., Morgan, T. E., et al. (1995). Clusterin (Apoj) Alters the Aggregation of Amyloid Beta-Peptide (a-Beta (1-42)) and Forms Slowly Sedimenting a-Beta Complexes That Cause Oxidative Stress. *Experimental Neurology, 136* (1), 22-31.

Ohler, B. (2007). Cantilever spring constant calibration using laser Doppler vibrometry. *Review of Scientific Instruments, 78* (6), 063701.

Paravastu, A. K., Leapman, R. D., Yau, W. M., & Tycko, R. (2008). Molecular structural basis for polymorphism in Alzheimer's beta-amyloid fibrils. *Proceedings of the National Academy of Sciences of the United States of America, 105* (47), 18349-18354.

Perutz, M. F., Finch, J. T., Berriman, J., & Lesk, A. (2002). Amyloid fibers are water-filled nanotubes. *Proceedings of the National Academy of Sciences of the United States of America, 99* (8), 5591-5595.

Reches, M., & Gazit, E. (2003). Casting metal nanowires within discrete self-assembled peptide nanotubes. *Science, 300* (5619), 625-627.

Rief, M., Gautel, M., Oesterhelt, F., Fernandez, J. M., & Gaub, H. E. (1997). Reversible unfolding of individual titin immunoglobulin domains by AFM. *Science, 276* (5315), 1109-1112.

Salvetat, J. P., Briggs, G. A. D., Bonard, J. M., Bacsa, R. R., Kulik, A. J., Stockli, T., et al. (1999). Elastic and shear moduli of single-walled carbon nanotube ropes. *Physical Review Letters, 82* (5), 944-947.

Sawaya, M. R., Sambashivan, S., Nelson, R., Ivanova, M. I., Sievers, S. A., Apostol, M. I., et al. (2007). Atomic structures of amyloid cross-beta spines reveal varied steric zippers. *Nature, 447* (7143), 453-457.

Scheibel, T., Parthasarathy, R., Sawicki, G., Lin, X. M., Jaeger, H., & Lindquist, S. L. (2003). Conducting nanowires built by controlled self-assembly of amyloid fibers and selective metal deposition. *Proceedings of the National Academy of Sciences of the United States of America, 100* (8), 4527-4532.

Selkoe, D. J. (2001). Alzheimer's disease: Genes, proteins, and therapy. *Physiological Reviews, 81* (2), 741-766.

Shackelford, J., Alexander, W., & Park, J. (1995). *CRC Practical Handbook of Materials Selection* (1st Ed ed.). Boca Raton, FL: CRC.

Shibayama, Y., Joseph, K., Nakazawa, Y., Ghebreihiwet, B., Peerschke, E. I. B., & Kaplan, A. P. (1999). Zinc-dependent activation of the plasma kinin-forming cascade by aggregated beta amyloid protein. *Clinical Immunology, 90* (1), 89-99.

Sneddon, I. N. (1965). The Relation between Load and Penetration in the Axisymmetric Boussinesq Problem for a Punch of Arbitrary Profile. *INt. J. Eng. Sci., 3*, 11.

Stine, W. B., Dahlgren, K. N., Krafft, G. A., & LaDu, M. J. (2003). In vitro characterization of conditions for amyloid-beta peptide oligomerization and fibrillogenesis. *Journal of Biological Chemistry, 278* (13), 11612-11622.

Strick, T., Allemand, J. F., Croquette, V., & Bensimon, D. (2000). Twisting and stretching single DNA molecules. *Progress in Biophysics & Molecular Biology, 74* (1-2), 115-140.

Sullan, R. M. A., Gunari, N., Tanur, A. E., Yuri, C., Dickinson, G. H., Orihuela, B., et al. (2009). Nanoscale structures and mechanics of barnacle cement. *Biofouling, 25* (3), 263-275.

Sweers, K., van der Werf, K., Bennink, M., & Subramaniam, V. (2011). Nanomechanical properties of alpha-synuclein amyloid fibrils: a comparative study by nanoindentation, harmonic force microscopy, and Peakforce QNM. *Nanoscale Research Letters, 6, 270.*

Tan, S. Y., & Pepys, M. B. (1994). Amyloidosis. *Histopathology, 25* (5), 403-414.

Toyama, B. H., & Weissman, J. S. (2011). Amyloid Structure: Conformational Diversity and Consequences. In R. D. Kornberg, C. R. H. Raetz, J. E. Rothman & J. W. Thorner (Eds.), *Annual Review of Biochemistry, Vol 80* (Vol. 80, pp. 557-585).

Tsigelny, I. F., Bar-On, P., Sharikov, Y., Crews, L., Hashimoto, M., Miller, M. A., et al. (2007). Dynamics of alpha-synuclein aggregation and inhibition of pore-like oligomer development by beta-synuclein. *Febs Journal, 274* (7), 1862-1877.

Tskhovrebova, L., Trinick, J., Sleep, J. A., & Simmons, R. M. (1997). Elasticity and unfolding of single molecules of the giant muscle protein titin. *Nature, 387* (6630), 308-312.

VanLandingham, M. R., Juliano, T. F., & Hagon, M. J. (2005). Measuring tip shape for instrumented indentation using atomic force microscopy. *Measurement Science & Technology, 16* (11), 2173-2185.

Vollrath, F., & Knight, D. P. (2001). Liquid crystalline spinning of spider silk. *Nature, 410* (6828), 541-548.

Wasmer, C., Lange, A., Van Melckebeke, H., Siemer, A. B., Riek, R., & Meier, B. H. (2008). Amyloid fibrils of the HET-s (218-289) prion form a beta solenoid with a triangular hydrophobic core. *Science, 319* (5869), 1523-1526.

Weisenhorn, A. L., Hansma, P. K., Albrecht, T. R., & Quate, C. F. (1989). Forces in Atomic Force Microscopy in Air and Water. *Applied Physics Letters, 54* (26), 2651-2653.

Westermark, G. T., Johnson, K. H., & Westermark, P. (1999). [1] Staining methods for identification of amyloid in tissue. In W. Ronald (Ed.), *Methods in Enzymology* (Vol. Volume 309, pp. 3-25): Academic Press.

Yu, J., Malkova, S., & Lyubchenko, Y. L. (2008). α-Synuclein Misfolding: Single Molecule AFM Force Spectroscopy Study. *Journal of Molecular Biology, 384* (4), 992-1001.

Zenhausern, F., Adrian, M., Tenheggelerbordier, B., Eng, L. M., & Descouts, P. (1992). DNA and Rna-Polymerase DNA Complex Imaged by Scanning Force Microscopy - Influence of Molecular-Scale Friction. *Scanning, 14* (4), 212-217.

Part 3

DNA, Chromatin and Membranes

8

Analyzing DNA Structure Quantitatively at a Single-Molecule Level by Atomic Force Microscopy

Yong Jiang and Yuan Yin
School of Chemistry and Chemical Engineering, Southeast University, Nanjing
P. R. China

1. Introduction

The atomic force microscope (AFM), one of the most popular types of scanning probe microscopy, was invented by Binnig *et al* [1] in 1986. After that, its quick development resulted in the commercial AFM available at 1989 to the biological and chemical researchers. Two decades after its invention, now it has become a standard measurement technique in multiple branches of science and technology. The AFM's advantage over other techniques stems from its ability to work in different environment. It can work in vacuum, liquid, or ambient, and in addition its high resolution and sensitivity to measure spatial sizes and forces, respectively. The technique thus not only provides sharp images of nonconductive surfaces at a resolution of nanometer scale, but also enables the measurements of intra- or inter-molecular forces at a resolution of pico-newton scale. These properties make AFM ideal for biological samples, especially for DNA molecules.

The schematic in Figure 1A illustrates the basic principles of the AFM operation. A sharp tip reads the profile of the sample by scanning the surface. The tip is attached to a cantilever that works as a spring pressing the tip against the sample. The vertical position of the tip is measured by a laser reflected from the cantilever to the position of sensitive photo detector (PSPD). Three important features of the AFM instrument are listed below. First, the position of the sample relative to the tip is controlled by the scanner and it can be done with accuracy better than 1 nm. Second, the tip may be made tremendously sharp or customized for the desired measurement. Third, the vertical displacement of the tip relative to the surface is determined with sub-nanometer precision. These three major features allow AFM to provide the topographic image with nanometer resolution.

Figure 1B illustrates the major operation modes of the AFM. The manner of the microscope operation corresponding to the attraction part of the tip-sample interaction potential is non-contact mode (NC-AFM) [3]. A breakthrough in the high-resolution AFM imaging was made with implementation of the NC-AFM mode, offering a unique tool for real space atomic-scale studies of surfaces and nanoparticles. The probe of NC mode does not contact the sample surface, but oscillates above the adsorbed fluid layer on the surface during scanning. Using a feedback loop to monitor changes in the amplitude due to attractive forces the surface topography can be measured. After tip-surface attraction force passes the minimum

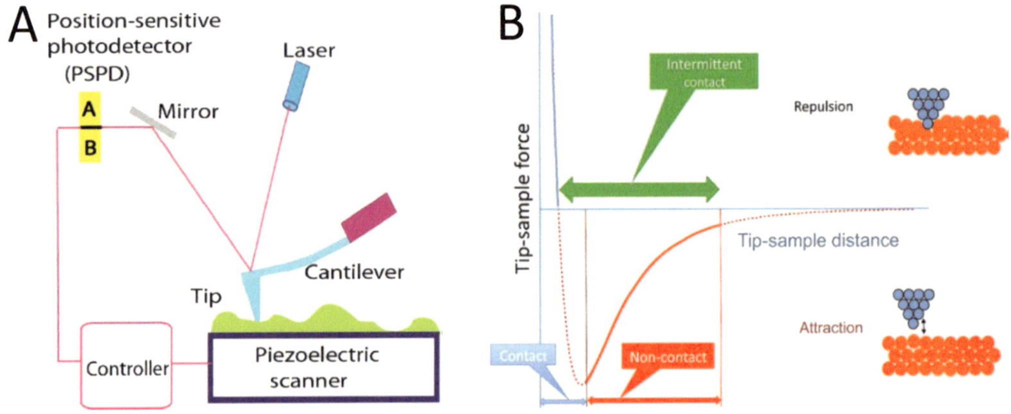

Fig. 1. (A) Schematic explaining the principles of AFM operation. The position of the tip relative to the sample is controlled by a piezoelectric scanner. The vertical displacement of the tip during scanning is detected using the optical lever principle, in which the position of the light spot on the position of sensitive photo detector (PSPD) is measured. (B) Scheme explains the operation modes of the AFM. A curve in the scheme shows the change of the tip-sample interaction depending on the distance between the apex of the tip and the sample. (Adapted and modified from reference [2], with permission)

on the potential curve, the repulsion interaction increases very fast, achieving large positive values in the very short range of the tip-sample distances. This scanning way is called contact mode. Since the interaction of the tip and the surface is so strong, the deformation of a soft sample typically occurs, and as the results of it, the soft sample may be damaged or moved by the sharp tip. Schematically, this deformation is occurred in the top right cartoon by displacement of the red spheres [3]. For hard samples at small tip-surface separation, the pressure created by the tip at the apex is so large that atoms can jump from tip to surface and vice versa. Therefore, contact mode of the AFM operation does not obtain reliable and stable images at atomic resolution for both soft and hard sample. In addition, damage or movement of soft biological samples can be made to the tip during approach or scanning process. Tapping modes with small pressure can obtain reliable and stable images at atomic resolution for any samples. The imaging of tapping Mode is alike to contact mode. However, in this mode the cantilever is oscillated at its resonant frequency. The probe lightly "taps" on the sample surface during scanning, contacting the surface at the bottom of its swing. By maintaining constant oscillation amplitude, a constant tip-sample interaction is maintained and an image of the surface is obtained. Tapping mode allows high resolution of samples that are easily damaged or loosely held to a surface, especially good for biological samples. As a summary, non-contact and tapping modes are two optional modes for DNA imaging.

Since the AFM physically interacts with the sample, the AFM can work as a force spectroscopy by stretching a single molecule between the tip and sample surface. If the spring constant of the cantilever is obtained, the AFM is an excellent force spectroscopy for probing the mechanical properties of individual molecules because it can measure their length and tension with nanometer (nM) and piconewton (pN) resolution, respectively. The working principle of an AFM force spectroscopy is shown in Figure 2. A laser is reflected

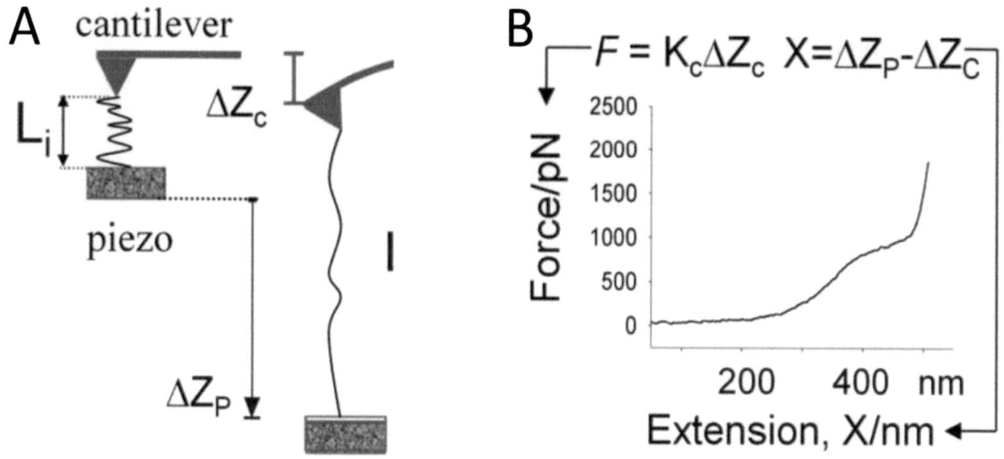

Fig. 2. AFM force spectroscopy: (A) Diagram of a single stretching experiment; (B) Example of a force extension curve, with definitions of force and extension. (Adapted and modified from reference [4], with permission)

off the back of the cantilever onto the center of the PSPD. The sample is fixed on the piezoelectric positioner and the molecules on the sample can attach to the tip by moving up the sample to physical contact it. The molecules are normally connected on the substrate or tip by nonspecific adsorption or designed chemical bond. In this way, the molecules form bridges between the substrate and the tip (Figure 2A). These molecules can be stretched and relaxed in a controlled manner by moving the substrate away and back from the tip. The stretched molecule exerts a mechanical force on the cantilever, thereby deflecting it. Because the force applied is much smaller than the chemical bond between the molecule and substrate or tip, the molecule will not detached from the substrate or tip during repeated stretching. This deflection is measured by the photodiode as a change in the voltage generated by the movement of the incident laser beam off of the photodiode center. The experimental result is a force-distance curve (force spectrogram) that reflects the elasticity of a single molecule, which for example was shown in Figure 2B.

In the last decade, AFM has proven to be one of most valuable techniques for the studies of DNA and the researches were mostly focused on the biological structure and dynamic processes of DNA [5-10]. However, AFM is normally used to gain qualitative results at a single-molecular level. By analyzing the topological structure of each DNA molecule from AFM images, the distributions of DNA with different configurations can be identified directly and easily. Due to this advantage, AFM imaging can also be ideal tool for quantifying DNA structure under a wide range of DNA amounts, concentrations and sizes that may not able to be handled by other methods. It has been demonstrated that AFM is capable of quantifying DNA plasmids with the amount less than 1 pico gram and the size up to 100 kilo base pairs. However, the application of AFM techniques in quantitative research is limited because of the lack of comparative studies with other traditional and well-established methods, such as gel electrophoresis. After we compared the results obtained by AFM with that obtained by gel electrophoresis [11-14], AFM was proven to be an accurate method in the identification and quantification of the DNA with different topological structures. Therefore, the purpose of this chapter is to present this single-molecule AFM imaging and force spectroscopy techniques that we developed for sensitive and quantitative analysis of DNA structure. We believe that this chapter will help to expand the application of AFM techniques in DNA research.

2. Materials and methods

2.1 Materials

pUC18, 2686 base pairs (bp), was isolated from *E. coli* and purified using the QIAFILTER plasmid maxi kit (QIAGEN Inc). pNEBR-R1 was purchased from New England Biolabs (Beverly, MA). Single-stranded poly(dA) was purchased from Sigma-Aldrich, Inc. (St. Louis, MO).

2.2 Sample preparation

For experiments in which the imaging buffer contains Mg^{2+}, freshly cleaved mica was used as DNA substrate directly. For experiments in which the imaging buffer did not have Mg^{2+}, 1-(3-Aminopropyl)-silatrane functionalyzed mica (APS-mica) was used for the binding of DNA molecules. APS-mica was prepared as described by Shlyakhtenko et al [15]. A drop of 10-50 μl of DNA solution (0.5-1 μg/ml) was deposited on the APS-mica surface at room temperature for 3 min. The sample was rinsed and air-dried before imaging. For AFM force spectroscopy, 80 μl of DNA solution (~60 ng/μl) in Tris-EDTA buffer (10 mM Tris+HCl, 1 mM EDTA, pH 8; Sigma-Aldrich, Inc), supplemented with 150 mM NaCl, was deposited onto a freshly evaporated gold surface. After the sample was incubated for 2-3 hours, it was gently rinsed 3-5 times with the buffer solution before test.

2.3 AFM imaging

AFM topographic images were taken using a Nanoscope IIIa MultiMode Scanning Probe Microscope (Veeco Instruments Inc) using Tapping mode with an E scanner. RTESP probes (Veeco) were used for imaging in air. The spring constant of AFM cantilevers was 20-80 N/m and their resonance frequency was 275-316 kHz. NP-S probes (Cantilever C) were used for imaging in solution. The spring constant of the cantilever was 0.32-0.64 N/m and their resonance frequency was 56-75 kHz. All of the images were collected at a scan rate of 2-3 Hz, a scan resolution of 512×512 pixels, and scan sizes of 1-5 μm.

2.4 Quantifying DNA structures from AFM images

The number of DNA with different configurations i.e. the damage, was quantified by a Poisson distribution $f(n;\lambda)=\lambda^n \times exp(-\lambda)/n!$ [16,17], based on percentages of supercoiled and relaxed DNA. The average number of damage per molecule, λ, can be obtained from $\lambda=-ln[f(\lambda;0)]$, where $f(\lambda;0)$ is the fraction of supercoiled (damage n=0) plasmids.

2.5 AFM force spectroscopy

For force spectroscopy measurements, we used nonspecific adsorption of DNA to fresh gold substrates [18] and untreated silicon nitride AFM probes (MLCT from Veeco). The cantilevers had a nominal spring constant of 10 mN/m and an actual spring constant between 10-20 mN/m, as determined by using the energy equipartition theorem [19]. 80 µl of ssDNA solution (~60 ng/µl) in Tris-EDTA buffer (10 mM Tris+HCl, 1 mM EDTA, pH 8; Sigma-Aldrich, Inc), supplemented with 150 mM NaCl, was deposited onto a freshly evaporated gold surface. After the sample was incubated for 2-3 hours, it was gently rinsed 3-5 times with the buffer solution.

3. Results and discussion

3.1 Analyzing DNA structure quantitatively at a single-molecule level by AFM

Plasmid DNA is broadly used as a model in DNA research because it has three different conformations: supercoiled forms, relaxed forms, and linear forms depending on structural modification such as single strand breaks (SSB) or double strand breaks (DSB) [11,20,21]. It is because intact plasmid DNA will relax to open circular form even though one SSB is introduced. Likewise, the ring-shaped plasmid will open and change to linear form if one double strand break takes place and more DSBs will fragment the plasmid to linear segments of shorter lengths. All these topological/lengths transformation of DNA are easy to resolve and quantify by gel electrophoresis [22-24] and AFM [7,8,25-29]. However, it is very important to know that some structural changes may occur in intact supercoiled DNA upon the binding of plasmids to the mica surface. This problem has been solved by Shlyakhtenko et al. who used APS-mica [15,30] instead of fresh-cleaved mica. The results revealed that the conformation of supercoiled DNA remains practically unchanged when DNA binds from high salt buffer solutions to the APS-mica. Unlike untreated mica, which is negatively charged and therefore demands a high concentration of divalent cations and a relatively low concentration of monovalent cations for a deposition of DNA, APS mica is positively charged and supercoiled DNA becomes immobilized quite effectively in the presence of high monovalent salts, and as a result, the topology of the DNA will not be affected.

A typical AFM image, shown in Figure 3A, presents the plectonemic supercoiled configuration of pUC18 molecules after they had been deposited on the APS-mica. Following methods developed earlier for electron microscopy and AFM imaging of supercoiled plasmids [20,26,31], the number of nodes, generated at visible crossover points (figure 3A), was counted within single DNA molecules, and the distribution of the number of nodes was shown in Figure 3B. For a given plasmid size, the number of supercoiled nodes typically follows Gaussian distribution and also shifts according to the type and the concentration of cation and deposition conditions [32]. In the case of pUC18, the same buffer with 100 mM NaCl was employed in all experiments, so this error can be eliminated. For intact pUC18, the average number of nodes is eight, and this is consistent with the previously reported value for a supercoiled DNA composed of 2686 base pairs [20,21,26,33]. 5% of the plasmids show fewer than six nodes, which might imply that these plasmids represent a background of damaged DNA in our sample after extraction and purification using the QiaFilter plasmid maxi kit. Further experiments, using T4 Endonuclease V to nick pUC18 plasmids which were exposed to UV radiation, support our criterion of five nodes as the borderline between damaged and undamaged DNA. In the following discussion, we suppose that pUC18 molecules with a number of nodes greater than five are intact, while the number of nodes equal to or less than five will be indicative of some structural alterations within supercoiled DNA. Based on this assumption, our pUC18 DNA samples have 95% of intact supercoiled DNA.

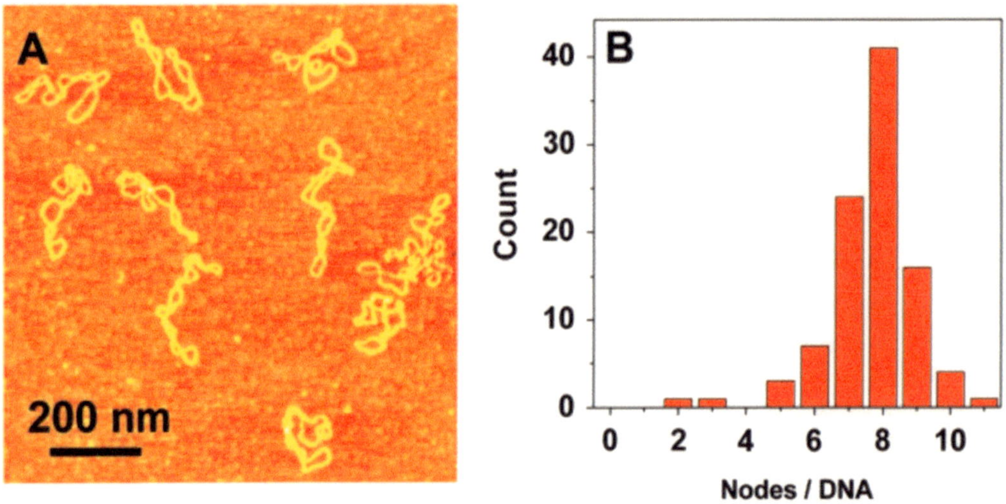

Fig. 3. (A) An tapping-mode AFM image of intact pUC18 plasmids adsorbed to APS-mica surface reveal their supercoiled topology. AFM was performed in tapping mode at a scan size 1×1 μm². (B) The frequency distribution of the number of supercoiled nodes in intact pUC18 plasmids (based on 21 AFM images). (Adapted and modified from reference [11], with permission)

Figure 4 shows the AFM images of pUC18 molecules exposed to UVB (302 nm) radiation. From Figure 4A and D, we discover that at a dose of 1.4 kJ/m², the configuration of DNA molecules did not change obviously as compared to the intact molecules shown in Figure 3A and B, with 95% of the plasmids having more than five supercoiled nodes. 5% of the plasmids have five or fewer nodes, which represent a background damage of our pUC18 DNA. In Figure 4B and C, pUC18 molecules were exposed to 165 kJ/m² and 660 kJ/m² of UVB radiation, respectively. Among molecules subjected to 165 kJ/m², 78%± 1% are relaxed circular plasmids and 16% are linear fragments (Figure 4B and E). At 660 kJ/m² of UVB radiation, this fraction, including fragments with an obviously reduced length, increased to 91% (Figure 4C and F). Therefore, our results suggest that UVB can cause significant degradation of DNA. The results of the three tests are graphically summarized in Figure 4 G.

One SSB is enough to relax a whole supercoiled plasmid, and the increasing size of the plasmid also increase our measurement sensitivity. To check this assumption, a bigger plasmid named pNEBR-R1 supercoiled DNA (10,338 bp) was irradiated with 29 J/m² of UVB and treated with T4 Endonuclease V. Figure 5 display a representative AFM image of these plasmids. 55% of pNEBR-R1 plasmids are in the relaxed circular form and 14% are in the linear form counted from similar images. In control experiments on pUC18 molecules, the percentages of supercoiled, relaxed circular and the linear form of DNA are 65%, 34% and 2%, respectively. From the percentage of supercoiled molecules, we evaluate that pNEBR-R1 plasmids contained 1.12 CPD/plasmid (λ=1.12), while for pUC18, the average number of CPD lesions per DNA plasmids is 0.4 (λ=0.4). So, increasing the size of the supercoiled plasmid by 3.8 fold (10338/2686) lead to a 2.8 fold (1.12/0.4) increase in damage detection sensitivity, which is consistent with our predictions.

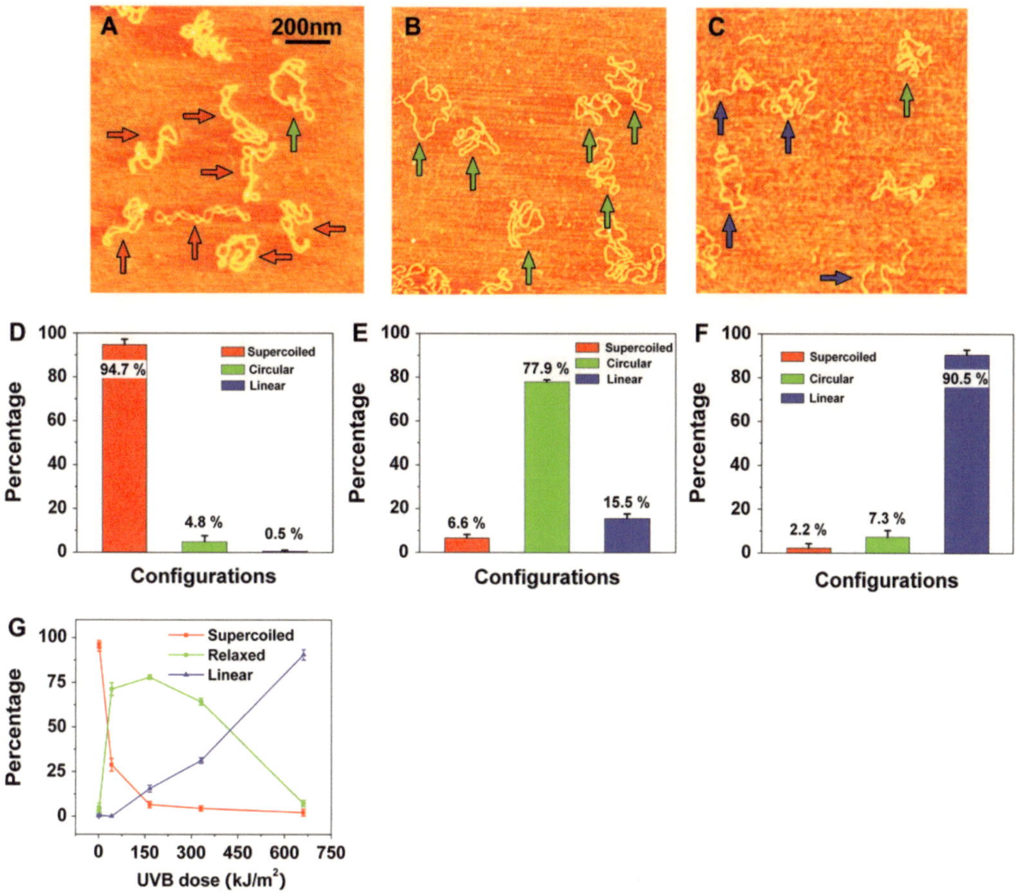

Fig. 4. AFM images of pUC18 molecules subjected to different doses of UVB radiation: (A) 1.4 kJ/m^2, (B) 165 kJ/m^2, (C) 660 kJ/m^2. Scan size in all the images is 1×1 μm^2. (D–F) Histograms of the occurrence of various configurations of pUC18 plasmids determined from the AFM images such as these shown in (A–C). (G) Percentages of different configurations of irradiated pUC18 as a function of UVB dose. Color code for the arrows, histogram and curves: red, supercoiled DNA; green, relaxed circular plasmids; blue, linear DNA. (Adapted and modified from reference [11], with permission)

Agarose gel electrophoresis is an extremely powerful, versatile, easy to use, sensitive, and quite rapid technique for quantitative DNA research, and contributed enormously to the progress of DNA damage and repair research. The three unique features of AFM that make it particularly suitable for quantitative DNA studies are a), the ability to examine individual DNA molecules and DNA protein complexes, b) molecules can be investigated under nearly in vivo conditions, and c), extremely small amounts of DNA and protein material are needed for the observation. To demonstrate this last point, 0.1 ml of a pUC18 plasmid solution containing the total amount of 1 pg of DNA (10 pg/ml) was coated over the mica surface and imaged at a scan size (5×5 μm^2). The AFM image, shown in Figure 6, captured four individual DNA molecules whose configuration was evaluated by scanning locally at a higher resolution. Thus, the amount of DNA need for this measurement is ~400 times less

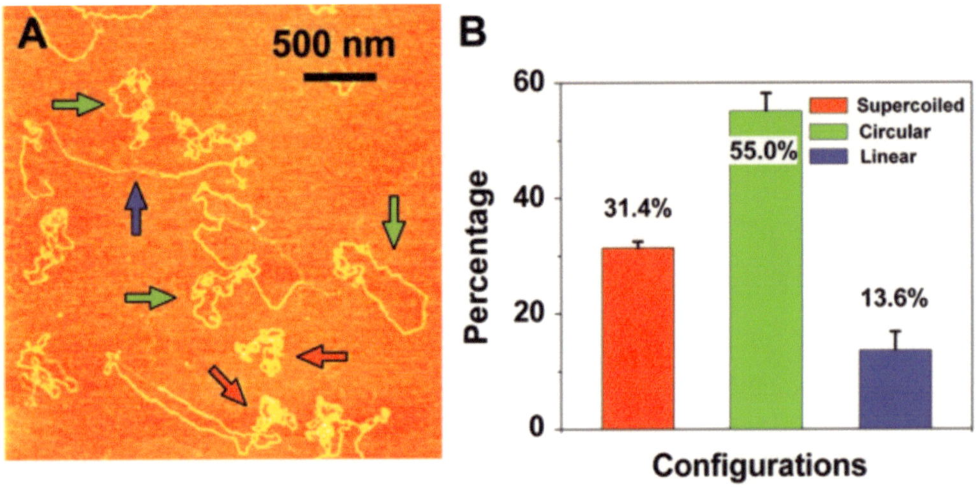

Fig. 5. Sensitivity of damage detection increases with plasmid size. (A) An AFM image of supercoiled plasmid pNEBR-R1 (10,338 base pairs) irradiated at 29 J/m^2 UVB. Scan size 3×3 μm^2. (B) Percentages of different configurations of pNEBR-R1 plasmids determined from AFM images such as these shown in A. (Adapted and modified from reference [11], with permission)

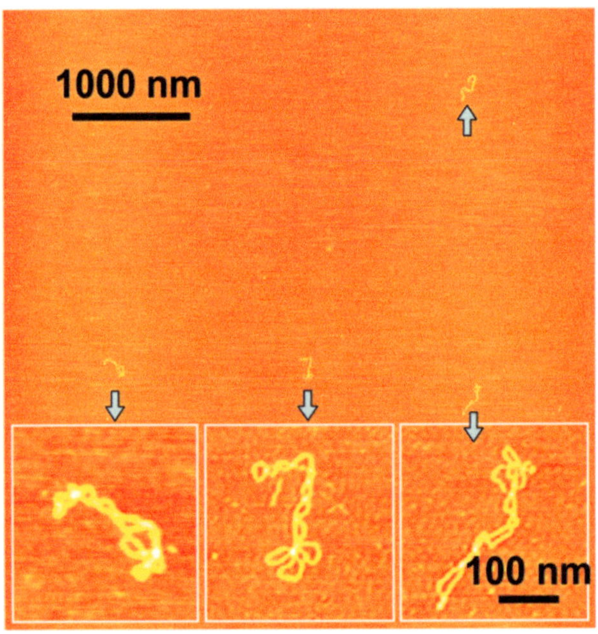

Fig. 6. An AFM image of intact pUC18 plasmids obtained from a sample that contained a total amount of 1 pg of DNA material. Scan size is 5×5 μm^2. The inset images obtained at a higher resolution show in detail the supercoiled structure of these plasmids. The scale bar for these inset images is 100 nm. The sample was prepared by spreading 0.1 ml of a 10 pg/ml solution of pUC18 on the APS-mica surface and incubating for 3 min. This assay requires extremely small amounts of DNA to evaluate damage. (Adapted and modified from reference [11], with permission)

than what is needed for the most sensitive gel electrophoresis assays presently [34], which amounts to ~1/5 of the DNA in a single cell. In some studies, it may be very useful to combine the advantages of gel electrophoresis with AFM imaging. Gel electrophoresis would separate the DNA into discrete bands, and the DNA extracted from a particular band would provide enough material for further examination by high resolution AFM imaging. It has been demonstrated that AFM is capable of quantifying DNA plasmids smaller than 100 kilo base pairs and total mass smaller than 1 pico-gram.

3.2 AFM method for DNA quantification is consistent with gel electrophoresis

Before comparing the accuracy of AFM imaging with gel electrophoresis, we need to calibrate both methods by working on a mixture with known composition. A mixture of supercoiled and linear pUC18 with a ratio of 1:1 was used as the reference sample, and was deposited on APS-mica for AFM imaging. From the image in Figure 7A, we can identify both supercoiled and linear forms clearly. Intact plasmid (labeled by letter "S") has a supercoiled configuration, while linear DNA (labeled by letter "L") has two clear ends. By counting the numbers of DNA in different structures in this image and different images on the same sample, the actual ratio of supercoiled and linear DNA on the mica surface was acquired. The result is summarized in Table 1. Supercoiled and linear DNA percentages were 50.1% and 48.1%, respectively, a ratio of linear/supercoiled DNA of 0.96 (the true value is 1 here). This means that the error is quite small, with no necessary calibration. It also means that the topological structures cannot be affected by DNA binding to mica during the sample preparation and AFM scanning process by sharp tips.

The ratio of different conformations (supercoiled, relaxed or linear forms) can be inferred to the numbers of SSB and DSB, which represent the level of DNA damage [15,17]. However, these three forms have the same sequence (molecular weight), so it is difficult to separate them by normal methods. Gel electrophoresis is one of the well-established methods to separate them since different topological structures have different radii of gyration and electrophoretic nobilities. DNA mobility of supercoiled DNA is much greater than that of its relaxed circular form. Therefore, it is significant to compare our results obtain by AFM imaging with the results obtained by gel electrophoresis assay.

We made the gel electrophoresis assay on the same DNA sample as used for AFM imaging. The relative amounts of DNA in various bands were quantified by measuring the intensities of each band in the gel photo. The gel is shown in Figure 7B and the results are summarized in Table 1, indicate a nonlinear relationship between the relative amounts and the band intensities of DNA in supercoiled forms versus linear forms. Supercoiled DNA is less fluorescent compared with circular and linear forms [20,30]. Therefore, quantification of supercoiled DNA by band intensity is much more complicated, compared to that of relaxed forms or linear forms.

In order to further test whether AFM imaging is an accurate method for DNA quantification with various topological configurations, the same DNA sample extracted from an agarose gel was used for AFM imaging. A mixture of supercoiled and relaxed pUC18 plasmids was chosen as model DNA. After the mixture was loaded on a gel electrophoresis, two bands which contain supercoiled DNA and relaxed DNA were separated as shown in Figure 8A. The DNA molecules in the supercoiled and relaxed DNA gel bands were extracted and purified back into solution separately for further AFM imaging. Figure 8B and C show the

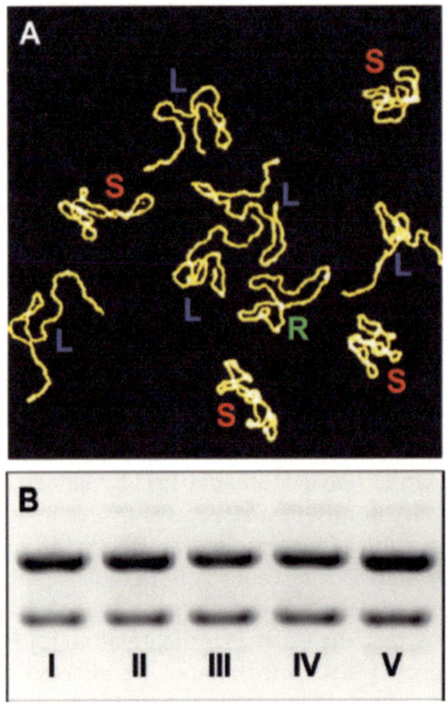

Fig. 7. (A) An AFM image showing the mixture of supercoiled and linear pUC18 DNA with the same weight ratio. Scan size is 1 × 1 μm². Color code: red, supercoiled DNA (S); green, relaxed circular plasmids (R); blue, linear DNA (L). (B) A photograph of the agarose gel showing the separated supercoiled and linear pUC18 bands on the same sample as shown in part A, with the same weight ratio. The gel was run with (I) *E. coli* Endonuclease IV reaction buffer, (II) *E. coli* Endonuclease IV enzyme and its reaction buffer, (III) *E. coli* Endonuclease V reaction buffer, (IV) *E. coli* Endonuclease V enzyme and its reaction buffer, (V) 10 mM Tris-HCl, 1 mM EDTA, and 100 mM NaCl buffer. The top bands in all lanes contain linear pUC18 while the bottom bands represent supercoiled DNA. The image was treated with flatten function in operation software (Veeco Inc.) to get rid of the background noise. (Adapted and modified from reference [13], with permission)

Band intensity	AFM	GEL		
		Tris, EDTA & NaCl	Endo-IV enzyme and its buffer	Endo-V enzyme and its buffer
Supercoiled%	50.1	32.6	32.2	38.4
Relaxed%	1.8	x	x	x
Linear%	48.1	67.4	67.8	61.6
Correction factor	0.96	2.07	2.10	1.60

"x" means undetectable

Table 1. Correction factor obtained from AFM and gel electrophoresis methods. (Adapted and modified from reference [13], with permission)

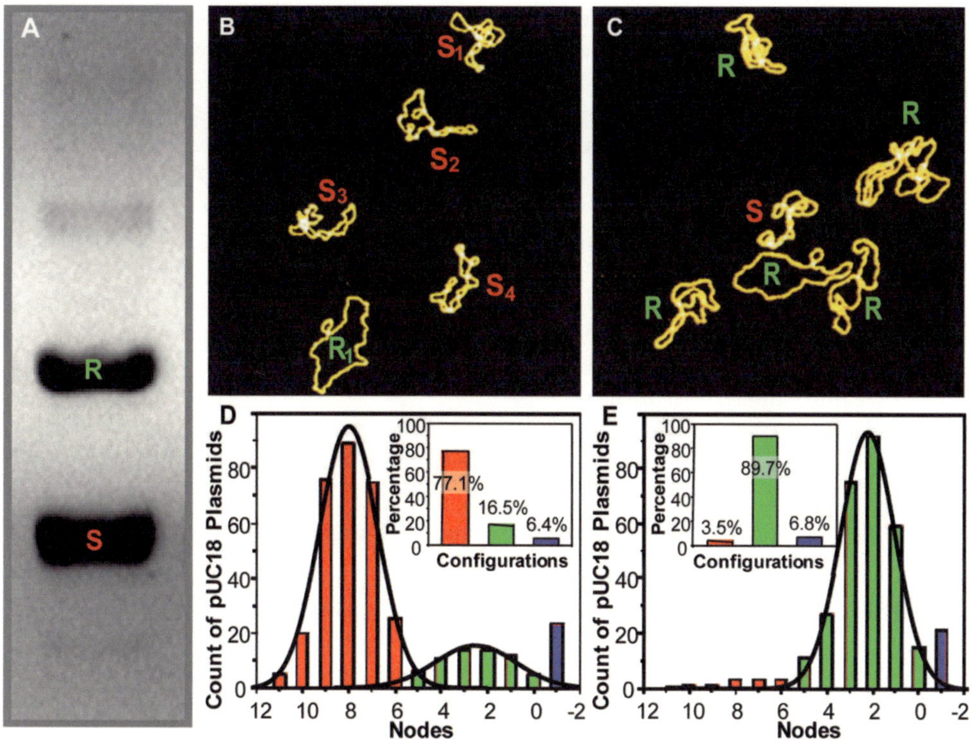

Fig. 8. (A) A photograph of the agarose gel showing separated supercoiled and relaxed pUC18 bands. AFM images of pUC18 DNAs that were extracted from agarose gel, (B) supercoiled band, and (C) relaxed band, as shown in part A. Scan size in both images is 1 × 1 μm^2. (D and E) Histograms showing the distributions of nodes of pUC18 plasmids counted from the AFM images such as those shown in parts B and C. The curves in the histogram show the Gaussian distribution fits. Inset figures show the histograms of the percentages of various conformations of pUC18 plasmids determined from the 6 nodes criterion. Color code: red, supercoiled DNA (S); green, relaxed circular plasmids (R); blue, linear DNA (L). The image was treated with flatten function in operation software (Veeco Inc.) to get rid of the background noise. (Adapted and modified from reference [13], with permission)

AFM images of these DNA obtained from supercoiled and relaxed DNA bands, respectively. Comparing Figure 8B with C, the conformations of DNA molecules are quite different. The DNA molecules obtained from the supercoiled band have significantly much more nodes (the number of visible crossover points in AFM images) than those from the relaxed band. Supercoiled and relaxed DNAs have obviously different node distributions as observed from this quantitative study as shown in Figure 8D and E. The plasmid molecules in the supercoiled band have about 6-11 nodes, while those in the relaxed band only have about 0-5 nodes [11]. These nodes count histograms were fitted with Gaussian distributions and 8.0±1.3 nodes (mean±standard deviation) was got for supercoiled DNA and 2.2±1.2 nodes for DNA in the relaxed band. According to these Gaussian distributions [11,13], the previous criterion [11] that we used to identify supercoiled and relaxed DNA is correct. The DNA molecules with more than 5 nodes can be considered as supercoiled, and those with 5 or less than 5 nodes are relaxed [11].

Moreover, according to this criterion, the distribution of percentages of various conformations of pUC18 plasmids was measured, and the results were shown as insets in Figure 8D and E. However, we found some deviations between AFM imaging and gel electrophoresis results. Only 77.1% of DNA extracted from the supercoiled band in the gel was actually supercoiled plasmids as shown in Figure 8B and D. Some relaxed molecules (16.5%) and even linear (6.4%) molecules were observed among the DNA extracted from the supercoiled band. These deviations may be caused by supercoiled DNA being damaged by the subsequent extraction processes and purification processes, and as a result degenerating into relaxed forms or linear forms. More significantly, from the AFM imaging results shown in Figure 8C and E, we can confirm small amounts (3.5%) of supercoiled molecules in our AFM images of the DNA extracted from the relaxed band. The number most likely represents the actual amount of supercoiled DNA in the relaxed band, since relaxed DNA cannot turn into supercoiled form automatically. The finding is direct evidence that gel electrophoresis may not be able to separate DNA entirely. Some supercoiled molecules will move to the "wrong" relaxed band, possibly due to molecular entanglement.

3.3 AFM can investigate the forces of the dynamic process of DNA

Besides AFM imaging, AFM force spectroscopy can also be used to analyze DNA quantitatively because it measures the relationship between molecular length and force, and has been used to examine the nanomechanics and mechanochemistry of DNA [36-38]. The technique has also proved unique in its ability to capture information about dynamic processes such as antigen-antibody complexes [39]. It can measure the length and tension of a single molecule with sub-nanometer (nM) and pico-newton (pN) resolution, respectively. A single DNA molecule was picked up by the AFM tip and stretched vertically in solution to determine it force-extension relationship [4].

Measurements of the force of DNA were carried out in solution, at room temperature, on an AFM instrument designed and equipped specifically for force spectroscopy measurements [40,41], as shown in Figure 9A. This instrument was built with a high accuracy piezoelectric *XYZ* stage equipped with three capacitive sensors, which offer an open-loop resolution of 0.1 nm in the *Z* axis and 1 nm in the *X* and *Y* axes. This instrument was also equipped with a commercial AFM head (Veeco Instruments Inc.). Untreated silicon nitride AFM cantilevers were used for picking up molecules and pulling measurements. The spring constant of each cantilever was measured in solution [19]. This measurement depended on attaching ssDNA molecules to the gold substrate and AFM tip by nonspecific adsorption, and this method has proved to be a simple, but effective method in previous DNA force spectroscopy studies [18,42]. For this methodology, the AFM tip picks up ssDNA fragments at random positions.

The force spectrograms, shown in Figure 9B, reveal two pronounced plateau features. The first plateau occurs at a force of 23 pN and overstretches the polynucleotide by about 80%. This lowforce plateau is very similar to the plateau theoretically predicted by Buhot and Halperin [43] based on their model of base-stacking interactions in poly(dA). The plateau likely represents the unwinding of the poly(dA) helix, and its force directly indicates the strength of base-stacking interactions among the adenines. The second plateau occurs at a force of about 113 pN and overstretches poly(dA) by an additional ~16%. We speculate that during this phase of base-unstacking, poly(dA) is still in the helical form, although this helix must be extended, and the high-force plateau represents the reorientation of bases, which is accompanied by the flip of the backbone bonds to new torsional states that increase the

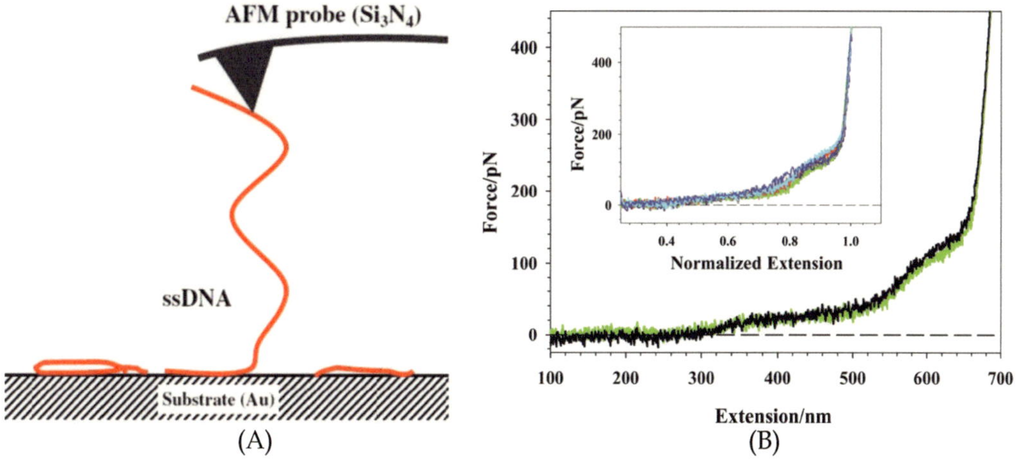

Fig. 9. (A). A schematic of single-molecule atomic force microscopy measurements of ssDNA molecules (the figure is not to scale). (B). typical force-extension measurement curves for poly(dA). The poly(dA) molecules were normalized corresponding to the longest molecule and the comparison between the stretching trace (green, online; gray, in print) and the relaxing trace (black). The inset plot shows the overlapping of six recorded force-extension curves of poly(dA) on a normalized extension basis. These recordings were obtained in different experiments on different poly(dA) molecules. (Adapted and modified from reference [35], with permission)

distance between the consecutive phosphates in a semidiscontinuous fashion. The reorientation of bases may, at higher forces, be also accompanied by a forced conformational transition in the deoxyribofuranose rings from their C3′ endo pucker (5.9 A° spacing between the neighboring phosphates) to a C2′ endo pucker (7A° spacing between the neighboring phosphates) [44,45]. Such a transition would produce an additional extension of the backbone chain up to 19%, which coincides with the width of the second plateau.

To research DNA methylation patterns, methylated single-stranded DNA molecules were linked to a glass substrate. An antibody was attached to the AFM tip that is specific towards 5-methylcytosine which has two free antigen-binding fragment arms (Figure 10a). Bringing the functionalized tip into contact with the DNA, two complexes formed between the two arms of the antibody and two 5-methylcytosines on the DNA.

Two characteristic force peaks was recorded by stretching the DNA-antibody complex, which they related to consecutive rupture events between the antibody arms and methylcytosines (Figure 10a) [46]. Since contacts between both the arms and various methylcytosines form randomly, the antibody arms may contact all possible pairs of methylated bases. The methylation patterns could then be obtained by analyzing the separations between force peaks. The first DNA oligomer examined by the group contained five equally spaced methylcytosines with three unmodified bases between neighbouring methylcytosines. It implies that there are four possible pairs in which the methylcytosines are separated by four nucleotide lengths: 3 pairs separated by 8 nucleotide lengths; 2 pairs that are separated by 12 nucleotide lengths and 1 pair separated by 16 nucleotide lengths (inset to Figure 10b). Hundreds of force spectroscopy measurements on this DNA sample

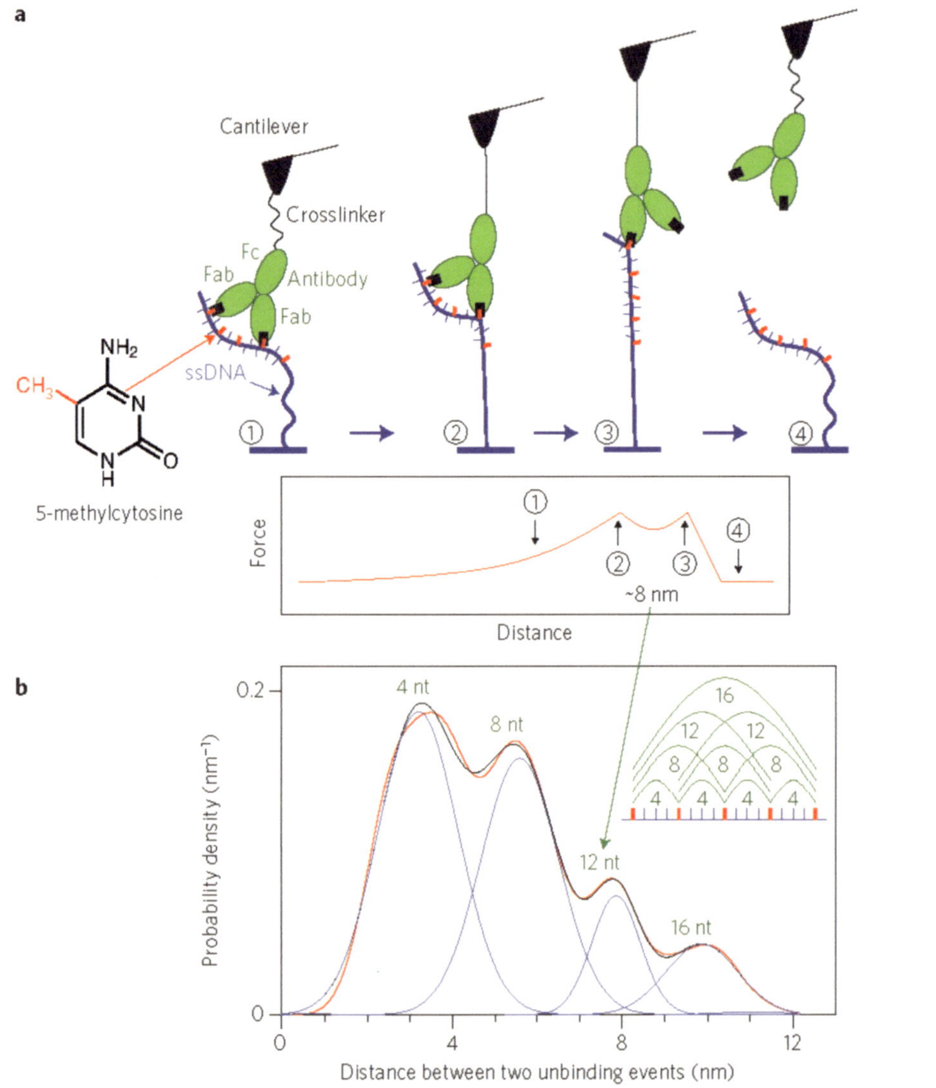

Fig. 10. A force-spectroscopy assay for detecting DNA methylation patterns. (A) Single-stranded DNA (ssDNA, blue lines) carrying methylated cytosines (red boxes; the chemical structure is shown in the inset) are coupled to a glass surface. The antibody (green) against 5-methylcytosine is tethered to the AFM cantilever tip, and the two arms bind to methylcytosines that are separated by a certain number of nucleotides (12 in this case). Panels 1–4 correspond to different stages during stretching of the antibody–DNA complex. These bonds break sequentially at stages 2 and 3, producing two characteristic force peaks in the force–extension curve (lower panel) that are separated by a distance equal to the spacing between two 5-methylcytidines in DNA. (B) Repeating this measurement numerous times produces a probability distribution of the distances between force peaks (red) that can be used to determine the methylation pattern. This distribution can be fitted by the sum of four Gaussian distributions (blue) of varying height that correspond to the different possible pairs of methylcytosines. (Adapted and modified from reference [46] with permission)

produced a relatively complex distribution of the spacing between two rupture events (Figure 10b). Notably, when the distribution was suitable for numerous Gaussian functions, four maxima at 4, 8, 12, and 16 nucleotides were identified. Furthermore, as expected, the relative amplitudes of these maxima were 4:3:2:1.

AFM can subject molecules to very high loads compared to other force measurement methods, such as optical or magnetic tweezers. The piezoelectric stages in AFMs can apply newtons of force, and the stiff cantilevers can detect large forces on the order of nanonewtons. Also, cantilevers and substrates can be functionalized with all types of chemistry, and that functionalization allows covalent bonds to form between the sample and the cantilever. On the contrary, optical and magnetic tweezers are limited by trap and magnetic field strength, respectively. The properties that make AFM so well suited for high force measurements are also what limit its function in the low force regime. The stiff cantilevers that can detect forces in the nanonewtons also exhibit much higher force noise, compared to the soft optical traps. Table 2 summarizes the force and spatial limits for these various force spectroscopy methods.

Method	Force range (N)	Spatial Resolution (m)	Adavantages
AFM	10^{-11}~10^{-7}	10^{-10}	High spatial resolution High applied forces
Magnetic Tweezers	10^{-14}~10^{-11}	10^{-8}	High force resolution Able to induce torque
Optical Tweezers	10^{-13}~10^{-10}	10^{-9}	High force resolution

Table 2. Force and spatial limits of common force spectroscopy methods. (Adapted and modified from reference [4], with permission)

4. Summary

AFM, which is normally used to gain qualitative results, can also be employed for quantitative research at a single-molecular level. By analyzing the numbers of DNA molecules with different topological configurations from AFM images, the distributions of DNA with different configurations can be identified directly. Based on this advantage, AFM imaging is ideal for quantifying DNA structure under a wide range of DNA amounts, concentrations and sizes that may not able to be handled by other methods. Atomic force microscopy is proven to be an accurate method in the identification and quantification of the plasmid with different topological structures, since these measurements are based on single-molecular observations. Thus, atomic force microscopy is a viable alternative to gel electrophoresis in the study of different DNA structures. The AFM force spectroscopy assay shows that AFM is also a very useful tool to analyze quantitatively the mechanical properties of individual DNA molecule. The structure of DNA, DNA-protein interaction and the dynamic processes that related to the mechanical properties can be measured accurately just by stretch single DNA between the substrate and the AFM tip.

5. Acknowledgements

We are grateful for the support of the National Natural Science Foundation of China (NSFC) to Y.J. uder Grant No. 21174029 and the startup fund from Southeast University to Y.J. under Grant No. 2009-81 and KJ2010479.

6. References

[1] Binnig, G., Quate, C. F. & Gerber, C. Atomic Force Microscope. *Physical Review Letters* 56, 930, doi:10.1103/PhysRevLett.56.930 (1986).

[2] Lyubchenko, Y. L. Preparation of DNA and nucleoprotein samples for AFM imaging. *Micron* 42, 196-206, doi:10.1016/j.micron.2010.08.011 (2011).

[3] Lauritsen, J. V. & Reichling, M. Atomic resolution non-contact atomic force microscopy of clean metal oxide surfaces. *J Phys Condens Matter* 22, 263001, doi:10.1088/0953-8984/22/26/263001 (2010).

[4] Rabbi, M. & Marszalek, P. E. Nanomechanics of nucleic acid structures investigated with AFM based force spectroscopy. *Ph.D. Dissertation of Duke University* (2010).

[5] Wang, H. *et al.* DNA bending and unbending by MutS govern mismatch recognition and specificity. *Proc Natl Acad Sci U S A* 100, 14822-14827, doi:10.1073/pnas.2433654100 (2003).

[6] Chen, L. W., Haushalter, K. A., Lieber, C. M. & Verdine, G. L. Direct visualization of a DNA glycosylase searching for damage. *Chemistry & Biology* 9, 345-350, doi:10.1016/s1074-5521(02)00120-5 (2002).

[7] Boichot, S. *et al.* Investigation of radiation damage in DNA by using atomic force microscopy. *Radiation Protection Dosimetry* 99, 143-145 (2002).

[8] Psonka, K., Brons, S., Heiss, M., Gudowska-Nowak, E. & Taucher-Scholz, G. Induction of DNA damage by heavy ions measured by atomic force microscopy. *Journal of Physics: Condensed Matter* 17, S1443-S1446, doi:10.1088/0953-8984/17/18/002 (2005).

[9] Lysetska, M. *et al.* UV light-damaged DNA and its interaction with human replication protein A: an atomic force microscopy study. *Nucleic Acids Res* 30, 2686-2691, doi:10.1093/nar/gkf378 (2002).

[10] Moreno-Herrero, F. *et al.* Mesoscale conformational changes in the DNA-repair complex Rad50/Mre11/Nbs1 upon binding DNA. *Nature* 437, 440-443, doi:10.1038/nature03927 (2005).

[11] Jiang, Y., Ke, C., Mieczkowski, P. A. & Marszalek, P. E. Detecting ultraviolet damage in single DNA molecules by atomic force microscopy. *Biophys J* 93, 1758-1767, doi:10.1529/biophysj.107.108209 (2007).

[12] Jiang, Y. *et al.* UVA generates pyrimidine dimers in DNA directly. *Biophys J* 96, 1151-1158, doi:10.1016/j.bpj.2008.10.030 (2009).

[13] Jiang, Y., Rabbi, M., Mieczkowski, P. A. & Marszalek, P. E. Separating DNA with different topologies by atomic force microscopy in comparison with gel electrophoresis. *J Phys Chem B* 114, 12162-12165, doi:10.1021/jp105603k (2010).

[14] Ke, C. *et al.* Nanoscale detection of ionizing radiation damage to DNA by atomic force microscopy. *Small* 4, 288-294, doi:10.1002/smll.200700527 (2008).

[15] Shlyakhtenko, L. S. *et al.* Silatrane-based surface chemistry for immobilization of DNA, protein-DNA complexes and other biological materials. *Ultramicroscopy* 97, 279-287, doi:10.1016/s0304-3991(03)00053-6 (2003).

[16] Lobachevsky, P. N., Karagiannis, T. C. & Martin, R. F. Plasmid DNA breakage by decay of DNA-associated auger electron emitters: Approaches to analysis of experimental data. *Radiation Research* 162, 84-95, doi:10.1667/RR3187 (2004).

[17] Sachs, R. K., Ponomarev, A. L., Hahnfeldt, P. & Hlatky, L. R. Locations of radiation-produced DNA double strand breaks along chromosomes: a stochastic cluster process formalism. *Mathematical Biosciences* 159, 165-187, doi:10.1016/s0025-5564(99)00019-x (1999).

[18] Rief, M., Clausen-Schaumann, H. & Gaub, H. E. Sequence-dependent mechanics of single DNA molecules. *Nature Structural Biology* 6, 346-349, doi:10.1038/7582 (1999).

[19] Florin, E. L. *et al.* SENSING SPECIFIC MOLECULAR-INTERACTIONS WITH THE ATOMIC-FORCE MICROSCOPE. *Biosensors & Bioelectronics* 10, 895-901, doi:10.1016/0956-5663(95)99227-c (1995).

[20] Cherny, D. I. & Jovin, T. M. Electron and scanning force microscopy studies of alterations in supercoiled DNA tertiary structure. *Journal of Molecular Biology* 313, 295-307, doi:10.1006/jmbi.2001.5031 (2001).

[21] Vologodskii, A. V. & Cozzarelli, N. R. CONFORMATIONAL AND THERMODYNAMIC PROPERTIES OF SUPERCOILED DNA. *Annual Review of Biophysics and Biomolecular Structure* 23, 609-643, doi:10.1146/annurev.bb.23.060194.003141 (1994).

[22] Folkard, M., Prise, K. M., Vojnovic, B., Brocklehurst, B. & Michael, B. D. Critical energies for ssb and dsb induction in plasmid DNA by vacuum-UV photons: an arrangement for irradiating dry or hydrated DNA with monochromatic photons. *International Journal of Radiation Biology* 76, 763-771, doi:10.1080/09553000050028913 (2000).

[23] Folkard, M., Prise, K. M., Turner, C. J. & Michael, B. D. The production of single strand and double strand breaks in DNA in aqueous solution by vacuum UV photons below 10 eV. *Radiation Protection Dosimetry* 99, 147-149 (2002).

[24] Chen, W. M., Blazek, E. R. & Rosenberg, I. THE RELAXATION OF SUPERCOILED DNA-MOLECULES AS A BIOPHYSICAL DOSIMETER FOR IONIZING-RADIATIONS - A FEASIBILITY STUDY. *Medical Physics* 22, 1369-1375, doi:10.1118/1.597420 (1995).

[25] Shlyakhtenko, L. S., Miloseska, L., Potaman, V. N., Sinden, R. R. & Lyubchenko, Y. L. Intersegmental interactions in supercoiled DNA: atomic force microscope study. *Ultramicroscopy* 97, 263-270, doi:10.1016/s0304-3991(03)00051-2 (2003).

[26] Bussiek, M., Mucke, N. & Langowski, J. Polylysine-coated mica can be used to observe systematic changes in the supercoiled DNA conformation by scanning force microscopy in solution. *Nucleic Acids Res* 31, doi:10.1093/nar/gng137 (2003).

[27] Murakami, M., Hirokawa, H. & Hayata, I. Analysis of radiation damage of DNA by atomic force microscopy in comparison with agarose gel electrophoresis studies. *Journal of Biochemical and Biophysical Methods* 44, 31-40, doi:10.1016/s0165-022x(00)00049-x (2000).

[28] Pang, D., Berman, B. L., Chasovskikh, S., Rodgers, J. E. & Dritschilo, A. Investigation of neutron-induced damage in DNA by atomic force microscopy: Experimental evidence of clustered DNA lesions. *Radiation Research* 150, 612-618, doi:10.2307/3579883 (1998).

[29] Pang, D., Rodgers, J. E., Berman, B. L., Chasovskikh, S. & Dritschilo, A. Spatial distribution of radiation-induced double-strand breaks in plasmid DNA as

resolved by atomic force microscopy. *Radiation Research* 164, 755-765, doi:10.1667/rr3425.1 (2005).

[30] Lyubchenko, Y. L. DNA structure and dynamics - An atomic force microscopy study. *Cell Biochemistry and Biophysics* 41, 75-98, doi:10.1385/cbb:41:1:075 (2004).

[31] Sperrazza, J. M., Register, J. C. & Griffith, J. ELECTRON-MICROSCOPY CAN BE USED TO MEASURE DNA SUPERTWISTING. *Gene* 31, 17-22, doi:10.1016/0378-1119(84)90190-2 (1984).

[32] Lushnikov, A. Y. *et al.* Interaction of the Zalpha domain of human ADAR1 with a negatively supercoiled plasmid visualized by atomic force microscopy. *Nucleic Acids Res* 32, 4704-4712, doi:10.1093/nar/gkh810 (2004).

[33] Lyubchenko, Y. L. & Shlyakhtenko, L. S. Visualization of supercoiled DNA with atomic force microscopy in situ. *Proc Natl Acad Sci U S A* 94, 496-501, doi:10.1073/pnas.94.2.496 (1997).

[34] SYBR Gold. *Clare Chenmical Research http://www.clarechemical.com/gold.htm.*

[35] Ke, C., Humeniuk, M., S-Gracz, H. & Marszalek, P. E. Direct Measurements of Base Stacking Interactions in DNA by Single-Molecule Atomic-Force Spectroscopy. *Physical Review Letters* 99, doi:10.1103/PhysRevLett.99.018302 (2007).

[36] Clausen-Schaumann, H., Seitz, M., Krautbauer, R. & Gaub, H. E. Force spectroscopy with single bio-molecules. *Current Opinion in Chemical Biology* 4, 524-530, doi:10.1016/s1367-5931(00)00126-5 (2000).

[37] Fisher, T. E., Marszalek, P. E. & Fernandez, J. M. Stretching single molecules into novel conformations using the atomic force microscope. *Nature Structural Biology* 7, 719-724, doi:10.1038/78936 (2000).

[38] Bustamante, C., Chemla, Y. R., Forde, N. R. & Izhaky, D. Mechanical processes in biochemistry. *Annual Review of Biochemistry* 73, 705-748, doi:10.1146/annurev.biochem.72.121801.161542 (2004).

[39] Kienberger, F., Ebner, A., Gruber, H. J. & Hinterdorfer, P. Molecular recognition imaging and force spectroscopy of single biomolecules. *Accounts of Chemical Research* 39, 29-36, doi:10.1021/ar050084m (2006).

[40] Lee, G. *et al.* Nanospring behaviour of ankyrin repeats. *Nature* 440, 246-249, doi:10.1038/nature04437 (2006).

[41] Marszalek, P. E., Oberhauser, A. F., Pang, Y. P. & Fernandez, J. M. Polysaccharide elasticity governed by chair-boat transitions of the glucopyranose ring. *Nature* 396, 661-664, doi:10.1038/25322 (1998).

[42] Clausen-Schaumann, H., Rief, M., Tolksdorf, C. & Gaub, H. E. Mechanical stability of single DNA molecules. *Biophys J* 78, 1997-2007, doi:10.1016/S0006-3495(00)76747-6 (2000).

[43] Buhot, A. & Halperin, A. Effects of stacking on the configurations and elasticity of single-stranded nucleic acids. *Physical Review E* 70, doi:10.1103/PhysRevE.70.020902 (2004).

[44] Olson, W. K. & Sussman, J. L. HOW FLEXIBLE IS THE FURANOSE RING .1. A COMPARISON OF EXPERIMENTAL AND THEORETICAL-STUDIES. *Journal of the American Chemical Society* 104, 270-278, doi:10.1021/ja00365a049 (1982).

[45] Daune, M. Molecular Biophyscis Structures in motion. *United States by Oxford University Press. New York*, 42-48 (1999).

[46] Zhu, R. *et al.* Nanomechanical recognition measurements of individual DNA molecules reveal epigenetic methylation patterns. *Nat Nanotechnol* 5, 788-791, doi:10.1038/nnano.2010.212 (2010).

9

Atomic Force Microscopy of Chromatin

Delphine Quénet[1], Emilios K. Dimitriadis[2] and Yamini Dalal[1*]
[1]*LRBGE/NCI/NIH, Bethesda*
[2]*LBPS/NIBIB/NIH, Bethesda*
USA

1. Introduction

Atomic force microscopy or scanning tunneling microscopy (AFM/STM) is a powerful single molecule tool for the visualization of biological materials at sub-nanometer resolution. AFM is versatile because it can directly measure physical properties due to its sensitivity at picoNewton force scales, thus enabling dissection of molecular forces. STM/AFM has been considered revolutionary since its discovery 32 years ago, and a mere 7 years after its invention, Binnig and Rohrer were awarded the Nobel Prize in Physics, along with Ruska, inventor of the first electron microscope. In subsequent years, AFM has evolved fast, with the range of applications for STM/AFM expanding to encompass all physical sciences. Despite it's popularity in physics, engineering, material and chemistry sciences, it has remained a less prominent tool for biologists, who are much more familiar with techniques like electron microscopy (EM), X-ray crystallography or nuclear magnetic resonance (NMR). The relatively low cost of the microscope, the ease of sample preparation, and the lack of any requirement for staining, freezing, excessive denaturation or preservation, should make AFM an ideal tool for laboratories interested in imaging and manipulating biological samples down to macromolecules at the nanoscale. In this chapter, we will discuss how AFM can be an effective high-resolution technique for structural and molecular interaction studies in biology.

2. Biophysical tools to characterize biological structures

Biophysical techniques like AFM, EM, X-ray crystallography and NMR are commonly used to determine ultra-structure of macromolecular complexes. The choice is often related to the availability of the tools as well as the skills required to operate them in a given laboratory. All of these techniques have distinct advantages and disadvantages for imaging of biological specimens, which should be considered before making a choice (Table 1).

2.1 Electron microscopy

EM is the preeminent and most mature high-resolution microscopy (Ruska, 1980) which uses a focused beam of electrons to generate a magnified and detailed image. Since the wavelength of electrons is orders of magnitude smaller than that of visible light, this method

* Corresponding Author

Technique	Electron microscopy	X-ray cristallography	NMR	AFM
Resolution	For SEM: 1 nm For TEM: 5 Å	0.2-3.5 Å	2-3.5 Å	1-5 nm (lateral) 0.1 nm (vertical)
Advantage	Magnification (max 50 000 000X for TEM)	Atomic resolution	Measurements in solution	Measurements in solution
Disadvantage	Sample preparation Expensive equipment	High quantity of purified crystal Time of preparation	Purification of molecule Time of acquisition	Immobilized sample
Observation	Fixed sample under vacuum	Crystal	Sample in solution	Sample in ambient air or in solution

Table 1. Comparison of biophysical techniques commonly used in biology.

is not limited by the diffraction limit of visible light (200 nm). Therefore, its resolution approaches Angstroms. However, the use of focused beam of electrons at high voltage (typically 40-100 kV) is destructive, and requires elaborate sample preparation and mounting techniques. To obtain a homogeneous and straight beam of electrons, EM is always performed under high vacuum, which requires elimination of liquids from the sample to be visualized. Nucleoprotein complexes have very low electron density (and thus are "invisible" by standard EM). Thus, visualization of such material requires fixation using glutaraldehyde, dehydration by drying or ethanol substitution, followed by shadowing or staining with heavy atom-containing reagents (e.g. gold, palladium, platinum, uranyl acetate, *etc.*). Heavy metals diffract electrons strongly, providing meaningful contrast so that sub-molecular details in nucleoprotein complexes can be revealed.

Two types of EM were developed, whose use depends on the sample and the purpose of imaging: transmission electron microscope (TEM) and scanning electron microscope (SEM). TEM is used for thin samples to generate two-dimensional, electron density maps of transmitted electrons. A collection of such images at a series of sample rotations can be used for 3-dimensional (3D) reconstruction of internal structures of a cell or macromolecular complexes (electron tomography). In contrast, images generated by SEM result from the capture of diffracted electrons, giving 3D details of the surface of the sample, typically used for cells, organelles, and other large structures.

Advances such as cryo-EM permit the visualization of samples embedded in a liquid lattice, requiring imaging at sub-zero temperatures (Lepault et al, 1983; Taylor & Glaeser, 1974). This technique lacks the high contrast offered by more traditional EM techniques involving fixation, shadowing and staining, and consequently requires extensive post-processing and image reconstruction from hundreds of identically oriented particles. However, cryo-EM does afford a native view of particles, and is a powerful tool for analysis of materials at very high resolution.

2.2 X-ray crystallography

X-ray crystallography is the highest resolution technique currently available for the determination of ultra-structure (Chiu, 1993). This method consists of illuminating a crystal composed of highly ordered particles created from *in vitro* ultra-pure components which must be all aligned in precisely the same orientation within a crystal lattice. A beam of X-rays is focused on the crystal to determine the 3D organization of atoms by subsequent analysis and molecular modeling of X-ray diffracted patterns. The major disadvantage of this method is the sample needs to be crystallized, requiring milligram quantities of complexes folded correctly at very high concentrations in non-physiological buffers. Since X-rays are destructive, each crystal can only be imaged once. While this technique is still the gold standard for obtaining precise location for every atom and molecule in a complex at Angstrom resolution, the complexes exist in a static conformation. Moreover, it is still very challenging to obtain useful crystals for classes of molecules like membrane proteins and intrinsically disordered proteins.

2.3 Nuclear magnetic resonance

NMR, like X-ray crystallography is used to derive 3D structure and dynamics of molecules (Chiu, 1993). Highly purified complexes in solution are exposed to a multidimensional magnetic field, exciting specific magnetic resonance of active nuclei in their environment. The resonance signatures, called chemical shifts, give the distances between atoms which enable the 3D reconstruction of the molecule. Time required to acquire and to analyze the signature is a major disadvantage of this technique. The resolution of the obtained structure depends on the size of the macromolecule with a limit to about 100 kDa. NMR relies on previously obtained structural models of the major parts of the complex, upon which the resonance shift can be mapped. One advantage of NMR is its ability to characterize intrinsically disordered proteins, which is not possible with X-ray crystallography.

2.4 Atomic force microscopy

In AFM, images are topographic maps of samples attached to a solid substrate (Binnig et al, 1986). They are obtained by scanning the surface of the samples with a nanometer-size tip etched at the end of a flexible cantilever (figure 1). Two unique capabilities distinguish the technology: (i) the ability to both image and perform co-localized force spectroscopy for the determination of a range of sample properties (mechanical, electrical, molecular recognition) and (ii) the ability to probe and image samples in ambient air conditions or under physiological fluids. These are accomplished by the tip-deflection of the cantilever being continuously monitored by a focused laser beam with accuracy of about 1-2 Å. The stiffness of the cantilever is estimated (the softest commercially available cantilevers have nominal stiffness around 0.005N/m), the force sensitivity is in a range of picoNewtons, which allows force interactions at single molecule level. A number of imaging modalities have been developed to accommodate the nature of the sample and the purpose of the investigation. The simplest one, called contact mode, has the cantilever contacting and scanning the sample with a preset small deflection while a feedback loop maintains the deflection constant (Figure 1). The other most common modality has the cantilever oscillating with preset amplitude near its resonance frequency and is named tapping mode (or non-contact mode or amplitude modulation feedback) (Figure 1). When the cantilever approaches the

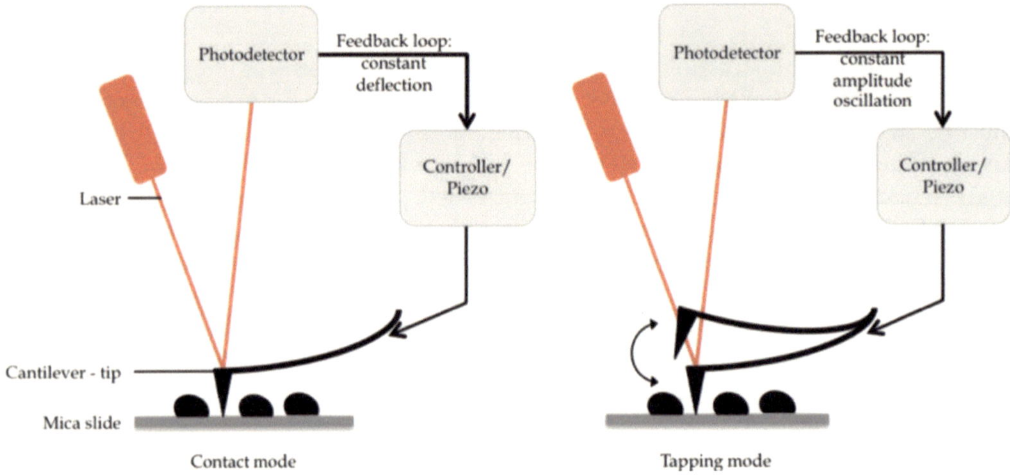

Fig. 1. Principle of atomic force microscopy.
In contact mode (left), the tip contacts the sample surface with a small cantilever deflection and the feedback loop maintains that deflection constant; this is equivalent to a constant force. In tapping mode (right), the input to the z-piezo-actuator is oscillatory and the photodetector output signal is analyzed into amplitude and phase of the cantilever oscillation. The feedback loop maintains the oscillation amplitude constant. The phase shift between input and output depends on sample properties.

sample, probe-sample interaction forces lead to a drop in amplitude and a small shift in resonance frequency. The feedback maintains the reduced amplitude of oscillation constant during the scan. To maintain the feedback parameter constant, the piezoelectric actuator that controls the motion of the cantilever has to follow the sample topography and hence generates the topographic image of the sample.

A great advantage of this method is that minimal sample preparation involved. AFM is normally performed under gentle physico-chemical conditions (physiological hydration, temperature, salt concentration) in air or in buffer, thus allowing biological samples to retain their native form during the experiment. More challenging, sometimes, is the attachment of the certain types of sample to the substrate; attachment has to be firm enough to permit stable imaging. Both substrate properties and sample solution composition are important in this respect.

3. Choice of AFM instrument modality and conditions for biological sample studies

The mode in which the AFM will be used depends entirely on the sample and on the objectives of the study. Biological samples, from tissues, and cells, and down to single molecules, present very different properties and require different handling.

The first issue to decide is whether imaging will be performed in ambient air or under fluid. For hydrated tissues (e.g. cartilage), biological membranes (e.g. supported lipid bilayers), and live cells, the choice of fluid environment is obvious. Because experimenters are interested in the functionality of biological samples under physiological conditions, fluid environment is also a better choice for molecular recognition studies (i.e., using tips coated with an antibody that recognizes its corresponding antigen on the sample) and for molecular pulling or force curve spectroscopy (for the study of the folding properties of proteins). One disadvantage of using fluid is the higher noise level compared to ambient air. So, if samples do not absolutely require the use of buffers, such as stably folded proteins, nucleic acids (DNA - Deoxyribonucleic acid or RNA - Ribonucleic acid), or nucleoprotein complexes, acquisition of data can be performed in air. It is generally well accepted that even after drying a significant level of hydration contain within molecules maintain samples in their native structure (Cantor & Schimmel, 1980; Garcia de la Torre, 2001). For both types of imaging, air or fluid, the most commonly used surface for the attachment of biological samples is freshly cleaved mica which is atomically flat, inert, and presents the most appropriate properties for AFM imaging.

A second choice, which is mainly dependent on the physico-chemical properties of the sample, is whether AFM will be performed in "contact" or "non-contact/tapping" mode. As briefly discussed above, these are the two basic modes for imaging. Imaging under fluid or air can be performed in either mode and the choice will depend on the firmness of attachment to the mica plate and on the stiffness of the sample. For example, supported lipid bilayers are usually quite robust and can equally well be imaged in contact and in tapping modes. On the other hand, live cells are usually rather soft and labile, requiring gentler forces such as those applied in tapping mode. For imaging in air, contact mode is most challenging due to the high capillary forces between the adsorbed water layers on tip and hydrated sample. Given the usual sensitivity of soft biological samples, imaging in air is always performed in tapping mode.

For imaging nucleic acids or chromatin in air, it is best to use rather stiff cantilevers in tapping mode. Commonly available tips made of single crystal silicon with resonance frequency in the range of 300 kHz, stiffness in the tens of N/m and tip radius of around 5-7 nm typically work well. For the highest resolution, the use of super-sharp cantilevers with a tip radius in the 1-2 nm range will enhance the acquisition. However, ambient humidity should be maintained at 60% rh to reduce tip-sample adhesion due to excessive surface hydration and the probability of tip contamination. In all cases, gentle tapping is recommended to avoid sample damage and tip contamination.

For these same types of samples in fluid, tapping mode is performed with much softer cantilevers. Softer cantilevers are also necessary for molecular recognition studies since the binding forces to be measured are in the range of picoNewtons. Such levels of force sensitivity can only be provided by very soft cantilevers. For example, the detection of 1 nm deflection resulting from 10 picoNewton force can easily be detected by cantilever stiffness of 0.01 N/m. It should be noted that imaging resolution under fluid will be lower than in air, because of higher noise, and because softer silicon-nitride cantilevers are less sharp than ones made of silicon. Stable tapping with the softest cantilever in the market (stiffness 0.005 N/m) may be challenging and often, a slightly stiffer cantilever (0.06-0.12 N/m) may give better results. Despite the two orders of magnitude stiffness differences among the cantilevers used under fluid, their resonance frequencies are all in the range of 10 kHz, primarily determined by the fluid mass displaced by the oscillation of the cantilever.

The quality of imaging is determined by the parameters described above, and by scanning parameters. A critical parameter is the free tapping amplitude, namely the amplitude of the cantilever oscillation when the tip is far from the sample and free of interactions. For samples like DNA and chromatin, this amplitude should be kept at ~5-30 nm, with lower amplitudes used for more fragile samples maintained under fairly low humidity. Even more critical is the amplitude set-point, which corresponds to the amplitude reduced by tip-sample interaction forces when tip reaches the sample. The set-point determines the tip-sample forces during scanning, and in tapping mode, a feedback loop attempts to keep this set-point constant. The speed of the scan should be kept low enough (~1-5 μm/sec), so that the feedback loop is given adequate time to work efficiently. The feedback gain parameters characterize the speed at which the mathematical control algorithms are attempting to follow the topography of the sample. These parameters are critical, but instrument and modality dependent. One can try increasing the gains as long as the feedback stays stable. The amplitude set-point also determines the force regime and magnitude of the tip-sample interaction forces. During sample engagement, as the cantilever approaches the sample, the interaction force first goes from zero through the long-range attractive van der Waals region, and if pushed closer to the sample, enters the repulsive region, wherein there is actual contact during the downward leg of the oscillation (Figure 2). For a given tapping frequency and set-point, the operating regime is also determined by the elasticity of the sample, but for single molecular complexes such as chromatin, it may be assumed that the sample is rather stiff, similar to the mica plate. Under these conditions, it is desirable to stay in the attractive region which applies lower forces to the sample and produces reliably accurate and high quality images. This is generally accomplished by choosing a set-point slightly lower than the free oscillation amplitude (90-95%). Tip-sample forces shift the cantilever resonance to lower frequencies causing a change of the free amplitude. Staying within the attractive regime is ensured by setting the oscillation frequency slightly lower than resonance of the tip. Upon engagement, the amplitude of oscillation decreases, reducing the chances of entering the repulsive regime.

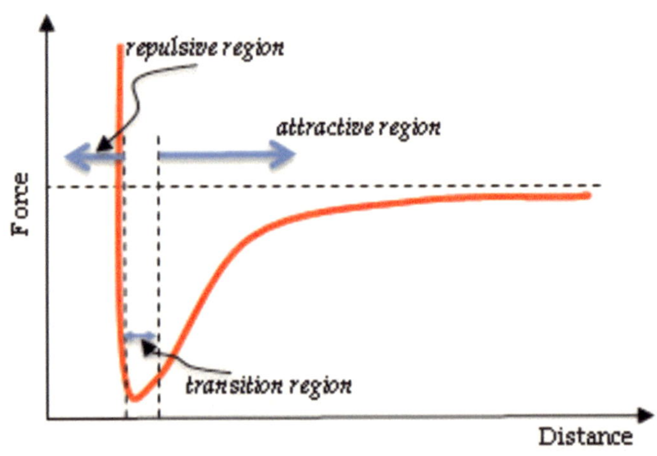

Fig. 2. Scanning force regimes in tapping mode.
Depending on the amplitude of free oscillation, the amplitude setpoint and the oscillation frequency relative to the resonance of the cantilever, the tip-sample force can be attractive or repulsive.

4. Sample preparation

The eukaryotic genome is a complex macromolecule, presenting a range of folding from 2 nm-wide DNA to 1.4 μm-wide chromosome. The nucleosome is the fundamental repeating structural unit of the chromosome and consists of 147 base pairs of DNA wrapped around an octamer of two copies of each histone proteins H2A, H2B, H3 and H4. Linker histone H1 stabilizes this structure through its binding to DNA. The distribution of nucleosomes along the DNA molecule leads to the formation of an 11 nm fiber, called "beads on a string", which can be folded into higher-order structures ranging from 30 nm to 100 nm fibers in the interphase nucleus, to quasi-crystalline chromosome during mitosis (Li & Reinberg, 2011). Chromatin structure is also dynamic, since it is regulated by reversible modifications such as DNA methylation, post-translational modifications of histones, and interactions with chromatin-binding factors (Kouzarides, 2007). Mechanisms involved in chromatin folding and biophysical characteristics of each level of genome organization have been extensively studied using AFM technology.

In contrast to relatively rigid samples encountered in solid-state or polymer physics, biological samples must be maintained in an appropriate environment that will protect them from degradation. For example, proteins are sensitive to proteases, and DNA or RNA will be cleaved by nucleases naturally present on human skin. In addition, the best environments for biological samples could be inappropriate for standard AFM manipulation and special modifications, and trade-offs have to be designed. Nevertheless, AFM still allows a higher flexibility than other techniques. Indeed, samples can be analyzed in air or in liquid, and in real time, for instance, to follow the modification of chromatin condensation, or in response to the addition of chromatin-binding protein. Below we will discuss appropriate use of sample preparation and buffers that best preserve structural information.

4.1 Mica slides preparation

Mica is a naturally occurring sheet silicate mineral with a hexagonal pseudo-crystal structure arranged in 1 nm thick layers. After cleaving using adhesive tape or a sharp scalpel, mica sheet presents an atomically flat surface, which is highly negatively charged, hydrophilic, chemically inert, and very stiff in the transverse direction. Thus, fresh cleaved mica constitutes an ideal surface for the attachment and topographic imaging of individual macromolecules. For AFM, grade 1 muscovite mica is preferred for its high purity and ease of cleaving.

The negatively charged mica offers strongly adsorbing support for positively charged samples but not negatively charged molecules, such as DNA. In addition, ionic conditions of the sample solution may alter attachment. In the presence of significant quantities of monovalent ions (e.g. Na^+ or K^+) charge screening prevents DNA from attaching to bare mica (Pastre et al, 2006; Pastre et al, 2003). Divalent ions (e.g. Mg^{2+}) presumably bridge negative charges on the sample and the mica, and are often and reliably used. However, in many cases the use of divalent is not recommended for functional reasons and chemical modification of the mica surface is necessary. The most common modification involves the use of silanes to produce a positively charged and hydrophobic mica surface with exposed amine groups. Several protocols for mica silanization, using generally 1-(3-aminopropyl)silatrane (APS) or 3-

aminopropyltriethoxysilane (APTES) have been developed (Figure 3) (Lyubchenko et al, 1992; Shlyakhtenko et al, 2003). The simplest method uses direct deposition of APS solution (300x dilution of 50 mM stock in ultra-pure water) onto the mica and incubation for a brief period (~30 minutes) before rinsing and drying the modified surface. An extension of these methods that also works reliably entails the treatment of silanized mica with 0.1% fresh-prepared glutaraldehyde for 5 min at room temperature, followed by careful rinsing with ultra-pure water and drying (Wang et al, 2002).

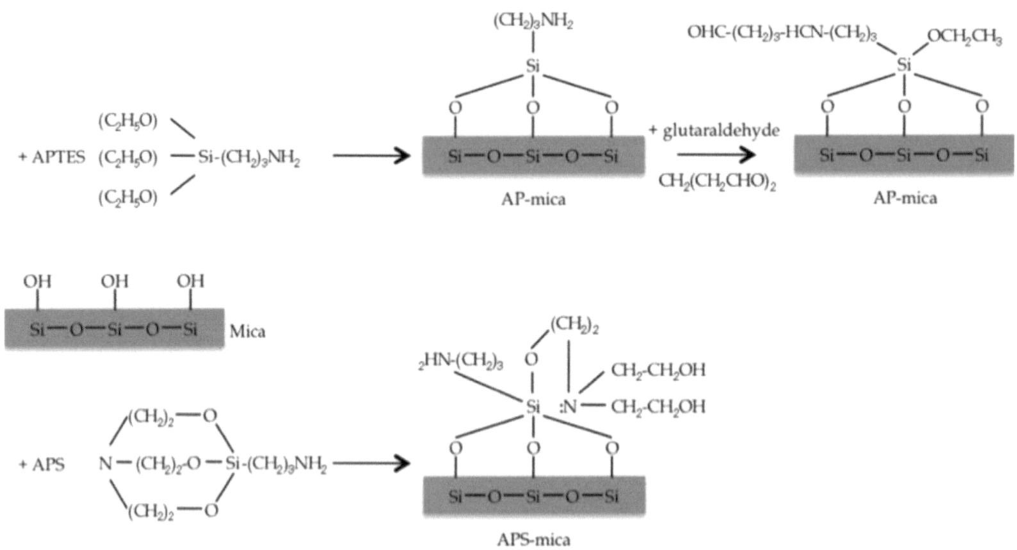

Fig. 3. Schema of modified mica surface by APS or APTES followed by glutaraldehyde treatment.

4.2 DNA preparation

DNA is a long polymer, whose the sub-unit is a nucleotide composed of a base, a sugar and a phosphate group. Two DNA strands are usually entwined in a double helix stabilized by hydrogen bonds between bases on the different strands. DNA can present different conformation: relaxed or coiled, or complex forms during cellular process such as replication or recombination, which may be visualized on AFM (Barattin & Voyer, 2011; Hamon et al, 2007; Hansma & Laney, 1996; Hansma et al, 1995; Lyubchenko et al, 1992; Shlyakhtenko et al, 2003).

DNA analysis takes place in a nuclease-free environment. All buffers used for the purification and the loading of DNA on the mica slide, must be sterile. In a typical protocol, 20-50 picograms of DNA is diluted in 5 mM HEPES buffer pH 7.5, 2 mM $MgCl_2$, and deposited on the fresh cleaved mica for 5-10 minutes. APS-mica itself is a very good substrate for DNA under physiological conditions, in the absence of divalent ions (Shlyakhtenko et al, 2003). Slides are gently rinsed three times with ultra-pure water to remove salts before drying in a stream of inert argon for analysis in air, or with the appropriate buffer to remove unattached objects for analysis in fluid.

4.3 *In vitro* and *in vivo* chromatin preparation

AFM is a useful tool for the characterization of chromatin structure by the extraction of information like the height, volume, position and movement of nucleosomes, the determination of the DNA wrapping handedness around the core histone complex, the association of chromatin-associated factors and changes in chromatin folding. Preparation of chromatin has to be performed in appropriate conditions of salts and temperature to best conserve the native state. Both chromatin extracted from nuclei (referred to as "*in vivo*" chromatin) or chromatin reconstituted *in vitro* from purified recombinant components can be analyzed equally well by AFM, allowing direct comparison. Here we described protocols used in our laboratory to examine chromatin structure by AFM.

4.3.1 Native chromatin extraction from various tissues/cell lines

The following protocol of native chromatin extraction has been adapted successfully in our lab for a range of samples including human cancer cell lines (such as HeLa, DLD1, SW480), non-carcinoma cells (HEK293), human tumors, mouse tissue, as well as Drosophila S2 and Kc cells cells (figure 4) (Dalal et al, 2005; Dalal et al, 2007; Dimitriadis et al, 2010; Wang et al, 2008).

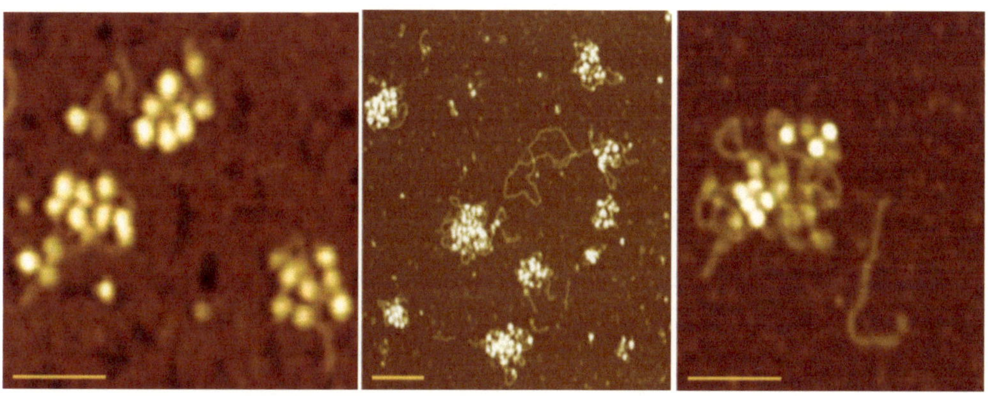

Fig. 4. Examples of topography images of native chromatin extracted from HeLa cells (unpublished data; scale bars 100 nm, Nanoscope, non-contact mode in air).

1. Tissues are disrupted and homogeneized by Dounce (no. A) strokes in standard chromatin buffer (60 mM KCl, 15 mM NaCl, 0.15 mM spermine, 0.5 mM spermidine, 15 mM 2-mercaptoethanol, 15 mM tris, pH7.4). For cell lines, cells are harvested from flasks by trypsinization.
2. Released cells either from tissue or flasks are washed three times with 1X PBS, 0.1% Tween.
3. Nuclei are extracted with TM2 Buffer (20 mM Tris pH8.0, 2 mM $MgCl_2$, 0.5 mM PMSF) supplemented with 0.5% Nonidet P40 (Sigma Cat#74385), and rinsed once with TM2 buffer.
4. Chromatin is digested by Micrococcal nuclease (Sigma Cat#N3755) at 0.2 units/mL final in the presence of a final concentration of 2 mM $CaCl_2$ at 37°C, and the reaction is stopped by addition of 10 mM EGTA. Incubation time depends on the size of the array expected, typically ranging from 30 seconds to obtain oligo-nucleosomal arrays to 10 minutes to obtain mononucleosomes.

5. After centrifugation 10 min 800 rpm at 4°C, the nuclear pellet is resuspended in low salt buffer (0.5X PBS, 5 mM EGTA, 0.5 mM PMSF) or high-salt buffer (0.35 M NaCl-supplemented 1X PBS, 5 mM EGTA, 0.5 mM PMSF) and incubated over night at 4°C on an end-over-end rotator.
6. Soluble extracted chromatin fibers are separated from remnant nuclei by spinning down the pellet by centrifugation 10 min 8000 rpm at 4°C.
7. Chromatin is deposited on APS-mica pre-treated with Mg^{2+} for 10-30 minutes. The mica is rinsed gently before drying in a gentle stream of inert argon. For fluid imaging, the mica is rinsed twice with 1X PBS to remove background unattached materials, and a thin layer of 1X PBS is added to the sealed imaging chamber prior to imaging. Care must be taken that the liquid does not dry while the AFM tip is engaged.

4.3.2 *In vitro* chromatin reconstitution by salt dialysis

Purified histones can be obtained by the expression of recombinant histones in *Escherichia coli*, followed by denaturation in urea and re-folding (Luger et al, 1997; Workman et al, 1991). An alternative popular method is the purification of native histones by hydroxyapatite extraction from chicken erythrocyte or HeLa nuclei (Bloom & Anderson, 1978; Stein, 1989). For chromatin reconstitution, DNA, such as negatively supercoiled plasmids or DNA fragments, are diluted at a final concentration of 200 mg/mL in 2 M NaCl, 10 mM Tris pH8.0, 1 mM EDTA and then mixed with purified histones at ratio ranging from 0.7-0.9 mg of histones/mg of pure DNA in 2 M NaCl, 10 mM Tris pH8.0, 1 mM EDTA, 0.5 mM PMSF. After 30 min incubation on ice, the sample is dialyzed 2-4 hrs at 4°C successively against 1/0.8/0.6/0.15 M NaCl diluted in 10 mM Tris pH 8.0, 1 mM EDTA, 0.5 mM PMSF. Supercoiling and nuclease assays are recommended to ensure that correct chromatin deposition has occurred. As for native chromatin, the sample is directly deposited on APS-mica pre-treated with Mg^{2+} for 10 min and mica slide is rinsed gently either before drying in a stream of inert argon or incubation in the appropriated buffer for liquid mode imaging.

4.4 Chromosome preparation

AFM has also been used for observation and structural analysis of bigger macromolecules like intact metaphase chromosomes (figure 5). The following protocol was developed for different cell lines such as HeLa cells (Hoshi et al, 2004; Ushiki & Hoshi, 2008).

Cells are treated with 0.1 mg/mL final concentration of colcemid for 12 hrs at 37°C. Cells are washed twice with 1X PBS before trypsinization. Trypsin activity is stopped by addition of complete medium when cells begin to lift off. Medium, PBS and trypsinized cells are collected in a conical tube and submitted to centrifugation 5 min 1000 rpm. Pellet of cells is resuspended drop-by-drop in 2 mL pre-warmed hypotonic buffer (75 mM KCl) and then additional 40 mL is added. After incubation at 37°C for 20 min, 5 drops of freshly prepared fixation solution (3:1 methyl alcohol/glacial acetic acid or Carnoy's solution) are added and chromosomes are harvest by centrifugation 5 min 1200 rpm. The chromosomes are washed three times with fixation solution and finally conserved at 4°C in this solution. Chromosomes are spread on fresh mica slide and observed after evaporation of the fixation solution. This protocol may be used for fluid analysis as described by Ushiki *et al.* (Ushiki & Hoshi, 2008).

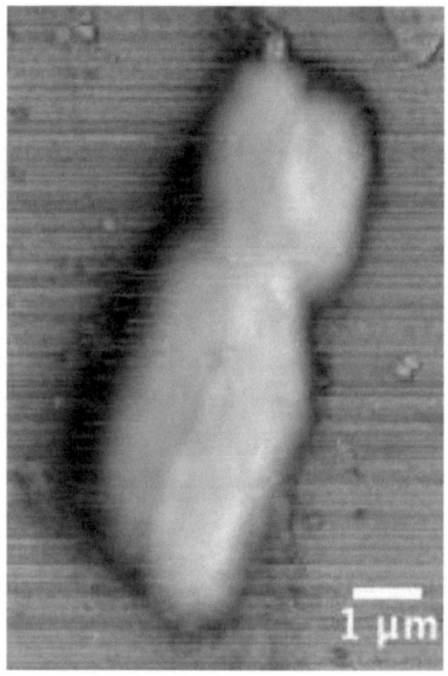

Fig. 5. Example of topography images of metaphase chromosomes extracted from HeLa cells (unpublished data; AFM: Agilent 5500, tapping mode in air).

5. Usual applications of AFM in biology

The major application of AFM in biology is the visualization of topography and the characterization of material properties via phase or other measurements. From the analysis of topography, information such as the height and volume of molecular complexes may be measured, allowing determination of stoichiometries and of 3D arrangement of oligomeric complexes. Phase imaging, namely the map of the phase difference between the piezo excitation and the cantilever tip response, informs of sample surface properties, like elasticity, charge and hydrophobicity. Although not quantitative, phase offers a possible measure for distinguishing regions on a sample and for molecular recognition when they cannot be differentiated by the topography (Hansma et al, 1997; Nagao & Dvorak, 1999; Zhao et al, 2010).

However a more robust approach for molecular identification can be achieved by probing antigen-antibody interactions with tips chemically functionalized to carry specific antibodies or other molecules that have specific binding partners on the sample. Consequently, AFM is a powerful technique for the structural study of complex macromolecular structures precisely because it can simultaneously provide visual, physical, electrostatic and chemical insights. Another important feature is the acquisition of real-time and kinetics sample information with the use of high-speed AFM (HS-AFM), which is able to acquire numerous images in a short period of time. Thus, DNA, chromatin and chromosome have been extensively studied using this technique, examples of which are provided below.

5.1 Topography analysis

5.1.1 Alternative DNA structure imaging

DNA is a flexible macromolecule which could present different conformations such as canonical B or alternative A and Z conformations, but also cruciform or triple helices, both observed during, and involved in, DNA replication, transcription and repair (Lebrun &

Lavery, 1997; Mills et al, 2002). AFM has been used to study the structure and the function of these conformations. Thus Shlyakhtenko *et al.* described continuous transition between two forms of cruciforms (Shlyakhtenko et al, 2000; Shlyakhtenko et al, 1998). The first cruciform presents a square planar structure with a 180° angle between the hairpin arms, whereas the second form displays an "X" conformation with bent main DNA strands. The transition between both forms may be performed by the recombinant protein RuvA, which specifically binds and unfolds cruciforms to convert them to an extended planar conformation. Further study has revealed the dynamic of cruciform structure like Hollyday junction (Mikheikin et al, 2006). This transition between both cruciform forms involving the coordination of arm movement for the parallel orientation of arm and the resolution of the structure, was also suggested by X-ray crystallography and FRET (Förster resonance energy transfer) (Hohng et al, 2004; Khuu et al, 2006). Interestingly, negative DNA supercoiling is important for the stabilization of the folded conformation.

DNA sequence may be involved in disease development like Huntington's, a neurodegenerative disorder, which results from the expansion of the CAG trinucleotides beyond 300 repeats in the Huntingtin gene (Finkbeiner, 2011). The analysis of DNA containing high number of CAG repeats by AFM revealed unusual and unexpected structures of the nucleic acid at this locus, structures like hairpins and loops, which may contribute to the neurodegeneration process *in vivo* (figure 6) (Duzdevich et al, 2011).

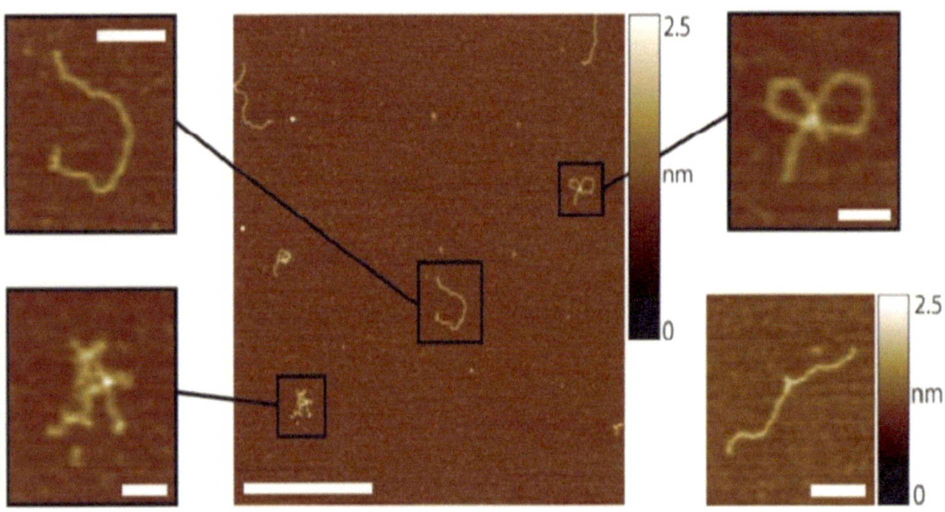

Fig. 6. DNA structure of CAG trinucleotides repetitions.
AFM study of CAG repeats fragments revealed linear normal DNA (upper left; scale bar 100 nm) and unexpected DNA structure such as unorganized (lower left; scale bar, 50 nm), folded (upper right; scale bar, 50 nm), or with protrusion (lower right; scale bar 100 nm). Inset, middle; scale bar 500 nm. From (Duzdevich et al, 2011) doi: 10.1371/journal.pone.0017119.g002.

5.1.2 Chromatin fiber folding

The formation of the 10 nm chromatin fiber has been explored using AFM. Particularly, the influence of DNA length and bending upon the efficiency of *in vitro* chromatin reconstitution using purified histones has been examined (Hizume et al, 2004). Results show that relaxed circular or positively supercoiled plasmids are not competent to form chromatin *in vitro*, whereas longer DNA with negative supercoiling strongly promotes the formation of nucleosomes. In addition, the efficiency of *in vitro* chromatin reconstitution using linearized DNA is lower than with circular plasmids. These observations confirm previous biochemical and biophysical studies, which showed that the negative supercoiled double helical nature of DNA was the form most preferred by nucleosomes (Germond et al, 1975; Luger et al, 1997; Simpson et al, 1985). This conformation also supports chromatin condensation and separation of DNA strands during replication.

5.1.3 Histone and higher folding

The importance of the N-terminal histone tail in chromatin structure has been also investigated (Hizume et al, 2009). *In vitro* chromatin reconstitution using tail-less histones is efficient, but interactions between histones are weaker than using full histones. Importantly, 30 nm chromatin fiber could not be formed after addition of linker histone H1, suggesting the role of histone tails, in collaboration with H1, is primarily to effect higher-order chromatin folding. These AFM-based results were independently confirmed by biophysical sedimentation studies (Gordon et al, 2005; Kan et al, 2007; McBryant et al, 2009).

5.1.4 Histone modifications and chromatin dynamics

A key regulator of chromatin dynamics is the post-translational modifications of histones. Ten different types of modifications have been described to date, including major types such as phosphorylation, methylation, and acetylation, and less common types such as ubiquitination, biotinylation, glycosylation, ADP-ribosylation and SUMOylation (Kouzarides, 2007). Acetylation is usually associated with more accessible and transcriptionally active chromatin, whereas methylation has been linked to chromatin condensation and transcriptional quiescence.

The role of biotinylation in chromatin structure was revealed to be related to higher condensation compared to non-biotinylated nucleosome using AFM as a tool (Filenko et al, 2011). This phenotype results from an increase of DNA turn around the octamer with 1.75 and 2 turns for non-biotinylated and biotinylated nucleosomes respectively (Figure 7). This result provides a mechanistic basis for a previously described role of biotinylation in gene silencing (Hassan & Zempleni, 2008). Thus, AFM is a sensitive tool to reveal subtle modifications of chromatin condensation.

5.1.5 Study of chromatin-binding protein function in DNA pathways

AFM was also used to characterize the role of chromatin-binding proteins in complex cellular pathways. These proteins may play a role as regulator of chromatin folding, like histone variants and post-translational modifications. They participate either in the relaxation or the condensation of chromatin. Several investigations focused on Parp-1 (Poly-ADP-ribose Polymerase-1) whose binding to single and double strand breaks triggers the decondensation through the synthesis of ADP-ribose polymer and initiates DNA repair (Hakme et al, 2008). Parp-1 is also involved in DNA transcription through its binding to alternative DNA structure at gene regulating domains (Soldatenkov et al, 2002). To better

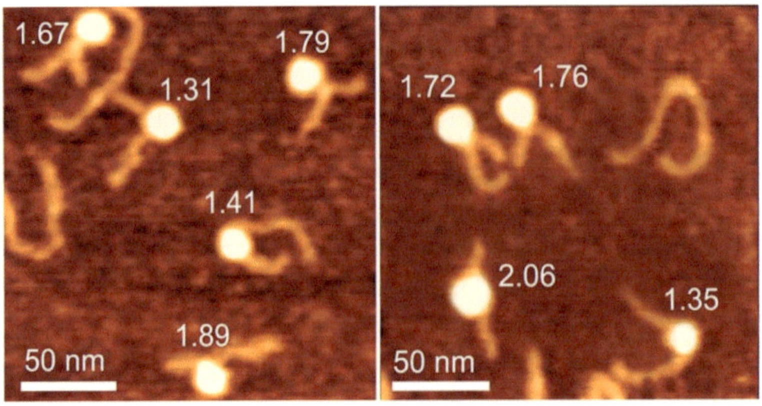

Fig. 7. Modification of *in vitro* nucleosome structure in response to biotinylation of histone H4. The effect of the post-translational modification of histone H4 (biotinylated) is analyzed by the determination of the number of DNA turns around histone octamers. On left, non-biotinylated nucleosome. On right, nucleosome containing biotinylated histone H4. From (Filenko et al, 2011) doi:10.1371/journal.pone.0016299.g003.

understand Parp-1 function in this pathway, the dynamic of chromatin structure, in the presence or absence of this factor, was investigated by AFM (Wacker et al, 2007). Condensation of *in vitro* reconstituted chromatin is observed in presence of Parp-1 in a concentration-dependent manner, like after addition of histone H1. The absence of N-terminal tail of histones does not affect this Parp-1 property. Further study showed that only the DNA binding domain of Parp-1 is required for chromatin compaction, whereas the addition of NAD^+ (nicotinamide adenine dinucleotide), substrate of Parp-1 for the synthesis of ADP-ribose polymer, reversed the chromatin condensation. Together, these data suggest a cooperative role of Parp-1 DNA binding domain and catalytic domain in regulation of chromatin dynamic. Again, AFM has proven a powerful tool for the investigation and confirmation of molecular mechanisms. Indeed, in Drosophila melanogaster and in mammals, Parp-1 is localized at silenced genes loci (e.g. Hsp70), which are expressed by the activation of Parp activity in response to the addition of NAD^+ or heat shock (Ouararhni et al, 2006; Tulin & Spradling, 2003).

Transcription has been extensively studied by AFM. The assembly of the bacterial RNA polymerase (RNAP) machinery and its progression on DNA after flow-through of nucleotides, were followed by AFM (Guthold et al, 1994; Kasas et al, 1997). Later, Crampton *et al.* analyzed the mechanism of RNAP collision, which results from discontinuous progression of RNAPs along DNA. Authors showed that collided RNAPs stayed associated with DNA with the retrogression of one of them (Crampton et al, 2006). These works demonstrated the interesting possibility of the *in vitro* study of processes in complex biological protein machinery by AFM.

Another example of DNA pathway analyzed by AFM is the V(D)J recombination, essential for the establishment of a large repertoire of adaptive immune T cells (Gellert, 2002). This mechanism consists of DNA fragments rearrangement in T cell receptor gene by endonuclease activity of RAG1/2 complex. These proteins recognize specific DNA motifs where they catalyze double-strand breaks and lead to the formation of a DNA loop to facilitate the next step of ligation. EM and AFM analysis of purified RAG1/2 complex binding to specific recombination motif revealed the stochiometry of the nucleo-protein complex and its structural organization (Figure 8) (Grundy et al, 2009).

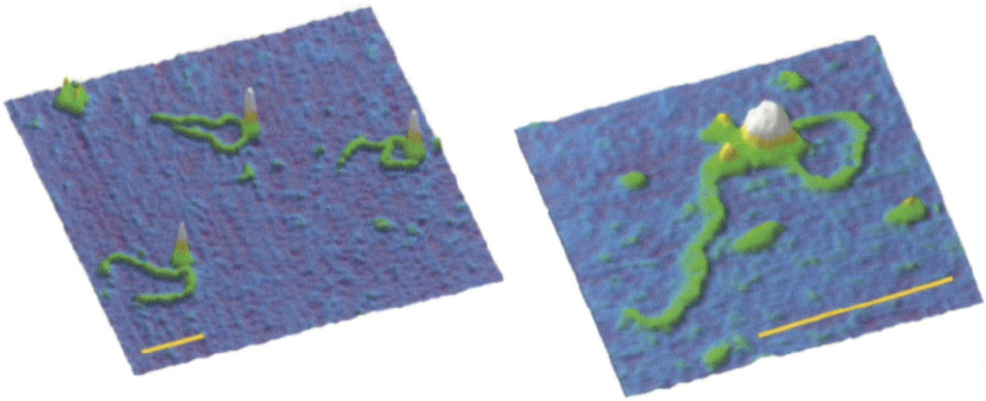

Fig. 8. Visualization of RAG1/2 complex loaded on DNA recombination motif by AFM. On the left, topography image reveals the 3-D arrangement of the complex. On the right, a tetramer of the proteins RAG1 and RAG2 bind two recombination signal sequences on DNA and lead to the formation of a DNA loop. (scale bars 100 nm). From (Grundy et al, 2009) doi: 10.1016/j.molcel.2009.06.022.

5.2 High Speed AFM

Beyond the standard commercial instruments, several configurations and capabilities have been developed and are being implemented offering new possibilities. The most powerful of these is the advent of HS- or video AFM. The major disadvantage of traditional AFM is the time required to acquire a high-resolution image. The speed for the acquisition is kept low (typically 1-2 lines/sec) to allow time for the feedback to follow the topography faithfully without affecting the sample or reducing the quality of the final image. Consequently, the time scale for obtaining an image ranges from a few minutes to several hours, which is far too slow for probing molecular kinetics, such as the movement of molecules, or the interaction between an enzyme and its substrate. To resolve this issue, HS-AFM was developed (Manalis et al, 1996).

5.2.1 Strategy of HS-AFM development

Different strategies have been explored for the buildup of HS-AFM. Humphris *et al.* conceived a new laser system, which focuses onto the back on the tip for a direct measurement of the height, whereas the laser deflection at the extremity of the tip is used for the feedback loop only (Humphris et al, 2011). In addition, VideoAFM (infinitesimal, Oxford, U.K.) has also been developed, wherein the increase of scan-time speeds results from quartz oscillation, and which can magnify the images at 1000X (Zhao et al, 2009). Another breakthrough strategy utilizes miniaturized cantilever with high resonance frequency (0.5-2 MHz) enabling faster response time (Ando et al, 2001). A scan stage was added to enhance spatial and temporal resolution for a capture of 10 images per second (1000 X 600 nm - 192 X 144 pixel).

5.2.2 Chromatin analysis by High-Speed AFM

The accessibility of DNA in the context of chromatin and the dynamic of nucleosome on a millisecond time scale were investigated using HS-AFM (Miyagi et al, 2011). Remarkably, a long-held speculation of how nucleosomal DNA can be accessed, which posits spontaneous wrapping/unwrapping at the entry and exit DNA of the nucleosomes was found to be accurate of single nucleosome oscillations (Li et al, 2005). Indeed, AFM studies revealed that spontaneous nucleosome unwrapping in the absence of ATP or any chromatin remodelers can occur *in vitro*, on a time a scale of less than 1 min. Furthermore, the study was able to identify kinetic steps in the process. First, the nucleosome was observed to slide along the DNA molecule until it was closer to its ends. Then, a transient state of unwrapping was observed, relaxing the DNA-octamer interactions, followed by the asymmetric unwrapping, which was revealed by the length increase of only one DNA arm but not the other.

Studies of nucleosome dissociation using HS-AFM also showed a second potential and alternative mechanism (Miyagi et al, 2011; Suzuki et al, 2010). Nucleosomes may translocate reversibly along the DNA molecule through a process of sliding (Miyagi et al, 2011). Interestingly, complete eviction of nucleosome by one-directional sliding mechanism happened if a non-denaturing detergent (i.e. CHAPS) was added in the medium. This mechanism occurred by translocation steps of around 10-15 nm (3/4 turn of DNA). In agreement with these observations, nucleosome may be evicted from chromatin fiber in two different forms. Suzuki *et al.* observed that nucleosome may dissociate in one step from the octameric form or sequentially in two equal small subunits, probably two tetramers (Suzuki et al, 2010).

In vitro chromatin assembly in presence of the histone chaperone NAP1 and the ATP-dependent motor protein ACF is still studied by HS-AFM (Torigoe et al, 2011). Nucleosome formation is performed in different steps with first a rapid formation of DNA-histones intermediate, before the wrapping of DNA around the octamer to form the nucleosome. This second step is slower and ATP-dependent. The binding of histones onto DNA is initiated by the deposition of H3-H4 and may require NAP1 but the histone chaperone does not stay associated.

The ability of HS-AFM to analyze kinetics is already established. EcoP15I is a type III restriction enzyme, which recognizes two inversely oriented non-palindromic sequences and generates double strand break. EcoP15I cutting activity depends on the presence and recognition of two restriction sites separated by 3500 base pairs. AFM analysis demonstrated that to reduce this distance and generate the break, a large DNA loop is formed between the two sites (Crampton et al, 2007). The acquisition of 1-3 images per second revealed the ATP-dependent translocation of EcoP15I along plasmid at a rate of 79 base pairs/s, leading to the accumulation of supercoiling. Similar experiment with the restriction enzyme EcoRII highlighted the importance of HS-AFM as tool to characterize the mechanism of search of second restriction site by these enzymes and their translocation along the DNA molecule (Gilmore et al, 2009).

5.3 Elastic and other material property measurement

The unique feature of AFM is that it can both image and measure forces at high resolution. The latter offers the possibility to measure material properties at the micro- and the nanoscale. One of the first applications of AFM was the measurement of elastic properties of microscopic biological structures, such as single cells and inhomogeneous tissues at microscopic scales. This is done by indenting the sample with the AFM probe and acquiring cantilever deflection *vs* displacement curves. Then, with mathematical models of contact mechanics, the elastic modulus of the sample (Young's modulus) is estimated (Dimitriadis et al, 2002; Lin et al, 2007a; Lin et al, 2007b). AFM is the only method that can map elastic properties at high resolution in ambient or under physiological condition. These elasticity maps can be correlated with topography to gain insights into the architecture that leads from the nanoscale to the macroscale properties of a tissue.

5.4 Receptor-ligand interaction

5.4.1 Strategy of coating

The AFM is also used for the chemical recognition of molecules. The technique requires the pre-coating of the AFM probe with a specific antibody against a protein of interest. Such functionalized probes are then used to scan the sample and map the corresponding target antigen. During the topography scan, the binding of the antibody with its antigen will be detected by the modification of the cantilever oscillation, generating a parallel image of antigen-antibody interaction hits (Hinterdorfer & Dufrene, 2006; Kamruzzahan et al, 2006; Raab et al, 1999; Stroh et al, 2004). The success of the recognition depends on the choice of this specific antibody and the quality of its coating.

Several protocols for covalently attaching such molecules to AFM probes exist in the literature, ranging from simple physisorption to complex chemistry that first attaches a spacer molecule to which the antibody is then covalently bound (Barattin & Voyer, 2011). Examples of chemical systems are glutathione/glutathione S-transferase, or Ni-NTA (nickel-nitrilotriacetic acid) -His6/GST-His6-tag-protein (Gamsjaeger et al, 2004; Schmitt et al, 2000; Yoshimura et al, 2006). The spacer gives the antibody freedom of movement to accommodate the fixed position and orientation of the antigen. A challenge to recognition is non-specific binding which requires carefully planned controls.

5.4.2 Examples of receptor-ligand analysis in the context of chromatin

This technique has been already used in the chromatin field, such as for the recognition of proteins within the centromeric histone variant nucleosome (Wang et al, 2008). In this study, the direct identification of CENH3 confirmed that CENH3 nucleosomes display mainly a tetrameric structure. This method of recognition was also used to follow assembly/disassembly of nucleosome during remodeling. Swi-Snf is an ATP-dependent nucleosome remodeling complex whose function was analyzed by recognition imaging using specific antibody against histone H2A (Bash et al, 2006). Incubation of *in vitro* reconstituted chromatin with Swi-Snf leaded to the release of histone H2A, suggesting that remodeling requires partial disassembly of the nucleosome.

As previously mentioned, the specificity of the antibody is a major factor of success for recognition. Lin *et al.* tested another system of recognition using DNA aptamers, to reduce cross-reactivity and enhance detection (Lin et al, 2007c). These nucleic acid molecules display similar properties to antibody such as their characteristic folding complementary to the structure of their target epitope (Bunka & Stockley, 2006; Colas, 2008). However, their small size and their nucleic composition facilitate their design and synthesis. DNA aptamers against histone H4 were used successfully with a high efficiency of recognition (85% compared to 48% for a commercial antibody) and limited cross-reactivity with the other histones. While this exciting alternative strategy has not been used in chromatin field, it continues to be investigated for the selection of strong affinity aptamers by the method of AFM-SELEX (Systematic Evolution of Ligands by an Exponential enrichment) (Miyachi et al, 2010).

6. Next generation AFM for the study of specific molecules in biological context *in situ*

An exciting new generation of AFM instruments is being developed and made available to the research community, which combines the power of structural analysis by AFM with simultaneous molecular identification of specific targets using immunofluorescence/confocal microscopy. Instruments now exist which combine AFM with epi-fluorescence, TIRF microscopy (total internal reflection fluorescence), high resolution Raman and infrared spectroscopy.

For chromatin studies, epi-fluorescence and TIRF are equivalent, since the chromatin samples will have to be immobilized to the mica surface. The combination of high resolution fluorescence microscopy with AFM (FIONA-AFM) allows the identification and the localization of fluorescent-tagged molecules such as proteins on topographic image. The strength of this technique was evaluated by the analysis of the interaction of the protein complex UvrA-UvrB, involved in the initiation of nucleotide excision repair pathway, with DNA, and the binding of RNAP on *Escherichia coli* DNA (Ebenstein et al, 2009; Fronczek et al, 2011). Both studies showed the correlation between optical and AFM signals, providing a proof of principle for combining structural details of multi-molecular complexes with dynamic information yielded by fluorescence.

Raman and infrared spectroscopies (Fourier Transform-Infrared Spectroscopy or Ft-IR) are vibrational techniques used for chemical identification. They give similar but complementary information since they use different regions of the spectrum. Standard Raman or FT-IR spectroscopies are diffraction limited. Therefore the resolution of Raman spectroscopy is in the 1 μm range while for FT-IR it is in the 5-10 μm range. Raman spectroscopy has the additional disadvantage of a weak signal requiring large samples and long acquisition times. Their combination with AFM is relatively recent but the technological advances hold great promise for label-free, single molecule identification. The sub-diffraction resolution of Raman spectroscopy is achieved by using the AFM tip, coated with Au, Pt or Ag to achieve Raman signal enhancement by orders of magnitude (Anderson & Pike, 2002). More recently, Neascu *et al.* demonstrated enhancement of over 10^9 to achieve single molecule sensitivity (Neacsu et al, 2006). Applications in biology are starting to appear more frequently and are expected to expand further in the future.

In the infrared range, a novel idea directly couples AFM with IR spectroscopy in a new photothermal technique called photothermal induced resonance (PTIR) (Yeo et al, 2008). A pulsed, tunable infrared laser is directed to the sample through a prism at a total reflection angle. Infrared absorption by the sample excites the cantilever through the contacting tip into resonance. Analysis of the ring-down signal of the cantilever maps the IR absorption spectrum. The method has demonstrated a resolution below 50-100 nm and applicability to a fluid environment (Dazzi et al, 2007; Dazzi et al, 2008).

7. Conclusion

As we have seen above, AFM is a versatile and powerful tool for biological studies. Several protocols are now perfectly established to characterize nucleoprotein complexes such as chromatin, or nucleic acid molecules (DNA or RNA). Applications range from observation of native complexes undergoing dynamic change to precise measurement of static physical dimensions. The panel of potential available studies results from the different modalities of the AFM by itself (e.g. non-contact/tapping vs. contact mode; ambient air vs. fluid; high-speed) and its combination with other biophysical method such as Raman spectroscopy. Newer applications permit combination of fluorescence imaging to single molecule measurement, thus finally bridging the resolution gap between light microscopy and electron microscopy. In consequence, the fast evolving nature of the technology continuously yields new applications for AFM researchers. Pre-existing AFM applications, and yet to be developed new tools, will continue to qualitatively and quantitatively enhance our capacity to study of dynamics and structure of biological materials.

8. Acknowledgement

We thank Dr. Marcin Walkiewicz for his comments of the manuscript.

9. References

Anderson MS, Pike WT (2002) A Raman-atomic force microscope for apertureless-near-field spectroscopy and optical trapping. *Review of Scientific Instruments* 73(3): 1198 - 1203

Ando T, Kodera N, Takai E, Maruyama D, Saito K, Toda A (2001) A high-speed atomic force microscope for studying biological macromolecules. *Proc Natl Acad Sci U S A* 98(22): 12468-12472

Barattin R, Voyer N (2011) Chemical modifications of atomic force microscopy tips. *Methods Mol Biol* 736: 457-483

Bash R, Wang H, Anderson C, Yodh J, Hager G, Lindsay SM, Lohr D (2006) AFM imaging of protein movements: histone H2A-H2B release during nucleosome remodeling. *FEBS Lett* 580(19): 4757-4761

Binnig G, Quate CF, Gerber C (1986) Atomic force microscope. *Phys Rev Lett* 56(9): 930-933

Bloom KS, Anderson JN (1978) Fractionation and characterization of chromosomal proteins by the hydroxyapatite dissociation method. *J Biol Chem* 253(12): 4446-4450

Bunka DH, Stockley PG (2006) Aptamers come of age - at last. *Nat Rev Microbiol* 4(8): 588-596

Cantor CR, Schimmel PR (1980) *Biophysical Chemistry: Part II: Techniques for the Study of Biological Structure and Function*.

Chiu W (1993) What does electron cryomicroscopy provide that X-ray crystallography and NMR spectroscopy cannot? *Annu Rev Biophys Biomol Struct* 22: 233-255

Colas P (2008) The eleven-year switch of peptide aptamers. *J Biol* 7(1): 2

Crampton N, Bonass WA, Kirkham J, Rivetti C, Thomson NH (2006) Collision events between RNA polymerases in convergent transcription studied by atomic force microscopy. *Nucleic Acids Res* 34(19): 5416-5425

Crampton N, Yokokawa M, Dryden DT, Edwardson JM, Rao DN, Takeyasu K, Yoshimura SH, Henderson RM (2007) Fast-scan atomic force microscopy reveals that the type III restriction enzyme EcoP15I is capable of DNA translocation and looping. *Proc Natl Acad Sci U S A* 104(31): 12755-12760

Dalal Y, Fleury TJ, Cioffi A, Stein A (2005) Long-range oscillation in a periodic DNA sequence motif may influence nucleosome array formation. *Nucleic Acids Res* 33(3): 934-945

Dalal Y, Wang H, Lindsay S, Henikoff S (2007) Tetrameric structure of centromeric nucleosomes in interphase Drosophila cells. *PLoS Biol* 5(8): e218

Dazzi A, Prazeres R, Glotin F, Ortega JM (2007) Analysis of nano-chemical mapping performed by an AFM-based ("AFMIR") acousto-optic technique. *Ultramicroscopy* 107(12): 1194-1200

Dazzi A, Prazeres R, Glotin F, Ortega JM, Al-Sawaftah M, de Frutos M (2008) Chemical mapping of the distribution of viruses into infected bacteria with a photothermal method. *Ultramicroscopy* 108(7): 635-641

Dimitriadis EK, Horkay F, Maresca J, Kachar B, Chadwick RS (2002) Determination of elastic moduli of thin layers of soft material using the atomic force microscope. *Biophys J* 82(5): 2798-2810

Dimitriadis EK, Weber C, Gill RK, Diekmann S, Dalal Y (2010) Tetrameric organization of vertebrate centromeric nucleosomes. *Proc Natl Acad Sci U S A* 107(47): 20317-20322

Duzdevich D, Li J, Whang J, Takahashi H, Takeyasu K, Dryden DT, Morton AJ, Edwardson JM (2011) Unusual structures are present in DNA fragments containing super-long Huntingtin CAG repeats. *PLoS One* 6(2): e17119

Ebenstein Y, Gassman N, Kim S, Weiss S (2009) Combining atomic force and fluorescence microscopy for analysis of quantum-dot labeled protein-DNA complexes. *J Mol Recognit* 22(5): 397-402

Filenko NA, Kolar C, West JT, Smith SA, Hassan YI, Borgstahl GE, Zempleni J, Lyubchenko YL (2011) The role of histone H4 biotinylation in the structure of nucleosomes. *PLoS One* 6(1): e16299

Finkbeiner S (2011) Huntington's Disease. *Cold Spring Harb Perspect Biol* 3(6)

Fronczek DN, Quammen C, Wang H, Kisker C, Superfine R, Taylor R, Erie DA, Tessmer I (2011) High accuracy FIONA-AFM hybrid imaging. *Ultramicroscopy* 111(5): 350-355

Gamsjaeger R, Wimmer B, Kahr H, Tinazli A, Picuric S, Lata S, Tampe R, Maulet Y, Gruber HJ, Hinterdorfer P, Romanin C (2004) Oriented binding of the His6-tagged carboxyl-tail of the L-type Ca2+ channel alpha1-subunit to a new NTA-functionalized self-assembled monolayer. *Langmuir* 20(14): 5885-5890

Garcia de la Torre J (2001) Hydration from hydrodynamics. General considerations and applications of bead modelling to globular proteins. *Biophys Chem* 93(2-3): 159-170

Gellert M (2002) V(D)J recombination: RAG proteins, repair factors, and regulation. *Annu Rev Biochem* 71: 101-132

Germond JE, Hirt B, Oudet P, Gross-Bellark M, Chambon P (1975) Folding of the DNA double helix in chromatin-like structures from simian virus 40. *Proc Natl Acad Sci U S A* 72(5): 1843-1847

Gilmore JL, Suzuki Y, Tamulaitis G, Siksnys V, Takeyasu K, Lyubchenko YL (2009) Single-molecule dynamics of the DNA-EcoRII protein complexes revealed with high-speed atomic force microscopy. *Biochemistry* 48(44): 10492-10498

Gordon F, Luger K, Hansen JC (2005) The core histone N-terminal tail domains function independently and additively during salt-dependent oligomerization of nucleosomal arrays. *J Biol Chem* 280(40): 33701-33706

Grundy GJ, Ramon-Maiques S, Dimitriadis EK, Kotova S, Biertumpfel C, Heymann JB, Steven AC, Gellert M, Yang W (2009) Initial stages of V(D)J recombination: the organization of RAG1/2 and RSS DNA in the postcleavage complex. *Mol Cell* 35(2): 217-227

Guthold M, Bezanilla M, Erie DA, Jenkins B, Hansma HG, Bustamante C (1994) Following the assembly of RNA polymerase-DNA complexes in aqueous solutions with the scanning force microscope. *Proc Natl Acad Sci U S A* 91(26): 12927-12931

Hakme A, Wong HK, Dantzer F, Schreiber V (2008) The expanding field of poly(ADP-ribosyl)ation reactions. 'Protein Modifications: Beyond the Usual Suspects' Review Series. *EMBO Rep* 9(11): 1094-1100

Hamon L, Pastre D, Dupaigne P, Le Breton C, Le Cam E, Pietrement O (2007) High-resolution AFM imaging of single-stranded DNA-binding (SSB) protein--DNA complexes. *Nucleic Acids Res* 35(8): e58

Hansma HG, Kim KJ, Laney DE, Garcia RA, Argaman M, Allen MJ, Parsons SM (1997) Properties of biomolecules measured from atomic force microscope images: a review. *J Struct Biol* 119(2): 99-108

Hansma HG, Laney DE (1996) DNA binding to mica correlates with cationic radius: assay by atomic force microscopy. *Biophys J* 70(4): 1933-1939

Hansma HG, Laney DE, Bezanilla M, Sinsheimer RL, Hansma PK (1995) Applications for atomic force microscopy of DNA. *Biophys J* 68(5): 1672-1677

Hassan YI, Zempleni J (2008) A novel, enigmatic histone modification: biotinylation of histones by holocarboxylase synthetase. *Nutr Rev* 66(12): 721-725

Hinterdorfer P, Dufrene YF (2006) Detection and localization of single molecular recognition events using atomic force microscopy. *Nat Methods* 3(5): 347-355

Hizume K, Nakai T, Araki S, Prieto E, Yoshikawa K, Takeyasu K (2009) Removal of histone tails from nucleosome dissects the physical mechanisms of salt-induced aggregation, linker histone H1-induced compaction, and 30-nm fiber formation of the nucleosome array. *Ultramicroscopy* 109(8): 868-873

Hizume K, Yoshimura SH, Takeyasu K (2004) Atomic force microscopy demonstrates a critical role of DNA superhelicity in nucleosome dynamics. *Cell Biochem Biophys* 40(3): 249-261

Hohng S, Joo C, Ha T (2004) Single-molecule three-color FRET. *Biophys J* 87(2): 1328-1337

Hoshi O, Owen R, Miles M, Ushiki T (2004) Imaging of human metaphase chromosomes by atomic force microscopy in liquid. *Cytogenet Genome Res* 107(1-2): 28-31

Humphris AD, Zhao B, Catto D, Howard-Knight JP, Kohli P, Hobbs JK (2011) High speed nano-metrology. *Rev Sci Instrum* 82(4): 043710

Kamruzzahan AS, Ebner A, Wildling L, Kienberger F, Riener CK, Hahn CD, Pollheimer PD, Winklehner P, Holzl M, Lackner B, Schorkl DM, Hinterdorfer P, Gruber HJ (2006) Antibody linking to atomic force microscope tips via disulfide bond formation. *Bioconjug Chem* 17(6): 1473-1481

Kan PY, Lu X, Hansen JC, Hayes JJ (2007) The H3 tail domain participates in multiple interactions during folding and self-association of nucleosome arrays. *Mol Cell Biol* 27(6): 2084-2091

Kasas S, Thomson NH, Smith BL, Hansma HG, Zhu X, Guthold M, Bustamante C, Kool ET, Kashlev M, Hansma PK (1997) Escherichia coli RNA polymerase activity observed using atomic force microscopy. *Biochemistry* 36(3): 461-468

Khuu PA, Voth AR, Hays FA, Ho PS (2006) The stacked-X DNA Holliday junction and protein recognition. *J Mol Recognit* 19(3): 234-242

Kouzarides T (2007) Chromatin modifications and their function. *Cell* 128(4): 693-705

Lebrun A, Lavery R (1997) Unusual DNA conformations. *Curr Opin Struct Biol* 7(3): 348-354

Lepault J, Booy FP, Dubochet J (1983) Electron microscopy of frozen biological suspensions. *J Microsc* 129(Pt 1): 89-102

Li G, Levitus M, Bustamante C, Widom J (2005) Rapid spontaneous accessibility of nucleosomal DNA. *Nat Struct Mol Biol* 12(1): 46-53

Li G, Reinberg D (2011) Chromatin higher-order structures and gene regulation. *Curr Opin Genet Dev* 21(2): 175-186

Lin DC, Dimitriadis EK, Horkay F (2007a) Robust strategies for automated AFM force curve analysis--I. Non-adhesive indentation of soft, inhomogeneous materials. *J Biomech Eng* 129(3): 430-440

Lin DC, Dimitriadis EK, Horkay F (2007b) Robust strategies for automated AFM force curve analysis-II: adhesion-influenced indentation of soft, elastic materials. *J Biomech Eng* 129(6): 904-912

Lin L, Hom D, Lindsay SM, Chaput JC (2007c) In vitro selection of histone H4 aptamers for recognition imaging microscopy. *J Am Chem Soc* 129(47): 14568-14569

Luger K, Rechsteiner TJ, Flaus AJ, Waye MM, Richmond TJ (1997) Characterization of nucleosome core particles containing histone proteins made in bacteria. *J Mol Biol* 272(3): 301-311

Lyubchenko YL, Jacobs BL, Lindsay SM (1992) Atomic force microscopy of reovirus dsRNA: a routine technique for length measurements. *Nucleic Acids Res* 20(15): 3983-3986

Manalis SR, Minne SC, Quate CF (1996) Atomic force microscopy for high speed imaging using cantilevers with an integrated actuator and sensor. *Appl Phys Lett* 68(6): 871-873

McBryant SJ, Klonoski J, Sorensen TC, Norskog SS, Williams S, Resch MG, Toombs JA, 3rd, Hobdey SE, Hansen JC (2009) Determinants of histone H4 N-terminal domain function during nucleosomal array oligomerization: roles of amino acid sequence, domain length, and charge density. *J Biol Chem* 284(25): 16716-16722

Mikheikin AL, Lushnikov AY, Lyubchenko YL (2006) Effect of DNA supercoiling on the geometry of holliday junctions. *Biochemistry* 45(43): 12998-13006

Mills M, Lacroix L, Arimondo PB, Leroy JL, Francois JC, Klump H, Mergny JL (2002) Unusual DNA conformations: implications for telomeres. *Curr Med Chem Anticancer Agents* 2(5): 627-644

Miyachi Y, Shimizu N, Ogino C, Kondo A (2010) Selection of DNA aptamers using atomic force microscopy. *Nucleic Acids Res* 38(4): e21

Miyagi A, Ando T, Lyubchenko YL (2011) Dynamics of nucleosomes assessed with time-lapse high-speed atomic force microscopy. *Biochemistry* 50(37): 7901-7908

Nagao E, Dvorak JA (1999) Phase imaging by atomic force microscopy: analysis of living homoiothermic vertebrate cells. *Biophys J* 76(6): 3289-3297

Neacsu CC, Dreyer J, Behr N, Raschke MB (2006) Scanning-probe Raman spectroscopy with single-molecule sensitivity. *Physical Review B* 73(19)

Ouararhni K, Hadj-Slimane R, Ait-Si-Ali S, Robin P, Mietton F, Harel-Bellan A, Dimitrov S, Hamiche A (2006) The histone variant mH2A1.1 interferes with transcription by down-regulating PARP-1 enzymatic activity. *Genes Dev* 20(23): 3324-3336

Pastre D, Hamon L, Landousy F, Sorel I, David MO, Zozime A, Le Cam E, Pietrement O (2006) Anionic polyelectrolyte adsorption on mica mediated by multivalent cations: a solution to DNA imaging by atomic force microscopy under high ionic strengths. *Langmuir* 22(15): 6651-6660

Pastre D, Pietrement O, Fusil S, Landousy F, Jeusset J, David MO, Hamon L, Le Cam E, Zozime A (2003) Adsorption of DNA to mica mediated by divalent counterions: a theoretical and experimental study. *Biophys J* 85(4): 2507-2518

Raab A, Han W, Badt D, Smith-Gill SJ, Lindsay SM, Schindler H, Hinterdorfer P (1999) Antibody recognition imaging by force microscopy. *Nat Biotechnol* 17(9): 901-905

Ruska E (1980) The early development of electron lenses and electron microscopy. *Microsc Acta Suppl*(Suppl 5): 1-140

Schmitt L, Ludwig M, Gaub HE, Tampe R (2000) A metal-chelating microscopy tip as a new toolbox for single-molecule experiments by atomic force microscopy. *Biophys J* 78(6): 3275-3285

Shlyakhtenko LS, Gall AA, Filonov A, Cerovac Z, Lushnikov A, Lyubchenko YL (2003) Silatrane-based surface chemistry for immobilization of DNA, protein-DNA complexes and other biological materials. *Ultramicroscopy* 97(1-4): 279-287

Shlyakhtenko LS, Hsieh P, Grigoriev M, Potaman VN, Sinden RR, Lyubchenko YL (2000) A cruciform structural transition provides a molecular switch for chromosome structure and dynamics. *J Mol Biol* 296(5): 1169-1173

Shlyakhtenko LS, Potaman VN, Sinden RR, Lyubchenko YL (1998) Structure and dynamics of supercoil-stabilized DNA cruciforms. *J Mol Biol* 280(1): 61-72

Simpson RT, Thoma F, Brubaker JM (1985) Chromatin reconstituted from tandemly repeated cloned DNA fragments and core histones: a model system for study of higher order structure. *Cell* 42(3): 799-808

Soldatenkov VA, Chasovskikh S, Potaman VN, Trofimova I, Smulson ME, Dritschilo A (2002) Transcriptional repression by binding of poly(ADP-ribose) polymerase to promoter sequences. *J Biol Chem* 277(1): 665-670

Stein A (1989) Reconstitution of chromatin from purified components. *Methods Enzymol* 170: 585-603

Stroh C, Wang H, Bash R, Ashcroft B, Nelson J, Gruber H, Lohr D, Lindsay SM, Hinterdorfer P (2004) Single-molecule recognition imaging microscopy. *Proc Natl Acad Sci U S A* 101(34): 12503-12507

Suzuki Y, Higuchi Y, Hizume K, Yokokawa M, Yoshimura SH, Yoshikawa K, Takeyasu K (2010) Molecular dynamics of DNA and nucleosomes in solution studied by fast-scanning atomic force microscopy. *Ultramicroscopy* 110(6): 682-688

Taylor KA, Glaeser RM (1974) Electron diffraction of frozen, hydrated protein crystals. *Science* 186(4168): 1036-1037

Torigoe SE, Urwin DL, Ishii H, Smith DE, Kadonaga JT (2011) Identification of a rapidly formed nonnucleosomal histone-DNA intermediate that is converted into chromatin by ACF. *Mol Cell* 43(4): 638-648

Tulin A, Spradling A (2003) Chromatin loosening by poly(ADP)-ribose polymerase (PARP) at Drosophila puff loci. *Science* 299(5606): 560-562

Ushiki T, Hoshi O (2008) Atomic force microscopy for imaging human metaphase chromosomes. *Chromosome Res* 16(3): 383-396

Wacker DA, Ruhl DD, Balagamwala EH, Hope KM, Zhang T, Kraus WL (2007) The DNA binding and catalytic domains of poly(ADP-ribose) polymerase 1 cooperate in the regulation of chromatin structure and transcription. *Mol Cell Biol* 27(21): 7475-7485

Wang H, Bash R, Yodh JG, Hager GL, Lohr D, Lindsay SM (2002) Glutaraldehyde modified mica: a new surface for atomic force microscopy of chromatin. *Biophys J* 83(6): 3619-3625

Wang H, Dalal Y, Henikoff S, Lindsay S (2008) Single-epitope recognition imaging of native chromatin. *Epigenetics Chromatin* 1(1): 10

Workman JL, Taylor IC, Kingston RE, Roeder RG (1991) Control of class II gene transcription during in vitro nucleosome assembly. *Methods Cell Biol* 35: 419-447

Yeo BS, Maedler S, Schmid T, Zhang W, Zenobi R (2008) Tip-enhanced Raman spectroscopy can see more: The case of cytochrome C. *Journal of Physical Chemistry B* 112(13): 4867-4873

Yoshimura SH, Takahashi H, Otsuka S, Takeyasu K (2006) Development of glutathione-coupled cantilever for the single-molecule force measurement by scanning force microscopy. *FEBS Lett* 580(16): 3961-3965

Zhao B, Howard-Knight JP, Humphris AD, Kailas L, Ratcliffe EC, Foster SJ, Hobbs JK (2009) Large scan area high-speed atomic force microscopy using a resonant scanner. *Rev Sci Instrum* 80(9): 093707

Zhao Y, Cheng Q, Qian M, Cantrell JH (2010) Phase image contrast mechanism in intermittent contact atomic force microscopy *Journal of Applied Physics* 108(9): 4311

10

Artificial and Natural Membranes

György Váró and Zsolt Szegletes
Institute of Biophysics, Biological Research Centre, Szeged
Hungary

1. Introduction

Non-cellular forms of life are not known on the earth. Starting with unicellular organisms, - such as bacteria - up to multicellular complex organisms, the basic building unit is the cell, surrounded by the cell membrane. The cell contains all the characteristics of life, having the genetic program to build up the structure and to keep it functioning.

Membranes are an essential structural component of living objects (Sybesma, 1977; Volkenstein, 1981). They are formed from different lipids and act as a selective barrier around the cell and cell organelles. The phospholipid bilayer is the basic structure of all biological membranes. Besides the phospholipids, some other lipids are generally present in the membrane, such as glycolipids and cholesterol. Many biological processes require membranes. Physically and chemically essential functions include metabolism and the process of the accumulation and usage of energy in the biological system.

An essential function of the membrane is to keep a well-defined chemical composition inside of the membrane at a limited volume, which is different from the outside. There are large concentration differences between the two sides. To build up and maintain this concentration difference, selective passive diffusion and selective active transport translocate biologically important molecules through the membrane. This is achieved by different channels and pumps built from a large variety of membrane proteins. The selectivity is achieved by the composition and structure of the transporter (Sybesma, 1977; Volkenstein, 1981).

Membrane proteins fall into two categories, depending on how they are bound to the membrane. One category is that of the peripheral proteins. They are loosely bound to the membrane through electrostatic interactions and they can be removed in lipid free-form by relatively mild treatments. In the second category are the integral proteins, embedded inside the membrane and often spanning it entirely. They are difficult to remove, having large hydrophobic domains, isolated with bound lipids. The integral membrane proteins occur in a wide variety of shapes. The most common formations are the α-helix and the β-sheet structures (Sybesma, 1977).

There are a large variety of structural possibilities and this is reflected in the very different properties and behaviour of the membrane proteins. Due to the lateral fluidity of the membrane, proteins are mobile in the surface and they can form aggregates. Large associations of proteins and lipids form rafts. By interacting with the proteins, new characteristic properties appear (Engel and Gaub, 2008).

Over the last decade, the atomic force microscope (AFM) has become an important tool in biology. Besides of high resolution imaging single molecule experiments were performed in native environments and important parameters of the studied objects were determined, such as micro-elasticity, viscosity, dielectric property, electric charge distribution and other important parameters (Muller et al., 1997a).

2. Sample holder surfaces

For the modelling of a biological system, it is becoming increasingly important to understand the physical properties of living objects. In order to achieve the goal of determining their mechanical parameters, a sample is fixed to a clean surface which is flat at the atomic level. The bonds should be strong enough to avoid the dragging of the tip but equally they should not cause structural alterations to the system (Santos and Castanho, 2004).

The most commonly used support for biological samples is muscovite mica (Muller et al., 1997a). Its composition is $(KF)_2(Al_2O_3)_3(SiO_2)_6(H_2O)$. Chemically it is relatively inert. The crystal structure is characterised by its layered structure. Along this layer, the cleavage yields an atomically flat surface (Figure 1, panel a). The cleaved surface has a net negative charge with an average surface charge density of -0.0025 C/m^2, which corresponds to 0.015 electrons per surface unit cell. By using different pre-treatments, the mica surface can fix a large variety of biological samples.

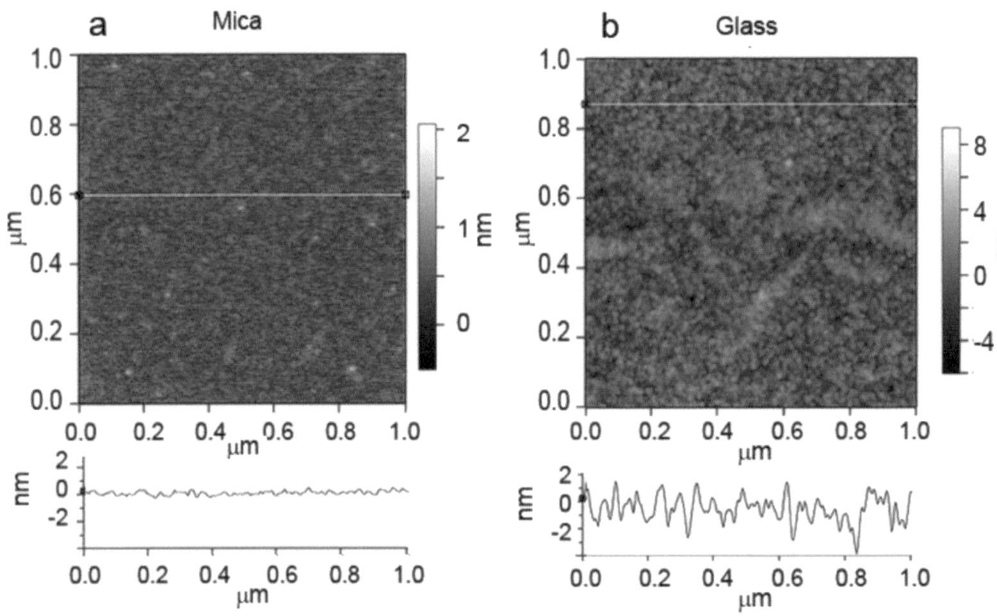

Fig. 1. High-resolution surface images of mica and glass - the materials most used by the AFM technique for membrane deposition.

Glass microscope slides or cover slips are frequently used as a transparent specimen support. The amorphous surface of the glass can be manipulated with chemical treatment, so as to fixate the biological probes (Muller et al., 1997a). Care should be taken to ensure that the glass surface roughness is about 1-2 nm (Figure 1, panel b), which is commensurable with the thickness of the membrane (Bálint et al., 2007a).

Highly oriented pyrolytic graphite (HOPG) is also used as a support for AFM probe if a conductive sample is prepared or a strongly hydrophobic flat surface is required for the sample preparation (Morris et al., 1999). Another possibility for manufacturing a conductive sample is by using vacuum-evaporated gold surface as the support. The gold surface binds thiols or disulphides, which can be used to covalently bind biological molecules (Muller et al., 1997a).

Nowadays, it is increasingly common to use a polished silicon wafer surface as a holder of the AFM sample. Its electrical and mechanical characteristics are well-known. Depending on the doping material used, the silicon can be positively or negatively charged (Morris et al., 1999; Bálint et al., 2007a).

The adhesion between the supporting medium and the sample strongly depends on the quality of the contact surfaces, a subject which has been intensively studied (Eastman and Zhu, 1996). It has been shown that the adhesive force can be accounted for by the van der Waals forces and the capillary forces between the contact surfaces (Eastman and Zhu, 1996).

3. Artificial membranes

Either artificial or natural membranes can be deposited on the above mentioned surfaces for AFM investigation. Artificially supported lipid membranes are model systems for the understanding of the phenomena occurring in the cell membrane. The most suitable methods for forming a supported lipid bilayer involve the Langmuir–Blodgett (LB) techniques and the fusion of lipid vesicles. LB films are formed when amphiphilic molecules interact with the air through an air-water interface. The overall effect is a reduction in the surface energy (or, equivalently, the surface tension of the water). By this method, a monolayer of lipids is compressed on an aqueous subphase. Compression/decompression isotherms are obtained by plotting the surface pressure as a function of the interfacial area. Such isotherms provide useful information about the physical state, the packing and the organisation of the lipid molecules(Dufrene et al., 1997; Rinia et al., 1999).

The LB technique allows the transferral of the monolayer of amphiphilic molecules onto a solid support - usually mica or silicon - at a constant surface pressure and a constant speed (Vie et al., 1998). If the solid support is hydrophilic - like mica - the lipid polar heads interact with the support, thus exposing the hydrophobic tails to the environment. To better mimic cellular membranes, a supported bilayer can be formed by transferring a second lipid layer onto the first mica-supported lipid monolayer. The second lipid monolayer transferred can be of different composition, thus yielding asymmetric supported lipid bilayers (Dufrene et al., 1997; Rinia et al., 1999).

The fusion of lipid vesicles on solid supports is the simplest method for preparing supported lipid bilayers (Brian and McConnell, 1984; HORN, 1984; Jass et al., 2000; Richter and Brisson, 2005). The fusion step is achieved by depositing the small unilamellar vesicle suspension onto freshly cleaved mica. Unlike LB deposition, the fusion method cannot be used to prepare asymmetric bilayers composed of two layers of a different nature. However, the fusion approach is remarkably simple, and the lateral mobility of the lipids is only slightly slower than in giant unilamellar vesicles (Przybylo et al., 2006), meaning that these membranes are biologically more relevant.

Multilayered polyelectrolyte films (Figure 2) prepared by the layer-by-layer consecutive adsorption method (Decher, 1997) became very popular over the past decade because of the numerous possible applications of the approach in various fields. They offer a simple and versatile tool and have surfaces with adjustable properties. These films can be functionalised with widely varying features, ranging from antifungal activity (Etienne et al., 2005) to anti-inflammatory properties (Schultz et al., 2005) to electro-optical devices (Eckle and Decher, 2001). By varying the electrolytes and/or the build-up conditions, the properties of the films -such as thickness (Shiratori and Rubner, 2000), cell adhesion (Richert et al., 2002), and protein adsorption (Gergely et al., 2004) - can be largely modified (Figure 3, panels a and b).

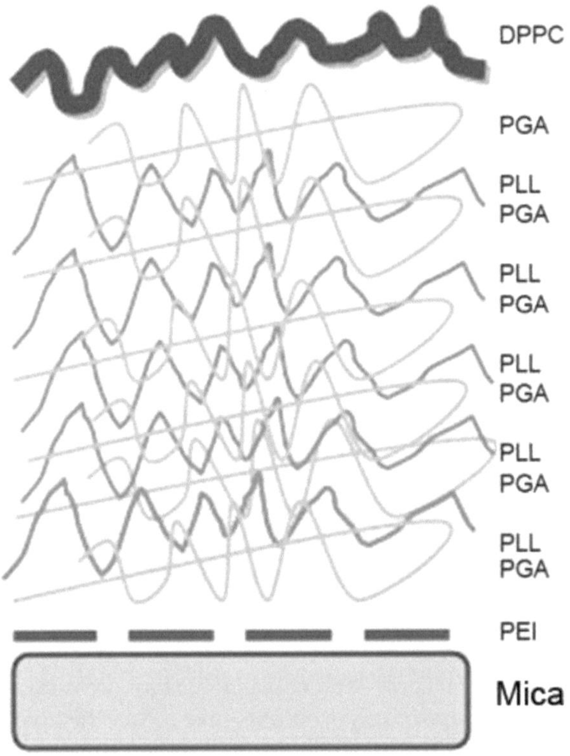

Fig. 2. Model of the structure and how the polyelectrolyte multilayer is deposited on a mica surface.

The build-up of the polyelectrolyte film began with poly(ethyleneimine) (PEI). Poly-(L-glutamic acid) (PGA)/poly(L-lysine) (PLL) polyelectrolyte film was adsorbed into the PEI-covered mica surface and then, on the surface of this film, a dipalmitoylphosphatidylcholine (DPPC) bilayer was created by the fusion of lipid vesicles. According to the AFM data, the surface roughness of the PGA/PLL film was considerably decreased by the lipid bilayer (Figure 3). In addition, the lipid surface completely closed the underlying PGA/PLL film. It seems that the forces which keep the DPPC bilayer together, in order to optimise the bilayer structure, can compress the extruding parts of the PGA/PLL films (Pilbat et al., 2007).

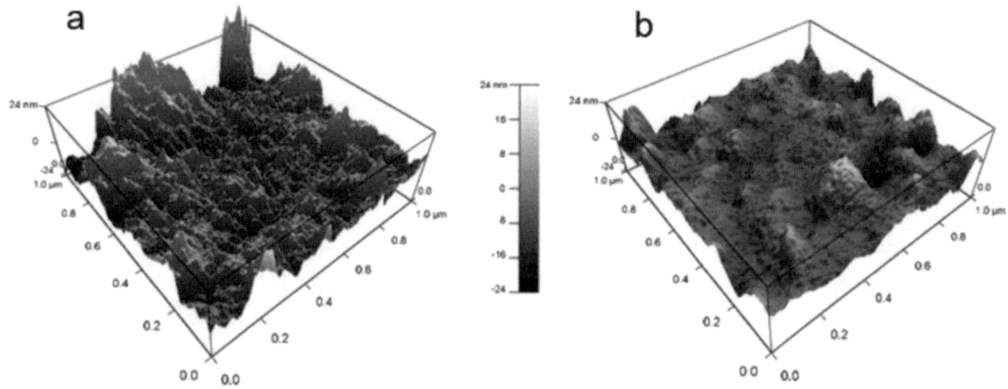

Fig. 3. High resolution image of the rough surface of polyelectrolytes (a) and its smoothed form when is covered with DPPC.

Depending on the components used, polyelectrolyte films may exhibit linear or exponential growth regimes (Lavalle et al., 2002; Gergely et al., 2004). Exponential growth requires the free diffusion of at least one of the film components in the interior of the film (Picart et al., 2002). Therefore, these films have less ordered structures than linearly growing films, which have been shown to be partially stratified with some interpenetration between neighbouring layers (Decher, 1997). Considering the extensively charged nature of the polyelectrolytes in these films, there is no chance for the direct incorporation of nonpolar, hydrophobic compounds into them. From the point of view of practical applications, however, it would be very useful if such compounds - e.g., different proteins, peptides and drugs - could be incorporated. For the incorporation of such protein molecules, lipid bilayers are needed at the very least (Figure 3b). If such bilayers were formed in the interior of polyelectrolyte films, they might be utilised as controllable internal barriers as well.

Supported lipid bilayers are readily adopted for high-resolution AFM imaging (Muller et al., 1997b; Goksu et al., 2009). A much more difficult problem is the determination of the mechanical properties of these membranes because - already at several nm indentation - the solid support is reached, thereby biasing the measured data.

4. Membrane proteins

Membrane proteins are involved in basic cellular functions, such as ion transport, energy or sensory stimuli transduction and information processing. Their large hydrophobic domains and their subunit structure make them able to assemble complicated structures, thus enabling them to fulfil this task. AFM provides the best tool for investigating the surface structure and mechanical properties of the membrane proteins in their native environment, which is in a physiological solution (Engel and Gaub, 2008). A great advantage of the AFM technique is that it allows individual molecules to be investigated in great detail. The high resolution imaging of the membrane provides information about the surface arrangement of the protein (Philippsen et al., 2002; Werten et al., 2002). It is possible to image the electrostatic potential of the membrane protein, such as the electrostatic potential of a transmembrane channel of the OmpF porin (Philippsen et al., 2002).

The most studied membrane protein is the bacteriorhodopsin (BR), a light-driven proton pump. It can be found in the purple membrane of *Halobacterium salinarum*. The purple membrane contains only 75% w/w BR and 25% lipids. By separating the purple membranes by centrifugation from the cell fragments, a clean membrane protein suspension can be obtained. The separated membrane patches are strongly packed with protein into a two-dimensional crystalline form (Lanyi, 2004a; Lanyi, 2004b). The BR, upon light excitation, goes through a photocycle and translocates a proton across the membrane (Oesterhelt, 1975).

A medium resolution AFM image shows the almost coin-like shape of the purple membrane patch (Figure 4). The height profile clearly shows the thickness of the membrane. On the high resolution image we can distinguish the hexagonal arrangement of the BR molecules in the membrane (Muller et al., 1995;Muller et al., 2000).

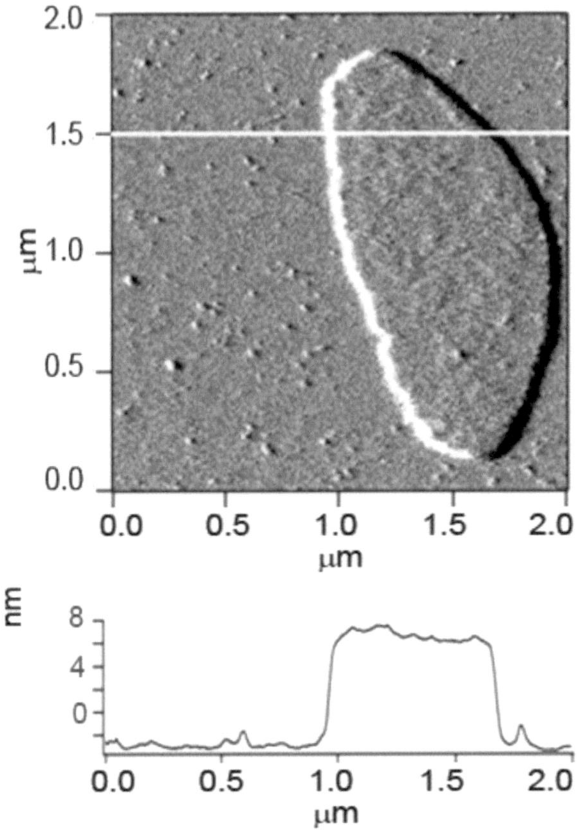

Fig. 4. The amplitude image and the height profile of a purple membrane from *Halobacterium salinarum*, deposited on mica. The image was taken in water.

A number of similar proteins were also imaged, such as the visual-rhodopsin (Fotiadis et al., 2003;Fotiadis et al., 2004), the chloride-pumping halorhodopsin (Persike et al., 2001) and the photosynthetic reaction centre of *Rhodopseudomonas viridis* (Scheuring et al., 2003;Scheuring et al., 2004). The common feature of all the imaged membrane proteins is their high density and the crystalline-like arrangement within their membranes. An image of an individual protein membrane is hard to obtain due to its strong interaction with the surrounding lipids (Dorogi et al., 2006).

An interesting question relates to how strong the proteins are which are bound in the membrane. To answer this, AFM experiments regarding pulling the protein were performed. The cantilever tip is chemically functionalised so as to bind to the protein. The tip is move above the membrane patch fixed to the sample compartment. By touching it to the membrane for a given time, the tip binds strongly to a protein in the membrane. By retracting the tip an increasing pulling force appears which for a moment reaches the level where a transmembrane segment of the protein is broken out. By pulling further, other membrane bounded parts of the protein can be removed. Through this, the whole binding force map of the protein is obtained (Oesterhelt et al., 2000; Janovjak et al., 2003; Janovjak et al., 2004; Ganchev et al., 2004).

5. Effect of small peptides on supported membranes

Antimicrobial peptides are host defence molecules produced by the innate immune system of organisms all across the evolutionary spectrum. They play a key role in the host defence system of many higher organisms (Boman, 1995). They were originally described in insects (Hultmark et al., 1980; Steiner et al., 1981) and plants (Fernandez de Caleya et al., 1972), and were subsequently identified in vertebrates (Lehrer et al., 1983; Ganz et al., 1985; Zasloff, 1987) as constituting a key component of the innate immune system. Most of the known antibacterial peptides are active against multiple microorganisms, such as viruses, bacteria, fungi and protozoa, and can be ascribed to one of three main groups: 1) α-helical peptides without cysteine, 2) peptides with three disulphide bonds, or 3) peptides rich in proline or tryptophan (Boman, 2003). AFM images of the changes on the membrane were monitored (Végh et al., 2011).

Indolicidin - encoded by a member of cathelicidin gene family and a cationic antimicrobial tridecapeptide amide - was isolated from cytoplasmic granules of bovine neutrophils (Selsted et al., 1992). It is one of the shortest known naturally-occurring antimicrobial peptides (Bowdish et al., 2005) and is toxic to both prokaryotes and eukaryotes (Falla et al., 1996; Bowdish et al., 2005). The high percentage of proline and tryptophan residues makes indolicidin a unique antimicrobial. Compared to α-helical antibiotic peptides, indolicidin is less able to dissipate the bacterial inner membrane potential and it forms smaller pores, yet it kills bacteria rapidly (Selsted et al., 1992). (Figure 5)

The purple membrane disks were deposited directly on a Ca^{2+} covered mica surface which is positively charged. In this case, the interaction of the purple membrane with indolicidin is quite specific. As it can be seen, indolicidin binds to the membrane. The edges were preferred (Figure 5), since the lipids are more accessible in those regions. Indolicidin attached to the membrane surface, especially on the border of membrane disk, but did not break the membrane's integrity. The surface area of the transient layer increased. This transient layer has about half the height (3-4 nm) of the purple membrane. Based on the height of the layer, it is probably a monolayer of lipids stabilised with indolicidin (Végh et al., 2011).

Understanding drug-cell or drug-membrane interaction is a key issue in current biophysical and pharmaceutical research (Balashev et al., 2001; Berquand et al., 2004; Van

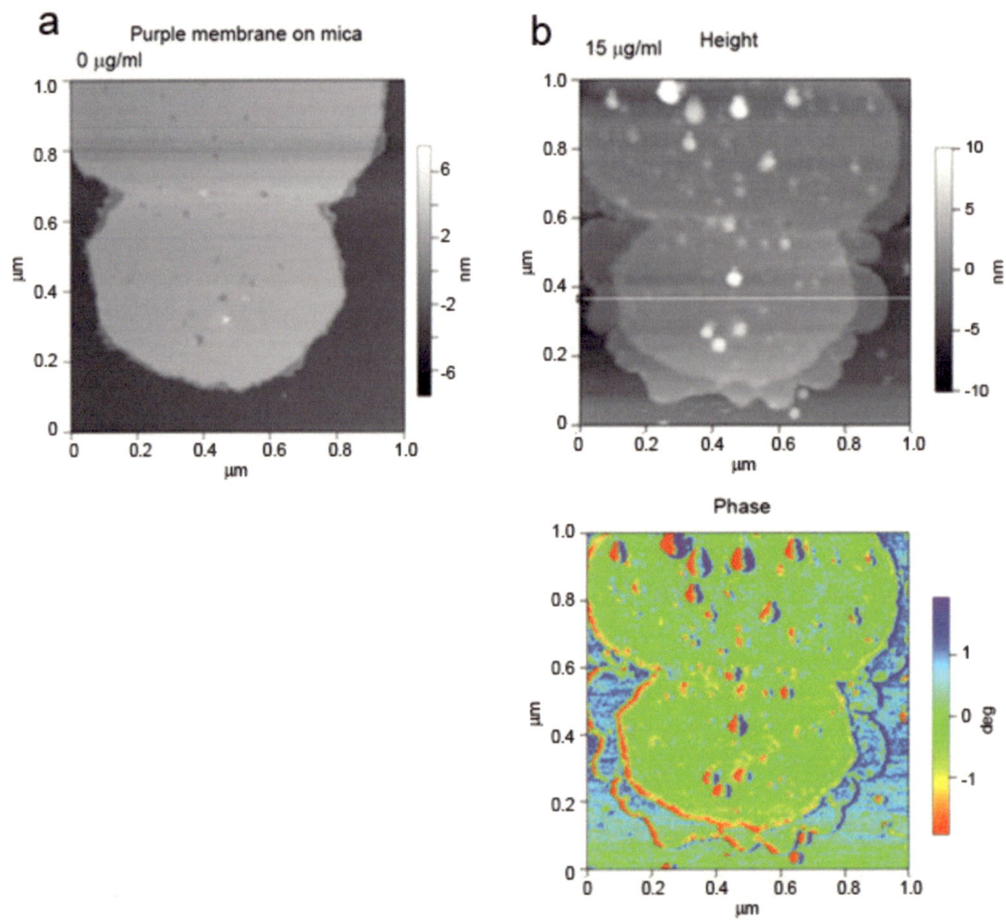

Fig. 5. The effect of the indolicidin on the purple membrane of *Halobacterium salinarum* (Végh et al., 2011) .

Vliet and Hinterdorfer, 2006). With AFM imaging, this interaction can be monitored in real-time at a high resolution (Berquand et al., 2004). With AFM it was possible to show the change of the cell elasticity when the membrane was cross-linked with an anti-cytoskeletal drug (Wu et al., 1998).

Lipid rafts are formed when large numbers of membrane proteins are interacting and aggregate on a closed configuration. The proteins inside the lipid raft can get new properties by interacting with others. An example of this are the bacteriorhodopsin in the purple membrane which interact with each other, regulating the photocycle (Tokaji, 1995; Dancsházy and Tokaji, 2000). As a matter of fact, the purple membrane packed with bacteriorhodopsin is a raft. There is a transition in the lipid composition and membrane protein density at the border of the raft, which can be detected by AFM (Poole et al., 2004; Johnston, 2009).

The membranes which are tightly-packed with protein give a good opportunity to observe the conformational change of the protein during its function (Lewis et al., 1996; Persike et al., 2000). Where there is a protein in the crystal lattice with a changed conformation, the surface symmetry is altered. Such an event was observed by the bleaching of the BR (Stahlberg et al., 2001; Braun et al., 2006). A drawback of the method is that the fast reversible processes of the conformational changes cannot be observed (Braun et al., 2006).

The instantaneous, fast conformational change of the bacteriorhodopsin was registered by an unusual arrangement of the AFM (Figure 6). The purple membranes were electrophoretically deposited in oriented-mode on a conducting cantilever (Figure 6, panel a). When the BR is excited by light, the protein goes through a photocycle, during which a conformational change occurs. The protein produces a volume change during the conformational motion which results in a deflection of the cantilever (Figure 6, panel b) (Bálint et al., 2007b).

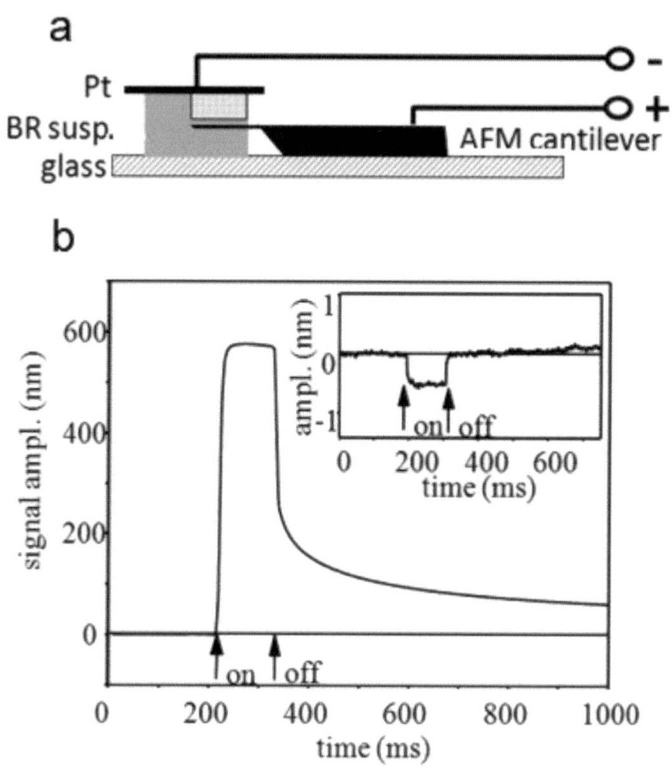

Fig. 6. The electrophoretic deposition of the purple membrane (a) and the deflection signal measured during illumination of the cantilever (b). The inset is a control signal measured with an empty cantilever (Bálint et al., 2007b) .

Several biological application of the AFM was presented. The study focused on a functionally important part of the living material, the lipid membrane. It was discussed how the membranes are deposited on a solid support for sampling and what kind of changes were observed during the measurements.

6. Acknowledgment

This work was supported by the National Science Fund of Hungary OTKA K81180 and by the COST Action TD1002.

7. References

Balashev K., Jensen T.R., Kjaer K., and Bjornholm T. (2001). Novel methods for studying lipids and lipases and their mutual interaction at interfaces. Part I. Atomic force microscopy. Biochimie 83:387-397.

Bálint Z., Nagy K., Laczkó I., Bottka S., Végh G.A., Szegletes Z., and Váró G. (2007a). Adsorption and self-assembly of oligodeoxynucleotides onto a mica surface. J. Phys. Chem. C 111:17032-17037.

Bálint Z., Végh G.A., Popescu A., Dima M., Ganea C., and Váró G. (2007b). Direct observation of protein motion during the photochemical reactio cycle of bacteriorhodopsin. Langmuir 23:7225-7228.

Berquand A., Mingeot-Leclercq M.P., and Dufrene Y.F. (2004). Real-time imaging of drug-membrane interactions by atomic force microscopy. Biochimica et Biophysica Acta-Biomembranes 1664:198-205.

Boman H.G. (1995). Peptide antibiotics and their role in innate immunity. Annu. Rev. Immunol. 13:61-92.

Boman H.G. (2003). Antibacterial peptides: basic facts and emerging concepts. J. Intern. Med. 254:197-215.

Bowdish D.M., Davidson D.J., Scott M.G., and Hancock R.E. (2005). Immunomodulatory activities of small host defense peptides. Antimicrob. Agents Chemother. 49: 1727-1732.

Braun T., Backmann N., Vogtli M., Bietsch A., Engel A., Lang H.P., Gerber C., and Hegner M. (2006). Conformational change of bacteriorhodopsin quantitatively monitored by microcantilever sensors. Biophys. J. 90:2970-2977.

Brian A.A. and McConnell H.M. (1984). Allogeneic stimulation of cytotoxic T cells by supported planar membranes. Proc. Natl. Acad. Sci. U. S. A. 81:6159-6163.

Dancsházy Z. and Tokaji Z. (2000). Blue light regeneration of bacteriorhodopsin bleached by continuous light. FEBS Lett. 476:171-173.

Decher G. (1997). Fuzzy nanoassemblies: Toward layered polymeric multicomposites RID E-7665-2011. Science 277:1232-1237.

Dorogi M., Bálint Z., Mikó C., Vileno B., Milas M., Hernadi K., Forro L., Váró G., and Nagy L. (2006). Stabilization effect of single-walled carbon nanotubes on the functioning of photosynthetic reaction centers. J. Phys. Chem. B 110:21473-21479.

Dufrene Y.F., Barger W.R., Green J.B.D., and Lee G.U. (1997). Nanometer-scale surface properties of mixed phospholipid monolayers and bilayers. Langmuir 13: 4779-4784.

Eastman T. and Zhu D.M. (1996). Adhesion forces between surface-modified AFM tips and a mica surface. Langmuir 12:2859-2862.

Eckle M. and Decher G. (2001). Tuning the performance of layer-by-layer assembled organic light emitting diodes by controlling the position of isolating clay barrier sheets RID E-7665-2011. Nano Letters 1:45-49.

Engel A. and Gaub H.E. (2008). Structure and mechanics of membrane proteins. Annual Review Of Biochemistry 77:127-148.

Etienne O., Gasnier C., Taddei C., Voegel J.C., Aunis D., Schaaf P., Metz-Boutigue M.H., Bolcato-Bellemin A.L., and Egles C. (2005). Antifungal coating by biofunctionalized polyelectrolyte multilayered films. Biomaterials 26:6704-6712.

Falla T.J., Karunaratne D.N., and Hancock R.E. (1996). Mode of action of the antimicrobial peptide indolicidin. J. Biol. Chem. 271:19298-19303.

Fernandez de Caleya R., Gonzalez-Pascual B., Garcia-Olmedo F., and Carbonero P. (1972). Susceptibility of phytopathogenic bacteria to wheat purothionins in vitro. Appl. Microbiol. 23:998-1000.

Fotiadis D., Liang Y., Filipek S., Saperstein D.A., Engel H.A., and Palczewski K. (2003). Atomic-force microscopy: Rhodopsin dimers in native disc membranes. Nature 421:127-128.

Fotiadis D., Liang Y., Filipek S., Saperstein D.A., Engel H.A., and Palczewski K. (2004). The G protein-coupled receptor rhodopsin in the native membrane. Febs Letters 564:281-288.

Ganchev D.N., Rijkers D.T.S., Snel M.M.E., Killian J.A., and Kruijff B. (2004). Strength of integration of transmembrane a-helical peptides in lipiid bilayers as determined by atomic force spectroscopy. Biochemistry 43:14987-14993.

Ganz T., Selsted M.E., Szklarek D., Harwig S.S., Daher K., Bainton D.F., and Lehrer R.I. (1985). Defensins. Natural peptide antibiotics of human neutrophils. J. Clin. Invest. 76:1427-1435.

Gergely C., Bahi S., Szalontai B., Flores P., Schaaf P., Voegel J.C., and Cuisinier F.J.G. (2004). Human serum albumin self-assembly on weak polyelectrolyte multilayer films structurally modified by pH changes. Langmuir 20:5575-5582.

Goksu E.I., Vanegas J.M., Blanchette C.D., Lin W.C., and Longo M.L. (2009). AFM for structure and dynamics of biomembranes. Biochim. Biophys. Acta 1788:254-266.

Horn R.G. (1984). Direct Measurement of the Force between 2 Lipid Bilayers and Observation of their Fusion. Biochim. Biophys. Acta 778:224-228.

Hultmark D., Steiner H., Rasmuson T., and Boman H.G. (1980). Insect immunity. Purification and properties of three inducible bactericidal proteins from hemolymph of immunized pupae of Hyalophora cecropia. Eur. J. Biochem. 106:7-16.

Janovjak H., Kessler M., Oesterhelt D., Gaub H.E., and Muller D.J. (2003). Unfolding pathways of native bacteriorhodopsin depend on temperature. Embo Journal 22:5220-5229.

Janovjak H., Struckmeier J., Hubain M., Kedrov A., Kessler M., and Muller D.J. (2004). Probing the energy landscape of the membrane protein bacteriorhodopsin. Structure 12:871-879.

Jass J., Tjarnhage T., and Puu G. (2000). From liposomes to supported, planar bilayer structures on hydrophilic and hydrophobic surfaces: an atomic force microscopy study. Biophys. J. 79:3153-3163.

Johnston L.J. (2009). Nanoscale imaging of domains in supported lipid membranes. Langmuir 23:5886-5895.

Lanyi J.K. (2004a). Bacteriorhodopsin. Annual Review of Physiology 66:665-688.

Lanyi J.K. (2004b). Transport mechanism in bacteriorhodopsin. Abstracts Of Papers Of The American Chemical Society 225:U521.

Lavalle P., Gergely C., Cuisinier F.J.G., Decher G., Schaaf P., Voegel J.C., and Picart C. (2002). Comparison of the structure of polyelectrolyte multilayer films exhibiting a linear and an exponential growth regime: An in situ atomic force microscopy study RID E-7665-2011. Macromolecules 35:4458-4465.

Lehrer R.I., Selsted M.E., Szklarek D., and Fleischmann J. (1983). Antibacterial activity of microbicidal cationic proteins 1 and 2, natural peptide antibiotics of rabbit lung macrophages. Infect. Immun. 42:10-14.

Lewis A., Rousso I., Khachatryan E., Brodsky I., Lieberman K., and Sheves M. (1996). Directly probing rapid membrane protein dynamics with an atomic force microscope: A study of light-induced conformational alterations in bacteriorhodopsin. Biophys. J. 70:2380-2384.

Morris V.J., Kirby A.R., and Gunning A.P. 1999. Atomic force microscopy for biologists. London, UK.

Muller D.J., Engel H.A., and Amrein M. (1997a). Preparation techniques for the observation of native biological systems with the atomic force microscope. Biosensors & Bioelectronics 12:867-877.

Muller D.J., Heymann J.B., Oesterhelt F., Moller C., Gaub H.E., Buldt G., and Engel H.A. (2000). Atomic force microscopy of native purple membrane. Biochimica Et Biophysica Acta-Bioenergetics 1460:27-38.

Muller D.J., Schabert F.A., Buldt G., and Engel H.A. (1995). ImagingPurple membrane in aqueous-solutions at subnanometer resolution by atomic-force microscopy. Biophys. J. 68:1681-1686.

Muller D.J., Schoenenberger C.A., Schabert F.A., and Engel H.A. (1997b). Structural changes in native membrane proteins monitored at subnanometer resolution with the atomic force microscope: A review. Journal Of Structural Biology 119:149-157.

Oesterhelt D. (1975). The purple membrane of Halobacterium halobium: a new system for light energy conversion. Ciba. Found. Symp.147-167.

Oesterhelt F., Oesterhelt D., Pfeiffer M., Engel H.A., Gaub H.E., and Muller D.J. (2000). Unfolding pathways of individual bacteriorhodopsins. Science 288:143-146.

Persike N., Pfeiffer M., Guckenberger R., and Fritz M. (2000). Changes in the surface structure of purple membrane upon illumination measured by atomic force microscopy. Colloids And Surfaces B-Biointerfaces 19:325-332.

Persike N., Pfeiffer M., Guckenberger R., Radmacher M., and Fritz M. (2001). Direct observation of different surface structures on high- resolution images of native halorhodopsin. Journal Of Molecular Biology 310:773-780.

Philippsen A., Im W.P., Engel H.A., Schirmer T., Roux B., and Muller D.J. (2002). Imaging the electrostatic potential of transmembrane channels: Atomic probe microscopy of OmpF porin. Biophys. J. 82:1667-1676.

Picart C., Mutterer J., Richert L., Luo Y., Prestwich G.D., Schaaf P., Voegel J.C., and Lavalle P. (2002). Molecular basis for the explanation of the exponential growth of polyelectrolyte multilayers. Proc. Natl. Acad. Sci. U. S. A. 99:12531-12535.

Pilbat A.M., Szegletes Z., Kóta Z., Ball V., Schaaf P., Voegel J.C., and Szalontai B. (2007). Phospholipid bilayers as biomembrane-like barriers in layer-by-layer polielectrolyte films. Langmuir 23:8236-8242.

Poole K., Meder D., Simons K., and Muller D. (2004). The effect of raft lipid depletion on microvilli formation in MDCK cells, visualized by atomic force microscopy. Febs Letters 565:53-58.

Przybylo M., Sykora J., Humpolickova J., Benda A., Zan A., and Hof M. (2006). Lipid diffusion in giant unilamellar vesicles is more than 2 times faster than in supported phospholipid bilayers under identical conditions. Langmuir : the ACS journal of surfaces and colloids 22:9096-9099.

Richert L., Lavalle P., Vautier D., Senger B., Stoltz J.F., Schaaf P., Voegel J.C., and Picart C. (2002). Cell interactions with polyelectrolyte multilayer films. Biomacromolecules 3:1170-1178.

Richter R.P. and Brisson A.R. (2005). Following the formation of supported lipid bilayers on mica: a study combining AFM, QCM-D, and ellipsometry. Biophys. J. 88:3422-3433.

Rinia H.A., Demel R.A., van der Eerden J.P., and de Kruijff B. (1999). Blistering of langmuir-blodgett bilayers containing anionic phospholipids as observed by atomic force microscopy. Biophys. J. 77:1683-1693.

Santos N.C. and Castanho M.A.R.B. (2004). An overview of the biophysical applications of atomic force microscopy. Biophysical Chemistry 107:133-149.

Scheuring S., Seguin J., Marco S., Levy D., Robert B., and Rigaud J. (2003). Nanodissection and high-resolution imaging of the Rhodopseudomonas viridis photosynthetic core complex in native membranes by AFM. Proc. Natl. Acad. Sci. U. S. A. 100: 1690-1693.

Scheuring S., Sturgis J.N., Prima V., Bernadac A., Levy D., and Rigaud J.L. (2004). Watching the photosynthetic apparatus in native membranes. Proc. Natl. Acad. Sci. U. S. A. 101:11293-11297.

Schultz P., Vautier D., Richert L., Jessel N., Haikel Y., Schaaf P., Voegel J.C., Ogier J., and Debry C. (2005). Polyelectrolyte multilayers functionalized by a synthetic analogue of an anti-inflammatory peptide, alpha-MSH, for coating a tracheal prosthesis. Biomaterials 26:2621-2630.

Selsted M.E., Novotny M.J., Morris W.L., Tang Y.Q., Smith W., and Cullor J.S. (1992). Indolicidin, a novel bactericidal tridecapeptide amide from neutrophils. J. Biol. Chem. 267:4292-4295.

Shiratori S.S. and Rubner M.F. (2000). pH-dependent thickness behavior of sequentially adsorbed layers of weak polyelectrolytes. Macromolecules 33:4213-4219.

Stahlberg H., Fotiadis D., Scheuring S., Remigy H., Braun T., Mitsuoka K., Fujiyoshi Y., and Engel H.A. (2001). Two-dimensional crystals: a powerful approach to assess structure, function and dynamics of membrane proteins. Febs Letters 504:166-172.

Steiner H., Hultmark D., Engstrom A., Bennich H., and Boman H.G. (1981). Sequence and specificity of two antibacterial proteins involved in insect immunity. Nature 292:246-248.

Sybesma,C. 1977. Membranes. *In* Biophysics An Introduction. Kluwer Academic Publisher, Dordrecht/Boston/London. 29-36.

Tokaji Z. (1995). Cooperativity-regulated parallel pathways of the bacteriorhodopsin photocycle. FEBS Lett. 357:156-160.

Van Vliet K.J. and Hinterdorfer P. (2006). Probing drug-cell interactions. Nanotoday 1:18-25.

Végh G.A., Nagy K., Bálin Z., Kerényi Á., Rákhely G., Váró G., and Szegletes Z. (2011). Effect of antimicrobial peptide-amide,indolicidin on biological membranes. J. Biomed. Biotechnol. doi:10.1155./2011/670589

Vie V., Van Mau N., Lesniewska E., Goudonnet J.P., Heitz F., and Le Grimellec C. (1998). Distribution of ganglioside G(M1) between two-component, two-phase phosphatidylcholine monolayers. Langmuir 14:4574-4583.

Volkenstein,M. 1981. Physique des membanes. *In* Biophysique. Moscou. 345-75.

Werten P.J.L., Remigy H.W., de Groot B.L., Fotiadis D., Philippsen A., Stahlberg H., Grubmuller H., and Engel H.A. (2002). Progress in the analysis of membrane protein structure and function. Febs Letters 529:65-72.

Wu H.W., Kuhn T., and Moy V.T. (1998). Mechanical properties of l929 cells measured by atomic force microscopy: Effects of anticytoskeletal drugs and membrane crosslinking. Scanning 20:389-397.

Zasloff M. (1987). Magainins, a class of antimicrobial peptides from Xenopus skin: isolation, characterization of two active forms, and partial cDNA sequence of a precursor. Proc. Natl. Acad. Sci. U. S. A. 84:5449-5453.

Part 4

Viral Physiology

11

Atomic Force Microscopy in Detection of Viruses

Norma Hernández-Pedro, Edgar Rangel-López, Benjamín Pineda and Julio Sotelo
Neuroimmunology Unit, National Institute of Neurology and Neurosurgery, Mexico City Mexico

1. Introduction

Properties of biological samples, such as DNA, proteins, components of bacterial surfaces and viruses have been studied extensively and provided the driving force for the outstanding progress of detection methods used in cell biology and physiology. Methods like magnetic twisting cytometry, laser-tracking microrheology, magnetic tweezers, the optical stretcher, and various cell indenters; have been used in the study of cell properties, however, imaging resolution has been low. Atomic Force Microscope (AFM) was developed by Binning, Quate and Gerber in 1986, and since its commercialization, AFM has been a powerful research tool in the scientific community, demonstrating its capability to provide images of biomolecules with high resolution. One of the most important benefits of AFM is the requirement of a minimal amount of sample to perform an accurate diagnostic. Also, AFM does not require staining, labelling, or samples coating, and it is possible to acquire images with minimal pre-treatment in a short time (sometimes minutes). AFM can also be used for real-time and high-resolution imaging of hydrated biological specimens ranging from single molecules to whole cells and tissues.

2. Fundamentals of atomic force microscopy (AFM)

AFM is a member of the family of probe microscopes used to scan and characterize surfaces. It generates topographical images from a variety of materials with resolutions of a nanometer (nm) fraction. AFM consists of a microscale rectangular or "V"-shaped cantilever **(Table 1)**, typically made of silicon or silicon nitride, with a sharp tip (probe) at its end, with a tip radius of curvature on the order of 50–100 nm. The tip is mounted at the end of a flexible cantilever that serves as a force sensor. The topography of a sample is obtained by measuring and modulating the interaction forces between the tip and the sample, by maintaining a constant tip-sample separation and using Hooke's Law ($F = -kx$ where F is force, k is the spring constant, and x is the cantilever deflection), the force between the tip and the sample are calculated and derive information about the surface of the sample. The movement of the cantilever is controlled in x, y, and z axis by piezoelectric crystals. A laser-based optical system is used to track the deflection of the cantilever with respect to the sample surface. As the tip encounters surface features, tiny disturbances in z cause the cantilever to bend. This movement is amplified by a laser beam focused on the backside of the cantilever that reflects onto a split photodiode, tracing the position of the cantilever.

Cantilever material	Silicon nitride[a]		Silicon[a]
Spring constant(k)	0.58, 0.32, 0.12, 0.06		20-100 N/m
Resonant frequency			200-400 kHz
Cantilever configuration	V-shaped		Single beam
Reflective coating	gold		Uncoated, aluminum
Tip shape	Pyramid	Sphere[b]glass/ polystyrene	Pyramid
Tip radius of curvature/diameter	20-60 nm	0.6-45 μm[b]	5-10 nm
Sidewall angles	35° on all four sides	NA	35° on all four sides

[a]Adapted from SPM Training Notebook (2003).
[b]Parameters from Novascan Technologies.
Abbreviation: NA, not applicable.

Table 1. The Most Common Cantilever Parameters

3. Contact and tipping mode to imaging of AFM

The two most common forms of AFM operation are contact and magnetic alternating current (Mac) tapping modes. In contact imaging, sample topography can be measured using constant-height or constant-force settings. In constant-height mode, the distance between the tip and the surface remains fixed during scanning, but the force between the tip and surface changes as the tip encounters surface features. Deflections in the position of the cantilever are used to create an image of the surface. In constant-force mode, the tip remains in contact with the sample using a known applied vertical force as the cantilever scans over the surface. Deflection of the cantilever signals a change in the voltage sent to the z piezo that is adjusted to maintain a constant interaction force between the tip and surface. This voltage sent to the z piezo is converted into height data to create the image. This type of imaging loses the true height information, but it presents more fine details of the sample than the height image because the feedback loop response is faster for correcting the position of the small cantilever. Contac mode is frequently used with hard inorganic surfaces, metals, and for high polymers (with high molecular weight) including polyethylene, silicone and polyurethane elastomers (Siedlecki and Marchant 1998), others uses include fixed cells, proteins, cell surfaces or low modulus biomaterials.

As do other, the Tapping Mode or Mac Mode prevent damage to the soft tip (i.e. on diamond, silicon carbide) is often used for observe molecules, cell surface samples and even dynamic process that occur *in vivo* (Hansma, Cleveland et al. 1994; Moreno-Herrero, Colchero et al. 2004). This method overcomes problems associated with friction, adhesion, electrostatic forces, and other difficulties that conventional AFM scanning methods by alternately placing the tip in contact with the surface to provide high resolution and then lifting the tip off the surface to avoid dragging the tip across the surface, avoiding sample damage by compressing, and tearing. The cantilever vibrates at its resonant frequency under an external electrical excitation, the feedback loop adjusts the oscillation amplitude to restore the original set point value, and a height image can be recorded (Putman, van der Werf et al. 1994; Schindler, Badt et al. 2000). The contrast of a phase image is directly dependent on the elastic properties of the sample.

Applications of Tapping Mode AFM in materials, biomaterials and biology sciences are constantly growing. The commercial technology has improved due to request of users and from experience in acquiring tapping mode data. Some studies show high resolution imaging of molecules such as proteins (Karrasch, Hegerl et al. 1994), channels and receptors on cell surfaces (Muller, Schabert et al. 1995), lipids (Anderton, Lou et al. 2011), and also has been used to imaging living cells; including yeast (Dhadwar, Bemman et al. 2003), neurons (Kondra, Laishram et al. 2009), endothelial cells, virus (Ohnesorge, Horber et al. 1997), and others. Furthermore, important applications of tapping mode include monitoring the action of drugs or other compounds on cells. **Figure 1**

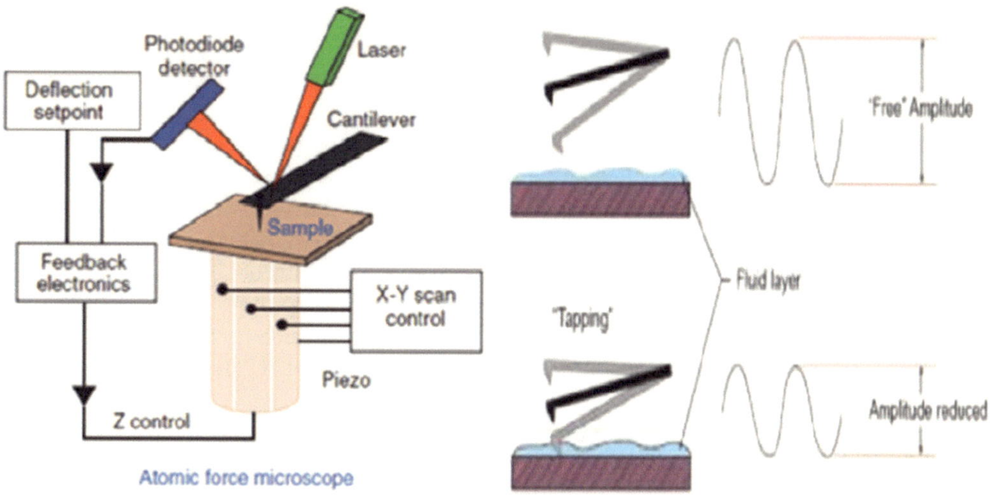

Fig. 1. **Contact mode and tapping mode AFM.** In contact mode imaging is obtained by raster scanning the cantilever and attached probe with respect to the sample surface. Shear forces are applied to the sample during scanning since the probe tip remains in constant contact. In tapping mode, the cantilever is oscillating vertically at high frequency during raster scanning. Interaction of the tip with the sample causes attenuation of the oscillation amplitude, which is used to monitor changes in sample height. Shear forces on the sample are negligible, because the lateral scanning movement of the probe occurs above the sample

4. Sample preparation and fixing

The critical steps in AFM are the sample preparation and surface immobilization, and this is considered the most important aspect to imaging living cells. To fixing the sample is necessary to attach the biomaterial to the sample holder. Substrates that are frequently used include glass cover slips, mica, highly ordered pyrolytic graphite, silicon oxide wafers, and atomically flat gold (Schneeweiss and Rubinstein 2007). The substrate used from AFM depends of the sample that one desires to measure for example, the majority of living cells such as smooth muscle cells, endothelial cells, and fibroblasts, attach well to classical substrates like polystyrene or glass. Other samples, such as those obtained from a cell culture dish, have used gelatine or an extracellular matrix protein like fibronectin and laminin, which can improve the cell attachment (Trache and Meininger 2008). In addition, the use of an adhesive is often required to fix nanoparticles on a substrate. The most common materials used to bond particles to the substrate are Poly-L-lysine, poly-D-lysine,

PEI (poly-ethyleneimide) or APTES (aminopropyltriethoxysilane) (Kasas and Ikai 1995; Wagner 1998; Dufrene 2000; Engel and Muller 2000).

Two drive mechanisms for tapping mode in fluids are available on the multimode AFM. The conventional method of driving the cantilever by acoustic excitation has been joined by a magnetic actuated drive (Putman, 1994). Acoustically driven oscillations of the cantilever in liquid on the multimode AFM occur by excitation of a piezo electric ceramic element in the cantilever holder; however, the sample can move and give erroneous information. The Magnetic Actuated Drive (MAD) mechanism uses an electromagnet in the fluid cell to create a magnetic field to drive specialized event. These probes are coated with a magnetic film (Co or Co/Cr) on the backside (only) to preserve the tip sharpness. It is somewhat easier to identify the resonant frequency of the cantilever when working with the magnetic drive, as the tune shows mainly only the resonant frequency oscillation of the probe. However, the magnetic coating on the backside of the cantilever can lead to the possibility of contamination of sensitive samples with soluble earth and transition metal ions (Revenko and Proksch 2000). Another example that has been developed to diminish the contamination and improve the measurement is the use of like isopore polycarbonate membrane with a pore size comparable to the cell size that is used in a concentrated cell suspension of single bacteria, yeast, or fungal cells under physiological conditions (Kasas and Ikai 1995; Dufrene 2000). Recently, other material like Nanoporous gold (NPG) has been developed for protein immobilization with better results due to its open bi-continuous structure, high surface-to-volume ratio, tunable porosity, chemical stability, and biocompatibility (Tan, Schallom et al. 2011).

5. Imaging

AFM images of biomolecules give structural information, as well as information about the material properties of the sample. It is a method with suitable advantages for the study of cell mechanics, by providing high sensitivity, spatial resolution and the ability to be used for real-time measurements (Kirmizis and Logothetidis 2010). The AFM is based on a direct bound to a surface by virtue of a change in local topography allowing a direct mechanical interaction between the probe and the sample. This ability allows the AFM to distinguish between a single monolayer of proteins bound to a surface and multiple layers that result from an interaction between members of an affinity pair. Images often show surface features that are invisible or barely visible in height images or amplitude images (Dufrene 2002).

Imaging surfaces at variables forces set points gives information about the compressibility of the surface as well as characterization of material properties and structure manipulation on the nanometer scale, and visualization and probing of single macromolecules. Some examples to structural parameters measured such as that contained in chromatin fibers (Daban 2011), reconstituted fibers of sequence-defined DNA and core histone octamers on gap junction membranes (Hoh, Lal et al. 1991). Other biomaterials as proteins, DNA molecules, protein-protein complexes, and DNA-protein complexes (Hansma, Sinsheimer et al. 1992; Murphy, Shannon et al. 2011; Shen, Bao et al. 2011) chromosomes (Jondle, Ambrosio et al. 1995; Daban 2011), and cells (Henderson, Haydon et al. 1992) and more recently single RNA molecules (Heus, Puchner et al. 2011) have been measured with AFM.

Other methods, like imaging in air, have been used to visualize cell nuclei disrupted *in situ* (Fritzsche, Schaper et al. 1994; Fritzsche, Schaper et al. 1995), reconstituted fibres of sequence-defined DNA and core histone octamers (Allen, Dong et al. 1993), and soluble chromatin fibres isolated from hypotonically lysed micrococcal nuclease-treated nuclei (Volkening and Spatz 2009). Inside cells there are some important factors such as the aqueous gel nature of the cytoplasm (Evans and Yeung 1989), heterogeneously distributed actin filaments, intermediate filaments, microtubules (Wang 1998), cell adhesiveness (Pourati, Maniotis et al. 1998), or the presence of nucleus and other organelles (Petersen, McConnaughey et al. 1982) which could affect the mechanical properties of the cells. **Table 2**

	Protein Structures	**Function**	**Citation**
Molecular motors	F-adenosine trip-hosphate (ATP) synthase rotors	Synthases use the energy of a transmembrane proton	Seelert et al., 2000 and Stahlberg et al., 2001
	The f29 rotary motor	Converts a mechanical rotation to atranslational movement of DNA	Simpson et al, 2000
Ion pumps and channels	Bacterio-rhodopsin	Converts the energy of "green" light(500–650 nm) into an electrochemical proton gradient	Haupts U et al 1999
	Halorhodopsin	showed neighbored tetramers to be orientated with their extra-cellular and cytoplasmic surface towards the membrane surface	Persike et al., 2001 and Kolbe et al., 2000
	Potassiumchannel	Stabilize membrane potential	van Huizen et al., 1999
Membrane channels	Aquaporin1 (AQP1)	Channel proteins that transport-ing water and other metabolites	Pohl et al., 2001
	Major intrinsic protein (AQP0)	Intrinsic protein expressed in eye lens fiber cells	Fotiadis et al., 2000
Proteinsinvol vedinto-pho-tosynthesis	Photosystem I	Oxygenic photosynthesis in cyanobacteria and plants	Fotiadis et al., 1998
	Light-harvesting-complex 2	Transfers excitation energy to thelight-harvesting complex 1	Scheuring et al., 2001
Toxins	Cholera toxin	Causes the enzymatic subunit to be clipped from the rest of the pro-teinand transferred into the cell	Mou et al., 1995; and Yang et al., 1993
	Cry1Aa	Forms toxic pores	Vie et al., 2001
	a-hemolysin	Create water-filled channels thatlead to cell death and lysis	Czajkowsky et al., 1998 and Song et al., 1996
	VacA	Induces vacuolation of acidic intracellular components	Czajkowsky et al., 1999 and Iwamoto et al., 1999
Chaperonins and protea-somes	GroE chaperone system	Chaperone machinery	Mou et al., 1996, 1996
	20 S proteasome	Degrades misfolded or regulatory proteins	Dorn et al., 1999
Cellulose		Unbranched polymer of glucose residues joined	Baker et al., 1997; Baker et al., 2000

Table 2. Some Applications of Atomic Force Microscopy

6. Virus detection by AFM

Historically, the optical microscope and the electron microscope (EM) have played a key role in the discovery and structural characterization of viral isolates (Biel and Gelderblom 1999; Hazelton and Gelderblom 2003). Today, EM is used mainly as a research tool and not in main stream routine diagnoses because it is not suited for high through-put analyses. For routine virus detection and monitoring the spread of disease, most available diagnostic methods rely almost exclusively on polymerase chain reaction (PCR) or enzyme-linked immunosorbent assay (ELISA). Identification and measurement of viral DNA or RNA is provided by PCR, whereas viral proteins and antiviral antibodies detection are made by ELISA (Belak and Thoren 2001; Henrickson 2004; Madeley 2004; Olofsson, Brittain-Long et al. 2011). The inconvenience of these techniques is that they do not measure complete particles and they are indirect indicators of viral load. Also, in conditions where viral latency has been established, the ability to directly monitor recurrences through the measurement of intact viral particles would be a great asset for the clinical setting. The early and correct diagnosis of viral infection is also relevant, especially in severe infections such as atypical herpes virus infections, in order to ensure effective treatment of the disease and prevention of complications (Hawrami and Breuer 1999; Pineda, Saniger et al. 2009). The use of new tools such as AFM could play an important role in the clinical or epidemiological setting when critical situations require a rapid diagnosis, for example the recent H1N1 influenza epidemic experienced in the United States and Mexico (Tian, Wang et al. 2011) where AFM could be the only method available that allows morphological identification by direct visualization of intact particles.

7. Viruses morphology

Viruses are grouped on the basis of size and shape, chemical composition, structure of the genome, and mode of replication. Viral genomes are surrounded and protected by a protein shell, the capsid. The type of capsid has been used to classify viruses in three main groups: Helical symmetry, Virus Core Structure and Icosahedral Symmetry. Some techniques, like X-ray diffraction and cryo-electron microscopy, have been used to determine the structure of viral capsids providing a good resolution. Nevertheless, the use of AFM has allowed the discovery of new structures, obtaining higher resolution, and physical characteristics of the capsid. In the next sections, we give some examples of AFM measurement according to their capsid classification.

7.1 Helical symmetry

A fundamental parameter for virus particles is their symmetry. Helical viruses are defined by their pitch; a single type of capsomer stacked around a central axis to form a helical structure and the protein of the coat has exactly the same orientation (Gelderblom 1996). The symmetric shapes allow to use the same component protein multiple times to create large structures from a minimum number of distinct protein species.

The Tobacco Mosaic Virus (TMV) has a variety of organized structures, such as the disk aggregate and helical rod, which play distinct roles in the genesis of the virus during infection (Sachse, Chen et al. 2007). This virus infects plants which will often displays developmental abnormalities that include stunting, leaf curling, and the loss of apical dominance. TheTMV is the typical member of the Tobamovirus genus in the Virgaviridae family and is one of the most studied viruses by AFM (Dawson, Beck et al. 1986). TMV virion, measured by AFM, consists of approximately 2,130 identical coat proteins helically wrapped around a 6.4 kb positive strand of genomic mRNA, making it an 18 nm diameter and 300 nm long rigid nanotube with a 4 nm diameter inner channel (Culver 2002; Michel, Ivanovska et al. 2006). Recently, other structures were identified in TMV by AFM, such as the satellite tobacco mosaic virus characterized by RNA helical segments, where, RNA base sequence, therefore, may be sufficient to encode the conformation of the encapsidated RNA even in the absence of coat proteins (Day, Kuznetsov et al. 2001).

Another important virus is influenza. This is a member of orthomyxoviridae family, and it has three members: influenza virus A, B, and C. Influenza A virus, both seasonal and pandemic, has the potential to cause rampant the devastation disease around the world. Influenza A uses its RNA during impregnation and causes a subsequent infection, which is characterized primarily by pulmonary affection that may advance to an acute pulmonary respiratory failure. Influenza type A is the most studied by AFM and some studies exhibit a surface topography that is characterized by rugged features and gear-like protuberances (Liu, Hu et al. 2008). Also, surface morphology is characterized by the presence of large nanoparticles, typically 120 to 250 nm wide at the base and 50 to 100 nm tall. Now, it is known that the influenza virus is a quasi-spherical object, approximately of 100 to 120 nm in diameter (Wickramasinghe, Kalbfuss et al. 2005).

Ebola and Marburg viruses are prime examples of emerging pathogens; they cause fatal hemorrhagic fever in humans. Identification of major determinants of the Ebola virus pathogenicity has been hampered by the lack of effective strategies for experimental mutagenesis. Recent discoveries suggest that filoviruses, along with other phylogenetically or functionally related viruses, utilize a complex mechanism of replication exploiting multiple cellular components including lipid rafts, endocytic compartments, and vacuolar protein sorting machinery (Aman, Bosio et al. 2003). The single-stranded negative-sense RNA genome is encased in a nucleocapsid complex, which consists of the following four viral proteins: the nucleoprotein (NP), the viral proteins (VP35 and VP30) and the polymerase (L). This complex is surrounded by a matrix consisting of VP40 and VP24, which is packaged by a lipid membrane envelope obtained during budding from the host cell. The envelope is composed of the glycoprotein (GP) protein, which is post-translationally cleaved by a furin protease into two fragments, GP1 and GP2, although this cleavage is not necessary for *in vitro* viral infection of cells (Wool-Lewis and Bates 1999; Neumann, Feldmann et al. 2002). Ebola fusion peptide interacts with living cells, and its capacity to induce cell fusion is decreased in cholesterol-depleted cells. Force spectroscopy based on AFM assays reveals a pattern of high affinity force when the Ebola fusion peptide interacts with membrane rafts. It is also observed that the peptide is able to induce aggregation of the lipid rafts, suggesting an important role for phosphatidylinositol and cholesterol during entry of the virus into the target cells (Suarez, Gomara et al. 2003).

7.2 Virus core structure

Except for helical nucleocapsids, little is known about the packaging or organization of the viral genome within the core. Small virions are simple nucleocapsids containing 1 to 2 protein species. The larger viruses contain within the core the nucleic acid genome complexed with basic proteins and are protected by a single- or double layered capsid or by an envelope (Gelderblom 1996).

Isolated human immunodeficiency virus (HIV) and HIV-infected human lymphocytes in culture have been imaged for the first time by atomic force microscopy. Purified virus particles spread on glass substrates are roughly spherical, reasonably uniform, though pleomorphic in appearance, and have diameters of about 120 nm. Similar particles are also seen on infected cell surfaces, but morphologies and sizes are considerably more varied, which is possibly a reflection of the budding process. The surfaces of HIV particles exhibit filaments of protein, presumably GP120, which do not physically resemble spikes. The protein filaments, which number about 100 per particle, have average diameters of about 200 A°, nonetheless, they have a large size variance. They likely consist of arbitrary associations of small numbers of GP120 monomers on the surface. Examining several hundred of virus particles, authors found no evidence that the GP120 monomers form trimmer based on three fold symmetry (Kuznetsov, Victoria et al. 2003).

Hepatitis B, is a virus consists of an inner nucleocapsid or core, surrounded by a lipid envelope containing virally encoded surface proteins, it is member of the taxonomic family hepadnaviridiae and still poses a major health threat; it causes hepatitis, liver cancer, and liver cirrhosis. Direct measurements with AFM revealed morphological changes upon maturation through induced and heat-/storage-incurred oxidative refolding. Particle uniformity and regularity was greatly improved, and protrusions formed by the protein subunits were more prominent on the surface of the mature particles. Decreased conformational flexibility in the mature surface antigen of Hepatitis B virus (rHBsAg) particles was demonstrated. Both the accessible hydrophobic cavities under native conditions and the changeable hydrophobic cavities upon denaturant-induced unfolding showed substantial decrease upon maturation of the rHBs Ag particles. These changes in the structural properties may be critical for the antigenicity and immunogenicity of this widely-used vaccine component (Zhao, Wang et al. 2006).

Vaccinia virus, a characterized member of the Poxviridaefamily, is unusual among most double-stranded DNA viruses in that both viral transcription and replication occur in the cytoplasm of the host cell (Condit, Moussatche et al. 2006). Poxviridaevirus is generally shaped like a brick or as an oval form, similar to a rounded brick because they are wrapped by the endoplasmic reticulum (Holowczak 1982). The virion is exceptionally large; its size is around 200 nm in diameter and 300 nm in length and carries its genome in a single, linear, double-stranded segment of DNA (Dales and T. 1981; Fenner, Wittek et al. 1989; Moss 1991). This virus has relevance because of its historical role in smallpox eradication, and its relatively benign tropism and is one of the largest viruses to replicate in humans are reasons that explains why is the most studied virus in this family. The viral DNA genome is linear, double stranded. The Copenhagen strain is 191 kbp in length and contains at least 266 open reading frames (Goebel, Johnson et al. 1990; Johnson, Goebel et al. 1993). Kuznetsov et al characterized the shape, dimensions, and general surface characteristics of hydrated vaccinia mature virus. The virus assumes a familiar rectangular shape upon dehydration while particles were pleomorphic with an outer surface design varying from the more regular, short, haphazardly, intersecting to railroad tracks topography. Removal of the outer lipid/protein membrane on vaccinia, a layer of 20 to 40 nm in thickness, was encountered that was composed of fibrous elements. Beneath this layer were the virus core and its prominent lateral bodies. The core, in addition to the lateral bodies, was composed of a thick, multilayered shell of proteins of several sizes and shapes. The shell was thoroughly permeated with pores, or channels. The DNA was readily visualized by AFM, revealing some regions to be "soldered" by proteins, others to be heavily complexed with protein, and yet other parts to apparently exist as bundled, naked DNA (Kuznetsov, Gershon et al. 2008). Also, the Poxviridae virus, characterized by AFM in an aqueous environment, shows a fairly regularly repeating pairs of rodshaped structures with a total width of 7-11 nm and a length of 60-90 nm (Ohnesorge, Horber et al. 1997).

In 2003, Malkin et al, described by AFM intact intracellular mature vaccinia virus (IMV), virions, as well as the chemical and enzymatic treatment products thereof. In their observations, they described virion cores, core-enveloping coats, and core substructures of the vaccinia virus. The AFM imaging of core substructures indicated an association of the linear viral DNA genome with a segmented protein sheath forming an extended around 16 nm-diameter filament with helical surface topography; enclosure of this filament within a 30 to 40-nm-diameter tubule which also shows helical topography; and enclosure of the folded, condensed 30 to 40-nm-diameter tubule within the core by a wall covered with peg-like projections. The size of the isolated virions was 70 to 100-nm-diameter particles (Malkin, McPherson et al. 2003).

7.3 Icosahedral symmetry

An icosahedron is a polyhedron having 20 equilateral triangular faces and 12 vertices. Lines through opposite vertices define axes of fivefold rotational symmetry: all structural features of the polyhedron repeat five times within each 360° of rotation about any of the fivefold axes. Lines through the centers of opposite triangular faces form axes of threefold rotational symmetry; twofold rotational symmetry axes are formed by lines through midpoints of opposite edges. An icosaheron (polyhedral or spherical) with fivefold, threefold, and twofold axes of rotational symmetry is defined as having 532 symmetry (Gelderblom 1996).

Various surfaces, proteins, and RNA are identifiable by AFM. Marek's disease virus (MDV) is one of the most potent oncogenic alpha herpes viruses, leads to highly contagious immunosuppressive and neoplastic disease in susceptible chickens and less commonly turkeys and quails (Federica Giardi, La Torre et al. 2009). It is the etiologic agent of Marek's disease (MD), which is a highly contagious malignant lymphoma that causes dullness with progression of T-lymphomas and finally ataxia and paralysis (Morimura, Ohashi et al. 1998). Di Bucchianico et al investigated the different structure of chromatin in chromosome aberrations due to MDV insertion. They found a duplication [78,WZ,dup(1p)(p22-p23)] and a deletion [78,WZ cht del(3)(q2.10)] of chromosomes 1 and 3 (Di Bucchianico, Giardi et al. 2010). The architecture of chromosomes observed by AFM can be related to the data obtained with classic banding techniques. Also, evidence the presence of chromatin bridges between sisters and deletions of chromatid regions. The deletions of the two chromatids have a size of 100 and 50 nm, respectively (Di Bucchianico, Giardi et al. 2011).

RNA molecules are other structures investigated by AFM, and this is important due to a small amount of RNA in icosahedrical viruses (Kuznetsov, Daijogo et al. 2005). Poliovirus and turnip yellow mosaic virus (TYMV) are monopartite viruses, containing a positive-strand RNA, which infects crucifers (broccoli, cauliflower, radishes, and several green vegetables) (Weiland and Dreher 1993). Kuznetsov et al, studied RNA in different conditions and found a uniform spherical inside of virion to approximately 20 nm. After 30 minutes to an hour, the spherical particles lose their integrity, assume an irregular banded fiber appearance, segment into secondary structural domains and finally single-stranded RNA connecting secondary structural domains (Kuznetsov, Daijogo et al. 2005).

Paramecium bursaria chlorella virus type 1 (PBCV-1) is a member of large group "Phycodnaviridae viruses" that infect eukaryotic cells. The highest resolution AFM images have revealed a protein surface network; an individual trimetric capsid protein as well as their subunits displayed about the central threefold axis. The shapes of the subunits and their arrangements are most consistent. This AFM study also provides information on the structure of the PBCV-1 that is involved in virus infection. A distinctive pentamer of five unique proteins occurs in fivefold vertex, along with another distinctive protein exactly in the center of the homopentamer. This apical protein is unusual in that it appears sensitive to mechanical force and retracts into the interior of the virion (Kuznetsov, Gurnon et al. 2005).

Mason–Pfizer monkey virus (M-PMV) is a type D retrovirus which pre-assembles immature capsids in the cytoplasm prior to transport to the host cell membrane where they are released. Maturation then takes place. Bacteria expressing M-PMV Gag protein, and various truncated forms of Gag, produce spherical particles within inclusion bodies, and these exhibit features suggestive of icosahedral symmetry (Nermut, Hockley et al. 1998). Particles of ΔProCANC, a fusion of capsid (CA) and nucleocapsid (NC) proteins of Mason–Pfizer monkey virus (M-PMV), which lacks the proline amino terminal, were reassembled *in vitro* and visualized by AFM. The particles, 83–84 nm in diameter, exhibited ordered domains based on trigonal arrays of prominent rings with center to center distances of 8.7 nm. Imperfect closure of the lattice on the spherical surface was affected by formation of discontinuities. The lattice is consistent only with plane group p3 where one molecule is shared between contiguous rings. There are no pentameric clusters or evidence that the particles are icosahedral. Tubular structures were also reassembled, *in vitro,* from two HIV fusion proteins, ΔProCANC and CANC. The tubes were uniform in diameter, 40 nm, but varied in length to a maximum of 600 nm. They exhibited left handed helical symmetry based on a p6 hexagonal net (Kuznetsov, Ulbrich et al. 2007).

Herpes viruses are a leading cause of human viral disease, after the influenza and cold viruses. They are capable of causing overt disease or remain silent for many years only to be reactivated. This reflects the creeping or spreading nature of the skin lesions caused by many herpes virus types. Herpes simplex virus type 1 (HSV1) virions encapsulate their 152 kbp double-stranded DNA genome in an icosahedral capsid that is surrounded by an amorphous protein layer, called the tegument, and a lipid-containing envelope. Assembly of herpes viruses is initiated in the nucleus where procapsids self-assemble around a protein scaffold and subsequently mature. Ross et al, determined structural changes during maturation of virus and DNA packaging by AFM. Atomic force microscopy experiments revealed that A and C capsids were mechanically indistinguishable, indicating that the presence of DNA does not account for changes in mechanical properties during capsid maturation (Roos, Radtke et al. 2009).

8. Solid-phase assay for detection of varicella zoster virus by AFM

We performed an study regarding the detection of varicella zoster virus using a novel Bionanotechnological approach that couples atomic force microscopy with high affinity solid phase capture of viral particles called Virichip® (Pineda, Saniger et al. 2009).

Many general features of virus architecture are readily apparent from a variety of studies; high resolution AFM allows the discrimination of viruses based on their size and shape in a process that does not require staining, fixing or other synthetic preparations. This technique has been used successfully to diagnose viral infections such as West Nile virus, herpes viruses, retroviruses and poxviruses. These enabling properties of AFM combined with solid phase immunocapture of virus particles make possible a multi-tiered detection and identification assay with potential use in rapid pathogen diagnosis.

Afterwards, Nettikadan et al, developed a solid phase and affinity substrate called Virichip® which consists in a microarray of viral proteins on a fresh gold-coated silicon surface; this is incubated with recombinant protein A/G to generate a surface capable to bind and orientate monoclonal antibodies. The first detection of virus using ViriChip platform and AFM was made to detect canine parvovirus virus-like particles (CPV), Coxsackie virus B3 Nancy (CB3), and one morphologically distinct linear helical virus, bacteriophage fd (Nettikadan, Johnson et al. 2003).

The rapid detection and identification of pathogens is critically important to minimize the transfer and spread of diseases and to devise and evaluate effective treatment strategies. For example, Varicela Zoster virus (VZV) detection is clinically important, however the techniques used to detect this disease have disadvantages, including false positive and negative results, the use of specialized and expensive equipment and the need of expert personal performance. At present, the serological methods for the detection of antibodies (either IgG or IgM) are sometimes used to confirm the diagnosis, however, patients who are immuno-supressed or immuno-compromised may have VZV infection without any detectable antibodies.

Varicella ViriChip® construction (VVC) is a sensitive, specific and quick method that allows the visualization of the virus, the specific detection by immunological means and the recovery of virus particles for further analysis. The method does not require additional steps, and a minimal quantity obtained from a vesicle fluid from cutaneous VZV lesions is a sufficient amount to discriminate between VZV and other common pathogens. Additionally, VVC allows sample transportation for further analysis and now Portable AFMs are already available (Pineda, Sanigeret al. 2009) (**see Figure 2**).

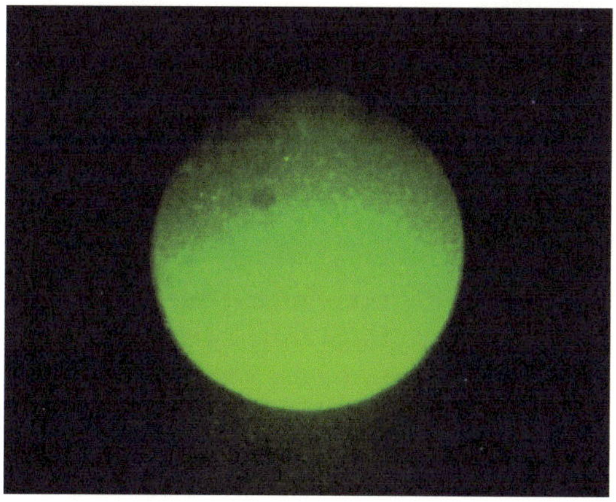

Fig. 2. **Virus distribution on the VVC.** Distribution of the virus in the VVC domain is indicated by the fluorescent antibodies against varicella zoster virus. The target area (circle) has a diameter of 600 μm.

The importance of Virichip is its ability to detect whole virus particles and identify them using two integrated sets of criteria without damaging the virus or its genome. First, the dimensional properties of the captured particles as determined by AFM should be in agreement with those for the *family* of viruses suspected, and second, the capture by a type specific antibody indicates positive type-specific interaction. The combination of these properties should permit placement of a virus within a *family*, sub-family and a serotype depending on the nature of the epitope recognized by the capture antibody[79]. Currently, the AFM has a sensitivity of 10^3 TCID50 μl^{-1}. In contrast, ELISA-based detection using the same antibodies has a detection limit of only 107 plaque forming units. Furthermore, although RT-PCR is reportedly more sensitive (−0.1 TCID50), RTPCR measures only the presence of RNA and provides no information as to the bioinfectivity in the sample or whether there are even virus particles present (Straub, Pepper et al. 1994; Metcalf, Melnick et al. 1995). The use of Virichip® allows the rapid detection of the virus and it requires a minimal quantity of sample. VVC allows the rapid detection of the virus and it diminishes the handling time, the risks of cross-contamination, and the probability of false positive results (**see Figure 3 and 4**).

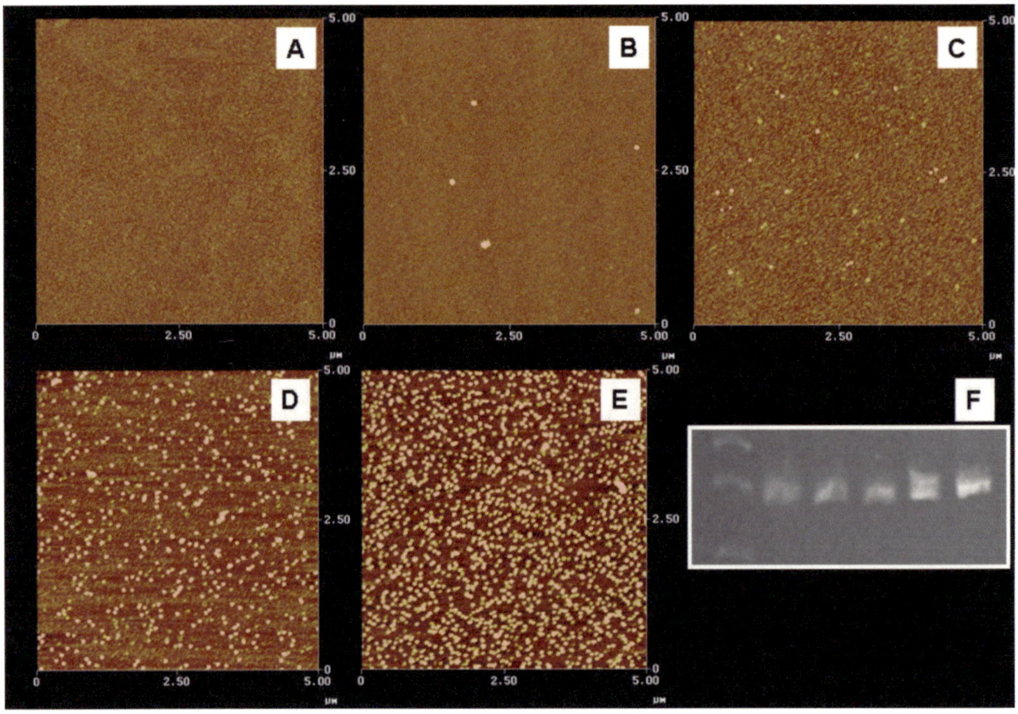

Fig. 3. **Tenfold serial dilutions of VZV over the chip surfaces and its correlation with conventional PCR.**Virus particles from 1μl of 10-fold serial dilutions ranging from 10^5 viral particles of VZV were captured on a chip and used as templates to determine the VVZ sensitivity comparing it to PCR. **(A)** 10^1 (1:100,000 dilution). **(B)** 10^2 (1:10,000 dilution). **(C)** 10^3 (1:1,000 dilution). **(D)** 10^4 (1:100 dilution). **(E)** 10^5 (1:10 dilution).**(F)** PCR amplification of each Virichip, from left to right: lane 1, molecular weight marker (MWM), lanes 2-6 show amplification of the virus chips containing from 10^1 to 10^5 copies of VZV. The signal intensity in the agarose 2% gel appeared to be proportional to the virus concentration. The sensitivity of this detection method was 10^2 viral particles/μl.

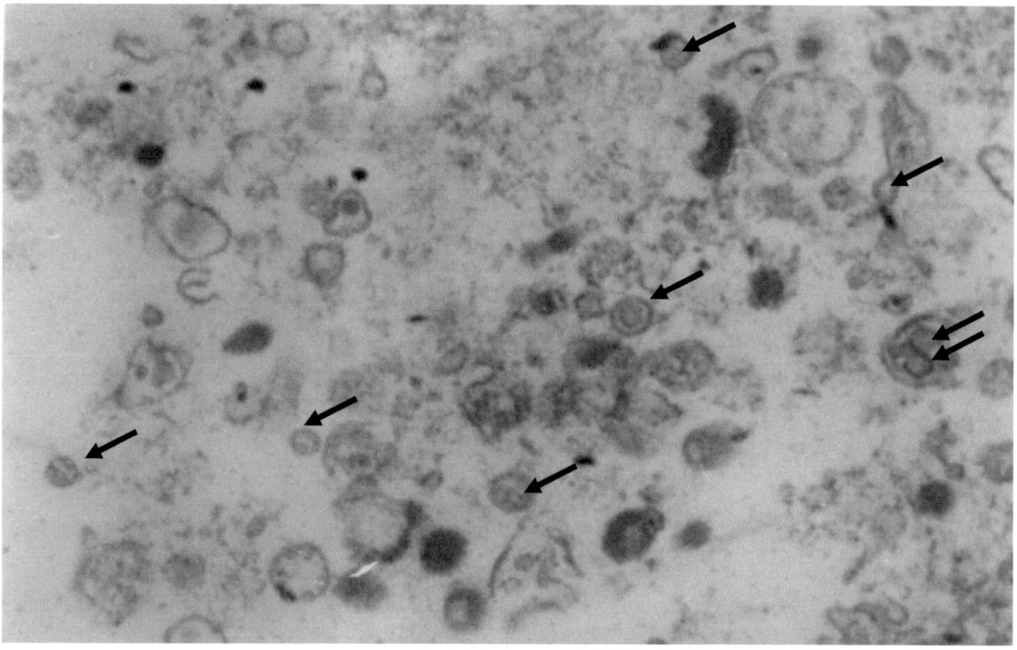

Fig. 4. **Electron microscopy appearances of VZV particles.**The viral particles were eluted from the ViriChip and concentrated by ultracentrifugation. The image shows enveloped and non-enveloped virions containing dense cores. The size of the virus with the capsomere ranges between 80-120 nm and with the envelope between 180-200 nm.

9. Conclusions

The AFM has many advantages as it is a simple and relatively inexpensive technique; it is more portable than SEM or TEM; requires a minimal quantity of sample for measurements, and can be linked with other molecular techniques, such as PCR or EM, with efficient results. The method does not damage the virus or its genome, allowing the detection of whole virus particles and the possibility to identify the family, sub-family, serotype and other complex structures. Also, the Virichip® allows the rapid detection of the VVZ, reduces handling time, risks of cross-contamination, and the probability to detect false positives; making it an attractive clinical diagnostic tool in the virology field. The combination the AFM visualization with immunocapture and molecular biology methods is a useful tool for the identification, determination of diagnosis, and the monitoring of many virus infections. The Virichip® is a novel and promising method that could be used to increase the acquaintance and treatment of diseases caused by virus infections.

10. References

Allen, M. J., X. F. Dong, et al. (1993). "Atomic force microscope measurements of nucleosome cores assembled along defined DNA sequences." Biochemistry 32(33): 8390-8396.

Aman, M. J., C. M. Bosio, et al. (2003). "Molecular mechanisms of filovirus cellular trafficking." Microbes Infect 5(7): 639-649.

Anderton, C. R., K. Lou, et al. (2011). "Correlated AFM and NanoSIMS imaging to probe cholesterol-induced changes in phase behavior and non-ideal mixing in ternary lipid membranes." Biochim Biophys Acta 1808(1): 307-315.

Belak, S. and P. Thoren (2001). "Molecular diagnosis of animal diseases: some experiences over the past decade." Expert Rev Mol Diagn 1(4): 434-443.

Biel, S. S. and H. R. Gelderblom (1999). "Diagnostic electron microscopy is still a timely and rewarding method." J Clin Virol 13(1-2): 105-119.

Condit, R. C., N. Moussatche, et al. (2006). "In a nutshell: structure and assembly of the vaccinia virion." Adv Virus Res 66: 31-124.

Culver, J. N. (2002). "Tobacco mosaic virus assembly and disassembly: determinants in pathogenicity and resistance." Annu Rev Phytopathol 40: 287-308.

Daban, J. R. (2011). "Electron microscopy and atomic force microscopy studies of chromatin and metaphase chromosome structure." Micron 42(8): 733-750.

Dales, S. and P. B. G. T. (1981). "Biology of poxviruses. Virology monographs." Springer-Verlag.

Dawson, W. O., D. L. Beck, et al. (1986). "cDNA cloning of the complete genome of tobacco mosaic virus and production of infectious transcripts." Proc Natl Acad Sci U S A 83(6): 1832-1836.

Day, J., Y. G. Kuznetsov, et al. (2001). "Biophysical studies on the RNA cores of satellite tobacco mosaic virus." Biophys J 80(5): 2364-2371.

Dhadwar, S. S., T. Bemman, et al. (2003). "Yeast cell adhesion on oligopeptide modified surfaces." Biotechnol Adv 21(5): 395-406.

Di Bucchianico, S., M. F. Giardi, et al. (2010). "Cytogenetic stability of chicken T-cell line transformed with Marek's disease virus: atomic force microscope, a new tool for investigation." J Mol Recognit.

Di Bucchianico, S., M. F. Giardi, et al. (2011). "Cytogenetic stability of chicken T-cell line transformed with Marek's disease virus: atomic force microscope, a new tool for investigation." J Mol Recognit 24(4): 608-618.

Dufrene, Y. F. (2000). "Direct characterization of the physicochemical properties of fungal spores using functionalized AFM probes." Biophys J 78(6): 3286-3291.

Dufrene, Y. F. (2002). "Atomic force microscopy, a powerful tool in microbiology." J Bacteriol 184(19): 5205-5213.

Engel, A. and D. J. Muller (2000). "Observing single biomolecules at work with the atomic force microscope." Nat Struct Biol 7(9): 715-718.

Evans, E. and A. Yeung (1989). "Apparent viscosity and cortical tension of blood granulocytes determined by micropipet aspiration." Biophys J 56(1): 151-160.

Federica Giardi, M., C. La Torre, et al. (2009). "Effects of transferrins and cytokines on nitric oxide production by an avian lymphoblastoid cell line infected with Marek's disease virus." Antiviral Res 81(3): 248-252.

Fenner, F., R. Wittek, et al. (1989). "The orthopoxviruses. ." Academic Press, Inc., New York, N.Y.

Fritzsche, W., A. Schaper, et al. (1994). "Probing chromatin with the scanning force microscope." Chromosoma 103(4): 231-236.

Fritzsche, W., A. Schaper, et al. (1995). "Scanning force microscopy of chromatin fibers in air and in liquid." Scanning 17(3): 148-155.

Gelderblom, H. R. (1996). "Structure and Classification of Viruses."

Goebel, S. J., G. P. Johnson, et al. (1990). "The complete DNA sequence of vaccinia virus." Virology 179(1): 247-266, 517-263.
Hansma, H. G., R. L. Sinsheimer, et al. (1992). "Atomic force microscopy of single- and double-stranded DNA." Nucleic Acids Res 20(14): 3585-3590.
Hansma, P. K., J. P. Cleveland, et al. (1994). Tapping mode atomic force microscopy in liquids, AIP.
Hawrami, K. and J. Breuer (1999). "Development of a fluorogenic polymerase chain reaction assay (TaqMan) for the detection and quantitation of varicella zoster virus." J Virol Methods 79(1): 33-40.
Hazelton, P. R. and H. R. Gelderblom (2003). "Electron microscopy for rapid diagnosis of infectious agents in emergent situations." Emerg Infect Dis 9(3): 294-303.
Henderson, E., P. G. Haydon, et al. (1992). "Actin filament dynamics in living glial cells imaged by atomic force microscopy." Science 257(5078): 1944-1946.
Henrickson, K. J. (2004). "Advances in the laboratory diagnosis of viral respiratory disease." Pediatr Infect Dis J 23(1 Suppl): S6-10.
Heus, H. A., E. M. Puchner, et al. (2011). "Atomic force microscope-based single-molecule force spectroscopy of RNA unfolding." Anal Biochem 414(1): 1-6.
Hoh, J. H., R. Lal, et al. (1991). "Atomic force microscopy and dissection of gap junctions." Science 253(5026): 1405-1408.
Holowczak, J. A. (1982). "Poxvirus DNA." Curr Top Microbiol Immunol 97: 27-79.
Johnson, G. P., S. J. Goebel, et al. (1993). "An update on the vaccinia virus genome." Virology 196(2): 381-401.
Jondle, D. M., L. Ambrosio, et al. (1995). "Imaging and manipulating chromosomes with the atomic force microscope." Chromosome Res 3(4): 239-244.
Karrasch, S., R. Hegerl, et al. (1994). "Atomic force microscopy produces faithful high-resolution images of protein surfaces in an aqueous environment." Proc Natl Acad Sci U S A 91(3): 836-838.
Kasas, S. and A. Ikai (1995). "A method for anchoring round shaped cells for atomic force microscope imaging." Biophys J 68(5): 1678-1680.
Kirmizis, D. and S. Logothetidis (2010). "Atomic force microscopy probing in the measurement of cell mechanics." Int J Nanomedicine 5: 137-145.
Kondra, S., J. Laishram, et al. (2009). "Integration of confocal and atomic force microscopy images." J Neurosci Methods 177(1): 94-107.
Kuznetsov, Y., P. D. Gershon, et al. (2008). "Atomic force microscopy investigation of vaccinia virus structure." J Virol 82(15): 7551-7566.
Kuznetsov, Y. G., S. Daijogo, et al. (2005). "Atomic force microscopy analysis of icosahedral virus RNA." J Mol Biol 347(1): 41-52.
Kuznetsov, Y. G., J. R. Gurnon, et al. (2005). "Atomic force microscopy investigation of a chlorella virus, PBCV-1." J Struct Biol 149(3): 256-263.
Kuznetsov, Y. G., P. Ulbrich, et al. (2007). "Atomic force microscopy investigation of Mason-Pfizer monkey virus and human immunodeficiency virus type 1 reassembled particles." Virology 360(2): 434-446.
Kuznetsov, Y. G., J. G. Victoria, et al. (2003). "Atomic force microscopy investigation of human immunodeficiency virus (HIV) and HIV-infected lymphocytes." J Virol 77(22): 11896-11909.

Liu, Y. F., K. X. Hu, et al. (2008). "[Study on the morphology of influenza virus A by atomic force microscopy]." Bing Du Xue Bao 24(2): 106-110.

Madeley, C. R. (2004). "Molecular and diagnostic clinical virology in real time." Clin Microbiol Infect 10(5): 471; author reply 471-472.

Malkin, A. J., A. McPherson, et al. (2003). "Structure of intracellular mature vaccinia virus visualized by in situ atomic force microscopy." J Virol 77(11): 6332-6340.

Metcalf, T. G., J. L. Melnick, et al. (1995). "Environmental virology: from detection of virus in sewage and water by isolation to identification by molecular biology--a trip of over 50 years." Annu Rev Microbiol 49: 461-487.

Michel, J. P., I. L. Ivanovska, et al. (2006). "Nanoindentation studies of full and empty viral capsids and the effects of capsid protein mutations on elasticity and strength." Proc Natl Acad Sci U S A 103(16): 6184-6189.

Moreno-Herrero, F., J. Colchero, et al. (2004). "Atomic force microscopy contact, tapping, and jumping modes for imaging biological samples in liquids." Phys Rev E Stat Nonlin Soft Matter Phys 69(3 Pt 1): 031915.

Morimura, T., K. Ohashi, et al. (1998). "Pathogenesis of Marek's disease (MD) and possible mechanisms of immunity induced by MD vaccine." J Vet Med Sci 60(1): 1-8.

Moss, B. (1991). "Vaccinia virus: a tool for research and vaccine development." Science 252(5013): 1662-1667.

Muller, D. J., F. A. Schabert, et al. (1995). "Imaging purple membranes in aqueous solutions at sub-nanometer resolution by atomic force microscopy." Biophys J 68(5): 1681-1686.

Murphy, P. J., M. Shannon, et al. (2011). "Visualization of recombinant DNA and protein complexes using atomic force microscopy." J Vis Exp(53).

Nermut, M. V., D. J. Hockley, et al. (1998). "Further evidence for hexagonal organization of HIV gag protein in prebudding assemblies and immature virus-like particles." J Struct Biol 123(2): 143-149.

Nettikadan, S. R., J. C. Johnson, et al. (2003). "Virus particle detection by solid phase immunocapture and atomic force microscopy." Biochem Biophys Res Commun 311(2): 540-545.

Neumann, G., H. Feldmann, et al. (2002). "Reverse genetics demonstrates that proteolytic processing of the Ebola virus glycoprotein is not essential for replication in cell culture." J Virol 76(1): 406-410.

Ohnesorge, F. M., J. K. Horber, et al. (1997). "AFM review study on pox viruses and living cells." Biophys J 73(4): 2183-2194.

Olofsson, S., R. Brittain-Long, et al. (2011). "PCR for detection of respiratory viruses: seasonal variations of virus infections." Expert Rev Anti Infect Ther 9(8): 615-626.

Petersen, N. O., W. B. McConnaughey, et al. (1982). "Dependence of locally measured cellular deformability on position on the cell, temperature, and cytochalasin B." Proc Natl Acad Sci U S A 79(17): 5327-5331.

Pineda, B., M. d. M. Saniger, et al. (2009). "Solid-phase assay for the detection of varicella zoster virus." Future Virology 4(6): 543-551.

Pourati, J., A. Maniotis, et al. (1998). "Is cytoskeletal tension a major determinant of cell deformability in adherent endothelial cells?" Am J Physiol 274(5 Pt 1): C1283-1289.

Putman, C. A., K. O. van der Werf, et al. (1994). "Viscoelasticity of living cells allows high resolution imaging by tapping mode atomic force microscopy." Biophys J 67(4): 1749-1753.

Revenko, I. and R. Proksch (2000). " Magnetic and acoustic tapping mode microscopy of liquid phase phospholipid bilayers and DNA molecules." J. Appl. Phys 87(1): 526-533.

Roos, W. H., K. Radtke, et al. (2009). "Scaffold expulsion and genome packaging trigger stabilization of herpes simplex virus capsids." Proc Natl Acad Sci U S A 106(24): 9673-9678.

Sachse, C., J. Z. Chen, et al. (2007). "High-resolution electron microscopy of helical specimens: a fresh look at tobacco mosaic virus." J Mol Biol 371(3): 812-835.

Schindler, H., D. Badt, et al. (2000). "Optimal sensitivity for molecular recognition MAC-mode AFM." Ultramicroscopy 82(1-4): 227-235.

Schneeweiss, M. A. and I. Rubinstein (2007). Metal Substrates for Self-assembled Monolayers. Encyclopedia of Electrochemistry, Wiley-VCH Verlag GmbH & Co. KGaA.

Shen, X. C., L. Bao, et al. (2011). "A simple and effective sample preparation method for atomic force microscopy visualization of individual DNA molecules in situ." Mol Biol Rep 38(2): 965-969.

Siedlecki, C. A. and R. E. Marchant (1998). "Atomic force microscopy for characterization of the biomaterial interface." Biomaterials 19(4-5): 441-454.

Straub, T. M., I. L. Pepper, et al. (1994). "Detection of naturally occurring enteroviruses and hepatitis A virus in undigested and anaerobically digested sludge using the polymerase chain reaction." Can J Microbiol 40(10): 884-888.

Suarez, T., M. J. Gomara, et al. (2003). "Calcium-dependent conformational changes of membrane-bound Ebola fusion peptide drive vesicle fusion." FEBS Lett 535(1-3): 23-28.

Tan, Y. H., J. R. Schallom, et al. (2011). "Characterization of protein immobilization on nanoporous gold using atomic force microscopy and scanning electron microscopy." Nanoscale 3(8): 3395-3407.

Tian, D., Y. Wang, et al. (2011). "A novel strategy for exploring the reassortment origins of newly emerging influenza virus." Bioinformation 7(2): 64-68.

Trache, A. and G. A. Meininger (2008). "Atomic force microscopy (AFM)." Curr Protoc Microbiol Chapter 2: Unit 2C 2.

Volkening, J. D. and S. J. Spatz (2009). "Purification of DNA from the cell-associated herpesvirus Marek's disease virus for 454 pyrosequencing using micrococcal nuclease digestion and polyethylene glycol precipitation." J Virol Methods 157(1): 55-61.

Wagner, P. (1998). "Immobilization strategies for biological scanning probe microscopy." FEBS Lett 430(1-2): 112-115.

Wang, N. (1998). "Mechanical interactions among cytoskeletal filaments." Hypertension 32(1): 162-165.

Weiland, J. J. and T. W. Dreher (1993). "Cis-preferential replication of the turnip yellow mosaic virus RNA genome." Proc Natl Acad Sci U S A 90(13): 6095-6099.

Wickramasinghe, S. R., B. Kalbfuss, et al. (2005). "Tangential flow microfiltration and ultrafiltration for human influenza A virus concentration and purification." Biotechnol Bioeng 92(2): 199-208.

Wool-Lewis, R. J. and P. Bates (1999). "Endoproteolytic processing of the ebola virus envelope glycoprotein: cleavage is not required for function." J Virol 73(2): 1419-1426.

Zhao, Q., Y. Wang, et al. (2006). "Maturation of recombinant hepatitis B virus surface antigen particles." Hum Vaccin 2(4): 174-180.

12

Force Microscopy – A Tool to Elucidate the Relationship Between Nanomechanics and Function in Viruses

J.L. Cuéllar and E. Donath
University of Leipzig
Germany

1. Introduction

Within the last 20 years nanotechnology has broadened our perspective of different well established disciplines. One of these is virology, which through the development of techniques for the manipulation of single nanoobjects has evolved and acquired a new direction giving birth to the new emerging field of physical virology. An excellent review on this has been recently published (Roos, et al., 2010). Viruses, originally conceived only as harmful parasites, causatives of disease are now being investigated from a single particle point of view. The intrinsic mechanical properties of individual viruses have started to be unveiled by means of ultrasensitive surface probe techniques such as Atomic force microscopy (AFM) (Roos & Wuite, 2009). The profiler device is an ultrasharp tip which is also being used for probing viruses with piconewton (10^{-12} N) loading forces.

From the materials science point of view viruses can be considered as highly ordered nanostructured assemblies usually composed by no more than a handful of different components. Viruses can be either non-enveloped or enveloped viruses. In a non-enveloped virus the genome being either DNA or RNA is encaged inside a quasi-spherical protein shell, the capsid. In an enveloped virus the capsid is additionally covered with a lipid bilayer which contains proteins. This lipid envelope stems usually from the cellular membrane of the host. The viral capsid is on one hand a protective barrier which allows save transportation of the genome against chemical hazards, mechanical deformation, and drastic changes in environmental conditions. On the other hand the capsid is designed by nature for being capable of cell entry and cargo release. The capsid self-assembles without requiring external energy. One of the remarkable features of viral capsids is their symmetry which is a consequence of self-assembly from identical subunits (Baker, et al., 1999). The shape of a wide range of viruses can be described by the quasi-equivalence principle (Caspar & Klug, 1962). In this concept the shape of viral capsids is composed of a network of hexagons forming the facets and connected by pentagons at the vertices of the resulting icosahedra. The triangulation number T used to classify viral shapes can be calculated from a walk between two neighboring pentagons over the shortest possible distance performing h steps in one direction and k steps in the other direction as shown in Fig. 1. In this particular example h equals 1 and k equals 2. T is then given by

$$T = h^2 + k^2 + h \cdot k = 1 + 4 + 2 = 7 \quad (1)$$

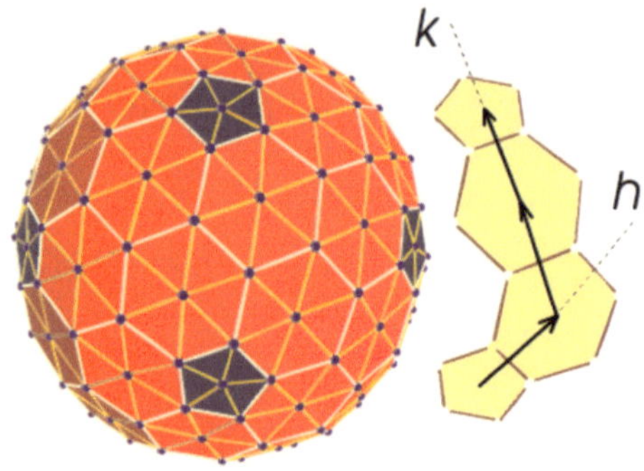

Fig. 1. Scheme of the Caspar & Klug construction for the calculation of triangulation numbers. With permission from (Siber, 2006).

However, there are some exceptions. For example, viruses within the family of Papovaviridae cannot be properly described by the Caspar & Klug principle. Recently developed concepts account for a wider gamma of features in viral capsid structure (Twarock, 2006).

Some viruses like the Tobacco mosaic virus require the presence of the genome for posterior capsid assembly (Fraenkel-Conrat & Williams, 1955). Other capsids, such as that of the Cowpea Chlorotic Mottle Virus (CCMV) may be reversibly assembled *in vitro* without the presence of the genome resulting in so-called virus-like particles (VLP) (Bancroft, et al., 1967). Empty capsids of several human viruses like papilloma virus, norovirus, rotavirus and Ebola virus have been used as vaccines (Nicollier-Jamot, et al., 2004, Schiller & Lowy, 2001, Warfield, et al., 2003) (Crawford, et al., 1999). Self assembly of viral capsids in the absence of the genome may lead to capsids with different triangulation numbers observing as a rule a reduced stability (White, et al., 1997). The surface of VLP´s can be engineered by bioconjugation approaches. As the position of every amino acid is known with subnanometer precision nanostructures with an unprecedented accurateness of the chemical properties of their surface can be fabricated. The use of viruses and VLPs extends well beyond medicine. Aided by modern genetic engineering techniques like the Baculo virus expression system the production of large amounts of recombinant proteins became possible (Ernst, et al., 1998, Kost & Condreay, 1999, Kost, et al., 2005). This has paved the way for using viral cages in nanotechnology, for example, as containers and templates for the assembly of hybrid materials (Graff, et al., 2002) (S. W. Lee, et al., 2003, Nam, et al., 2006). Viruses and VLP´s are currently being used as basic elements in electronic devices, as nanoreactors for catalysis, platforms for surface functionalization and display systems (Fischlechner & Donath, 2007, Fischlechner, et al., 2006, Singh, et al., 2006, Uchida, et al., 2007, Vriezema, et al., 2005).

The structural and material properties of viruses including their mechanical properties have developed through millions of years of interacting evolution with their hosts. Following the enormous progress in molecular virology, exploring their mechanical properties in relation to function is of great importance for understanding the biology of viruses. AFM could reveal the mechanics during the first steps of viral entry. A nanoindentation experimental setup can uncover internal structural transformations. In most cases, it is not known how the capsid gets destabilized at the final stage of infection and how this is correlated with the release of the genome. This chapter focuses thus on the application of force microscopy as a novel powerful technique as applied to virology. Nanoindentation experiments may help to answer questions like how soft, hard or fragile is a single wild type virus or an empty viral capsid? How elastic or how stable are these assemblies under external applied forces? Do their material properties resemble similarities with those of macroscopic materials? Which external environmental conditions can change their mechanical properties? And finally, what can their mechanical properties tell us about their mechanism of infection. Also the newly developed field of single receptor-virus interactions is briefly introduced.

2. Mechanical properties of lipid layers and vesicles

With atomic force microscopy, the material properties of single nanoobjects can be probed directly after they have been localized with imaging. After positioning the cantilever above the desired object repeated approach-retraction cycles can be performed by controlling the movement of the piezo-crystal in the z direction. The tip is pressed against the sample until a predetermined cantilever deflection is attained. After an eventual dwell time the cantilever is retracted completing one approach-retraction cycle. With the cantilever spring constant the originally recorded deflection values can be converted into force. Finally, forces vs. separation curves are obtained. In commercial devices this procedure is usually provided by a software option. Force vs. separation curves provide a wealth of information about the details of interaction of the tip with the sample and the mechanical properties in the nanoscale (Capella & Dietler, 1999). In the force-mode the AFM tip can be used as an indenting tool to test deformability and compliance of soft homogeneous, layered or composite nanomaterials (Bhushan, 2007, Radmacher, et al., 1995). The Young modulus can be obtained from indentation experiments applying the Hertz model (Hertz, 1882). Refinements of this model take account for the finite thickness of layers on solid supports.

Of special interest for virus related studies are the mechanical behavior of supported lipid bilayers and the indentation of lipid vesicles, since supported lipid layers form a constitutive part of enveloped viruses. When the tip starts to compress the bilayer, repulsion is observed. If the load gets sufficiently large the tip may puncture the bilayer overcoming the intermolecular forces holding the lipid molecules together. The associated breakthrough forces have been measured (Loi, et al., 2002, Pera, et al., 2004, Richter & Brisson, 2003). After breakthrough, as a rule, regular desorption plateaus upon retraction can be observed. They are associated with pulling tethers of lipids connecting the tip with the substrate. The tips can be modified to control their interaction with lipid membranes. Dufrene and Schneider studied the mechanical behavior of supported bilayers in some detail (Dufrene, et al., 1998) At forces below 5 nN the lipid bilayer behaves as an elastic film. Repulsion was attributed to steric and hydration forces as well as to the elastic response after contact. The observed hardness was 108 Nm^{-2}. Distances traveled by the AFM tip within jumps into the substrate were of the order of ~ 6-7nm, which is close to the value of the bilayer thickness. Their studies established a connection between mechanical properties of lipid bilayers with the interaction forces between the lipid molecules within the bilayer and stressed their importance for adhesion of cells and membrane fusion. Recently, more sophisticated theoretical and experimental approaches have been undertaken to extract mechanical parameters like the bending rigidity κ and the surface tension σ from indentation experiments (Norouzi, et al., 2006, Steltenkamp, et al., 2006). The mechanics of various vesicle structures has also been studied. When a small spherical vesicle of the size of the order of viruses is being indented at least at larger indentations the volume cannot be conserved as the area of the vesicle membrane can only slightly increase because of the high stretching resistance of bilayers. The elastic properties of cholinergic synaptic vesicles were first reported by the group of Hansma (Garcia, et al., 1998, Laney, et al., 1997). For Indentations of about 10 nm on vesicles with diameters of about 110 nm with AFM tips with a radius of 11-23 nm, Young moduli of 2-13 x 10^5 Pa were calculated. Studies on synaptic vesicles and their interaction with the Synapsin protein were also reported (Awizio, et al., 2007). Their stiffness was 0.2 pN/nm and the Young modulus was 75 kPa applying Reissner´s theory of deformation of thin elastic shells (Reissner, 1952). The deformation of closed shells depends significantly on whether the shells are empty or filled, because the response is given by an interplay of out of plane bending and in plane stretching that arises at the point of compression. The response of the material to the applied force is thus governed by its intrinsic elastic (Y) and bending (κ) material properties. When sufficiently high loading forces are applied buckling may occur (Helfer, et al., 2001, Tamura, et al., 2004). Buckling is an instability phenomenon which further complicates the analysis of indentation experiments. Liang et al. investigated the mechanical response of Egg yolk Phosphatidylcholine unilamellar vesicles by nanoindentations (Liang, et al., 2004). It was found that force distance curves showed two breakthrough forces which was interpreted as the puncturing the upper and lower bilayer of the vesicle. Values for the bending and Young modulus of 0.21×10^{-19} J and 1.97×10^6 Pa were reported using the Hertz model. The application of the Hertz to closed thin shells is, however, problematic. As an example of a biological vesicle the elastic properties of Clathrin-coated vesicles have been measured (Jin & Nossal, 2008, Jin, et al., 2006). A bending rigidity of about 285 k_bT was calculated for these protein-reinforced vesicles with diameters of about 100 nm. Delorme et al. fabricated hollow faceted polyhedrons from a mixture of cationic surfactants. The shape of them resembled that of viruses (Delorme, et al., 2006). Localized indentations in faces or vertexes exhibited pronounced differences in stiffness. Using the Reissner model a Young´s modulus of 180 MPa and a bending rigidity of 450 k_BT were obtained. Interestingly, concepts from continuum mechanics apply quite well to deformations in assembled nanostructured materials formed by subunits if they show a fluid behavior at the individual scale.

3. Imaging viruses and capsids with AFM

Atomic force microscopy has proved to be an efficient tool for imaging of soft nanomaterials in the dry state as well as under liquid conditions. Even though experimental techniques like X-ray diffraction, Scanning electron microscopy and Cryo-Transmission electron microscopy provide a wealth of information from external and internal features of virus morphology and structure with nearly atomic resolution, samples often require artificial staining or fixation methods which can be problematic with regard to virus characterization in the native state. With AFM viruses can be imaged under physiological conditions within minutes (Malkin, et al., 2002). AFM is thus as a complementary tool for the immediate identification of pathogens. Structural and morphological changes of the virus can be monitored in response to a change of the environmental conditions as the media can be exchanged during the experiment. Another major advantage is that only minimal amounts of the sample are required for imaging. 50-100 µl of a concentrated sample are more than sufficient. The preparation of a virus sample for AFM imaging is straightforward. First, appropriate attachment of the viral particles to the substrate is required since shear forces present an unavoidable risk during scanning with the AFM tip even with soft cantilevers. This can be accomplished by proper selection of the substrate to ensure sufficient adhesion of the viruses or VLP´s. For example, the substrate can be coated with polymers or it can be made more hydrophobic by silanization (Zhao, et al., 2006). Viruses can be also covalently attached to previously functionalized surfaces. Anti-viral antibodies (McDonnell, et al., 2002) and patterned surfaces have been employed (Howorka, et al., 2009). However, it has to be taken into account that adhesion forces if strong enough could lead to flattening of VLP´s. This may lead to a subsequent underestimation of the diameter of the virus (Cuellar, et al., 2010). In the context of imaging it is thus advisable to study the affinity of the viruses to the surface, because if the attachment is too weak imaging might induce detachment. In the opposite case of a rather strong interaction the virus envelopes might be deformed or even destroyed. A related problem is, that the applied loading forces during imaging have to be kept as low as possible in order to reduce deformation of the virus shell. Imaging hollow VLP´s has to be performed with particular care. The absence of the genome renders them even more susceptible to deformation. In this case tapping mode should be preferred because shear forces and contact times with the sample are largely reduced (Moller, et al., 1999). Glass and mica are the most common substrates for particle immobilization as AFM is concerned. Both surfaces are easily available and are rather flat. While glass normally required mild cleaning procedures through well established protocols, mica has to be only cleaved (pulled apart) with the help of a commercial adhesive tape. This produces a molecularly flat and clean surface ready to use. In AFM imaging a superior subatomic resolution can be reached as far as height is concerned, but its lateral resolution is much lower being limited by the accuracy of the piezo scanner and the shape and dimensions of the tip. Even the sharpest AFM tip has a finite tip radius of the order of 10 nm. Therefore pits and slots with characteristic dimensions of the tip radius cannot be imaged. Furthermore, convolution caused by the tip size and shape leads to an overestimation of the width and makes measurements of shape of spherical objects below the equator impossible (Banin, et al., 2002). As a rule of thumb, for viruses, the measured width has been reported to be 2 to 5 times that of the real particle (Kuznetsov, et al., 2001). Enveloped viruses are more difficult to image than non-enveloped ones because the space between the soft lipid envelope and the capsid core is usually filled with a soft matrix protein layer which enhances the compliance of the virus and also increases the possibility of disruption of the surface by the tip while imaging. Also if the size of the capsid is much smaller than the entire particle, the capsid may be free to move inside the viscous matrix protein resulting in a further enhanced compliance of the virus. Viruses can be imaged both in the dry state (air) as well as under physiological conditions (liquid). Imaging in the dehydrated state is generally easier, and the resolution is higher but it has to be taken into account that during dehydration, the virus may loose mechanical stability and strength leading to shrinkage and collapse into oblong or flattened shapes because of strong capillary forces occurring during evaporation of the liquid. Crystallization of salt is another difficulty associated with drying from physiological solutions. Imaging in dry state can be advantageous in certain situations, for example, when information of the general architecture of a virus is in the focus rather than the mechanical properties of the virus itself. Image acquisition can start right after placement of the sample under the AFM scanner since the sample must not be incubated to reach equilibrium due thermal motion within the fluid prior to imaging. However, important features of a virus can be only revealed under at least near physiological conditions, where the virus particle retains all its natural properties.

AFM has been applied to characterize the surface of tobacco mosaic virus, and the interaction with its genome for the full and partial coated case (Drygin, et al., 1998). The host-virus interaction was studied with Pox virus on living cells (Ohnesorge, et al., 1997). A detailed characterization of morphological and structural aspects of several plant, insect and animal viruses was undertaken by the group of A. McPherson. The successful attachment of a large amount of viral particles to flat substrates and their posterior growth into 2 and 3D crystals by a vapor diffusion approach permitted to investigate their nucleation mechanism into highly packed hexagonal lattices (Malkin, et al., 2002, McPherson, et al., 2003). It was found that sometimes aberrant sized virions where incorporated within the lattices, inducing defects on the surface and breaking the symmetry of the crystal. Tapping mode AFM yielded images of small viruses of about 28 nm with molecular resolution. Images of Brome mosaic virus and Turnip yellow mosaic virus showed the individual capsomers (see figure 2). However in other cases, like the satellite tobacco mosaic virus and the insect tipula Iridescent virus, the molecular details could not be resolved but the faceted shapes of the capsids were recognized.

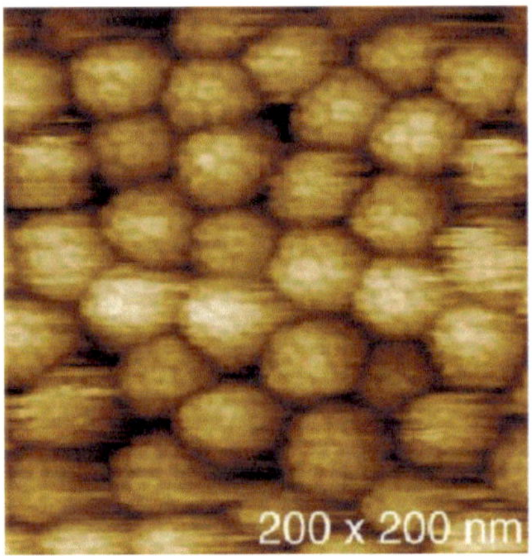

Fig. 2. High resolution AFM images of Brome mosaic virus. Capsomers at the surface can be identified. With permission from (Kuznetsov, et al., 2001).

They also studied animal viruses of relevance for health like Vaccinia, HIV, Herpes simplex virus and Murine Leukemia virus. Their external morphological features where comparable to those obtained by electron microscopy, and moreover, the internal structure of these viruses could be uncovered by using detergents to remove the lipid envelope, using proteolytic enzymes, low pH exposure or assisted particle disruption.

Decomposition of Herpes simplex virus allowed for identification of structural elements in every layer (Malkin, et al., 2002). Elongated glycoproteins protruding 10 to 25 nm out the surface of the enveloped particle were detected. When the envelope was removed with detergents pentons and hexons forming the capsomers could be identified. Remarkable high resolution AFM images of wild type Herpes virus and a pentonless empty version of the capsids of the same virus were obtained after treatment with Urea (Sodeik, et al., 2009). Finally, the treatment of the virus with a strong ionic detergent like sodium dodecyl sulfate (SDS) induced extrusion of the viral DNA which was clearly seen in the AFM images. Images of the surface at high magnification of wild type Murine Leukemia virus and Human immunodeficiency virus revealed dense arrangements of protein tufts on their surface (McPherson, et al., 2004, McPherson, et al., 2004). For HIV, the protrusions on the surface of the envelope have been associated with aggregates of the gp120 protein. Blebs protruding out of the surface were observed and have been identified as being scars from the budding process of the virus. After detergent treatment a capsid size of 35 to 40 nm was determined from AFM images. The envelope formed a 35 nm thick layer around the capsid (McPherson, et al., 2005). The size distribution of MLV and HIV VLP´s was not consistent with a homogeneous population of VLP´s. The particle size ranged from 120 - 170 nm and 100 - 160 nm, respectively. These broad distributions in virus size may be a product of deviations in the self assembly process of the capsid proteins. This is more likely to occur in empty capsids where the genome is not involved during particle formation, because it is known that the genome forms the scaffold for assembly and induces stability.

The multilayered architecture of Vaccinia virus has been investigated in hydrated and dehydrated conditions. It was found that the outer corona with embedded proteins and its respective proteinaceous lateral bodies characteristic for this virus were clearly visible (McPherson, et al., 2008). Exposure of these virions to proteases yielded empty cores which when dried resembled flattened sacs with pancake shapes. From this study it was further concluded that the encased genome was moderately condensed within the capsid, rather than being in a dense and compact state. The group of P. Hinterdorfer investigated the topography and RNA release of Human Rhinovirus onto mica surfaces under physiological conditions (Hinterdorfer, et al., 2004). It was shown that polygonal subunits with sizes of about 3 nm could be discerned in individual particles and that exposure of the virions to acidic conditions lead to RNA release. The absence of loop formation of the RNA molecule in the case of partial release suggested that the observed features of release induced by acid conditions may be related to the mechanism of genome release from the viral capsid upon infection.

The capability of AFM to resolve fine topographical features at the surface of the viral particle strongly depends on the radius of the apex of the tip and on the particular molecular architecture on the external capsid surface. A sharper tip is obviously advantageous for imaging small pits and protrusions at the viral surface. Theoretically it should be possible to visualize the hexameric and pentameric arrangements of proteins within capsomers or the localization of spike proteins at the surface. Nevertheless, for viruses which have crowded proteins coronas with only narrow molecular canyons, like Norovirus and Cowpea Chlorotic Mottle virus, high resolution images at the surface are limited by the geometrical constraints of the tip (Cuellar, et al., 2010, Knobler, et al., 2006). In these cases, with typical commercial Silicon Nitride tips with a radius of about 15 nm the viruses appear as hemispherical caps as shown in figure 3. With the fast advancement of AFM technology, these limitations will be improved by the use of sharper probes fabricated

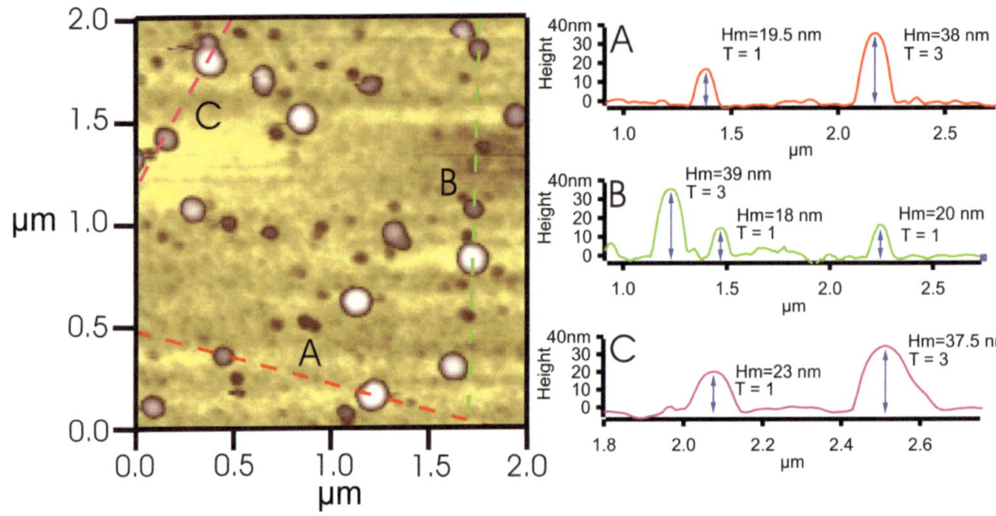

Fig. 3. Height image of coexisting Norovirus-like particles with T = 1 and T = 3 capsid number. The capsids appear as hemispherical caps without discernible substructure.

for example from carbon nanotubes. Nonetheless the positions of the symmetrical five, three and two-fold capsid axes with respect to the substrate was distinguishable with the current tips even for one of the smallest viruses like the Parvovirus minute virus of mice (MVM) with a average size of only about 25 nm (Pablo, et al., 2006). Refined studies on the protein organization of influenza A virus in neutral an low pH have been recently reported (Le Grimellec, et al., 2010). A clear honey comb organization of activated spike proteins at low pH was noticed possibly related to the initial steps of viral fusion with the endosomal membrane.

The two key steps of infection, membrane fusion during entry of the virus into the cell and release by budding may be explored by AFM. Fusion of enveloped viruses with membranes is usually a pH triggered mechanism that can be studied using supported lipid bilayers. AFM Images of fused Rubella-like particles onto lipid coated colloids have been reported in the context of engineering authentic viral building blocks on colloids (Fischlechner, et al., 2007). The particles appear as distinctive objects of smaller size than the original particles embedded into the lipid layer when imaged onto a solid substrate. The uptake of nanoparticles by cells via endocytosis has been followed by AFM (Labhasetwar & Vasir, 2008). These results encourage the use of AFM as a perspective technique to explore the entry mechanisms of a variety of non-enveloped viruses for which little is known. The process of viral budding has been recorded for several enveloped viruses in a real-time frame sequence (McPherson, et al., 2003). Massive numbers of virions have been seen appearing at the cell surface as shown in figure 4. Moreover, the interesting topographic changes a cell suffers at different stages of infection can be monitored, as has been done for West Nile virus and corona virus in Vero cells (J. W. M. Lee & Ng, 2004). An increase of filopodia formation was observed following infection by West Nile virus, accompanied by actin filament formation in the periphery of the infected cell membrane. Magnified cellular regions showed how newly formed viruses where transported into cell filopodia within sacs or envelopes. Cells infected with severe acute respiratory syndrome-associated corona virus

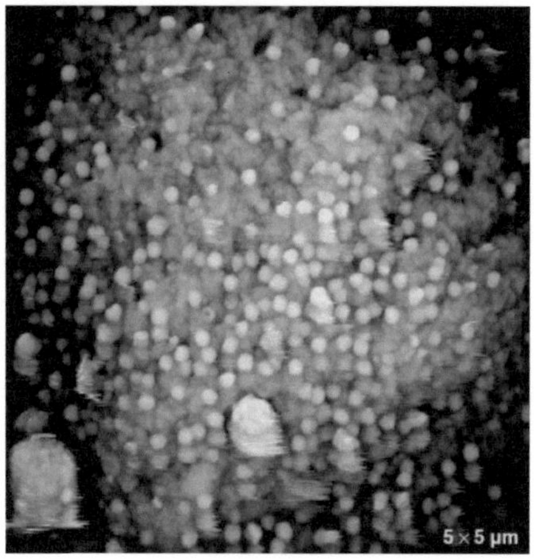

Fig. 4. AFM image of a massive number of HIV particles budding out the surface of a virus infected H9 human fibroblast in culture. With permission from (Kuznetsov, et al., 2004)

showed thickening at the edges of their pseudopodia, which are likely to be responsible for the extrusion of incipient particles (Ng, et al., 2004). The budding of retroviruses has been demonstrated (Rousso & Gladnikoff, 2008, Rousso, et al., 2009). The budding process of Moloney murine leukemia virus was continuously visualized as viral particles emerged out from the membrane within a time period of about 48 minutes. Budding dynamics of viral particles was observed to occur at two different rates. It was also found that budding take place at indifferent sites onto the cell membrane. Their subsequent study on budding of the HIV showed how the infection process alters the internal organization of the cell cytoskeleton in the immediate regions of virus release. This demonstrated that assembly and budding of retroviruses are a cytoskeleton mediated processes.

4. Nanointdentation studies in viruses and capsids

The mechanical properties of individual viruses and VLP´s can be obtained in a straightforward way from nanoindentation experiments. The force vs separation curves yield effective spring constants as a function of the applied force. The effective spring constant is a combination of the spring constants of the cantilever and that of the viral particle. This cantilever-capsid system can be treated as two springs in series. The spring constant of the employed cantilever is determined before by pressing it onto a hard surface and by analyzing its thermal noise spectrum in solution. The point stiffness or spring constant of the capsid itself can be thus obtained as follows $k_{Cap} = (k_{Cant} * k_{Eff})/(k_{Cant} - k_{Eff})$. The spring constant of the capsid depends both on the fundamental elastic material properties such as Young modulus and Poisson number as well as on the shape of the object and on the way how the force is applied. Extracting the elastic properties of the material itself from the experimentally obtained spring constants is a rather challenging task, especially in the case of more complicated geometries, where analytically tractable formulas are not available. Furthermore, there is always an uncertainty whether the tip was pressed onto the center of the nanoparticle or whether it was displaced from it by an unknown distance. It has also to be considered that in the case of facetted viral particles the mechanical response will be different depending on whether the tip was pressed onto a vertex or a facet. Although the point stiffness already provides a mechanical feature of the capsid, it is nevertheless desirable to extract the fundamental elastic parameters of the capsid material itself. From the theory of elasticity it is known that the complete description of elastic deformations of bodies requires knowledge of two elastic constants related to the properties of the material itself. In most cases these two parameters are given by the Young modulus Y and the Poisson ratio μ. For example, the tensile strength of materials is usually characterized in terms of the Young modulus which provides a direct measure of the hardness of the material under consideration. The Young modulus is the ratio of stress applied to the face of a body with constant cross section to the resulting strain. Poisson´s number represents the negative ratio of the relative change in thickness to the strain being the relative change in length. In order to derive the Young modulus of virus particles or capsids some simplifying assumptions have to be made. Quite often the particle is approximated as a closed thin shell where the radius is much larger than shell thickness. This allows using the well elaborated theory of deformation of thin shells (Landau & Lifshitz, 1986). For small deformations ξ of the order of the shell thickness, d, applied on a spherical shell of radius R by a point loading force F a linear response is predicted. This linearity with the applied force is given by

$$F = \frac{\alpha \cdot Y \cdot d^2 \cdot \xi}{R} \tag{2}$$

here α is a proportionality factor close to unity which has been derived for viral capsids by means of a finite element analysis (Gibbons & Klug, 2007). Most studies related to mechanics of viral shells apply thin shell theory and/or numerical finite element analysis to interpret experimental Data (see figure 5) (Kasas & Dietler, 2008). The virus capsid is considered as a homogeneous elastic material with Hookean behavior.

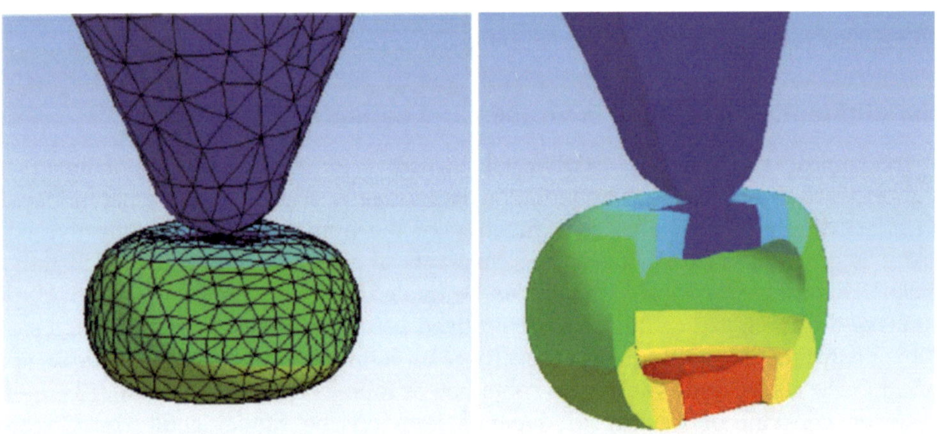

Fig. 5. Scheme of finite element analysis to model the compression of a shell by an AFM tip. With permission (Kasas & Dietler, 2008).

The first nanoindentation experiments on VLP´s were conducted by Ivanovska et al. on the φ29 bacteriophage capsid (Ivanovska, et al., 2004). The life cycle of this phage is rather interesting. The capsid is first assembled and then connected to a molecular motor which is used to pack the genome inside the assembled capsid. It has been shown that the capsid can withstand internal pressures as high as 60 bar (Smith, et al., 2001). This stored pressure is subsequently used as an energy reservoir to provide the driving force for the infection process. After the virus attaches to a specific receptor at the surface of the bacterium a molecular gate opens and the genome is forced into the interior of the bacterium. Indentations on the φ29 capsids showed an elastic behavior at small loading forces. A bimodal distribution for the capsid stiffness was found, which was attributed to the inhomogeneous structural features in the capsid protein structure. Deformations of up to about 30% of the total height of the capsid observed a linear response. Repetitive indentations showed full recovery of the shell. Indentations with higher loading forces of about 2.8 nN led to a nonlinear behavior which usually terminated with a sudden collapse of the shell. Consecutive indentations finally resulted in breakage of the shell indicating induced fatigue of the material. A Young modulus of 1.8 GPa was found which is within the range of hard plastics. Two years later, the mechanical properties of the empty and wild type CCMV were investigated at different pH values.

The idea behind this was that the CCMV capsid shows a reversible expansion as a function of pH, which is thought to be caused by mutual electrostatic repulsion between internal residues of the capsid proteins (Michel, et al.,2006). It was found that the radial swelling was accompanied by a softening of the capsid material. In the swollen state at pH 6, the capsid responded linearly for deformations up to 70% of the capsid diameter followed by complete recovery. At pH 5, a three-fold increase in the capsid stiffness together with a drastic drop in the force was observed, which indicated a structural failure of the shell. The RNA containing capsid displayed a similar elastic behavior with a slight but yet measurable increase in stiffness. A single point mutation in the capsid increased its stiffness from 140 to 190 MPa. This is an important finding concerning the design of nanostructured materials with tunable properties. Stiffness values of the order of 10^2 MPa are comparable to soft plastics like Teflon.

For DNA - carrying viruses, an increase in stiffness of the native virus compared with the empty capsid can be expected, because the crowded inner state of its genome will resist externally induced compressions. This has been demonstrated for λ-phages (Evilevitch, et al.,2011, Ivanovska, et al.,2007). The virus was twice as strong as an empty capsid. A linear response of the capsid without hysteresis to the applied force was observed with fully reproducible elastic behavior for indentations of about 25% of the capsid radius. A critical maximal threshold force of 0.8 nN was required to break an empty capsid while 1.6 nN were needed to break DNA - filled capsids. This threshold force for rupturing empty λ-phage capsids is about half the value required to break the φ29 phage capsids. The capsid material had a Young modulus of 1.0 GPa. This study proved that viruses acquire structural support and stability against indentations due the internal osmotic pressure generated by the hydrated state of the highly packed genome within the capsid. Wild type minute virus of mice showed a similar reinforcement (Carrasco, et al.,2006). High resolution imaging and indentations performed precisely at the two, three and five-fold axes of the DNA-filled and empty viral capsids, permitted to discern an anisotropic behavior in the stiffness of capsid. Empty capsids showed an isotropic force response. It was therefore concluded that internal DNA interactions at specific sites of the capsid wall contributed differently to this mechanical reinforcement, decreasing the bending of the capsid wall during external induced deformations by the AFM tip. Replacement of a single amino acid was sufficient to remove specific non-covalent interactions between the DNA molecule and sixty equivalent binding sites within the capsid wall (Carrasco, et al., 2008).

The DNA-filled Herpes simplex virus-1(HSV-1) appeared to be the strongest virus tested to date by AFM nanoindentations. The envelope-free capsid could withstand maximal compression forces of about 6 nN (Liashkovich, et al.,2008). Mechanical failure of the DNA containing capsids was observed at loading forces of about 9 nN. This failure resulted in expulsion of the genome. For these large viral capsids of about 120-130 nm in diameter deformations slightly below the shell thickness (~16 nm) were linear, however, irreversible capsid damage was observe for forces above 7 nN. A noticeable decrease of stiffness observed for empty capsids was attributed to the absence of nucleic acids. Other data did not imply a difference in the stiffness and threshold breaking forces between empty and DNA-filled capsids (Roos, et al., 2009). One reason for this discrepancy concerning the influence of the content on capsid stiffness may be due to the presence of certain amount of tegument still attached to the particles. The presence of this tegument could probably reinforce the capsid resistance against deformation.

The first nanoindentation studies on mechanical properties of animal and enveloped viruses were performed by Kol et al. Murine Leukemia virus (MLV) and Human immunodeficiency virus (HIV) (Kol, et al.,2006, Kol, et al.,2007). The focus of this work was on detecting internal morphological alterations that these viruses undergo during the maturation process as a requirement for infectivity. A drastic change in the measured stiffness in both viruses between their mature and immature state was indeed observed. The stiffness of the MLV decreased three-fold and that of HIV more than 14-fold upon maturation, respectively. The mature shell of the MLV became brittle upon repetitive compression and by application of large loading forces. The higher stiffness of HIV particles in the immature state was attributed to the presence of a specific viral envelope protein cytoplasmic tail domain, since finite element calculations suggested that removal of this domain would result in an 8-fold decrease of the Young´s modulus of the particle. The decrease in stiffness goes along with a decrease in shell thickness during maturation. The authors conclude that the regulation of retroviral mechanical properties plays an important role in the life cycle of these viruses. They are stiff during viral budding and need to become soft during entry. In the above mentioned work, an eventual influence of the lipid envelope on the mechanical properties of viruses and VLP´s has been not taken into account. Recently, the mechanical properties of Rubella-like particles (RLPs) have been investigated (Cuellar, et al., 2012). Rubella viruses are enveloped viruses with a relatively thick matrix layer located between the envelope and the capsid (Risco, et al., 2003). Instead of a single linear regime, two consecutive linear force responses were obtained upon indentation. It was supposed that the first is related to the mechanical response of the envelope while in the second one the deformation is transmitted to the capsid (Figure 7C). It was found that RLP´s are very soft and can thus be easily deformed by external forces. Even when the particles were imaged with the lowest possible loading forces below 100 pN and with very soft cantilevers with a stiffness of 0.01 N/m the RLP´s were noticeably compressed during imaging. This followed from a comparison with indentation measurements which revealed the height at the first contact, which was comparable to electron microscopy data. The spring constant corresponding to the steeper linear regime was about 0.017 N/m. This is a quite small value compared with other viruses suggesting that the RLP´s represent rather soft particles. In a coming publication, the influence of membrane deformation and osmotic pressure due the entrapped matrix protein between capsid and envelope on the mechanical properties of RLP´s will be discussed.

AFM nanoindentation and imaging experiments with hepatitis B virus (HBV) capsids together with mass spectrometry of the HBV proteins showed that the proteins assemble into discernible T = 3 and T = 4 capsids (see figure 6) (Uetrecht, et al.,2008). The Young moduli of both structure variants were very close being in the range comparable to soft plastic materials. The capsids observed irreversible deformation for indentation forces close to 1 nN. Our own work on Norovirus (NV) virus-like particles showed a relationship between stiffness and size on one hand and the pH value on the other hand (Cuellar, et al., 2010). It was concluded that these changes are related to a modulation of non-covalent interactions among the capsomers by the pH. This pH dependence of the stiffness may play a role for infectivity. The Norovirus-like particles showed a remarkable elastic behavior upon repetitive indentations even for high loads as high as 8 nN, where the capsid was totally compressed and, nevertheless, the deformations were fully reversible upon retraction. Nonetheless, in certain occasions a progressive failure pattern developed in the force curves upon consecutive compressions. Even in this case the slope and the initial point of contact remained unchanged. The recovery of the particle stiffness after total compression suggests an inbuilt self-healing capacity of these capsids against externally induced deformations.

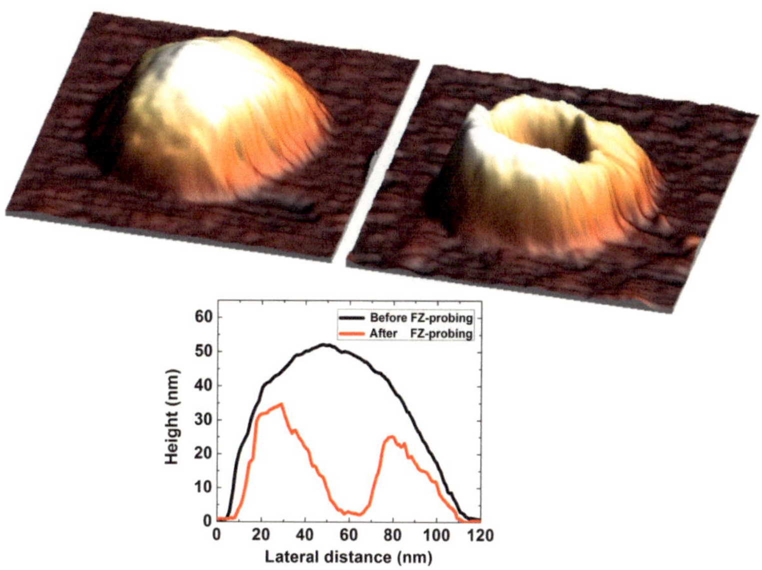

Fig. 6. A virus before and after indentation. Indentation with 4.5 nN resulted in capsid damage (right). The lower image provides height profiles across the capsid. With permission, W. H. Roos, G. J. L. Wuite, Nanoindentation studies reveal material properties of viruses. Adv. Mat., 2009, Vol. 21, 1187-1192

In parallel with experiments theoretical approaches have been developed to study the shape and deformation of viral capsids by taking into account both external loading forces and internal osmotic pressure exerted by the genome (Buenemann & Lenz, 2008, Zandi & Reguera, 2005, Zandi, et al., 2004). The indentation by an AFM tip has been simulated providing an understanding of the ongoing dislocation and the loss of stability on a molecular level (Ahadi, et al., 2009, Arkhipov, et al., 2009, Roos, et al., 2010, Vliegenthart & Gompper, 2007, Vliegenthart & Gompper, 2006, Zink & Grubmuller, 2009).

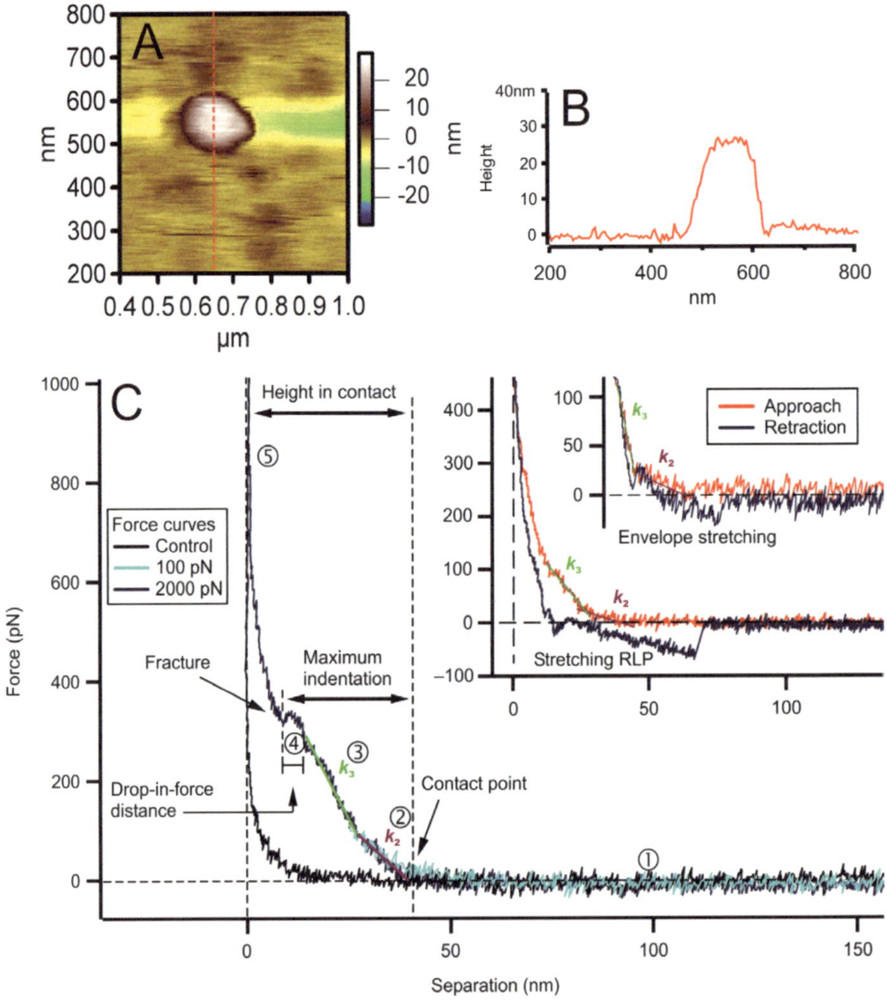

Fig. 7. Indentations on Rubella-Like particles. A and B show a height image of an RLP and its respective profile. In C, approach curves for small (light blue) and large (dark blue) indentations together with the control curve (black) are shown. The two insets show magnifications of approach and retraction curves for small loading forces.

An important parameter is the dimensionless Föppl-von Kármán number. It characterizes the balance between stretching and bending energies for large deflections of thin plates. If it becomes too large buckling occurs. It can thus be used to predict viral shapes and buckling transitions under high loads (Klug, et al., 2006, Lidmar, et al., 2003, Siber, 2006, Siber & Podgornik, 2009).

5. Force spectroscopy of receptor-virus interactions

In recent years, force spectroscopy has been applied for studying virus-host interactions at the level of single molecules. In this special AFM technique the properties of the single molecules themselves or their interaction with receptors are probed. A variety of chemical functionalization approaches permit the firm attachment of molecules of interest to AFM tips to test their interaction with surfaces. Most of the original studies of this later known as single molecule force spectroscopy (SMFS) technique were devoted to investigate the minute forces required for single polymer stretching or adsorption (Hugel, et al., 2001, Hugel & Seitz, 2001). The group of Gaub was the first, who have successfully applied this approach to measure bond breakage for individual ligand-receptor interactions. For example, the work required for unbinding can be quantified (Florin, et al., 1994, Grandbois, et al., 1999, Moy, et al., 1994). Typically, forces of about 2 nN were required for bond dissociation in single covalent silicon-carbon pairs, while one of the strongest known and commonly used non-covalent biological complexes that of stretptavidin-biotin resist only about 257 pN before rupture occurs. In this way, the doors to the field of single molecular recognition spectroscopy were open as was shown by subsequent studies on the affinity between individual antibody-antigen pairs (Allen, et al., 1997, Browning-Kelley, et al., 1997, Hinterdorfer, et al., 1996) . No less interesting is the force mapping of cellular receptors directly at the cell surface (Gunning, et al., 2008). Such studies could identify regions with a high or low density of specific receptors (Horton, et al., 2002). Thereby, the evident potential of using the AFM tip together with the cantilever as a fishing device for testing individual binding forces between viral particles and cell surface receptors is evident. Likewise, the mechanical aspects behind the fusion process of single viral particles with cells can be studied (Skehel & Wiley, 2000). The experimental setup is straightforward. Effective immobilization of one of the test molecules to the AFM tip is required while the complementary molecule can be properly fixed to a flat substrate, onto a spherical colloid or can even be part of the surface of a cell. Stable decoration of the AFM tip with proteins and virions has been frequently carried out by means of heterobifunctional crosslinker molecules with reactive groups to amines like N-hydroxysuccinimide (NHS) esters which provide strong bridging via amide bond formation (Riener, et al., 2003). This covalent linkage has been further improved by adding poly(ethylene)glycol linkers providing flexibility and freedom of movement to the bound particle [(Hinterdorfer, et al., 1996). For sufficiently small interaction forces, this approach ensures long term measurements of repetitive approach-retraction cycles without loss of the binding complex. The kinetics of single bond formation and dissociation can be theoretically described as initially proposed by Kramers, extended later by Bell, and finally refined by Evans & Ritchie (Bell,1978, Evans&Ritchie,1997, Hanggi, et al.,1990). This concept describes the physics of bond rupture induced by an externally assisted pulling force. One of the major results of these theories is that it provides an expression for the mean rupture force required to break the bond as a function of the applied pulling force. The predicted logarithmic increase in the rupture force with the rate of pulling has indeed been frequently observed for different binding molecular systems (Evans, 2001, Hanley, et al., 2003, Noy, 2008, Sulchek, et al., 2005).

Applications in virology are still scarce. To date, measurements and quantitative analysis of single virus-receptor interactions have been carried out only for the HIV virus and the human Rhinovirus (HRV). Not only was the single binding interaction of the HIV-1 gp120 viral protein with its co-receptor CD4, CCR5 and CXCR4 at the surface of the cell studied in detail, but also the dynamics at the initial state of fusion as well as its inhibition (Chang, et al., 2005, Dobrowsky, et al., 2008). Their results showed that maximal bond strengths within the binding pocket gp120-CD4 were about 26 pN at pulling rates of 200 pN/s, and increased to 35 pN for pulling rates of 500 pN/second. The bond had a lifetime of 0.27 seconds with an interaction length of 0.34 nm. After 0.3 seconds a decrease in tensile strength was observed which indicates a subsequent weakening of the bond. This destabilization of the bond was attributed to a conformational change that gp120 experiences when binding to the CCR5 receptor immediately before fusion. The free energy of the initial gp120-CD4 bond formation was 6.7 k_BT. It decreased to 3.9 k_BT during the destabilization phase to later increase to 7.6 k_BT after anchoring to CCR5. The use of molecules that could block fusion, but that do not interfere with the binding interaction between CD4 and CCR5, suggested that the apparent weakening of the initial bond between gp120 and CD4 was likely related to a conformational transition of the gp120-CD4 bond toward binding to CCR5.

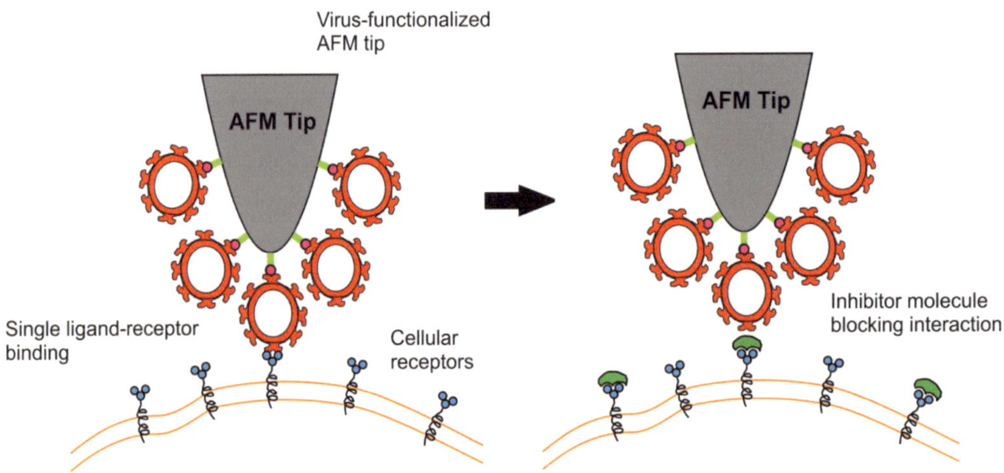

Fig. 8. Scheme of single virus-receptor binding measurements. Left: Specific binding between a virus epitope and a receptor. Right: An inhibitor molecule is used to block the interaction.

Hinterdorfer and coworkers have studied the binding of single human Rhino viruses to its lipoprotein (LDLR) receptor at the cell surface (Hinterdorfer, et al., 2008, Kienberger, et al., 2010). The viral particles were probed against receptor functionalized surfaces and living cells. Their applied protocol for virus attachment to the AFM tip resulted in a densely packed homogeneous monolayer of virions covering the tip and cantilever surface. They observed a time-dependent bond strength reinforcement as a result of consecutive binding of receptor molecules. Forces of about 82 pN were necessary for a single HRV-LDLR unbinding event; however analysis of multimodal force spectra showed peaks at 149, 203 and 273 pN for contact times of 31 milliseconds. It was thus determined that HRV can bind to up to 4 bonds at the initial state of attachment. In both studies the results are interpreted assuming that only one single viral particle being attached at the apex of the AFM tip interacted with the receptors. The pioneering work of these two groups undoubtedly has demonstrated that force spectroscopy is a rather useful tool for virology as it provides insight into the initial steps of virus binding and entry uncovering the mechanics of recognition, and entry in a time resolved fashion. This technique could also help to reveal details of the more intricate multistep binding processes that some other viruses undertake during cell entry. An interesting system worth of studying would be that of rotavirus or Herpex simplex virus A. It is known that these two viruses have to bind to more than two receptors before entry, however the details of binding leading finally to virus entry are far from being understood (Lopez & Arias, 2004, Lycke, et al., 1991). Research into this perspective direction has just started. Understanding the first steps of virus entry may be of considerable importance for development of novel antiviral drugs. Nanomedicine, for example, promises to develop precise and flexible methods of pathogen detection against emerging and fast spreading diseases. Biosensors based on single molecule technologies could offer alternative solutions to tackle future challenges. Progress in the selective immobilization of molecular targets allows for the fabrication of micro- and nano-patterned surfaces. This may eventually lead to the fabrication of biosensor platforms, which are expected to magnify the capabilities of force spectroscopy toward the implementation of ultrasensitive virus assays (Donath, 2009).

6. Viral mechanics and the infection cycle

Understanding the material properties of viruses and capsids and their changes at various stages of their infection cycle could establish a link between structure and function. An outstanding review regarding mechanical properties of viral capsids and their biological implications has been given by W.H. Roos et al. (Roos, et al., 2007). Research into this exciting direction is still in its beginnings. It was shown that the retroviruses MLV and HIV switch from a stiff to a soft structure during maturation. This may have a direct impact on infectivity (Kol, et al., 2006, Kol, et al., 2007). A stiffer particle could probably facilitate engulfment of the capsid by the bilayer during budding. On the contrary, a softer particle would be able to tolerate deformation facilitating penetration during cell entry. The DNA-anisotropic mechanical reinforcement observed in the MVM (Carrasco, et al., 2006), lead to the proposition that the lower rigidity measured at the fivefold axes where the capsid pores are located, could possibly have an adaptive biological role useful for posterior infectivity. The exceptional mechanical stability found for the HSV-1 virus might be a key factor for the survival during transport over long distances of the axonal cytoplasm where is exposed to mechanical stresses by molecular motors before it reaches its final point for cargo release (Liashkovich, et al., 2008). The reported mechanical stability and self-healing mechanism in Norovirus capsids (Cuellar, et al., 2010) with regard to drastic changes in pH may be an essential requirement for infection. To succeed as a pathogen the capsid has to survive the highly acidic pH in the stomach and become infectious under the weakly basic conditions within the ileum. The measured softening and loss of stability of the capsid at higher pH values could have a direct relation to the virus entry and RNA release. In the case of phages nanoindentation experiments have shown that the mechanical support, provided by the internal highly packed genome to the whole particle, contributes to their survival to shear stresses experienced by the capsid during adhesion to the surface of bacteria. Phages as well as probably other viruses have been optimized by nature for maximum capacity of storage limited only by the mechanical strength of the shell (Roos, et al., 2007, Roos & Wuite, 2009).

7. Acknowledgment

Own work presented in this chapter was supported by a grant from the Deutsche Forschungsgemeinschaft (DFG) DO 410/4-1. L. Cuellar was a fellow of CONACYT, Mexican Council of Science.

8. References

Ahadi, A., Colomo, J. & Evilevitch, A. (2009). Three-Dimensional Simulation of Nanoindentation Response of Viral Capsids. Shape and Size Effects. *Journal of Physical Chemistry B*, Vol. 113, No. 11, (Mar 19), pp. 3370-3378, ISSN 1520-6106.

Allen, S., Chen, X. Y., Davies, J., Davies, M. C., Dawkes, A. C., Edwards, J. C., Roberts, C. J., Sefton, J., Tendler, S. J. B. & Williams, P. M. (1997). Detection of Antigen-Antibody Binding Events with the Atomic Force Microscope. *Biochemistry*, Vol. 36, No. 24, (Jun 17), pp. 7457-7463, ISSN 0006-2960.

Arkhipov, A., Roos, W. H., Wuite, G. J. L. & Schulten, K. (2009). Elucidating the Mechanism Behind Irreversible Deformation of Viral Capsids. *Biophysical Journal*, Vol. 97, No. 7, (Oct 7), pp. 2061-2069, ISSN 0006-3495.

Awizio, A. K., Onofri, F., Benfenati, F. & Bonaccurso, E. (2007). Influence of Synapsin I on Synaptic Vesicles: An Analysis by Force-Volume Mode of the Atomic Force Microscope and Dynamic Light Scattering. *Biophysical Journal*, Vol. 93, No. 3, (Aug), pp. 1051-1060, ISSN 0006-3495.

Baker, T. S., Olson, N. H. & Fuller, S. D. (1999). Adding the Third Dimension to Virus Life Cycles: Three-Dimensional Reconstruction of Icosahedral Viruses from Cryo-Electron Micrographs. *Microbiology and Molecular Biology Reviews*, Vol. 63, No. 4, (Dec), pp. 862-922, ISSN 1092-2172.

Bancroft, J. B., Hills, G. J. & Markham, R. (1967). A Study of Self-Assembly Process in a Small Spherical Virus - Formation of Organized Structures from Protein Subunits in Vitro. *Virology*, Vol. 31, No. 2, pp. 354-379, ISSN 0042-6822.

Banin, U., Ebenstein, Y. & Nahum, E. (2002). Tapping Mode Atomic Force Microscopy for Nanoparticle Sizing: Tip-Sample Interaction Effects. *Nano Letters*, Vol. 2, No. 9, (Sep), pp. 945-950, ISSN 1530-6984.

Bhushan, B. editor. *Springer Handbook of Nanotechnology, 39. Mechanics of Biological Nanotechnology*. Springer, 2007, p. 1199 - 1222.

Browning-Kelley, M., E., Wadu-Mesthrige, K., Hari, V. & Liu, G. Y. (1997). Atomic Force Microscopic Study of Specific Antigen/Antibody Binding. *Langmuir*, Vol. 13, No. 2, pp. 343–350, ISSN 0743-7463.

Buenemann, M. & Lenz, P. (2008). Elastic Properties and Mechanical Stability of Chiral and Filled Viral Capsids. *Physical Review E*, Vol. 78, No. 5, (Nov), pp. 051924, ISSN 1539-3755.

Capella, B. & Dietler, G. (1999). Force-Distance Curves by Atomic Force Microscopy. *Surface Science Reports*, Vol. 34, No. 1, pp. 1-104, ISSN 0167-5729.

Carrasco, C., Carreira, A., Schaap, I. A. T., Serena, P. A., Gomez-Herrero, J., Mateu, M. G. & Pablo, P. J. (2006). DNA-Mediated Anisotropic Mechanical Reinforcement of a Virus. *Proceedings of the National Academy of Sciences of the United States of America*, Vol. 103, No. 37, (Sep 12), pp. 13706-13711, ISSN 0027-8424.

Carrasco, C., Castellanos, M., de Pablo, P. J. & Mateu, M. G. (2008). Manipulation of the Mechanical Properties of a Virus by Protein Engineering. *Proceedings of the National Academy of Sciences of the United States of America*, Vol. 105, No. 11, (Mar 18), pp. 4150-4155, ISSN 0027-8424.

Caspar, D. L. D. & Klug, A. (1962). Physical Principles in Construction of Regular Viruses. *Cold Spring Harbor Symposia on Quantitative Biology*, Vol. 27, No. pp. 1-24, ISSN 0091-7451.

Chang, M. I., Panorchan, P., Dobrowsky, T. M., Tseng, Y. & Wirtz, D. (2005). Single-Molecule Analysis of Human Immunodeficiency Virus Type 1 Gp120-Receptor Interactions in Living Cells. *Journal of Virology*, Vol. 79, No. 23, (Dec), pp. 14748-14755, ISSN 0022-538X.

Crawford, S. E., Estes, M. K., Ciarlet, M., Barone, C., O'Neal, C. M., Cohen, J. & Conner, M. E. (1999). Heterotypic Protection and Induction of a Broad Heterotypic Neutralization Response by Rotavirus-Like Particles. *Journal of Virology*, Vol. 73, No. 6, (Jun), pp. 4813-4822, ISSN 0022-538X.

Cuellar, J. L., Fischlechner, M., Koehler, G., Uxa, L. & Donath, E. Mechanical Properties of Rubella-Like Particles: Modulation of the Capsid Elasticity by the Envelope. University of Leipzig, Institute of Medical Physics and Biophysics, 2012, unpublished.

Cuellar, J. L., Meinhoevel, F., Hoehne, M. & Donath, E. (2010). Size and Mechanical Stability of Norovirus Capsids Depend on Ph: A Nanoindentation Study. *Journal of General Virology*, Vol. 91, No. (Oct), pp. 2449-2456, ISSN 0022-1317.

Delorme, N., Dubois, M., Garnier, S., Laschewsky, A., Weinkamer, R., Zemb, T. & Fery, A. (2006). Surface Immobilization and Mechanical Properties of Catanionic Hollow Faceted Polyhedrons. *Journal of Physical Chemistry B*, Vol. 110, No. 4, (Feb 2), pp. 1752-1758, ISSN 1520-6106.

Dobrowsky, T. M., Zhou, Y., Sun, S. X., Siliciano, R. F. & Wirtz, D. (2008). Monitoring Early Fusion Dynamics of Human Immunodeficiency Virus Type 1 at Single-Molecule Resolution. *Journal of Virology*, Vol. 82, No. 14, (Jul), pp. 7022-7033, ISSN 0022-538X.

Donath, E. (2009). Biosensors Viruses for Ultrasensitive Assays. *Nature Nanotechnology*, Vol. 4, No. 4, (Apr), pp. 215-216, ISSN 1748-3387.

Drygin, Y. F., Bordunova, O. A., Gallyamov, M. O. & Yaminsky, I. V. (1998). Atomic Force Microscopy Examination of Tobacco Mosaic Virus and Virion Rna. *FEBS Letters*, Vol. 425, No. 2, (Mar 27), pp. 217-221, ISSN 0014-5793.

Dufrene, Y. F., Boland, T., Schneider, J. W., Barger, W. R. & Lee, G. U. (1998). Characterization of the Physical Properties of Model Biomembranes at the Nanometer Scale with the Atomic Force Microscope. *Faraday Discussions*, Vol. 111, No. pp. 79-94, ISSN 0301-7249.

Ernst, W., Grabherr, R., Wegner, D., Borth, N., Grassauer, A. & Katinger, H. (1998). Baculovirus Surface Display: Construction and Screening of a Eukaryotic Epitope Library. *Nucleic Acids Research*, Vol. 26, No. 7, (Apr 1), pp. 1718-1723, ISSN 0305-1048.

Evans, E. (2001). Probing the Relation between Force—Lifetime—and Chemistry in Single Molecular Bonds. *Annual Review of Biophysics and Biomolecular Structure*, Vol. 30, No. pp. 105-128, ISSN 1056-8700.

Fischlechner, M. & Donath, E. (2007). Viruses as Building Blocks for Materials and Devices. *Angewandte Chemie-International Edition*, Vol. 46, No. 18, pp. 3184-3193, ISSN 1433-7851.

Fischlechner, M., Reibetanz, U., Zaulig, M., Enderlein, D., Romanova, J., Leporatti, S., Moya, S. & Donath, E. (2007). Fusion of Enveloped Virus Nanoparticles with Polyelectrolyte-Supported Lipid Membranes for the Design of Bio/Nonbio Interfaces. *Nano Letters*, Vol. 7, No. 11, (Nov), pp. 3540-3546, ISSN 1530-6984.

Fischlechner, M., Toellner, L., Messner, P., Grabherr, R. & Donath, E. (2006). Virus-Engineered Colloidal Particles - a Surface Display System. *Angewandte Chemie-International Edition*, Vol. 45, No. 5, pp. 784-789, ISSN 1433-7851.

Florin, E. L., Moy, V. T. & Gaub, H. E. (1994). Adhesion Forces between Individual Ligand-Receptor Pairs. *Science*, Vol. 264, No. 5157, (Apr 15), pp. 415-417, ISSN 0036-8075.

Fraenkel-Conrat, H. & Williams, R. C. (1955). Reconstitution of Active Tobacco Mosaic Virus from Its Inactive Protein and Nucleic Acid Components. *Proceedings of the National Academy of Sciences of the United States of America*, Vol. 41, No. 10, pp. 690–698, ISSN 0027-8424.

Garcia, R. A., Laney, D. E., Parsons, S. M. & Hansma, H. G. (1998). Substructure and Responses of Cholinergic Synaptic Vesicles in the Atomic Force Microscope. *Journal of Neuroscience Research*, Vol. 52, No. 3, (May 1), pp. 350-355, ISSN 0360-4012.

Gibbons, M. M. & Klug, W. S. (2007). Nonlinear Finite-Element Analysis of Nanoindentation of Viral Capsids. *Physical Review E*, Vol. 75, No. 3, (Mar), pp. 031901, ISSN 1539-3755.

Graff, A., Sauer, M., Van Gelder, P. & Meier, W. (2002). Virus-Assisted Loading of Polymer Nanocontainer. *Proceedings of the National Academy of Sciences of the United States of America*, Vol. 99, No. 8, (Apr 16), pp. 5064-5068, ISSN 0027-8424.

Grandbois, M., Beyer, M., Rief, M., Clausen-Schaumann, H. & Gaub, H. E. (1999). How Strong Is a Covalent Bond? *Science*, Vol. 283, No. 5408, (Mar 12), pp. 1727-1730, ISSN 0036-8075.

Gunning, A. P., Chambers, S., Pin, C., Man, A. L., Morris, V. J. & Nicoletti, C. (2008). Mapping Specific Adhesive Interactions on Living Human Intestinal Epithelial Cells with Atomic Force Microscopy. *FASEB Journal*, Vol. 22, No. 7, (Jul), pp. 2331-2339, ISSN 0892-6638.

Hanley, W., McCarty, O., Jadhav, S., Tseng, Y., Wirtz, D. & Konstantopoulos, K. (2003). Single Molecule Characterization of P-Selectin/Ligand Binding. *Journal of Biological Chemistry*, Vol. 278, No. 12, (Mar 21), pp. 10556-10561, ISSN 0021-9258.

Helfer, E., Harlepp, S., Bourdieu, L., Robert, J., MacKintosh, F. C. & Chatenay, D. (2001). Buckling of Actin-Coated Membranes under Application of a Local Force. *Physical Review Letters*, Vol. 87, No. 8, (Aug 20), 0031-9007.

Hertz, H. (1882). Ueber Die Berührung Fester Elastischer Körper. *Journal für die Reine und Angewandte Mathematik*, Vol. 92, No. pp. 156-171.

Hinterdorfer, P., Baumgartner, W., Gruber, H. J., Schilcher, K. & Schindler, H. (1996). Detection and Localization of Individual Antibody-Antigen Recognition Events by Atomic Force Microscopy. *Proceedings of the National Academy of Sciences of the United States of America*, Vol. 93, No. 8, (Apr 16), pp. 3477-3481, ISSN 0027-8424.

Hinterdorfer, P., Kienberger, F., Zhu, R., Moser, R. & Blaas, D. (2004). Monitoring Rna Release from Human Rhinovirus by Dynamic Force Microscopy. *Journal of Virology*, Vol. 78, No. 7, (Apr), pp. 3203-3209, ISSN 0022-538X.

Hinterdorfer, P., Rankl, C., Kienberger, F., Wildling, L., Wruss, J., Gruber, H. J. & Blaas, D. (2008). Multiple Receptors Involved in Human Rhinovirus Attachment to Live Cells. *Proceedings of the National Academy of Sciences of the United States of America*, Vol. 105, No. 46, (Nov 18), pp. 17778-17783, ISSN 0027-8424.

Horton, M., Charras, G. & Lehenkari, P. (2002). Analysis of Ligand-Receptor Interactions in Cells by Atomic Force Microscopy. *Journal of Receptor and Signal Transduction Research*, Vol. 22, No. 1-4, (Feb-Nov), pp. 169-190, 1079-9893.

Howorka, S., Pollheimer, P. D., Kastner, M., Ebner, A., Blaas, D., Hinterdorfer, P. & Gruber, H. J. (2009). Receptor Arrays for the Selective and Efficient Capturing of Viral Particles. *Bioconjugate Chemistry*, Vol. 20, No. 3, (Mar), pp. 466-475, ISSN 1043-1802.

Hugel, T., Grosholz, M., Clausen-Schaumann, H., Pfau, A., Gaub, H. & Seitz, M. (2001). Elasticity of Single Polyelectrolyte Chains and Their Desorption from Solid Supports Studied by Afm Based Single Molecule Force Spectroscopy. *Macromolecules*, Vol. 34, No. 4, (Feb 13), pp. 1039-1047, 0024-9297.

Hugel, T. & Seitz, M. (2001). The Study of Molecular Interactions by Afm Force Spectroscopy. *Macromolecular Rapid Communications*, Vol. 22, No. 13, (Sep 18), pp. 989-1016, ISSN 1022-1336.

Ivanovska, I., Carrascosa, J., Schmidt, C. & Wuite, G. (2004). Breaking Viral Shells: A Scanning Force Microscopy Study of the Mechanical Properties of Empty and Full Bacteriophage Capsids. *Biophysical Journal*, Vol. 86, No. 1, (Jan), pp. 478a-478a, ISSN 0006-3495.

Jin, A. J. & Nossal, R. (2008). Mechanical Rigidity of Clathrin Triskelions, Cages and Coated Vesicles. *Biorheology*, Vol. 45, No. 1-2, pp. 92-93, ISSN 0006-355X.

Jin, A. J., Prasad, K., Smith, P. D., Lafer, E. M. & Nossal, R. (2006). Measuring the Elasticity of Clathrin-Coated Vesicles Via Atomic Force Microscopy. *Biophysical Journal*, Vol. 90, No. 9, (May), pp. 3333-3344, ISSN 0006-3495.

Kasas, S. & Dietler, G. (2008). Probing Nanomechanical Properties from Biomolecules to Living Cells. *Pflugers Archiv-European Journal of Physiology*, Vol. 456, No. 1, (Apr), pp. 13-27, ISSN 0031-6768.

Kienberger, F., Zhu, R., Rankl, C., Gruber, H. J., Blaas, D. & Hinterdorfer, P. (2010). Atomic Force Microscopy Studies of Human Rhinovirus: Topology and Molecular Forces. *Methods in Enzymology, Vol 475: Single Molecule Tools, Pt B*, Vol. 474, No. pp. 515-539, ISSN 0076-6879.

Klug, W. S., Bruinsma, R. F., Michel, J. P., Knobler, C. M., Ivanovska, I. L., Schmidt, C. F. & Wuite, G. J. L. (2006). Failure of Viral Shells. *Physical Review Letters*, Vol. 97, No. 22, (Dec 1), pp. 228101, ISSN 0031-9007.

Knobler, C. M., Michel, J. P., Ivanovska, I. L., Gibbons, M. M., Klug, W. S., Wuite, G. J. L. & Schmidt, C. F. (2006). Nanoindentation Studies of Full and Empty Viral Capsids and the Effects of Capsid Protein Mutations on Elasticity and Strength. *Proceedings of the National Academy of Sciences of the United States of America*, Vol. 103, No. 16, (Apr 18), pp. 6184-6189, ISSN 0027-8424.

Kol, N., Gladnikoff, M., Barlam, D., Shneck, R. Z., Rein, A. & Rousso, I. (2006). Mechanical Properties of Murine Leukemia Virus Particles: Effect of Maturation. *Biophysical Journal*, Vol. 91, No. 2, (Jul 15), pp. 767-774, ISSN 0006-3495.

Kol, N., Shi, Y., Tsvitov, M., Barlam, D., Shneck, R. Z., Kay, M. S. & Rousso, I. (2007). A Stiffness Switch in Human Immunodeficiency Virus. *Biophysical Journal*, Vol. 92, No. 5, (Mar 1), pp. 1777-1783, ISSN 0006-3495.

Kost, T. A. & Condreay, J. P. (1999). Recombinant Baculoviruses as Expression Vectors for Insect and Mammalian Cells. *Current Opinion in Biotechnology*, Vol. 10, No. 5, (Oct), pp. 428-433, ISSN 0958-1669.

Kost, T. A., Condreay, J. P. & Jarvis, D. L. (2005). Baculovirus as Versatile Vectors for Protein Expression in Insect and Mammalian Cells. *Nature Biotechnology*, Vol. 23, No. 5, (May), pp. 567-575, 1087-0156.

Kuznetsov, Y. G., Malkin, A. J., Lucas, R. W., Plomp, M. & McPherson, A. (2001). Imaging of Viruses by Atomic Force Microscopy. *Journal of General Virology*, Vol. 82, No. (Sep), pp. 2025-2034, 0022-1317.

Kuznetsov, Y. G., Victoria, J. G., Low, A., Robinson, W. E., Fan, H. & McPherson, A. (2004). Atomic Force Microscopy Imaging of Retroviruses: Human Immunodeficiency Virus and Murine Leukemia. *Scanning*, Vol. 26, No. 5, (Sep-Oct), pp. 209-216, ISSN 0161-0457.

Labhasetwar, V. & Vasir, J. K. (2008). Quantification of the Force of Nanoparticle-Cell Membrane Interactions and Its Influence on Intracellular Trafficking of Nanoparticles. *Biomaterials*, Vol. 29, No. 31, (Nov), pp. 4244-4252, ISSN 0142-9612.

Landau, L. D. & Lifshitz, E. M. *Theory of Elasticity*. Oxford: Butterworth - Heinemann, 1986.

Laney, D. E., Garcia, R. A., Parsons, S. M. & Hansma, H. G. (1997). Changes in the Elastic Properties of Cholinergic Synaptic Vesicles as Measured by Atomic Force Microscopy. *Biophysical Journal*, Vol. 72, No. 2, (Feb), pp. 806-813, ISSN 0006-3495.

Le Grimellec, C., Giocondi, M. C., Ronzon, F., Nicolai, M. C., Dosset, P., Milhiet, P. E. & Chevalier, M. (2010). Organization of Influenza a Virus Envelope at Neutral and Low Ph. *Journal of General Virology*, Vol. 91, No. (Feb), pp. 329-338, ISSN 0022-1317.

Lee, J. W. M. & Ng, M. L. (2004). A Nano-View of West Nile Virus-Induced Cellular Changes During Infection. *Journal of Nanobiotechnology*, Vol. 2, No. 6.

Lee, S. W., Lee, S. K. & Belcher, A. M. (2003). Virus-Based Alignment of Inorganic, Organic, and Biological Nanosized Materials. *Advanced Materials*, Vol. 15, No. 9, (May 2), pp. 689-692, ISSN 0935-9648.

Liang, X. M., Mao, G. Z. & Ng, K. Y. S. (2004). Probing Small Unilamellar Eggpc Vesicles on Mica Surface by Atomic Force Microscopy. *Colloids and Surfaces B-Biointerfaces*, Vol. 34, No. 1, (Mar 1), pp. 41-51, 0927-7765.

Liashkovich, I., Hafezi, W., Kuhn, J. E., Oberleithner, H., Kramer, A. & Shahin, V. (2008). Exceptional Mechanical and Structural Stability of Hsv-1 Unveiled with Fluid Atomic Force Microscopy. *Journal of Cell Science*, Vol. 121, No. 14, (Jul 15), pp. 2287-2292, ISSN 0021-9533.

Lidmar, J., Mirny, L. & Nelson, D. R. (2003). Virus Shapes and Buckling Transitions in Spherical Shells. *Physical Review E*, Vol. 68, No. 5, (Nov), pp. 051910, ISSN 1539-3755.

Loi, S., Sun, G., Franz, V. & Butt, H. J. (2002). Rupture of Molecular Thin Films Observed in Atomic Force Microscopy. Ii. Experiment. *Physical Review E*, Vol. 66, No. 3, (Sep), pp. 031602, ISSN 1539-3755.

Lopez, S. & Arias, C. F. (2004). Multistep Entry of Rotavirus into Cells: A Versaillesque Dance. *Trends in Microbiology*, Vol. 12, No. 6, (Jun), pp. 271-278, ISSN 0966-842X.

Lycke, E., Johansson, M., Svennerholm, B. & Lindahl, U. (1991). Binding of Herpes-Simplex Virus to Cellular Heparan-Sulfate, an Initial Step in the Adsorption Process. *Journal of General Virology*, Vol. 72, No. (May), pp. 1131-1137, ISSN 0022-1317.

Malkin, A. J., Plomp, M. & McPherson, A. (2002). Application of Atomic Force Microscopy to Studies of Surface Processes in Virus Crystallization and Structural Biology. *Acta*

Crystallographica Section D-Biological Crystallography, Vol. 58, No. (Oct), pp. 1617-1621, ISSN 0907-4449.

Malkin, A. J., Plomp, M., Rice, M. K., Wagner, E. K. & McPherson, A. (2002). Rapid Visualization at High Resolution of Pathogens by Atomic Force Microscopy - Structural Studies of Herpes Simplex Virus-1. *American Journal of Pathology*, Vol. 160, No. 6, (Jun), pp. 1959-1966, ISSN 0002-9440.

McDonnell, L., Moloney, M. & O'Shea, H. (2002). Immobilisation of Semliki Forest Virus for Atomic Force Microscopy. *Ultramicroscopy*, Vol. 91, No. 1-4, (May), pp. 275-279, ISSN 0304-3991.

McPherson, A., Kumetsov, Y. & Gershon, P. D. (2008). Atomic Force Microscopy Investigation of Vaccinia Virus Structure. *Journal of Virology*, Vol. 82, No. 15, (Aug), pp. 7551-7566, ISSN 0022-538X.

McPherson, A., Kuznetsov, Y. G., Low, A. & Fan, H. (2004). Atomic Force Microscopy Investigation of Wild-Type Moloney Murine Leukemia Virus Particles and Virus Particles Lacking the Envelope Protein. *Virology*, Vol. 323, No. 2, (Jun 1), pp. 189-196, ISSN 0042-6822.

McPherson, A., Kuznetsov, Y. G., Low, A. & Fan, H. (2005). Atomic Force Microscopy Investigation of Isolated Virions of Murine Leukemia Virus. *Journal of Virology*, Vol. 79, No. 3, (Feb), pp. 1970-1974, ISSN 0022-538X.

McPherson, A., Kuznetsov, Y. G., Malkin, A. & Plomp, M. (2003). Macromolecular Crystal Growth as Revealed by Atomic Force Microscopy. *Journal of Structural Biology*, Vol. 142, No. 1, (Apr), pp. 32-46, ISSN 1047-8477.

McPherson, A., Kuznetsov, Y. G., Victoria, J. G., Low, A., Robinson, W. E. & Fan, H. (2004). Atomic Force Microscopy Imaging of Retroviruses: Human Immunodeficiency Virus and Murine Leukemia. *Scanning*, Vol. 26, No. 5, (Sep-Oct), pp. 209-216, ISSN 0161-0457.

McPherson, A., Kuznetsov, Y. G., Victoria, J. G. & Robinson, W. E. (2003). Atomic Force Microscopy Investigation of Human Immunodeficiency Virus (Hiv) and Hiv-Infected Lymphocytes. *Journal of Virology*, Vol. 77, No. 22, (Nov), pp. 11896-11909, ISSN 0022-538X.

Moller, C., Allen, M., V, E., Engel, A. & Muller, D. J. (1999). Tapping-Mode Atomic Force Microscopy Produces Faithful High-Resolution Images of Protein Surfaces. *Biophysical Journal*, Vol. 77, No. 2, (Aug), pp. 1150-1158, ISSN 0006-3495.

Moy, V. T., Florin, E. L. & Gaub, H. E. (1994). Intermolecular Forces and Energies between Ligands and Receptors. *Science*, Vol. 266, No. 5183, (Oct 14), pp. 257-259, ISSN 0036-8075.

Nam, K. T., Kim, D. W., Yoo, P. J., Chiang, C. Y., Meethong, N., Hammond, P. T., Chiang, Y. M. & Belcher, A. M. (2006). Virus-Enabled Synthesis and Assembly of Nanowires for Lithium Ion Battery Electrodes. *Science*, Vol. 312, No. 5775, (May 12), pp. 885-888, ISSN 0036-8075.

Ng, M. L., Lee, J. W. M., Leong, M. L. N., Ling, A. E., Tan, H. C. & Ooi, E. E. (2004). Topographic Changes in Sars Coronavirus-Infected Cells During Late Stages of Infection. *Emerging Infectious Diseases*, Vol. 10, No. 11, (Nov), pp. 1907-1914, ISSN 1080-6040.

Nicollier-Jamot, A., Ogier, A., Piroth, L., Pothier, P. & Kohli, E. (2004). Recombinant Virus-Like Particles of a Norovirus (Genogroup Ii Strain) Administered Intranasally and

Orally with Mucosal Adjuvants Lt and Lt(R192g) in Balb/C Mice Induce Specific Humoral and Cellular Th1/Th2-Like Immune Responses. *Vaccine*, Vol. 22, No. 9-10, (Mar 12), pp. 1079-1086, ISSN 0264-410X.

Norouzi, D., Muller, M. M. & Deserno, M. (2006). How to Determine Local Elastic Properties of Lipid Bilayer Membranes from Atomic-Force-Microscope Measurements: A Theoretical Analysis. *Physical Review E*, Vol. 74, No. 6, (Dec), pp. 061914, ISSN 1539-3755.

Noy, A. (2008). Strength in Numbers: Probing and Understanding Intermolecular Bonding with Chemical Force Microscopy. *Scanning*, Vol. 30, No. 2, (Mar-Apr), pp. 96-105, ISSN 0161-0457.

Ohnesorge, F. M., Horber, J. K. H., Haberle, W., Czerny, C. P., Smith, D. P. E. & Binnig, G. (1997). Afm Review Study on Pox Viruses and Living Cells. *Biophysical Journal*, Vol. 73, No. 4, (Oct), pp. 2183-2194, ISSN 0006-3495.

Pablo, P. J., Carrasco, C., Carreira, A., Schaap, I. A. T., Serena, P. A., Gomez-Herrero, J. & Mateu, M. G. (2006). DNA-Mediated Anisotropic Mechanical Reinforcement of a Virus. *Proceedings of the National Academy of Sciences of the United States of America*, Vol. 103, No. 37, (Sep 12), pp. 13706-13711, ISSN 0027-8424.

Pera, I., Stark, R., Kappl, M., Butt, H. J. & Benfenati, F. (2004). Using the Atomic Force Microscope to Study the Interaction between Two Solid Supported Lipid Bilayers and the Influence of Synapsin I. *Biophysical Journal*, Vol. 87, No. 4, (Oct), pp. 2446-2455, ISSN 0006-3495.

Radmacher, M., Fritz, M. & Hansma, P. K. (1995). Imaging Soft Samples with the Atomic-Force Microscope - Gelatin in Water and Propanol. *Biophysical Journal*, Vol. 69, No. 1, (Jul), pp. 264-270, ISSN 0006-3495.

Reissner, E. (1952). Stress Strain Relations in the Theory of Thin Elastic Shells. *Journal of Mathematics and Physics*, Vol. 31, No. 2, pp. 109-119, ISSN 0097-1421.

Richter, R. P. & Brisson, A. (2003). Characterization of Lipid Bilayers and Protein Assemblies Supported on Rough Surfaces by Atomic Force Microscopy. *Langmuir*, Vol. 19, No. 5, (Mar 4), pp. 1632-1640, ISSN 0743-7463.

Riener, C. K., Kienberger, F., Hahn, C. D., Buchinger, G. M., Egwim, I. O. C., Haselgrubler, T., Ebner, A., Romanin, C., Klampfl, C., Lackner, B., Prinz, H., Blaas, D., Hinterdorfer, P. & Gruber, H. J. (2003). Heterobifunctional Crosslinkers for Tethering Single Ligand Molecules to Scanning Probes. *Analytica Chimica Acta*, Vol. 497, No. 1-2, (Nov 14), pp. 101-114, ISSN 0003-2670.

Risco, C., Carrascosa, J. L. & Frey, T. K. (2003). Structural Maturation of Rubella Virus in the Golgi Complex. *Virology*, Vol. 312, No. 2, (Aug 1), pp. 261-269, ISSN 0042-6822.

Roos, W. H., Bruinsma, R. & Wuite, G. J. L. (2010). Physical Virology. *Nature Physics*, Vol. 6, No. 10, (Oct), pp. 733-743, ISSN 1745-2473.

Roos, W. H., Gibbons, M. M., Arkhipov, A., Uetrecht, C., Watts, N. R., Wingfield, P. T., Steven, A. C., Heck, A. J. R., Schulten, K., Klug, W. S. & Wuite, G. J. L. (2010). Squeezing Protein Shells: How Continuum Elastic Models, Molecular Dynamics Simulations, and Experiments Coalesce at the Nanoscale. *Biophysical Journal*, Vol. 99, No. 4, (Aug 18), pp. 1175-1181, ISSN 0006-3495.

Roos, W. H., Ivanovska, I. L., Evilevitch, A. & Wuite, G. J. L. (2007). Viral Capsids: Mechanical Characteristics, Genome Packaging and Delivery Mechanisms. *Cellular and Molecular Life Sciences*, Vol. 64, No. 12, (Jun), pp. 1484-1497, ISSN 1420-682X.

Roos, W. H., Radtke, K., Kniesmeijer, E., Geertsema, H., Sodeik, B. & Wuite, G. J. L. (2009). Scaffold Expulsion and Genome Packaging Trigger Stabilization of Herpes Simplex Virus Capsids. *Proceedings of the National Academy of Sciences of the United States of America*, Vol. 106, No. 24, (Jun 16), pp. 9673-9678, ISSN 0027-8424.

Roos, W. H. & Wuite, G. L. (2009). Nanoindentation Studies Reveal Material Properties of Viruses. *Advanced Materials*, Vol. 21, No. 10-11, (Mar 20), pp. 1187-1192, 0935-9648.

Rousso, I. & Gladnikoff, M. (2008). Directly Monitoring Individual Retrovirus Budding Events Using Atomic Force Microscopy. *Biophysical Journal*, Vol. 94, No. 1, (Jan 1), pp. 320-326, ISSN 0006-3495.

Rousso, I., Gladnikoff, M., Shimoni, E. & Gov, N. S. (2009). Retroviral Assembly and Budding Occur through an Actin-Driven Mechanism. *Biophysical Journal*, Vol. 97, No. 9, (Nov 4), pp. 2419-2428, ISSN 0006-3495.

Schiller, J. T. & Lowy, D. R. (2001). Papillomavirus-Like Particle Based Vaccines: Cervical Cancer and Beyond. *Expert Opinion on Biological Therapy*, Vol. 1, No. 4, (Jul), pp. 571-581, 1471-2598.

Siber, A. (2006). Buckling Transition in Icosahedral Shells Subjected to Volume Conservation Constraint and Pressure: Relations to Virus Maturation. *Physical Review E*, Vol. 73, No. 6, (Jun), ISSN 1539-3755.

Siber, A. & Podgornik, R. (2009). Stability of Elastic Icosadeltahedral Shells under Uniform External Pressure: Application to Viruses under Osmotic Pressure. *Physical Review E*, Vol. 79, No. 1, (Jan), ISSN 1539-3755.

Singh, P., Gonzalez, M. J. & Manchester, M. (2006). Viruses and Their Uses in Nanotechnology. *Drug Development Research*, Vol. 67, No. 1, (Jan), pp. 23-41, ISSN 0272-4391.

Skehel, J. J. & Wiley, D. C. (2000). Receptor Binding and Membrane Fusion in Virus Entry: The Influenza Hemagglutinin. *Annual Review of Biochemistry*, Vol. 69, No. pp. 531-569, ISSN 0066-4154.

Smith, D. E., Tans, S. J., Smith, S. B., Grimes, S., Anderson, D. L. & Bustamante, C. (2001). The Bacteriophage Phi 29 Portal Motor Can Package DNA against a Large Internal Force. *Nature*, Vol. 413, No. 6857, (Oct 18), pp. 748-752, 0028-0836.

Sodeik, B., Roos, W. H., Radtke, K., Kniesmeijer, E., Geertsema, H. & Wuite, G. J. L. (2009). Scaffold Expulsion and Genome Packaging Trigger Stabilization of Herpes Simplex Virus Capsids. *Proceedings of the National Academy of Sciences of the United States of America*, Vol. 106, No. 24, (Jun 16), pp. 9673-9678, ISSN 0027-8424.

Steltenkamp, S., Muller, M. M., Deserno, M., Hennesthal, C., Steinem, C. & Janshoff, A. (2006). Mechanical Properties of Pore-Spanning Lipid Bilayers Probed by Atomic Force Microscopy. *Biophysical Journal*, Vol. 91, No. 1, (Jul), pp. 217-226, ISSN 0006-3495.

Sulchek, T. A., Friddle, R. W., Langry, K., Lau, E. Y., Albrecht, H., Ratto, T. V., DeNardo, S. J., Colvin, M. E. & Noy, A. (2005). Dynamic Force Spectroscopy of Parallel Individual Mucin1-Antibody Bonds. *Proceedings of the National Academy of Sciences of the United States of America*, Vol. 102, No. 46, (Nov 15), pp. 16638-16643, ISSN 0027-8424.

Tamura, K., Komura, S. & Kato, T. (2004). Adhesion Induced Buckling of Spherical Shells. *Journal of Physics-Condensed Matter*, Vol. 16, No. 39, (Oct 6), pp. L421-L428, ISSN 0953-8984.

Twarock, R. (2006). Mathematical Virology: A Novel Approach to the Structure and Assembly of Viruses. *Philosophical Transactions of the Royal Society a-Mathematical Physical and Engineering Sciences*, Vol. 364, No. 1849, (Dec 15), pp. 3357-3373, ISSN 1364-503X.

Uchida, M., Klem, M. T., Allen, M., Suci, P., Flenniken, M., Gillitzer, E., Varpness, Z., Liepold, L. O., Young, M. & Douglas, T. (2007). Biological Containers: Protein Cages as Multifunctional Nanoplatforms. *Advanced Materials*, Vol. 19, No. 8, (Apr 20), pp. 1025-1042, ISSN 0935-9648.

Vliegenthart, G. A. & Gompper, G. (2007). Mechanical Properties of Icosahedral Virus Capsids. *Journal of Computer-Aided Materials Design*, Vol. 14, No. pp. 111-119, ISSN 0928-1045.

Vliegenthart, G. A. & Gompper, G. (2006). Mechanical Deformation of Spherical Viruses with Icosahedral Symmetry. *Biophysical Journal*, Vol. 91, No. 3, (Aug), pp. 834-841, ISSN 0006-3495.

Vriezema, D. M., Aragones, M. C., Elemans, J. A. A. W., Cornelissen, J. J. L. M., Rowan, A. E. & Nolte, R. J. M. (2005). Self-Assembled Nanoreactors. *Chemical Reviews*, Vol. 105, No. 4, (Apr), pp. 1445-1489, ISSN 0009-2665.

Warfield, K. L., Bosio, C. M., Welcher, B. C., Deal, E. M., Mohamadzadeh, M., Schmaljohn, A., Aman, M. J. & Bavari, S. (2003). Ebola Virus-Like Particles Protect from Lethal Ebola Virus Infection. *Proceedings of the National Academy of Sciences of the United States of America*, Vol. 100, No. 26, (Dec 23), pp. 15889-15894, ISSN 0027-8424.

White, L. J., Hardy, M. E. & Estes, H. K. (1997). Biochemical Characterization of a Smaller Form of Recombinant Norwalk Virus Capsids Assembled in Insect Cells. *Journal of Virology*, Vol. 71, No. 10, (Oct), pp. 8066-8072, ISSN 0022-538X.

Zandi, R. & Reguera, D. (2005). Mechanical Properties of Viral Capsids. *Physical Review E*, Vol. 72, No. 2, (Aug), 1539-3755.

Zandi, R., Reguera, D., Bruinsma, R. F., Gelbart, W. M. & Rudnick, J. (2004). Origin of Icosahedral Symmetry in Viruses. *Proceedings of the National Academy of Sciences of the United States of America*, Vol. 101, No. 44, (Nov 2), pp. 15556-15560, ISSN 0027-8424.

Zhao, Y., Mahajan, N., Long, S., Wang, Q. & Fang, J. (2006). Stability of Virus Nanoparticles on Substrates under Applied Load with Atomic Force Microscope. *Micro & Nano Letters*, Vol. 1, No. 1, (Jul), pp. 1-4, ISSN 1750-0443.

Zink, M. & Grubmuller, H. (2009). Mechanical Properties of the Icosahedral Shell of Southern Bean Mosaic Virus: A Molecular Dynamics Study. *Biophysical Journal*, Vol. 96, No. 4, (Feb 18), pp. 1350-1363, ISSN 0006-3495.

Part 5

Cellular Physiology

13

Single-Molecule Force Microscopy: A Potential Tool for the Mapping of Polysaccharides in Plant Cell Walls

Julian C. Thimm[1], Laurence D. Melton[2] and David J. Burritt[1]
[1]*The Department of Botany, The University of Otago, Dunedin*
[2]*Food Science Programmes, School of Chemistry Sciences, University of Auckland, Auckland*
New Zealand

1. Introduction

Plant cells are surrounded by a polysaccharide-rich cell wall that, as well as being a supporting structure (O'Neill & York, 2003), plays important roles in plant growth and development, and in the protection of plants from both biotic and abiotic stresses (Bowles, 1990). Plant cell walls are also of global economic importance, with the cell walls of food crops being of great nutritional value, while those of agricultural crops are important as a renewable resource for the textile and building industries, and increasingly as a sustainable source of fuel (O'Neill & York, 2003).

2. The plant cell wall

2.1 Plant cell wall structure

The primary plant cell wall is a three-dimensional assembly of the polysaccharides, cellulose, pectin and hemicelluloses together with water, minerals and some structural glycoproteins. Atomic force microscopy (AFM) of *Arabidopsis thaliana* leaf cell walls showed the cellulose exists as microfibrils (Davies & Harris, 2003). AFM of living celery parenchyma tissue showed the cellulose microfibrils exist in highly ordered parallel array (Thimm et al., 2000). While AFM on isolated cell walls from celery and cucumber hypocotyls that were kept hydrated showed the cellulose microfibrils were undulating in a roughly parallel manner (Thimm et al., 2009; Marga et al., 2005). Moreover, each cellulose microfibril is surrounded by matrix material (presumably pectin and hemicelluloses) that keeps the celluloses uniformly spaced apart (Marga et al., 2005; Thimm et al., 2000; Thimm et al., 2009). Small angle X-ray scattering of hydrated celery collenchyma cell walls also showed uniform spacing of cellulose microfibrils (Kennedy et al., 2007). Solid-state ^{13}C nuclear magnetic resonance spectroscopy (NMR) indicated that in mung bean hypocotyls less than 10% of the surface of cellulose microfibrils has xyloglucan adhering to it (Bootten et al., 2004) and a recent three-dimensional solid-state NMR study of *Arabidopsis thaliana* cell walls supported this finding and also showed somewhat more pectin than xyloglucan adhered to cellulose (Dick-Perez et al., 2011). Indeed, Zykwinska et al. (2007) have previously shown arabinan and galactan side chains of pectin are bound to cellulose. This leads to two possible models for the primary cell wall. In the first cellulose microfibrils are held apart at a uniform distance by a limited number of xyloglucan crosslinks that are reinforced by more indirect crosslinks via the pectin matrix (Bootten et al., 2004; O'Neill & York, 2003). It is pertinent to note that xyloglucan has been found covalently linked to pectin in cell walls (Popper & Fry, 2008). In the alternative model the cellulose micofibrils are embedded in a matrix of pectin and hemicelluloses some of which adhere strongly to the cellulose but others interact with those bound to cellulose and the interactions diminish with the distance from cellulose (Cosgrove, 2001; Talbott & Ray, 1992). In other words a layer of other cell wall polysaccharides, of decreasing density, surrounds each cellulose rod and there is no direct cross-linking between cellulose microfibrils.

However, it is important to note the structures of the primary plant cell walls detailed above are just models, developed from a wealth of information provided by studies that have conducted chemical analyses of isolated cell walls or independently imaged isolated, or more rarely intact cell walls (Thimm et al., 2009). Hence cell wall architecture and chemistry have yet to be fully reconciled.

The chemical composition of plant cell walls is usually studied by first isolating cell walls from the plant tissues to be analysed, and then sequential extraction techniques are used to fractionate the main polysaccharide groups that make up the cell wall (Thimm et al. 2009). While isolated cell wall polysaccharides can be analysed using chemical methods or by cytochemical staining to visualise the polysaccharide types and gather information about their quantity and location, they do not give a true picture of the cell wall in its undisturbed state (Carpita et al., 1996; Thimm et al., 2002; Vian & Roland, 1991).

2.2 Imaging the plant cell wall of higher plants

While imaging techniques such as transmission electron microscopy (TEM), field emission scanning electron microscopy (FESEM) and contact mode atomic force microscopy (AFM) can provide valuable information on the appearance, arrangement and structural dimensions of cell wall components (Hansma et al., 1997; Li, 1999; Thimm et al., 2002; Thimm et al., 2009), only limited chemical information can be obtained. For example, when using AFM, the contrast mechanism used to obtain an image is the force between the tip and the sample, and many samples produce the same force, thus it is difficult to reliably determine the chemical groups that are imaged. However, single-molecule force spectroscopy (SMFS), a technique where AFM tips are modified by the addition of specific molecules has the potential to provide both structural and chemical information (Mueller et al., 2009a & 2009b).

3. Atomic force microscopy as a tool for studying plant cell walls

3.1 Contact mode AFM

Contact mode AFM is a non-destructive imaging technique by which images with nanometer resolution can be obtained, and is therefore ideal for studying cell wall structure. In this mode a sharp stylus or tip is scanned across the surface of a sample and the force between the tip and sample is measured at a series of points. A colour or grey scale is assigned to each force, and then a map of colours displays an ``image'' of the surface (Thimm et al., 2000). This form of AFM has been used to examine isolated cell wall material from plants including apple, water chestnut, potato, carrot (Kirby et al., 1996a & 1996b) cotton (Pesacreta et al., 1997) and celery (Thimm et al., 2009), and in the "intact walls" of celery parenchyma cells (Thimm et al., 2002) and single *Zinnia elegans* tracheary elements (Lacayo et al., 2010). For a recent review of the application of AFM and other scanning probe microscopy techniques potentially useful for the study of plant cell walls see Yarbrough et al. (2009). While providing useful structural information this technique does not provide any chemical information regarding the structures observed.

3.2 Chemical and single-molecule AFM

Ducker et al. (1992) demonstrated that the forces between colloid particles could be measured by attaching a colloid particle to the end of an AFM cantilever. In biological systems, this approach has been adapted to estimate bond strength between different biological molecules such as ligands and receptors (You & Yu, 1999), antigen antibody binding (Nyquist et al., 2000), receptor binding (Raiteri et al., 1999), and the molecular assembly of biomolecules (Kossek et al., 1998, Perrin et al., 1999).

The principle of sensor force measurement involves attaching one type of molecule to the AFM tip and binding another molecule to a surface. The tip is moved towards the surface until the molecules interact. This has been demonstrated for biotin-streptavidin (Florin et al., 1994), avidin-biotin (Moy et al., 1994), for cell-cell interactions (Antonik et al., 1997), cell-adhesion proteoglycans (Dammer et al., 1995; Misevicz, 1999) and antigen-antibody systems (Dammer et al., 1996; Hinterdorfer et al., 1996). This technique can also be used to gain chemical information from the surfaces of structural components isolated from cells or from the surfaces of living cells (Mueller et al. 2009a & 2009b). For example, Gad et al. (1997) used gold-coated tips functionalized with concanavalin A to map the cell wall polysaccharides of living microbial cells.

Single-molecule force sensors can also be used to resolve topographical information (Muller et al., 2009a & 2009b). Force mapping is a force sensing technique where a small area is raster force probed. Each force curve can potentially be identified and a force map generated, showing for example the distribution of cell wall polysaccharides as mentioned above. When using single-molecule force microscopy, the probe is not in physical contact with the surface, but instead uses the attractive/repulsive part of the force curve, whereby the cantilever is purely force driven. We used a variant of this technique, with sugars attached to the tip of the cantilever, in an attempt to map the distribution of polysaccharides in the parenchyma cell walls of celery epidermal peels, produced as described in Thimm et al. (2000). In the following sections we present some preliminary findings regarding the development of sensors to both image and to determine the chemical characteristics of celery parenchyma cell walls.

4. A system for single-molecule force microscopy of celery (*Apium graveolens* L.) parenchyma cell walls using glycoside probes

4.1 The celery cell wall

Thimm et al. (2002) isolated the primary walls of celery parenchyma cells and their polysaccharide components were characterized by glycosyl linkage analysis, cross-polarization magic-angle spinning solid-state ^{13}C nuclear magnetic resonance (CP/MAS ^{13}C

NMR) and X-ray diffraction. The cell walls consisted of mainly cellulose (43 mol%) and pectic polysaccharides (51 mol%), made up of rhamnogalacturonan (28 mol%), arabinan (12 mol%) and galactan (11 mol%), with only smalls amounts of xyloglucan (2 mol%) and xylan (2 mol%) detected in the cell walls. Solid-state ^{13}C NMR signals were consistent with the constituents identified by glycosyl linkage analysis and allowed the walls to be divided into three domains, based on the rigidity of the polymers. Cellulose (rigid) and rhamnogalacturonan (semi-mobile) polymers responded to the CP/MAS ^{13}C NMR pulse sequence and were distinguished by differences in proton spin relaxation time constants. The arabinans, the most mobile polymers, responded to single-pulse excitation (SPE), but not CP/MAS ^{13}C NMR. From solid-state ^{13}C NMR of the cell walls the diameter of the crystalline cellulose microfibrils was determined to be approximately 3 nm while X-ray diffraction of the cell walls gave a value for the diameter of approximately 2 nm.

4.2 Sensor design

Glucose and galactose were chosen as sensor molecules as cellulose is a polymer of glucose and is one of the main structural components in the celery cell wall, while galactose is an important component of celery pectins (Thimm et al., 2002). The two main types of probes used in conventional AFM experiments are either silicon-nitride (pyramidal) or silicon (ultralever). Sugar groups can be covalently attached directly to the silanol or silolamine surface groups on commercial tips, or the commercial tip can be coated in a thin film that is convenient for further reactions. Gold is a useful film because a broad spectrum of groups can be attached to gold via thiol linkages. Thiols are well known to adsorb under mild conditions onto gold surfaces (Biebuyck & Whitesides, 1994; Fritz et al., 1996; Liu et al., 1994, Nyquist et al., 2000) and thiol adsorption is strong enough to use sugar-thiols as sensors, for these reasons we chose to use gold-coated tips.

Most interactions in biological systems depend on the orientation of the molecules. Therefore, forces between the sensor and the surface can only be detected if the sensor is able to align itself unhindered relative to the surface molecule. A carbon spacer chain was introduced to ensure that the sensor molecule had enough flexibility to sample different orientations relative to the sample. The chain-length of the spacer between the sugar ring-system and the probe determines its flexibility or ability to rotate freely, and a spacer of C4-carbons between the interacting sugar ring and the thiol-group was found to be sufficient for probing plant cell wall extracts and surfaces (Thimm, 2000).

4.3 Synthesis of glycoside-sensors and attachment of glycoside-sensors to gold-coated cantilevers

The synthetic approach for the derivatisation of thiobutyl-glycosides with a C4-spacer (butyl-spacer) can be found in Thimm (2000) and the probes used are shown in Figure 1.

To avoid contamination of the gold-coated AFM cantilevers, all sensor attachment procedures were conducted in a laminar flow cabinet, in 9 cm polystyrene petri dishes. A glass-slide was cut to fit inside a petri dish and 30 min prior to sensor attachment, distilled ethanol was poured around the glass-slide and the dish was covered to saturate the atmosphere with ethanol vapour. The cantilevers were placed onto the glass-slide and 3-4 drops of a dilute ethanolic solution (1 to 5 mmol) of the thio-glycosides was placed onto the gold-coated cantilever and the petri dish was covered. If the sample appeared to be drying

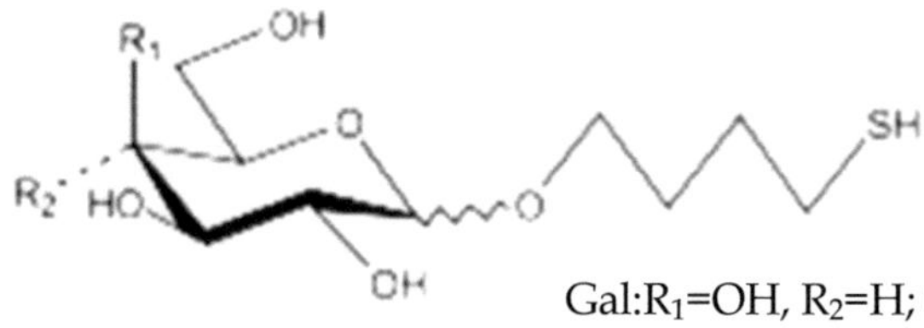

Gal:R_1=OH, R_2=H; Glc:R_1=H, R_2=OH

Fig. 1. The probes used in the experiments detailed below

out within the incubation time, a drop of distilled ethanol was added. The surfaces were then carefully washed with ethanol and then deionised water, and stored wet. Force experiments were conducted where glycoside-sensors were used to probe gold-coated surfaces, to which glycosides were attached, to the determine if the sensors were sufficiently coated with thio-glycosides and to determine the functionality of the system (Thimm, 2000).

5. Force mapping celery cell wall fractions

5.1 Cell wall fractionation

As discussed in section 3 plant cell walls can be studied by selectively fractionating the polysaccharide groups that make up the wall, using sequential extractions, so that each fraction can be studied in more detail (Melton & Smith, 2005). Water-soluble pectins are extracted with boiling water or cold HEPES buffer, while less-methylated pectins, held in the wall with calcium bridges, are solubilised with calcium chelating agents such cyclohexane-trans-1,2-diaminetetraacetic acid (CDTA). Esterified pectins, and some hemicelluloses are extractable with weak alkali (sodium carbonate, Na_2CO_3). Hemicelluloses and some branched pectins are extracted with 1M KOH, while 4M KOH is used to extract more hemicelluloses, including xylogucans, and additional branched pectins (Siddiqui, 1989a and 1989b). The insoluble final residue is largely cellulose, with any remaining hemicelluloses and some complex pectins (Percy et al., 1997, Redgwell et al., 1997; Thimm et al., 2009).

We used force mode AFM, using the glycoside-sensors detailed in the last section, to probe the cell wall components isolated/extracted from celery parenchyma cells as described by Thimm et al. (2009). The components probed were the final insoluble residue largely composed of cellulose, water-soluble pectins (referred to as the HEPES fraction) and the esterified pectins, and some hemiceluloses (referred to as the carbonate fraction). Briefly a dilute (1-4 mg/mL) 20 % ethanolic suspension of each component was adsorbed onto freshly cleaved mica and allowed to dry in air for up to 20 min. To avoid floating particles the sample was careful rinsed with 1-2 mL dionized water (Thimm et al., 2009). The cell wall components were then probed using glycoside-sensors and force curves generated for the cell wall components detailed above.

5.2 The final insoluble residue (cellulose)

To determine if the force curves associated with the final residue were largely due to the chemical properties of cellulose, a standard (Whatman cellulose, CF11) was probed and the force curves compared to those of the insoluble final residue. The force curves for both the

CF11 and the final insoluble residues were similar (Figure 2). The force curves showed jumps starting at 8 to 8.3 nm distance and less defined jumps at 3 to 3.1 nm and 2 to 2.3 nm distance. The force curves generated when the final insoluble residue was probed with either a galactoside or glucoside sensor showed no clear differences (Figure 3).

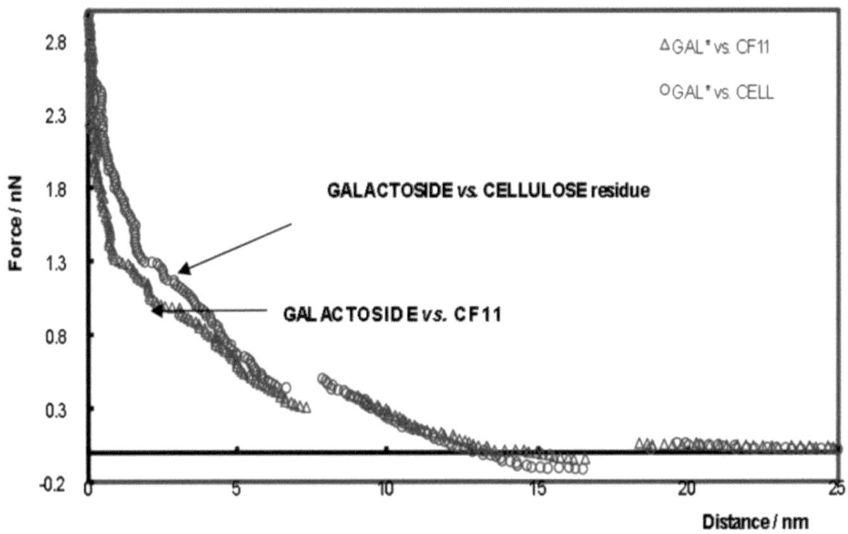

Fig. 2. Force-distance plots for a galactoside-sensor vs. the final cell wall residue (largely cellulose) and a galactoside-sensor vs. cellulose CF11.

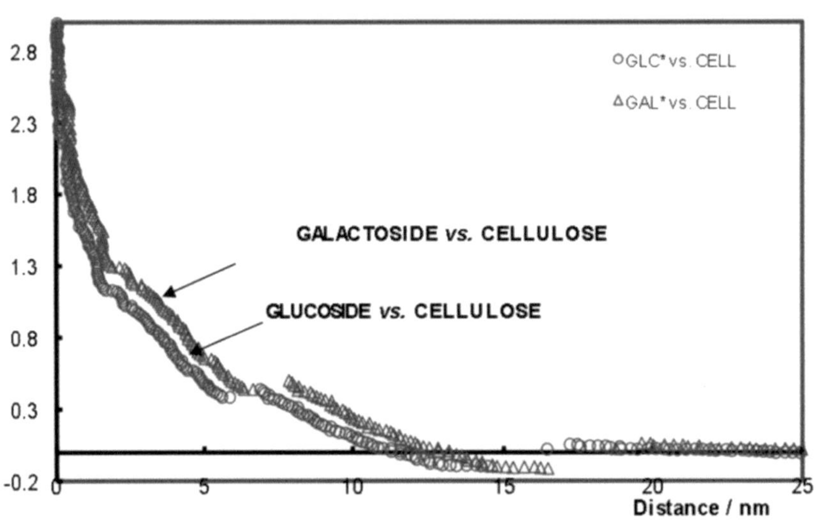

Fig. 3. Force-distance plots for galactoside- and glucoside-sensor vs. the final cell wall residue (largely cellulose).

5.3 Water-soluble pectins (the HEPES fraction)

Figure 4 shows a force-distance plot for a glucoside-sensor vs. the HEPES fraction. Jumps are observed at 49 ± 2 , 42 ± 2 (weak), 37.5 ± 2, 23.3 ± 1, 13.5 ± 1, 6.1 ± 0.5 (weak), 3.1 ± 0.1 and 1.7 nm ± 0.2.

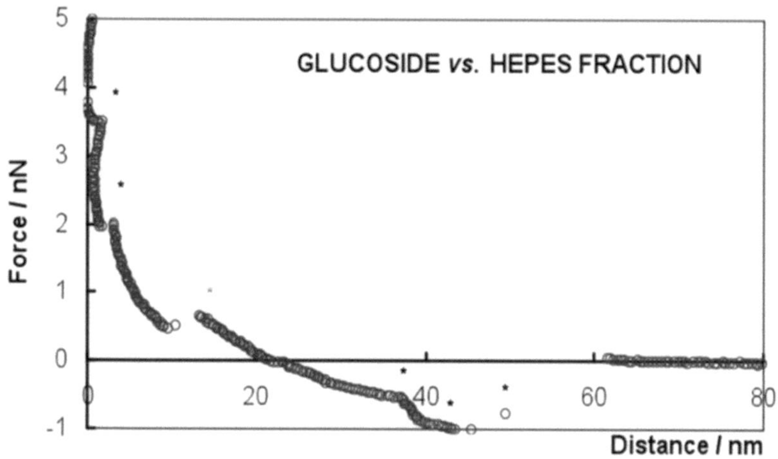

Fig. 4. A force-distance plot for a glucoside-sensor vs. the HEPES fraction. No differences were observed between the glucoside- and galactoside-sensors. Jumps are indicated by an *.

As with the final cell wall residue (cellulose) the glucoside- and galactoside-sensors showed only minor differences in their respective force curves and so could not be used as individual sensors to distinguish galactoses from glucoses and vice versa.

5.4 Esterified pectins and some hemicelluloses (the carbonate fraction)

Figure 5 shows a force-distance plot for a glucoside-sensor vs. the carbonate fraction. Two distinct jumps were observed at 16.5 nm ± 1 (with a displacement force of 0.2 nM ± 0.1) and at 2.9-3.2 nm (0.1 nN ± 0.05). Two weak repulsions at 5.4 ± 0.1 and 9.2 nm ± 0.7 were also observed, but these were often not well resolved.

5.5 Mixture of fractions

Force mapping experiments were also conducted on mixtures of the three cell wall components in an attempt to simulate an *in situ* system. This experiment attempted to determine if cell wall polysaccharides could be identified, by their force curves, in a complex mixture and if the results could then be used to generate a polysaccharide distribution map. A mixture of the three cell wall components (1:1:1 w/w) were adsorbed onto a mica sheet and the sheet was force mapped using a glucoside-sensor. Figure 6 shows a polysaccharide distribution map of such a mixture, showing the distribution of the three cell wall components, identified based on their force curves.

For one sample of mixed components, 242 force curves were generated. Of these, 78 counts (32 %) were for cellulose, possibly indicating that cellulose could readily be detected on the surface, possibly as a result of swollen microfibrils that are larger and hence were more easily detected that the other cell wall components.

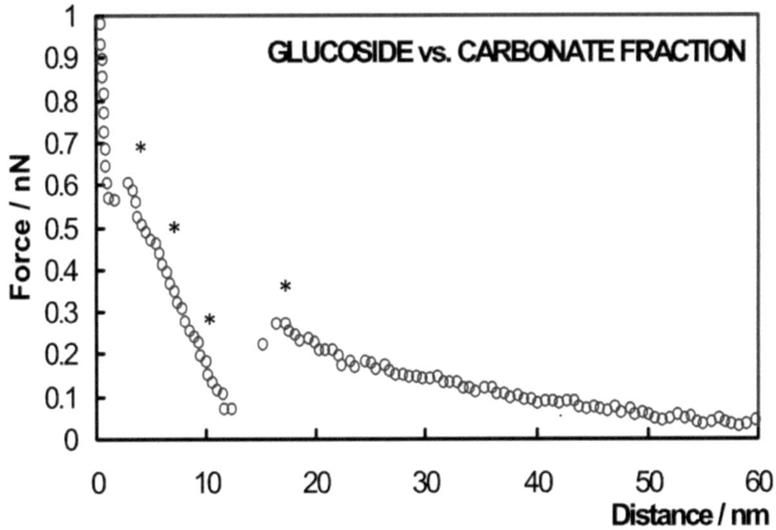

Fig. 5. A representative force-distance plot for a glucoside-sensor vs. the carbonate fraction. Jumps are indicated by an *.

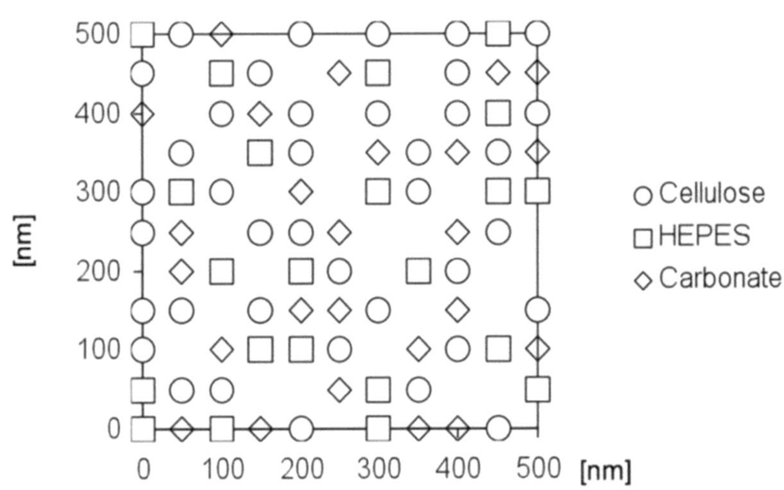

Fig. 6. A force curve distribution map of three cell wall components adsorbed onto a mica sheet and force mapped using glucoside-sensor.

The HEPES fraction was detected 44 times (18 %). This result was unexpectedly low and may have indicated preferred adsorption of the HEPES polysaccharides to the mica surface. Mica (muscovite) is a potassium aluminium silicate hydroxide fluoride that exposes silicate oxygen atoms at the surface, resulting in a negative charge in water. This charge might induce the preferred adsorption of particular polysaccharides from the polysaccharide mixture. Once the first species is adsorbed onto mica, their properties might drive the aggregation of the next layer. It is possible that the HEPES fraction adheres more quickly to the mica than the other cell wall components. The other cell wall components could then form a second or third layer on top of the HEPES fraction and thus it would be less accessible to the sensor, which probes only the surface.

The carbonate fraction was only detected slightly more frequently (21 %) than the HEPES fraction. This pectic material might show a similar behaviour as the HEPES fraction and hence compete for mica surface space. Adsorption to mica is possibly through the formation of electrostatic bonds with the uronic acids of the HEPES fraction. Greater branching and methyl-esterification of the carbonate fraction could result in a reduced ability to compete for mica, even though the sodium carbonate extraction might have caused saponification of methyl-esters to some degree. Another possible explanation might be that the three cell wall components aggregate in solution prior to adsorption to the mica.

A large number (70 counts (29 %) of 242 force curves) of force curves could not be identified. One factor contributing to this was the surface of the polysaccharide mixture seemed to be very rough for force experiments. During raster scanning, forces were probed in regions consisting of gaps or raised regions of the surface. Another explanation might be that forces that could not be assigned are a direct result of intermolecular aggregation of the three cell wall components in solution, resulting in new unidentified force profiles. The distribution maps for the three cell wall components showed an even distribution covering most of the scanned region. No accumulation of individual cell wall components at particular areas was observed.

6. Force mapping the celery cell wall *in situ*

6.1 Imaging using force mode

Figure 7 shows an AFM deflection image of a celery epidermal peel *in situ*, captured in force mode, using a glucoside sensor. Force mode was used to image the cell in order to prevent or minimize contamination of the sensor by reducing physical contact with the surface. The force mode images of the cell wall of celery parenchyma epidermal peels are not as sharp or defined as previously published contact mode images (Thimm et al., 2000).

6.2 Force mapping the surface *in situ*

Prior to force mapping the cell wall, a force mode image was captured and was used to guide the probe (reading x, y coordinates in nm) when force mapping the surface *in situ*. For the image shown in Figure 7, 126 force curves were generated, from different points on the sample and the structural identity of each point was determined by comparison to the forces curves generated from the isolated cell wall components. For each component of the wall, an example of a force curve from the *in situ* experiments is shown below, compared to the isolated cell wall components, cellulose (Figure 8), HEPES (Figure 9) and carbonate (Figure 10).

Of the 126 force curves generated *in situ* using the glucoside-sensor, 53 (42 %) could be attributed to cellulose, 9 (7 %) could be attributed to HEPES fraction polysaccharides and 13 (10 %) could be attributed to carbonate fraction polysaccharides. Of the 126 curves, 51 (41 %) could not be identified. The large number of forces that could not be assigned could be due to the presence of non-polysaccharide material, to aggregated polysaccharides or to

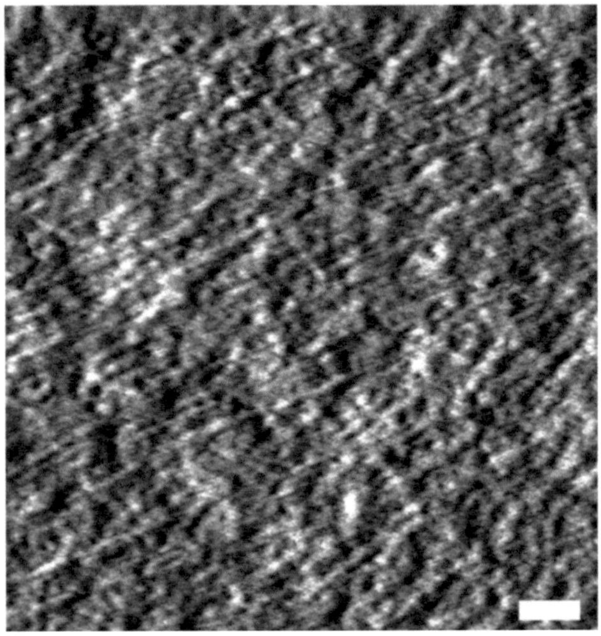

Fig. 7. AFM force mode deflection image of celery epidermal peels in situ captured using a glucoside sensor (scan size 2 μm, scale bar 200 nm, height scale 5 nm)

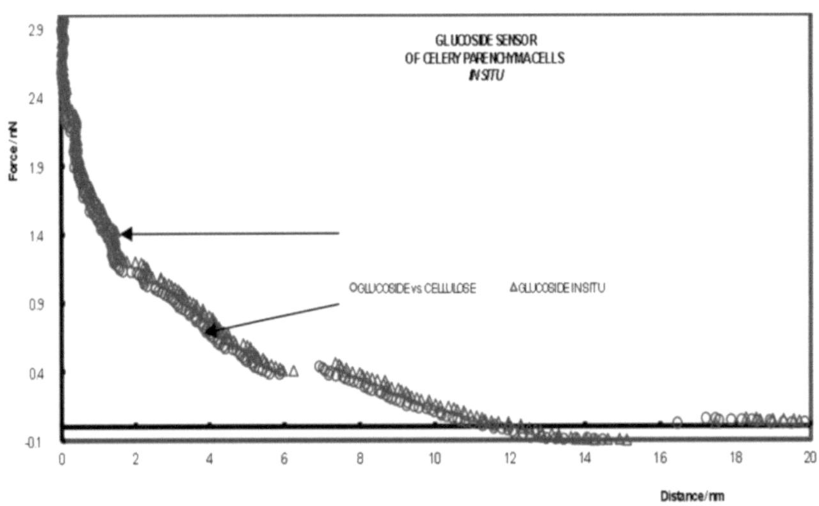

Fig. 8. Representative force-distance plots, using a glucoside-sensor, showing two over laid force curves. One for celery parenchyma cells *in situ* and the second for the cell wall final residue (mainly cellulose).

polysaccharide components of the cell wall for which no reference force curves were available. Most of the force curves that could not be identified showed a strong exponential repulsive behaviour, which could be due to the presence of high molecular weight polymers or aggregates.

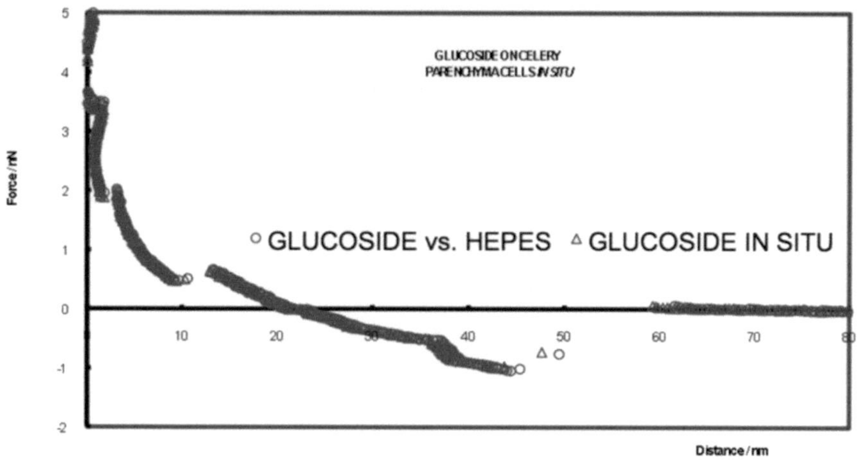

Fig. 9. Representative force-distance plots, using a glucoside sensor, showing two over laid force curves. One for celery parenchyma cells *in situ* and the second for HEPES fraction.

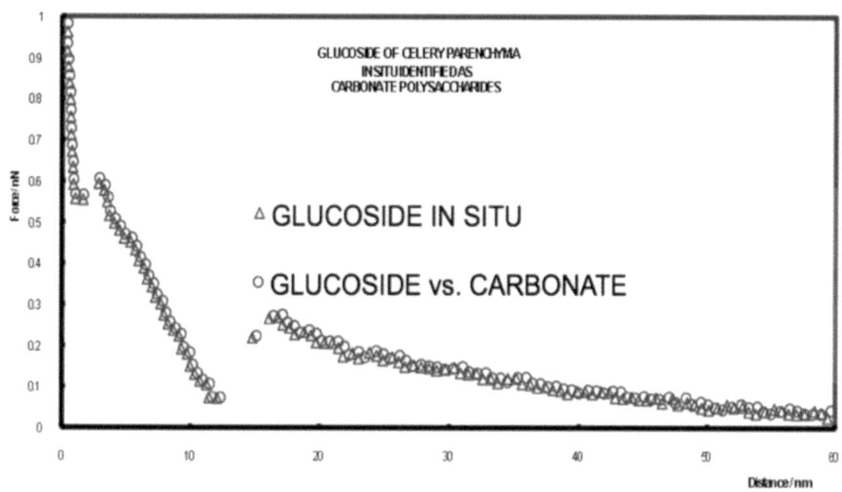

Fig. 10. Representative force-distance plots, using a glucoside-sensor, showing two over laid force curves. One for celery parenchyma cells *in situ* and the second for the carbonate fraction.

By overlaying data points of the force maps for each identified cell wall component, with the force mode AFM deflection image in Figure 7, an image of the wall *in situ* with some chemical information could be generated (Figure 11). Force curves identified as belong to the final cell wall residue did appear to be localised more frequently on the raised microfibril like structures clearly seen in Figure 11. However, no distinct pattern of localisation of the three cell wall components to any particular area of the image was consistently observed.

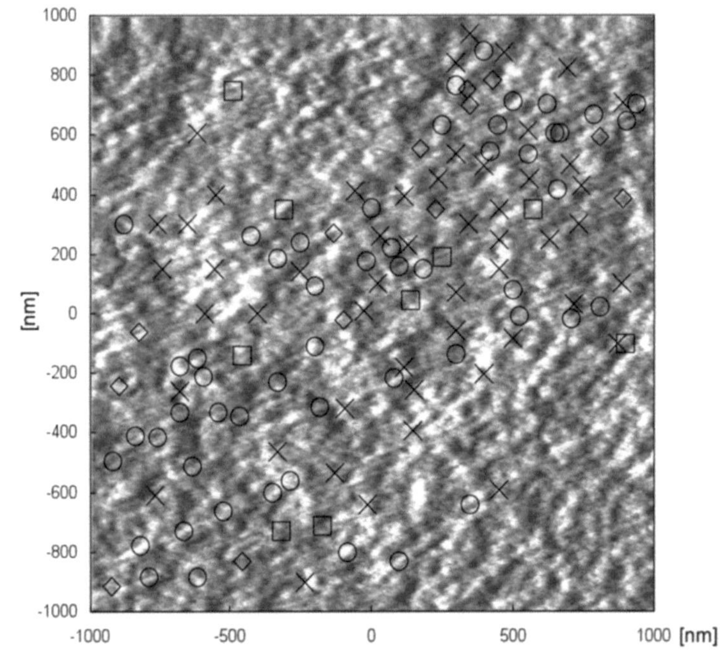

Fig. 11. A map of a celery epidermal cell wall *in situ*, showing the cell wall component distribution (cellulose, circle; HEPES, square; carbonate, diamond; unassigned forces, X).

7. Conclusions

The use of force curves generated by single molecule sensors is potentially a useful way that information about the chemical nature, the strength of interactions, and possibly the molecular arrangement of complex biological structures can be deduced (Gad et al., 1997; Hansma et al., 1997; Li et al., 1998; Li et al., 1999; Marzalek et al., 1998; Osada et al., 1999; Okabe et al., 2000; Rief et al., 1997). To date a few attempts have been made to force probe intact plant cell walls *in situ*. The approach taken in our investigation demonstrates the potential for using single molecule force microscopy to study plant cell wall chemistry and structure and opens up a variety of possible uses, depending on the type of sensor chosen. By probing, using the glucoside-sensors, the three celery cell wall components (HEPES fraction, carbonate fraction and the final residue) in isolation and a mixture of them, we have shown that individual cell wall components can be distinguished in a complex mixture.

When force mode imaging, using glucoside-sensors, was combined with force curve identification, it was possible to map the distribution of cell wall components in celery epidermal peels *in situ*. However, while a cell wall component distribution map of celery epidermal peels *in situ* was obtained, showing the chemical information overlaid over a topographical AFM force mode image, the HEPES and carbonate fraction polysaccharides did not show any regular or ordered distribution. Only force curves identified as belong to the final cell wall residues showed some localisation, appearing more frequently on the raised microfibril-like structures.

For celery, the chemical resolution of the force map was limited to the number of calibration standards produced. We used only three polysaccharide extracts (HEPES fraction, carbonate fraction and the final cellulose residue). The quality and/or purity of the fractions used as standards is unknown, because it is not known how many different types of polysaccharides are present in, for example, the HEPES or carbonate fraction. More sophisticated extraction and purification methods could be used to produce cell wall standards to generate force curves that could be interpreted in more detail.

By increasing the number of calibration standards a larger number of forces could be identified. Ideally polysaccharides that are highly purified or synthesised, to give molecules of known composition, molecular arrangement and linkage type (e.g. xyloglucan, xylan) could be used. A different approach might be to mimic polysaccharide structures in the plant cell wall by synthesising identified structural elements of, for example, polysaccharide sidechains of pectin (galactans and arabinans). Their conformation, strength and fingerprint forces could then be studied systematically.

In the present study, a number of forces could not be identified. One explanation for this was the lack of calibration standards, but another important factor might be the interaction of polysaccharides in solution and *in situ*. Aggregation of polysaccharides has been observed for xyloglucan and cellulose as well as pectin sidechains and cellulose (Pauly et al., 1999; Whitney et al. 1995 & 1999; Zykwinska et al., 2007) and this could influence the force curve observed. Force measurements of calibration standards (e.g. hemicelluloses such as xyloglucan and xylan, pectins such as homogalacturonan, arabinan, galactan or arabinogalactan) need to be made of polysaccharides mixed in solution prior to adsorption on to a mica surface. In addition, further experiments need to be conducted to determine what influences polysaccharide aggregation might have on the observed force curves.

8. References

Antonik, M.D.; D'Costa, N.P.; Hoh J.H. (1997). A biosensor based on micromechanical interrogation of living cells. *IEEE Engineering in Medicine & Biology Society*. Vol.16, 66-72.

Biebuyck, H.A; Whitesides, G.M. (1994). Self organization of organic liquids on patterned self-assembled monolayers of alkanethiolates on gold. *Langmuir*, Vol.10, 2790-2793.

Bootten, T.J.; Harris; P.J., Melton, L.D.; Newman, R.H. (2004). Solid-state ^{13}C-NMR spectroscopy shows that xyloglucan in the primary cell walls of mung beans (*Vigna radiata* L.) occur in different domains: a new model for xyloglucan-cellulose interactions in the cell wall. *Journal of Experimental Botany*, Vol.55, 571-583.

Bowles, D.J. (1990). Defence-related proteins in higher plants. *Annual Review of Biochemistry*, Vol.59, 873-907

Carpita, N.C.; McCann, M.; Griffing, L.R.; (1996) The plant extracellular matrix: news from the cell's frontier. *Plant Cell*, Vol 8, 1451-1463.

Cosgrove D.J. (2001). Wall structure and wall loosening. A look backwards and forwards. *Plant Physiology*, Vol.125, 131-134.

Dammer, U.; Hegner, M.; Anselmetti, D.; Wagner, P.; Dreier, M.; Huber, W.; Guntherodt, H.J. (1996). Specific antigen and antibody interactions measured by atomic force microscopy. *Biophysical Journal*, Vol.70, 2437-2441.

Dammer, U.; Popescu, O.; Wagner, P.; Anselmetti, D.; Guentherodt, H.J.; Misevic, G.N. (1995). Binding strength between cell adhesion proteoglycans measured by force microscopy. *Science*, 267, Vol.1173-1175.

Davies, L.M.; Harris, P.J. (2003) Atomic force microscopy of microfibrils in primary cell walls. *Planta,* Vol.217, 283-289.

Dick-Perez, M.; Zhang, Y.; Hayes, J.; Salazar, A.; Zabotina, O.A.; Hong, M. (2011). Structure and interactions of plant cell-wall polysaccharides by two- and three-dimensional magic-angle-spinning solid-state NMR. *Biochemistry,* Vol.50, 989-1000.

Ducker, W.A.; Senden, T.J.; Pashley, R.M. (1992). Measurement of forces in liquids using a force microscope. *Langmuir,* Vol.8, 1831-1836.

Florin, E.L.; Moy, V.T.; Gaub, H.E. (1994). Adhesion forces between individual ligand receptor pairs. *Science,* Vol.264, 415-417.

Fritz, M.C.; Hähner, G.; Spencer, N.D. (1996). Self-assembled hexasaccharides: surface characterisation of thiol-terminated sugars adsorbed on a gold surface. *Langmuir,* Vol.12, 6074-6082.

Gad, M.; Itoh, A.; Ikai, A. (1997) Mapping cell wall polysaccharides of living microbial cells using atomic force microscopy. *Cell Biology International,* Vol.21, 697-706.

Hansma, H. G.; Kim, K. J.; Laney, D. E.; Garcia, R. A.; Argaman, M.; Allen, M. J.; Parsons, S. M. (1997). Properties of biomolecules measured from atomic force microscope images: a review. *Journal of Structural Biology,* Vol.119, 99-108.

Hansma, H.G.; Hoh, H.J. (1994). Biomolecular imaging with the atomic force microscope. *Annual Review of Biophysics & Biomolecular Structure,* Vol.23, 115-139.

Hinterdorfer, P.; Baumgartner, W.; Gruber, H.J.; Schilcher, K.; Schindler, H. (1996). Detection and localization of individual antibody-antigen recognition events by atomic force microscopy. *Proceedings of the National Academy of Sciences of the United States of America,* Vol.93, 3477-3481.

Kennedy, C.J.; Sturcova, A.; Jarvis M.C.; Wess, T.J. (2007). Hydration effects on spacing of primary-wall cellulose microfibrils: a small angle X-ray scattering study. *Cellulose,* Vol.14, 401-408.

Kirby, A.R.; Gunning, A.P.; Morris, V.J. (1996a). Imaging polysaccharides by atomic force microscopy. *Biopolymers,* Vol.38, 355-366.

Kirby, A.R.; Gunning, A.P.; Waldron, K.W.; Morris, V.J.; Ng A. (1996b). Visualization of plant cell walls by atomic force microscopy. *Biophysical Journal,* Vol.70, 1138-1143.

Kossek, S.; Padeste, C.; Tiefenauer, L.X.; Siegenthaler, H. (1998) Localisation of individual biomolecules on sensor surfaces. *Biosensors & Bioelectronics,* Vol.13, 31-43.

Lacayo, C.I.; Malkin, A.J.; Holman, H.N.; Chen, L.A.; Ding, S-Y.; Hwang, M.S.; Thelen, M.P. (2010) Imaging Cell Wall Architecture in Single *Zinnia elegans* Tracheary Elements. *Plant Physiology,* Vol.154, 121-133.

Li, H.B.; Rief M.; Oesterhelt, F.; Gaub, H.E.; Zhang, X.; Shen, J. (1999) Single-molecule force spectroscopy on polysaccharides by AFM-nanomechanical fingerprint of alpha-(1,4)-linked polysaccharides. *Chemical Physics Letters,* Vol.305, 197-201.

Li, H.B.; Rief, M.; Oesterhelt, F.; Gaub, H.E. (1998). Single-molecule force spectroscopy on xanthan by AFM. *Advanced Materials,* Vol.10, 316-319.

Li, M.Q. (1999). Scanning probe microscopy (STM/AFM) and applications in biology. *Applied Physics (A) Materials Science and Processing,* Vol.68, 255-258.

Liu, Y.; Wu, T.; Fennell, E.D. (1994). Lateral force microscopy study on the shear properties of self assembled monolayers of dialkylammonium surfactant on mica. *Langmuir,* Vol.10, 2241-2245.

Marga, F.; Grandbois, M.; Cosgrove, D.J.; Baskin, T.I. (2005) Cell wall extension results in the coordinate separation of parallel microfibrils: evidence from scanning electron microscopy and atomic force microscopy. *Plant Journal,* Vol.43, 181-190.

Marszalek, P.E.; Oberhauser, A.F.; Pang, Y-P. Fernandez J.M. (1998). Polysaccharide elasticity governed by chair-boat transisitions of the glucopyranose ring. *Nature,* Vol.396, 661-664.

Melton, L.D.; Smith, B.G. (2005). Isolation of plant cell walls and fractionation of cell wall polysaccharides. In: Wrolstad, R. (Ed.), Handbook of Food Analytical Chemistry: Water, Proteins, Enzymes, Lipids and Carbohydrates. Wiley- Interscience, New Jersey, pp. 697-719.

Misevicz, G.N. (1999) Molecular self-recognition and adhesion via proteoglycan interactions as a pathway to multicellularity: Atomic force microscopy and color coded bead measurements in sponges. *Microscopy Research and Technique,* Vol.44, 304-309.

Morris, V.J.; Gunning, A.P.; Gunning, A.P.; Kirby, A.R.; Round, A.; Waldron, K.; Ng, A. (1997). Atomic force microscopy of plant cell walls, plant cell wall polysaccharides and gels. *International Journal of Biological Macromolecules,* Vol.21, 61-66.

Morris, V.J.; Kirby, A.R.; Gunning, A.P. (1999). Atomic force microscopy for biologists, Imperial College Press.

Moy, V.T.; Florin E.L.; Gaub H.E. (1994). Intermolecular forces and energies between ligands and receptors. *Science,* Vol.266, 257-259.

Mueller, D.J.; Helenius, J.; Alsteens, D.; Dufrene, Y.F. (2009a) Force probing surfaces of living cells to molecular resolution. *Nature Chemical Biology,* Vol.5, 383-390.

Mueller, D.J.; Krieg, M.; Alsteens, D.; Dufrene, Y.F. (2009b) New frontiers in atomic force microscopy: analyzing interactions from single-molecules to cells. *Current Opinion in Biotechnology,* Vol.20, 4-13.

Nyquist, R.M.; Eberhardt, A.S.; Silks, L.A.; Li, Z.; Yang, X.; Swanson, B.I. (2000). Characterisation of self-assembled monolayers for biosensor applications. *Langmuir,* Vol.16, 1793-1800.

O'Neill, M.A.; York,W.S. (2003). The composition and structure of plant primary cell walls. In: Rose, J. K. C. (Ed.), The Plant Cell Wall. Blackwell, Oxford. pp.1-54.

Okabe, Y.; Akiba, U.; Fujihira M. (2000). Chemical force microscopy of -CH_3 and -COOH terminal groups in mixed self-assembled monolayers by pulsed-force-mode atomic force microscopy. *Applied Surface Science,* Vol.157, 398-404.

Osada, T.; Takezawa, S.; Itoh, A.; Arakawa, H.; Ichikawa, M.; Ikai, A. (1999). The distribution of sugar chains on the vomeronasal epthelium observed with an atomic force microscope. *Chemical Senses,* Vol.24, 1-6.

Pauly, M.; Albersheim, P.; Darvill, A.; York, W.S. (1999). Molecular domains of the cellulose/xyloglucan network in the cell walls of higher plants. *Plant Journal,* Vol.20, 629-639.

Percy, A.E.; Melton, L.D.; Jameson, P.E. (1997). Xyloglucan and hemicelluloses in the cell wall during apple fruit development and ripening. *Plant Science,* Vol.125, 31-39.

Perrin, A.; Theretz, A.; Lanet, V.; Vialle, S.; Mandrand, B. (1999) Immunomagnetic concentration of antigens and detection based on a scanning force microsocpe. *Journal of Immunological Methods,* Vol.224, 77-87.

Pesacreta T.C., Carlson L.C. and Triplett BA (1997). Atomic force microscopy of cotton fiber cell wall surfaces in air and water: quantitative and qualitative aspects. *Planta,* Vol.202, 435-442.

Popper, Z.A.; Fry, S.C. (2008). Xyloglucan-pectin linkages are formed intra-protoplasmically, contribute to wall assembly, and remain stable in the cell wall. *Planta,* Vol.227, 781-794.

Raiteri R., Nelles G., Butt H.J., Knoll W. and Skladal P. (1999). Sensing of biological substances based on the bending of microfabricated cantilevers. – Sensors and Actuators B-Chemical 61: 213-217.

Redgwell, R.J.; Fischer, M.; Kendal, E.; Macrae, E.A.; (1997). Galactose loss and fruit ripening - high-molecular-weight arabinogalactans in the pectic polysaccharides of fruit cell walls. *Planta,*Vol. 203, 174-181.

Rief, M.; Oesterhelt, F.; Heymann, B.; Gaub H.E. (1997). Single molecule force spectroscopy on polysaccharides by atomic force microscopy. *Science,* Vol.275, 1295-1297.

Siddiqui, I.R., 1990a. Studies on vegetables. Investigation of water, oxalate, and sodium hydroxide soluble celery (*Apium graveolens*) polysaccharides: Celery arabinogalactan. *Journal of Agriculture & Food Chemistry,* Vol.38, 38-41.

Siddiqui, I.R., 1990b. Studies on vegetables. Investigation of water, oxalate, and sodium hydroxide soluble celery (*Apium graveolens*) polysaccharides: Pectic polysaccharides. *Journal of Agriculture & Food Chemistry,* Vol.38, 70-74.

Talbott, L.D.; Ray, P.M. (1992) Molecular size and separability features of pea wall polysaccharides. Implications for models of primary wall structure. *Plant Physiology,* Vol.92, 357-368.

Thimm, J.C. (2000) The plant cell wall architecture of celery (*Apium graveolens* L). Ph.D. Thesis, The University of Otago, Dunedin, New Zealand.

Thimm, J.C.; Burritt, D.J.; Ducker, W.A.; Melton, L.D (2009) Pectins influence microfibril aggregation in celery cell walls: An atomic force microscopy study. *Journal of Structural Biology,* Vol.168, 337-344.

Thimm, J.C.; Burritt, D.J.; Ducker, W.A.; Melton, L.D. (2000) Celery (Apium graveolens) parenchyma cell walls examined by atomic force microscopy: effect of dehydration on cellulose microfibrils. *Planta,* Vol.212, 25-32.

Thimm, J.C.; Burritt, D.J.; Sims, I.M.; Newman, R.H.; Ducker, W.A.; Melton, L.D. (2002). Celery (*Apium graveolens* L.) parenchyma cell walls: Cell walls with minimal xyloglucan. *Physiologia Plantarum,* Vol.116, 164-171.

Vian, B.; Roland, J.C. (1991). Affinodetection of the sites of formation and of the further distribution of polygalacturonans and native cellulose in growing plant-cells. *Biology of the Cell,* Vol.71, 43-55.

Whitney, S.; Brigham, J.; Darke, A.H.; Reid, J.S.G.; Gidley M.J. (1995). *In vitro* assembly of cellulose/xyloglucan networks: Ultrastructural and molecular aspects. *Plant Journal,* Vol.8, 491-504.

Whitney, S.E.C.; Gothard, M.G.E.; Mitchell, J.T.; Gidley, M.J. (1999). Roles of cellulose and xyloglucan in determining the mechanical properties of primary plant cell walls. *Plant Physiology,* Vol.121, 657-663.

Yarbrough, J.M.; Himmel, M.E.; Ding, S-Y. (2009). Plant cell wall characterization using scanning probe microscopy techniques. Biotechnology for Biofuels, Vol.2, 17, doi:10.1186/1754-6834-2-17.

You, H. X.; Yu, L. (1999). Atomic force microscopy imaging of living cells: progress, problems and prospects. *Methods in Cell Science,* Vol.21, 1-17.

Zykwinska, A.; Thibault, J.F.; Ralet, M.C. (2007). Organization of pectic arabinan and galactan side chains in association with cellulose microfibrils in primary cell walls and related models envisaged. *Journal of Experimental Botany,* Vol.58, 1795-1802.

14

AFM and Cell Staining to Assess the *In Vitro* Biocompatibility of Opaque Surfaces

Christopher L. Frewin, Alexandra Oliveros,
Edwin Weeber and Stephen E. Saddow
University of South Florida
USA

1. Introduction

Although many current biomedical devices have been able to assist millions of people, there are still many critical needs to be addressed. Many individuals need constant diagnostics, controlled and targeted delivery of drugs, or even the replacement of motor and sensory functions. Many of the current biomedical systems that perform these functions are large, non-transportable, cumbersome or, more importantly, they cannot be in contact with the body for extended amounts of time. One solution is to utilize micro-electromechanical machines, or MEMS. With the same processes used to create computer chips, we can now generate a variety of micron sized machines which are designed to deliver drugs, detect physiological changes, and even electrically interface with cells. These micron to nanometer sized devices can potentially be implanted into the body with minimal invasiveness. There is, however, a very important issue which in turn needs to be addressed before their widespread clinical use can come to realization.

A major difficulty of long-term implantable MEMS devices is the body's inflammatory response to foreign materials. This has been termed the property of biocompatibility which is summarized as a material's ability not to illicit a negative physiological response while maintaining the devices designed functionality within the body environment (D. F. Williams, 2008). Materials need to be screened and verified for their biocompatibility before use within the human body. One problem is that many of the materials implemented in MEMS devices are opaque, which are difficult to examine for biocompatibility using traditional methods. For example, total internal reflection fluorescence (TIRF) measures the cell/ surface interface within 200 nm; however this technique nominally requires evanescent and internal reflection wave generation (Easley IV et al., 2008). Confocal microscopy generates point illumination of a sample through a combination of filters, beam splitters, and gratings to eliminate out-of-focus light, thereby detecting light within a specific focal plane, and raster scanning can then be used to generate detailed two and three dimensional images (Booth et al., 2008). Confocal microscopes are very expensive, and many of the models used typically in biology labs are designed with inverted microscopes not suitable for opaque substrates. Many fluorescent light microscopes suffer from the same limitations.

Atomic force microscopy (AFM) uses a laser reflected off a cantilever to gather quantitative morphological surface information, can image cells an opaque surfaces, and nominally costs much less than a confocal microscope. It can provide information on cell spread and morphology on almost any surface. With this ability, the AFM can be used to investigate cellular activity on opaque materials. This chapter is dedicated to showing some of the methodologies we have developed to investigate biocompatibility of novel carbon materials.

1.1 Cellular to surface interactions

Examining the biocompatibility of a material for use in a medical device begins through the use of quantitative and qualitative techniques. These techniques have been collected into the International Standards Organization's (ISO) 10993 standards (ISO-10993-1, 2009; ISO-10993-5, 2009; ISO-10993-6, 2007). For *in vitro* testing, one of the most important qualifications is the interaction of cells on the surface of the material. Fig. 1 shows the process of cell attachment, which are mediated by the interactions between cell-surface integrin receptors and extra cellular matrix (ECM) proteins adsorbed on the substrate, in which the wettability, roughness, and charge of the surface play important roles (Lee, M.H. et al., 2005; McClary et al., 2000; Underwood et al., 1993). A biocompatible substrate will allow cells to perform required chemical processes on the materials surface, such as specific signal transduction responses, that lead to cell attachment and proliferation (Juliano & Haskill, 1993; Miyamoto et al., 1995).

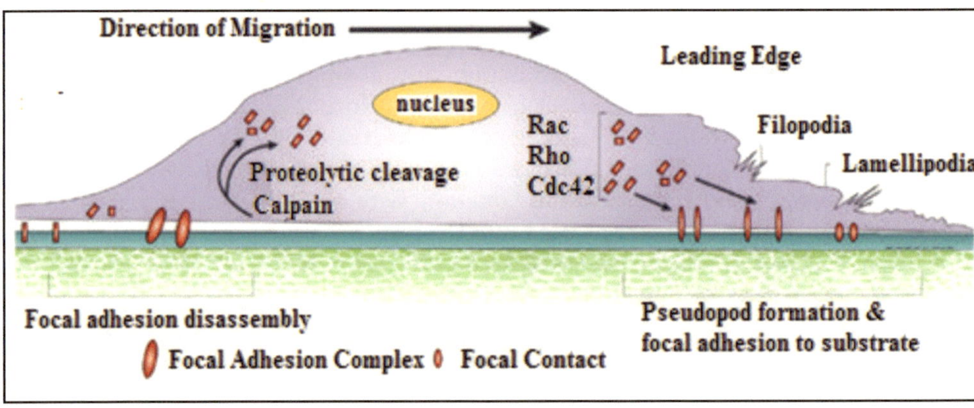

Fig. 1. A cartoon representation of cellular attachment factors to a substrate. The attachment involves focal adhesion complexes and contacts, filopodia, and lamellipodia (Frame et al., 2002).

Another measurement of surface biocompatibility is to evaluate the extension of lamellipodia or filopodia from motile cells onto a substrate surface (Levitan & Kaczmarek, 2002). Microtubule-filled growth cones, the backbone for dendritic spines and axons, are guided by the spike like filopodia and the membrane like lamellipodia (Levitan & Kaczmarek, 2002). The latter are attracted and repulsed by chemical and contact-mediated cues which influence how the structures connect to the outside world (Levitan & Kaczmarek, 2002). If an external surface is repulsive to the cells, these features will not couple with the surface and are retracted back into the central core, but if the substance is attractive, they couple strongly with the surface and new actin fibers flow to the leading edge (Levitan & Kaczmarek, 2002). Through the monitoring of lamellipodia or filopodia structures, a surface can be considered permissive to the cells if it produces attractive actions, and non-permissive if it repels them (Levitan & Kaczmarek, 2002).

1.2 Techniques used for study

For this chapter, we use three general methods to test our materials. Our first method was using MTT (3-(4,5-Dimethylthiazol-2-yl)-2,5-diphenyltetrazolium bromide) assay to quantitatively measure cellular viability/cytotoxicity on the materials. Our second method was AFM measurements to assess cellular morphology changes and lamellipodia/ filopodia permissiveness. Finally, we use immunohistochemistry to examine focal point adhesion and the actin mesh within cells on our substrates.

1.2.1 MTT assay

Cell viability/ cytotoxicity on the tested substrates were quantified using MTT assays. This proliferation assay was developed by Mossman and modified by Coletti et al. for bulk materials (Coletti et al., 2007; Mosmann, 1983). We take three 8 x 10 mm samples of the testing material, place them into a 12 or 24 well plate, and seed a predetermined number of cells (determined experimentally by previously producing 70 - 90% confluence layer) on each material and control. The cells are incubated at 37 °C, 5% CO_2, and 95% relative humidity for the time of the test without changing media. MTT, a chemical which is yellow in color, is added to each well (Mosmann, 1983). MTT is only metabolized by living mitochondria, with purple formazan as a by-product. We remove the remaining media carefully as to not disturb the formazan crystals, remove the samples from the wells, and place them into a 24 plate well (Coletti et al., 2007). This prevents corruption of the assay by adding formazan from cells attached to the polystyrene well to the formazan from material attached cells. Dimethyl sulfoxide, or DMSO, dissolves the purple formazan and is quantified by using a spectrophotometer measuring a wavelength of 500 to 600 nm (Mosmann, 1983). The MTT tests were repeated in triplicate for each tested material. The results from the MTT assays were normalized with respect to the control readings and expressed as the sampling distribution of the mean ($\bar{x}$) ± standard error of the mean (σ_M).

1.2.2 AFM techniques for live and fixed whole cells

This method was first reported in (Frewin et al., 2009b). AFM measurements are made using a Park Systems XE-100 AFM. Cells were seeded on each of the substrates within a 12 or 24 well plate incubated for at least 48 hours. The AFM of living cells was performed first within phosphate buffered solution, PBS, and provided the basis for a quantification of cell height, total surface area of the cell, angle of attachment, and the present extension of the lamellipodia/filopodia. The cells were then fixed using 4% paraformaldehyde for 20 minutes, which immobilized the lamellipodia and filopodia, and the cells were again measured using AFM. The measurements were repeated at least 3 times within each scan area, and are expressed as ratios or percentages to provide a basis for comparison. Analysis of the AFM images was performed with Park Systems XEI image analysis software as shown in Fig. 2(a).

Although the topographical measurement provided by AFM will not image the internal actin meshwork associated with lamellipodia and filopodia, these structures can still be identified and measured. It is the consensus view that filopodia are the cell vanguard for probing the local environment which is then followed by the generation of lamellipodia (Gordon-Weeks, 2004). By examining the sections of the outer extremities of the cell, we identified the spike-like

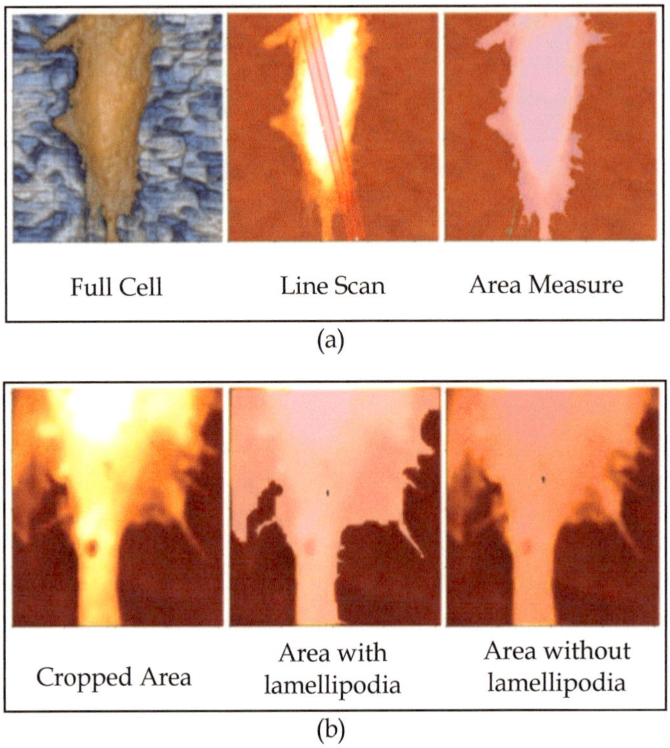

Fig. 2. Selection of 45 x 45 µm AFM micrographs utilized for cell permissiveness on the substrates. (a) From left to right: an enhanced color AFM micrograph of a cell, a line evaluation to determine cell height and angle of attachment, and a surface area measurement. (b) From left to right: a cropped 10 x 10 µm section of the AFM micrograph depicting filopodia/ lamellipodia, a full area measurement and an area measurement of the cell body eliminating the filopodia/ lamellipodia (Frewin et al., 2009b)

filopodia structures, as shown in Fig. 2(b). Lamellipodia are known to be a thin membrane layer 100 - 200 nm thick and parallel to the substrate surface (Gordon-Weeks, 2004). XEI area analysis was used on both living and fixed cell observations, normalized as a percentage of total cell attachment area, and the subsequent loss (or gain) percentage in area was used to quantitatively express the cell permissiveness to the substrate.

1.2.3 Immunohistological staining

To provide a clear picture of cellular attachment to a surface, we used immunofluorescence in one of our tests to examine the focal points and the actin cytoskeleton. We fixed the cells on our material using 4% paraformaldehyde, followed by a permeabilization and general antibody blocking for 2 hours with horse serum. The samples were then incubated with the primary antibody V4505 Monoclonal mouse anti-vinculin antibody (1:1000) in 4 °C overnight. The following day, we will conjugated the primary antibodies with goat anti mouse Alexa fluor 488 (1:250) for 2 hours at room temperature. We added rhodamine phalloidin (1:100) and ProLong® Gold antifade reagent with DAPI to stain the nucleus of the cells. The samples were viewed and recorded using a Leica DM2000 microscope with

EL6000 external light source. Microscope images were taken using a Canon Powershot S5 IS equipped with a Martin Microscope MM99 adapter.

2. Neuronal cellular interactions with opaque surfaces

The central nervous system, or CNS, is one of the most complicated systems in the body and consists of a dense network of neurons and glial cells. Implantation of a biomedical device into the CNS allows direct interaction with neural cells and effectively bypasses the blood-brain barrier. These devices can interact electrically with the CNS, be utilized as a platform for delivery of drugs, neural factors, proteins, genetic material, or even other cells to the CNS. These devices therefore can potentially repair a CNS system damaged by glial scarring due to trauma or disease (Stichel & Müller, 1998). Unfortunately, the construction materials for these devices activate microglia and astrocytes which begin to the process of gliosis, also referred to as the glial scaring (Fawcett & Asher, 1999).

The CNS response to chronic implantation is one of the greatest difficulties facing the widespread clinical incorporation of neutrally interfaced devices (Donoghue, 2008; Polikov et al., 2005). Not only is this reaction medically unsuitable, but neural implant (NI) devices which are electrode based are extremely vulnerable to changes in impedance and fail to function typically within months to a few years after glial encapsulation (Polikov et al., 2005; Rousche & Normann, 1998; J. C. Williams et al., 1999). Silicon (Si), a favored material for NI, is not chemically resistant and has been shown to consistently cause gliosis (Polikov et al., 2005; Rousche & Normann, 1998; J. C. Williams et al., 1999). Neural interfaces using SiO_2 and Si_3N_4 have shown gliosis also, but polyimide, a chemically resistive polymer material has shown excellent biocompatibility (Boppart et al., 1992; Rousche et al., 2001). Although this material offers excellent biocompatibility, displaying a fibroblast adherence, growth, and spread comparable to polystyrene, it has major drawbacks that hinder its acceptance as the material of choice for NI devices (Lee, K. K. et al., 2004). The material has a relatively high water uptake which decreases electrical impedance, and it is a very flexible material which add complications during NI implantation (Polikov et al., 2005).

A semiconductor material, silicon carbide (SiC), may offer a different approach to the generation of implantable neural MEMS devices. SiC has excellent mechanical properties, as it is incredibly hard but also possesses excellent elastic properties (Kordina & Saddow, 2004). SiC is chemically inert to acids, alkalis, and salts, does not absorb water and expand in liquid environments, and can be fashioned with many of the same processes used in the Si industry (Kordina & Saddow, 2004). More importantly, single crystal SiC is a semiconductor and therefore offers an alternative to Si as platform for the realization of NI devices.

Single crystal SiC has many different crystalline stacking sequences called polytypes, and each of these polytypes displays different electrical and mechanical properties. Although some literature exists on the biocompatibility of amorphous (a-SiC) and polycrystalline (poly-SiC), single crystal SiC needed more investigation (Kalnins et al., 2002; Li et al., 2005; Rosenbloom et al., 2004). This subsection reports on previously published research evaluating biocompatibility of cubic silicon carbide, 3C-SiC, nanocrystalline diamond (NCD), and silicon (Si) with immortalized neural cell lines (Frewin et al., 2009b). Cell treated polystyrene (PSt) and amorphous glass serve as negative and positive reaction control materials respectively.

2.1 Methods and materials

The samples used in this work were as follows: commercial (100) Si and (111) Si; (100) 3C-SiC and (111) 3C-SiC (growth process detailed in (Locke et al., 2009; Reyes et al., 2006)); NCD (process detailed in (Kumar et al., 2000)); amorphous glass cover slips; sterile Corning CellBIND® treated polystyrene. The Si and 3C-SiC were n-doped, possessing a negative bulk charge, and the NCD has intrinsic, or semi-insulating, doping. All samples were diced into dimensions of 8 mm x 10 mm. After dicing, the semiconductor and glass samples were ultrasonically cleaned in solvent baths of acetone, methanol, and isopropanol for 5 minutes each to remove dicing particulates and disinfect the surfaces. The semiconductor samples cleaned using the our standard cleaning process detailed in (Coletti et al., 2007; Frewin et al., 2009b). All H_2O was de-ionized (DI) with $\rho > 16$ MΩ cm. The PSt samples were cut with sterile scalpels within a class II A/B3 biological safety cabinet. All samples were placed into 70% (v/v) ethanol to prevent both bacterial growth and surface oxidation.

Two neural cell lines from American Type Culture Collection (ATCC) were used for this study; H4 human neuroglioma (#HTB-148), and PC12 Rat pheochromocytoma (#CRL-1721). The H4 cell line is derived from CNS glial cells and the PC12 is a neural modeling cell derived from the adrenal gland. The H4 cell line was cultured in advanced Dulbecco's Modified Eagle's Medium (DMEM) without L-glutamine supplemented with 10% fetal bovine serum (FBS), 2.2 mM L-glutamine, and 1% penicillin-streptomycin. The PC12 line was grown in Kaighn's F-12K Media supplemented with 2.5 % FBS, 15% horse serum, and 1% penicillin-streptomycin. The cells were cultured in Corning CellBIND® 75 mm^2 flasks to approximately 90% confluence, trypsinized, and enumerated using a hemocytometer.

Each sample was placed into a well of a 12-well plate. 1×10^5 H4 cells and 5×10^5 PC12 cells were seeded in each well followed with the addition of 3 ml of the appropriate media. After 96 hours, the MTT assay was performed in accordance with the procedures outlined in section 1.3.1. Amorphous glass was not tested in the MTT analysis due to numerous performance negative reports (Hench & Wilson, 1986). AFM procedures are detailed in 1.3.2.

2.2 Results

The MTT analysis results for both the H4 and PC12 cell lines are displayed in Fig. 3. The H4 cell line shows a viability level of approximately 80% ± 5% as compared to the PSt control for all samples excluding (111) Si, which performed at 108% ± 9%. The PC12 line indicates the 3C-SiC samples and (111) Si possess a proliferation greater than 90% of the PSt control, while the NCD and (100) Si possess proliferations of 46% and 55% percent, respectively. Fig. 4 displays selected AFM micrograph scans of the H4 and PC12 cell lines incubated on each of the tested substrates, and Table 1 summarizes the measurements of cellular morphology.

During the AFM measurement of both cell lines deposited on the various substrates, the Si surface was observed to suffer physical damage. Fig. 5 displays AFM scan micrographs of the semiconductor substrates before and after the cells had been deposited for a time of 48 hours. For each of the substrates seeded with cells, any cellular remnants and extracellular proteins were completely removed through the piranha cleaning method. Fig. 5a displays an AFM micrograph of the Si surface after the initial RCA cleaning, showing a surface marred by only a few nm deep polishing scratches, and it possesses a surface

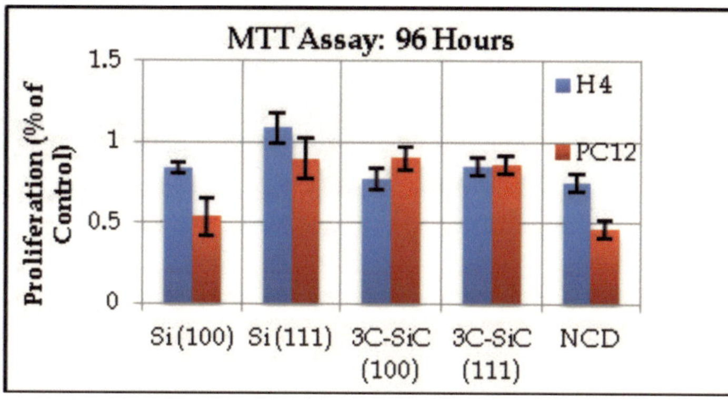

Fig. 3. The combined results of the MTT assay with the H4 and PC12 on our materials. The bars represent the SDM, $\bar{x}$, with error bars indicating the SEM, σ_M (Frewin et al., 2009b).

Cell Interaction with Substrate	Negative Interaction → → Positive Interaction				
H4 Cell Line	**Glass**	**PSt**	**Si**	**NCD**	**3C-SiC**
Live Cell Height/ Area (10^{-3} µm^2)	7.04	5.40	3.11	3.82	4.58
Angle of Attachment (°)	23.80	30.60	15.20	13.80	16.30
% Area: Lamellipodia/Filopodia Reduction	27.00	13.50	10.00	8.10	-0.30*
PC12 Cell Line	**Glass**	**NCD**	**Si**	**3C-SiC**	**PSt**
Live Cell Height/ Area (10^{-3} µm^2)	6.85	5.88	5.14	4.80	2.65
Angle of Attachment (°)	31.20	29.90	31.50	25.80	22.60
% Area: Lamellipodia/Filopodia Reduction	24.80	19.50	10.20	4.50	-3.30*

Table 1. Values for the cell-surface interaction measured with AFM (Frewin et al., 2009b).

root mean square (RMS) roughness, r_q in 5 x 5 µm of 0.137 nm. The surface of the Si after the cell deposition (not shown) indicates many large elliptical depressions approximately 100 - 200 µm long which roughly correlate to the shapes of the H4 or PC12 cells. The surface within the depressions, which is displayed in Fig. 5b, shows numerous small, rounded pits with diameters of 500 to 700 nm and ranging from 30 to 70 nm deep. These features increased 5 x 5 µm r_q to 18 nm RMS.

3C-SiC and NCD are known to be chemically inert materials and they therefore do not display the changes seen on the surface of the Si substrates. The surface of 3C-SiC, displayed in Fig. 5c & 5d show a rough, mosaic surface due to planar defects caused by the 20% lattice mismatch between 3C-SiC and Si, but no pitting or cellular damage. The deposited NCD shows the microcrystalline grain structures across the surface. The 3C-SiC has a 5 x 5 µm r_q of 2.46 nm RMS before and after cell seeding. NCD has much more surface variation as indicated by the differences in Fig. 5e and 5f, and shows 5 x 5 µm scan size r_q of 17.79 nm RMS and 13.42 nm RMS before and after cell seeding.

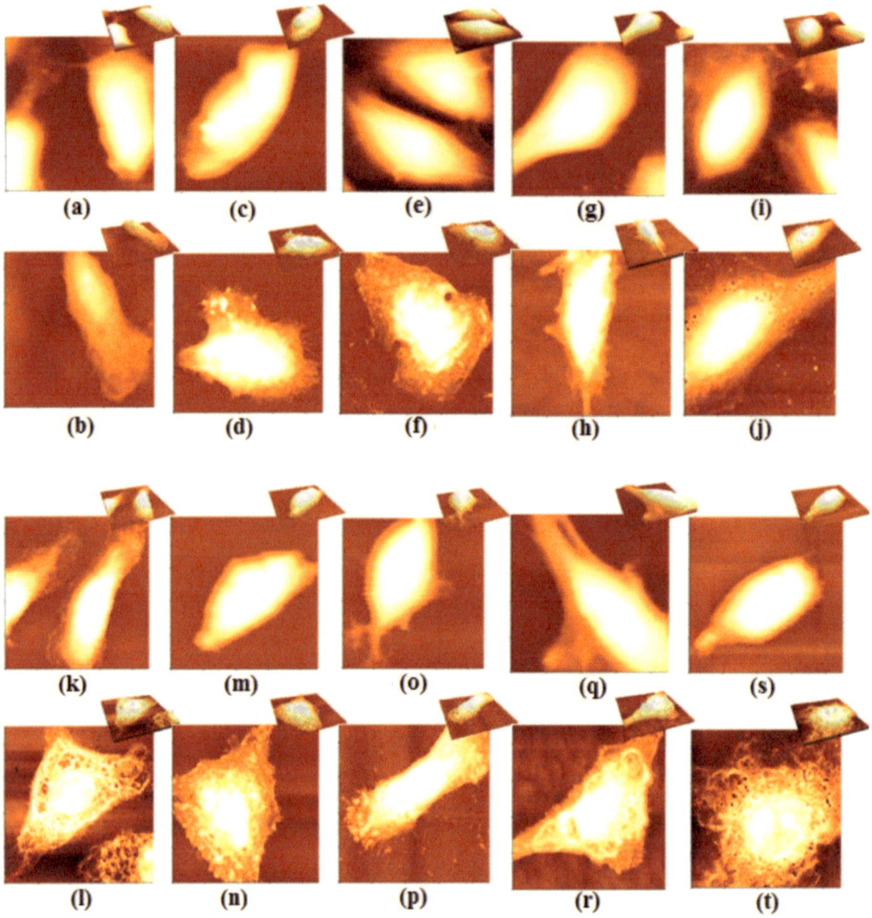

Fig. 4. 45 x 45 µm AFM micrograph of H4 andPC12 cells on the substrates. (a), (c), (e), (g), and (i) are live H4 cells measured in PBS deposited on PSt, glass, Si, 3C-SiC, and NCD respectively. (b), (d), (f), (h), and (j) are have been fixed on PSt, glass, Si, 3C-SiC, and NCD. (k), (m), (o), (q), and (s) are live PC12 cells measured in PBS deposited on PSt, glass, Si, 3C-SiC, and NCD respectively. (l), (n), (p), (r), and (t) are have been fixed on PSt, glass, Si, 3C-SiC, and NCD (Frewin et al., 2009b).

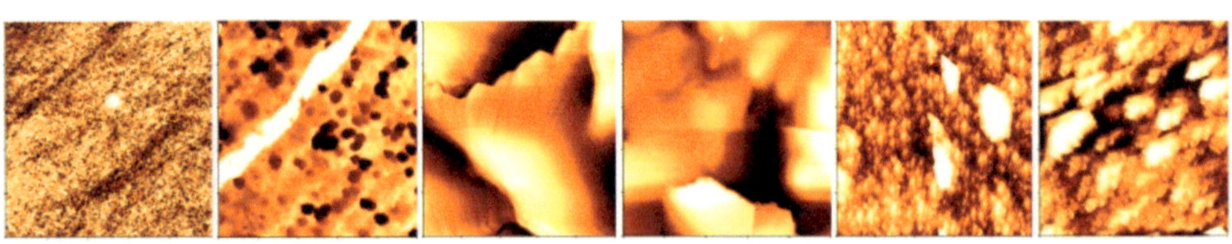

Fig. 5. 5 x 5 µm AFM micrographs of the surfaces of the three tested semiconductors. (a) and (b) are Si, (c) and (d) are 3C-SiC, and (e) and (f) are NCD before and after removal of cells. Note that Si shows signs of surface modification where NCD and 3C-SiC are relatively unchanged (Frewin et al., 2009b).

2.3 Discussion

This study focused on gaining insight of the biocompatibility of bare, untreated substrates with immortalized neuronal cell lines, and primarily used two factors to determine the level of biocompatibility. MTT assays, shown in Fig. 3, were used to determine cell proliferation and viability, and the AFM measurements, compiled in Table 1 and Fig. 4, were used to determine cell morphology for information on cell to substrate interaction and the permissiveness of the substrate. Cell proliferation and subsequent membrane attachment on substrates is dependent on a complex combination of physical, electrical, and chemical reactions which are influenced by both surface and bulk substrate properties and the cell membrane structure (Kumari et al., 2002; Richards, 1996). Cellular attachment to a substrate involves the absorption of proteins within the media serum to its surface, followed by cellular membrane integrin interactions (Rouhi, 1999). Subsequent membrane attachment, membrane spread, and cellular growth are controlled by internal cellular cues initiated by integrins, and it has been demonstrated that the response is heavily mediated by the surface wet-ability and surface charge (Kim et al., 2001; Rouhi, 1999). Hydrophilic and charged surfaces allow fibronectin (Fn), an extracellular protein which allows cell membrane to surface binding, to unravel and elongate as it is absorbed onto the surface, whereas hydrophobic surfaces show Fn is absorbed in its natural, compact, and rounded form (Bergkvist et al., 2003). Cells show little reactivity with Fn in solution, so elongation is one important factor for cell membrane reactions to occur (Bergkvist et al., 2003). Furthermore, cell charge and surface wet-ability have been indicated as very influential factors for both surface interaction and neurite growth and guidance. Growth cone formation and filopodia/ lamellipodia guidance have been shown to favor a more hydrophobic surface (Clark et al., 1993). Neurite formation and extension are also influenced by substrate charge, with this growth favoring positive charge over negative charge, and neutral charges produce almost no neurite outgrowth (Fine et al., 1991; Makohliso et al., 1993).

PSt treated through oxygenation for optimal cell attachment was used as a normalizing control for the MTT assay test and as a comparison for cell attachment in the AFM analysis. Proliferation of the H4 and PC12 was higher than the tested substrates with the exception of (111) Si for the PC12. The level of attachment of the cells to the PSt substrate showed some variation in that the AFM analysis indicated that the PC12 showed a low surface profile and large surface area spread for the cell membrane, while the H4 have a large angle of attachment, a subsequent high surface profile, and less surface area membrane attachment. The lamellipodia permissiveness was also much better for the PC12 than the H4 on this surface. This material has been shown to be normally hydrophilic, as indicated by (Kim et al., 2001), and the Corning data sheet provides a H_20 contact angle of 12.3° - 16.3°. This material has been also shown to often possess a negative surface charge (Bergkvist et al., 2003). The hydrophilic surface and the negative charge of this material would allow for elongation of the attached proteins, and therefore could be a reason the cells have high proliferation. The negative charge could also be a reason for the improved cell attachment and lamellipodia extensions for the PC12, as was also found with (Fine et al., 1991). However (Makohliso et al., 1993) showed evidence that CNS neurite growth was more sensitive to charge and favored a more positively charged environment, and this may be a reason for the decreased H4 and lamellipodia attachment.

The untreated amorphous glass substrate surface was evaluated in this study as it is more hydrophobic than 3C-SiC and slightly less hydrophobic than Si, PSt and NCD, respectively as seen by (Sklodowaka et al., 1999) which reports a contact angle of 51.05°. Amorphous glass would also not provide a net substrate charge as it is an insulating material but any charges that contact the surface would remain in place. The AFM analysis shows that both cells tend to greatly minimize their contact with this substrate and have little lamellipodia surface attachment, although cells on this substrate displayed large areas of lamellipodia probing, which is consistent with past observations (Bergkvist et al., 2003). The neutral charged surface could be a large factor in inhibiting the neurite expansion, as was shown by previous studies (Fine et al., 1991; Makohliso et al., 1993).

Both faces of Si have shown a measured contact angle of 65.85° (Coletti et al., 2007), indicating a weakly hydrophobic surface. The samples were doped n-type providing a negative charge potential within the bulk of the material. The H4 showed good viability for both Si surfaces. The PC12 results indicated poor cell viability for (100) Si, but excellent cell viability for (111) Si, while the AFM indicates a high cell profile, large angle of attachment, and a moderate lamellipodia attachment. As Si is hydrophobic, and the samples possess negative potential, the differences between the reactions of the cells to the PSt may be due to their chemical properties. The evidence may be displayed in Fig. 5d which indicates some chemical reaction on the Si has occurred when cells are present. Also, studies have indicated the presence of Si compounds present in the CNS (Birchall & Chappell, 1988). Both cell lines have much higher proliferation on the (111) Si face than the (100) Si face, which may be due to the available dangling surface bonds. The lower viability of the PC12 on (100) Si is not so easily explained, but the lower attachment quality shown by the AFM analysis indicates Si is not entirely favorable for this cell. The reaction of the cell and the substrate may be forming silicic acid, which can have a negative effect on the cell viability when present in large quantities (Carlisle, 1986). The moderate lamellipodia attachment to Si is most likely due to the negative charge of the substrate, and mirrors the results seen by (Fine et al., 1991; Makohliso et al., 1993), but attachment of the lamellipodia may have been altered due to the hydrophobic substrate surface (Clark et al., 1993).

Both faces of 3C-SiC, unlike Si, have high proliferation values for both cell lines when compared with the PSt control, and the surface, shown in Fig. 5e, showed no adverse effects of surface degradation through cellular interaction on the surface. The AFM indicated that the H4 have good cellular spread, low profile, and excellent lamellipodia permissiveness. A low angle of attachment, moderate cell spread, and a relatively good level of lamellipodia attachment was also observed for the PC12. The same difference in viability that was observed in the Si crystalline planes also exists with 3C-SiC. (Coletti et al., 2007) have shown the USF 'as grown' 3C-SiC has a contact angle of 52.53°, and (Yakimova et al., 2007) indicates that SiC contains both hydrophilic and hydrophobic sites due to its alternating elemental surface. It should be noted that these substrates are negatively charged, although at a level much lower than the Si substrates. The fact that this substance is hydrophilic and has viability levels comparable to the hydrophobic Si, along with the observation that there is a similar viability contrast between the crystal orientations, suggests that there may be competing bonding principals. One hypothesis is Si is the prevalent membrane bonding site on 3C-SiC and Si substrates, but the patchy C surface bonds slightly decrease the attachment sites, and thus viability, on 3C-SiC. However, the bonds involved for these cells are relatively strong, as indicated by the flattened cell profiles. Like PSt and Si, the negative material charge and presence of hydrophobic sites on 3C-SiC would generate good lamellipodia extension, but the greater attachment of the lamellipodia may be due to the hydrophobic sites on the surface caused by the patchy C bonding sites.

Intrinsic NCD shows a good level of viability, cellular membrane expansion, and attachment with the H4. Alternatively, the high cell profile and poor viability shows the PC12 does not favor NCD. The H4 shows a moderate level of lamellipodia attachment, and the PC12 line shows a very poor level of lamellipodia attachment. NCD has been shown by (Ostrovskaya et al., 2007) (via contact angle measurements of 75° - 95°) to be a hydrophobic surface which is mainly due to the large amount of sp2 bonded graphitic defects along the crystal grain boundaries. As the NCD is intrinsic, there should be no appreciable surface charge level, but random charges may be present along defect boundaries, and the underlying n-type Si substrate may produce capacitive effects. The PC12 follows the previous studies of (Kim et al., 2001; Rouhi, 1999) which show a low cellular viability and attachment due to a hydrophilic surface. The low lamellipodia attachment may be due to the intrinsic charge as was seen in (Fine et al., 1991; Makohliso et al., 1993). The H4 cell line, however, does not follow previous observations. Further exploration into the surface properties of NCD and how this material interacts with extracellular proteins would be necessary to determine reasons for the observed level of viability.

2.4 Conclusion

This initial study of neural cell interaction with 3C-SiC and NCD has provided evidence that these materials may be suitable for use in a NI device, but further investigation is needed to examine the neuron cell reaction on these substrates. 3C-SiC indicated that both cell lines used in this study showed a relatively high level of cellular viability as compared to PSt that has been treated for optimal cell viability. Cell morphology results showed that the cells attach very well to 3C-SiC, and. it has excellent lamellipodia permissiveness which is an important quality for NI devices. Furthermore, the chemical resilience of 3C-SiC demonstrates that this material resists the surface degradation that was observed on the Si surfaces. The as-grown NCD showed good viability and moderate permissiveness for the H4 cell line, but has a poor performance with the PC12 line. Future experiments need to be conducted to better understand the cellular membrane molecular interaction with the surfaces of 3C-SiC, Si, and NCD as many questions regarding substrate charge and protein reactivity remain unresolved.

3. Cellular interactions with Self-Assembled Monolayer (SAM) surfaces

An ideal biosensor would consist of a biocompatible material that could be functionalized to achieve a specific aim, such as detection of target bio-molecules or promotion of specific protein attachment (Vahlberg et al., 2005). Self assembled monolayers (SAM) modified surfaces yield inorganic/organic interfaces which can be used to tailor the surface properties of SiC to achieve a specific aim. Previous studies of SAM formation on Si, glass, and gold surfaces have proven many of these surfaces are highly biocompatible, with corresponding increases in cell adhesion which facilitated the identification of protein adsorption (Kapur & Rudolph, 1998; Low et al., 2006; Mrksich & Whitesides, 1996). SAMs are composed of organic molecules that are covalently immobilized on the surface of the semiconductor via suitable linker groups (Catellani & Cicero, 2007; Stutzmann et al., 2006). In general, hydrogen (H) or hydroxide (OH) terminated surfaces provide the reactive sites necessary to obtain high quality monolayers. Hydrosilylation and silanization are two common surface functionalization processes used extensively on Si substrates (Linford & Chidsey, 1993; Stutzmann et al., 2006), and SAMs have been analyzed in detail, with suppression or enhancement of cell spreading and proliferation depending on the SAM molecular end-group (Faucheux et al., 2004). In this section, we report on the results of our study on the biocompatibility of SAM surface-functionalized hexagonal silicon carbide, 6H-SiC, where the SAM surfaces produced both hydrophobic and hydrophilic surfaces. The biocompatibility was assessed through the AFM and MTT assay techniques detailed in 1.3.1 and 1.3.2.

3.1 Methods and materials

Two (0001) 6H-SiC 3.43° off-axis, n-type, 420 µm thick were diced into 5 x 5 mm die. First, we performed hydrogen etching in order to obtain well-ordered, atomically flat surfaces with reduced surface defect densities (Frewin et al., 2009a). The samples were cleaned as described in section 2.1. followed by a 5% diluted HF dip that results in OH termination of the surface (Li et al., 2005).

After cleaning and etching the samples, alkylation of (0001) 6H-SiC was performed by reaction of the hydroxylated surfaces with 1-octadecene for 120 min at 200°C under Ar. The samples were then ultrasonically cleaned in hexane, chloroform, and methanol for 10 min each (Schoell et al., 2008; Sharp et al., 2008). The silanization reactions were performed by immersing the samples in 10% APDEMS (or APTES) in anhydrous toluene for 90 min at room temperature in an N_2 environment, followed by ultrasonic cleaning in toluene and isopropanol for 20 min each (Schoell et al., 2008). After SAM formation, the samples were placed in 70% (v/v) ethanol to prevent bacterial growth.

Static water contact angle measurements were performed using a KSV CAM101 system from KSV Instruments. A 3 µl droplet of DI water was deposited on three different samples for each of the surfaces prepared. The droplet contact angle was determined by measuring the angles between the baseline of the drop and the tangent of the same. In addition, AFM topography measurements of the surfaces were performed.

We utilized the two ATCC neural cell lines, H4 and PC12, for this investigation. The same culture methods in 2.1, were used. The experimentally determined MTT assay cell seeding concentration was $5x10^5$ cells/ml for both the H4 and PC12 cell lines. The same amount of cells were seeded on samples and placed in 12 well plates for the evaluation.

3.2 Results

The results of this study have been previously reported in (Oliveros et al., 2009). Static water contact angle (SWCA) measurements give an idea of the degree of hydrophobicity and hydrophilicity of the functionalized substrates. Table 2 contains the SWCA and RMS roughness values for the surfaces tested. We observed a hydrophobic surface for the 1-octadecene-treated sample, consistent with methyl molecular end-groups (Schoell et al., 2008; Sharp et al., 2008). The APDEMS and APTES surfaces were moderately hydrophilic, similar to the expected values for amino end-groups (Schoell et al., 2008). The untreated sample exhibited hydrophilic behavior, consistent with a native oxide. Surface topography analysis with AFM showed a very smooth surface following etching and prior to functionalization (~ 0.3 nm RMS). The 1-octadecene-treated surface showed a similar topography to the pre-functionalized 6H-SiC surface, no aggregates (See Fig 6 b). On the

Substrate	Surface Roughness[1] (r_q, nm RMS)	Contact angle (°)[2]
6H-SiC H_2 etched	0.30	19 ± 2
6H-SiC with Octadecene	0.26	110 ± 5
6H-SiC with APDEMS	0.36	48 ± 4
6H-SiC with APTES	0.53	54 ± 2

[1] RMS is the mean of 5 scans over a 5 μm x 5 μm.

[2] Contact angle is the mean of 3 measurements for a 3 uL H_2O droplet on different surfaces.

Table 2. SAM characterization via AFM and water contact angle analysis (Oliveros et al., 2009).

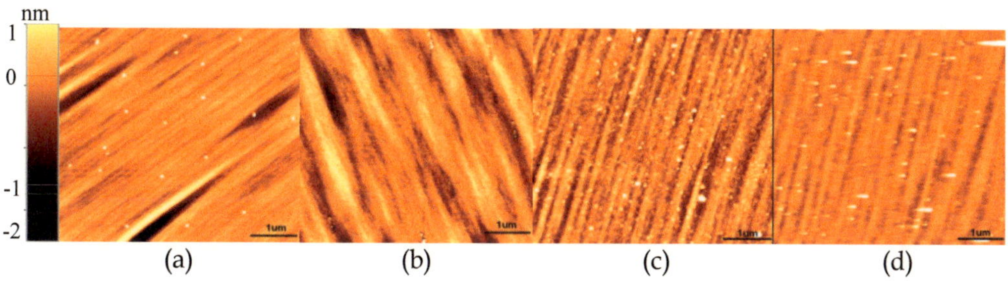

Fig. 6. 5 μm x 5μm AFM micrographs of (a) 6H-SiC, (b) 6H-SiC after alkylation, (c) 6H-SiC APDEMS and (d) 6H-SiC APTES. AFM data taken in tapping mode (Oliveros et al., 2009).

other hand, the APDEMS and APTES functionalized surfaces show some signs of polymerization, most likely due to homogeneous methoxy cross-linking, which were observed as particulates and a difference of r_q with respect to the 6H-SiC substrate (see Fig. 6c & 6d).

MTT assays were performed and normalized to the PSt control to quantify the cell viability on (0001) 6H-SiC without surface treatment and functionalized with the three SAM compounds. Fig. 7 indicates both cell lines show similar viability trends; however, the PC12 show lower levels of relative proliferation. For the H4 seeded on unmodified 6H-SiC, we obtained proliferation of only 31 ± 1% relative to PSt. The cell viability increased for the 1-octadecene functionalized surface by 240 ± 3% relative to the untreated surface, whereas the APDEMS and the APTES treated surfaces showed dramatic increases in cell proliferation, exceeding the untreated surface value by 670 ± 4% and 850 ± 5%, respectively. The PC12 cells displayed a lower proliferation on 6H-SiC of only 38 ±3% relative to PSt. The 1-octadecene functionalized surface results with the H4 show a 171 ± 3% increase of proliferation relative to untreated 6H-SiC. The APDEMS functionalized surface yielded a 320 ± 4% proliferation to the 6H-SiC, whereas cell proliferation for APTES increased 480 ± 4%. More importantly, these results show a statistically significant degree of higher cell proliferation than previous studies done with PC12 cells on porous Si (Low et al., 2006) and SAMs on Si and glass substrates (Faucheux et al., 2004).

Insight into the cell morphology was obtained via AFM analysis. Fig. 8a - 8h displays selected AFM micrographs of the H4 for both the unmodified and SAM-modified surfaces. Fig. 8i - 8p shows representations of the AFM micrographs recorded for the PC12. Although some subtle differences in cell morphology exist, both cell lines exhibited similar trends. For the bare 6H-SiC and 1-octadecene modified surfaces, AFM micrographs showed elongated

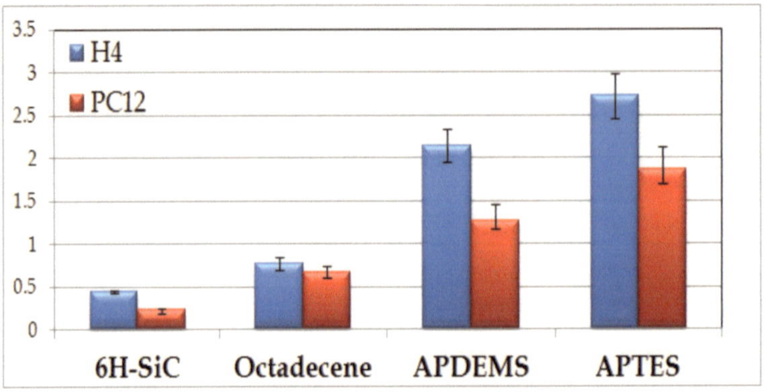

Fig. 7. Relative viability of the H4 and PC12 on the (0001) 6H-SiC as a function of surface termination as determined by MTT assay. The results are expressed as SDM ($\bar{x}$) and SEM (σ_M) and normalized to the PSt readings (Oliveros et al., 2009).

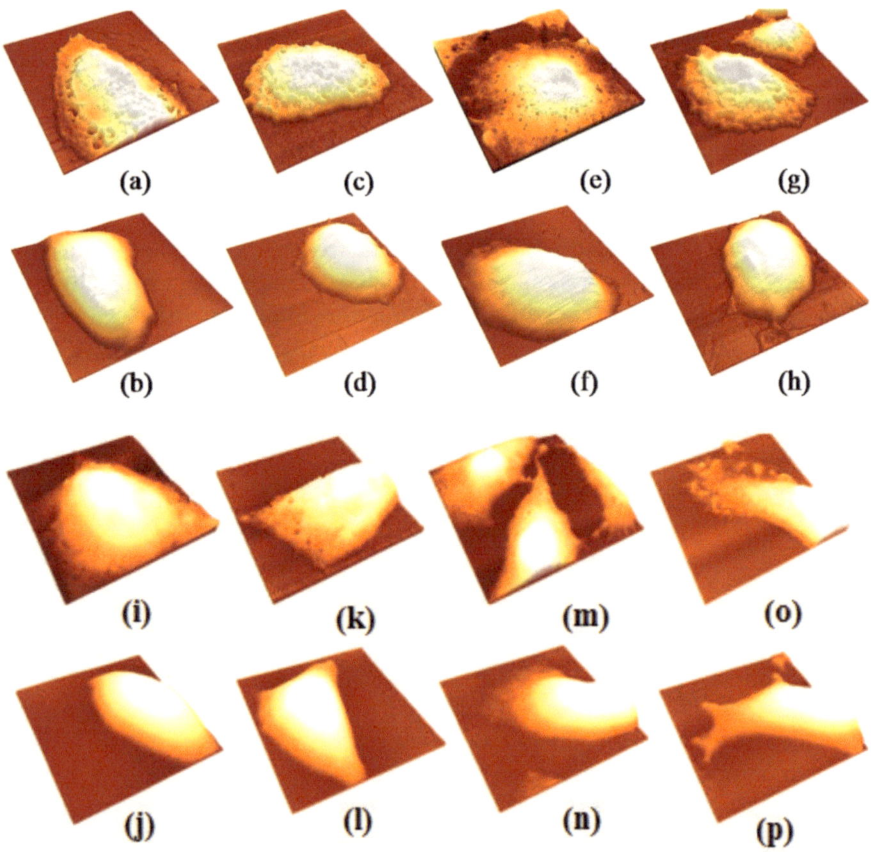

Fig. 8. 45µm x 45µm AFM micrographs for H4 (a – h) & PC12 (i – p) that are fixed (top row) and live (bottom row). (a, b, i, & j) are untreated 6H-SiC, (c, d, k, & l) are 6H-SiC after with 1-octadecene, (e, f, m, & n) are 6H-SiC with APDEMS, and (g, h, o, & p) are 6H-SiC with APTES (Oliveros et al., 2009).

or rounded cells with few focal points, filopodia, and lamellipodia extensions. Indeed, the lamellipodia areas seen on those surfaces were not significant with respect to the total cellular areas (Fig. 8). Conversely, on the APDEMS and APTES treated surfaces, we observed elongated and flattened cells that expanded over large surface areas, suggesting good attachment and consistent with the high proliferation observed using MTT assays (Fig. 7). Additionally, there was evidence of focal point attachment, filopodia and lamellipodia extensions, as well as intercellular interaction. These results compliment the MTT assays which showed greater proliferation on these surfaces compared to the untreated and 1-octadecene modified 6H-SiC surfaces.

3.3 Discussion

Cell attachment and proliferation on surfaces are the products of many chemical processes occurring between the cell membrane and the underlying substrate in contact with the cell. This involves chemical, morphological, and electrical properties of the surface, as well as cell protein-receptor binding and internal cellular reactions, all of which affect the cell-biomaterial interaction (Dan, 2003; Mrksich et al., 1996). Furthermore, ECM protein adsorption on the substrate, which can occur much more rapidly than cell adhesion, is a key step in the mechanism of cell attachment and spreading (Iwata & Arima, 2007; Ostuni et al., 1999). In general, cell attachment and proliferation are considered to occur in three stages: I) protein adsorption onto the substrate from the cell medium, II) attachment and spreading of cells on the protein-modified surface and, III) remodeling of the surface by the cells through cellular protein generation (Ostuni et al., 1999). Modification of surfaces with SAMs is thought to primarily impact the first stage, since hydrophobic, electrostatic, and chemical interactions between molecular end-groups and proteins in the growth medium significantly alter the orientation, composition, and amount of attached proteins, along with the strength of adhesion (Iwata & Arima, 2007; Ostuni et al., 1999).

Here, we have modified (0001) 6H-SiC surfaces, which are hydrophilic in their untreated state (~19° SWCA), with 1-octadecene, which possesses hydrophobic methyl endgroups (~100° SWCA), and APDEMS and APTES, which possess mildly hydrophilic amine endgroups (~50° SWCA). Cell proliferation was significantly higher on the amine terminated SAMs compared to the methyl terminated SAMs and untreated. These findings are in accordance with results obtained on amino terminated SAMs on other substrates by (Faucheux et al., 2004; Lee, M.H. et al., 2005; Low et al., 2006).

Morphological evaluation of cells provides another criterion to determine permissiveness, cellular attachment, and spreading. Elongated and flat cells that are spread out on the surface give an indication of positive cell-surface interactions (Tresco et al., 1998). On the other hand, large cell height to area ratios (corresponding to cell somata which are far from the substrate), cell clumps, cells of round shape with small interfacial areas, and/or few lamellipodia extensions, are all symptomatic of low substrate permissiveness (Coletti et al., 2007; Frewin et al., 2009b).

In this work, the cell morphology evaluation on untreated 6H-SiC and 1-octadecene modified 6H-SiC showed, in general, rounded cell shape and a few elongated flat cells. Additionally, few lamellipodia and filopodia extensions were observed, with evidence on the 1-octadecene treated surface that cell bodies avoid contact with the surface. This is an indication that, although the cells might attach to the substrate following gravitational settling from the medium, they do not find the appropriate conditions to spread and proliferate on the surface. In previous studies using other cell lines on alkylsilane-modified Si surfaces, similar cell morphologies were observed (Faucheux et al., 2004; Lee, M.H. et al., 2005; McClary et al., 2000).

AFM measurements of cells on both APDEMS and APTES treated surfaces showed significantly more elongation and spreading than on the untreated and 1-octadecene treated surfaces. The spreading and elongation were significantly more pronounced on the APTES functionalized surfaces. Indeed, the cells on the APTES surface exhibited a variety of shapes which were predominantly elongated. Such cell morphologies indicate spreading, short cell body-surface separations, and high adhesion to the surface similar to those reported by (Frewin et al., 2009b) for cells seeded on PSt and 3C-SiC. Additionally, we saw indications of microtubule and actin filament extensions on most of the cells seeded on the APDEMS and APTES treated substrates. These findings are similar to the cell morphology and cell spreading reported for rat hippocampal neurons (Stenger et al., 1993), PC12, epithelial (Low et al., 2006), and human fibroblast cells (Faucheux et al., 2004) on different amino-terminated surfaces. An additional study, which utilized fluorescence interference contrast microscopy, also demonstrated short cell-surface distances (~ 40 nm) of neurons of the dorsal root ganglia from rats on APTES-treated surfaces (Tiefenauer et al., 2001).

It has previously been demonstrated that very little protein adsorption, and essentially no fibronectin or vitronectin adsorption, occurs on non-ionic hydrophilic surfaces, such as the untreated 6H-SiC studied here (Faucheux et al., 2004). Conversely, significant protein adsorption, including fibronectin and vitronectin adsorption, occurs on both moderately hydrophobic (e.g. NH_2-terminal) and highly hydrophobic (e.g. CH_3-terminal) surfaces. However, for the case of hydrophobic surfaces, fibronectin receptor function is impaired due to poor fibronectin cell-binding domain accessibility (Faucheux et al., 2004; McClary et al., 2000). Furthermore, competitive adsorption of non-binding proteins, such as serum albumin, reduces the coverage of the ECM proteins which are important for cell spreading and proliferation on hydrophobic surfaces (McClary et al., 2000; Tresco et al., 1998). Thus, in terms of wettability, moderately hydrophilic surfaces provide a balance which allows significant ECM protein adsorption while retaining appropriate integrin function.

In addition to protein adsorption, direct cell-surface interactions should also be considered. It has been previously reported that cells show a tendency to attach to positively charged surfaces (Dan, 2003; Van Damme et al., 1994) and that surface charge may modulate cell attachment and spreading, as found by (Tresco et al., 1998) in their study of thiols, amines, and quaternary amines. In principle, such an effect could contribute to the differences in cell proliferation observed on untreated, CH_3 and NH_2 terminal surfaces (Tresco et al., 1998). In order to affirm that the behavior of the cells presented above is general to other cell types, and to ascertain the roles of electrostatic forces and surface chemistry, additional studies on surface-modified SiC will be required.

3.4 Conclusion

Although SiC has already seen some implementation in modern medical implants (Li et al., 2005), and previous studies have suggested that SiC is biocompatible with different cell lines (Coletti et al., 2007; Frewin et al., 2009b; Li et al., 2005), little research has been devoted to enhancing its biocompatibility via surface modification. In this work, we examined the possibility of increasing cellular proliferation and attachment on the (0001) Si face of 6H-SiC with PC12 and H4 using SAM with terminal methyl and amino groups. Our observations confirmed the influence of the substrate on viability and permissiveness, which were significantly better for the amino terminated surfaces compared to the alkyl terminated surfaces. Indeed, significant increases of cell proliferation were obtained using mildly hydrophilic amino-terminal monolayers; the APTES (APDEMS) modified surfaces exhibited an increase by a factor of ~5x (~3x) for the PC12 and ~8x (~6x) for the H4 with respect to untreated 6H-SiC. Only a moderate increase of the cell viability was observed on hydrophobic 1-octadecene modified surfaces.

This study indicates that the application of SAMs on 6H-SiC can greatly increase cell viability and substrate permissiveness while providing the ability to modify specific surface properties (Stutzmann et al., 2006). This method allows for direct control of the wettability along with surface reactivity and charge which can directly mediate cell adhesion and spreading.

4. Cellular interactions on graphene

Carbon allotropes, specifically carbon nanotubes (CNTs) and graphene have proven to be promising candidates for biological implants as they potentially combine good biocompatibility with excellent chemical resistance (Chen et al., 2008). Even though CNTs have been studied and applied in tissue engineering and biosensing (Yang et al., 2010), there are still some concerns regarding their biocompatibility (Pumera, 2009). On the other hand, although graphene is considered to be a relatively new material, it is well known for its exceptional electrical, thermal and mechanical properties (Geim & Novoselov, 2007), as well as for its high sensitivity to chemical environments (Novoselov et al., 2007). While graphene is an appealing candidate for biomedical applications its biocompatibility must first be assessed and established.

There are different ways to prepare graphene, such as mechanical cleaving, chemical synthesis, epitaxial growth on SiC, and CVD (chemical vapor deposition) on metals. Each process yields graphene with different electrical, optical and morphological properties. In Factors such as the interaction with the substrate, the presence of impurities, and the physical edge of the structure, as well as ultimately the number of layers formed, define the final properties of graphene (Geim & Novoselov, 2007). The epitaxial growth of graphene on SiC in an Ar environment produces high quality films with large domains and good thickness control, with the additional advantage of not having to physically transfer the graphene film to an insulating substrate (Emtsev et al., 2009).

To date, only a few reports discuss the biocompatibility of chemically prepared graphene derivatives (Agarwal et al., 2010; Chen et al., 2008). Recently a study of the biocompatibility of single layer graphene produced by CVD on Cu using human osteoblasts and mesenchymal stromal cells has reported better cell proliferation and morphology compared as to SiO_2/Si surfaces (Kalbac et al., 2010). 6H-SiC has been shown to be biocompatible (Coletti et al., 2007) but it has not been reported if the graphitization of this surface will present a similar behavior. This subsection presents our initial assessment of the biocompatibility of epitaxial graphene on (0001) 6H-SiC (Oliveros et al., 2011).

4.1 Methods and materials

The graphene films were epitaxially grown on (0001) 6H-SiC substrates. Initially, the 6H-SiC samples were H_2 etched in order to obtain a well ordered surface (Frewin et al., 2009a). Subsequently, graphitization was performed under an Ar environment at annealing temperature between 1600 and 1700 °C (Emtsev et al., 2009). The quality and thickness of the graphene films were evaluated by angle-resolved photoemission spectroscopy (ARPES) and X-ray photoelectron spectroscopy (XPS) as in (Coletti et al., 2010; Riedl et al., 2009). AFM and SWCA were used to assess the surface morphology and wettability of SiC and graphene. The SWCA was performed using the methods outlined in 3.1.

Prior to cell seeding the graphene surfaces were cleaned of possible air contamination by performing thermal annealing under an Ar atmosphere at 700°C in a chemical vapor deposition (CVD) reactor. For one set of samples (A) cell seeding was performed without any further surface treatment. Another set of samples (B) had an additional disinfection step via immersion in ethanol. The different surface treatment methods were considered with the intention of learning if the ethanol dip would change the cell morphology and proliferation. The 6H-SiC surfaces were HF dipped to remove the native oxide, annealed under the same conditions as graphene, and finally ethanol dipped.

For the cell morphology analysis and viability assays, human keratinocyte cells (HaCaT) were counted and plated at a density of 3.0×10^4 cells/cm^2 in DMEM supplemented with 10% FBS and incubated for 72 hours. A 5 μM solution of CMFDA (5-chloromethylfluorescein-diacetate) cell tracker dye was used to examine cell morphology analysis via fluorescent microscopy (Coletti et al., 2007), and AFM measurements (1.3.2) were performed on fixed cells to evaluate the filopodia and lamellipodia extensions. Viability evaluation was performed using MTT assays (1.3.1). Immunoflourescence was performed at 48 hours (1.3.3) to investigate focal attachment and the actin cytoskeleton of the HaCaT.

4.2 Results

Characterization of the epitaxial graphene and 6H-SiC surfaces was performed to assess the surface properties prior to cell seeding. In Fig. 9a we report the dispersion of the π-bands around the K-point of the graphene Brillouin zone measured via ARPES for a typical sample used in this work. The π-bands linear dispersion and the displacement of the Fermi level above the Dirac point of circa 0.42 eV are characteristic features of monolayer graphene epitaxially grown on (0001) SiC. Also the C1s XPS spectrum reported in Fig. 9b confirms the monolayer nature of the adopted graphene films. The analysis of the graphene surface topography with AFM (see Fig. 9c) showed indication of large continuous terraces, on average 3.6 ± 2 μm long with a step height of 6.3 ± 3.6 nm, which is larger than the original H_2 etched 6H-SiC substrate terraces (data not shown) consistent with (Emtsev et al., 2009).

The SWCA measured for graphene cleaned by methods A and B were 87.3° ± 9.5° and 94.9° ± 3.2°, respectively. These results confirm the hydrophobicity of graphene (Wang et al., 2009) and demonstrate that ethanol disinfection did not change the water affinity of the surface significantly. For 6H-SiC the SWCA was 47°.2 ± 3°, confirming the hydrophilic character of the surface in support of previous reported data (Coletti et al., 2007).

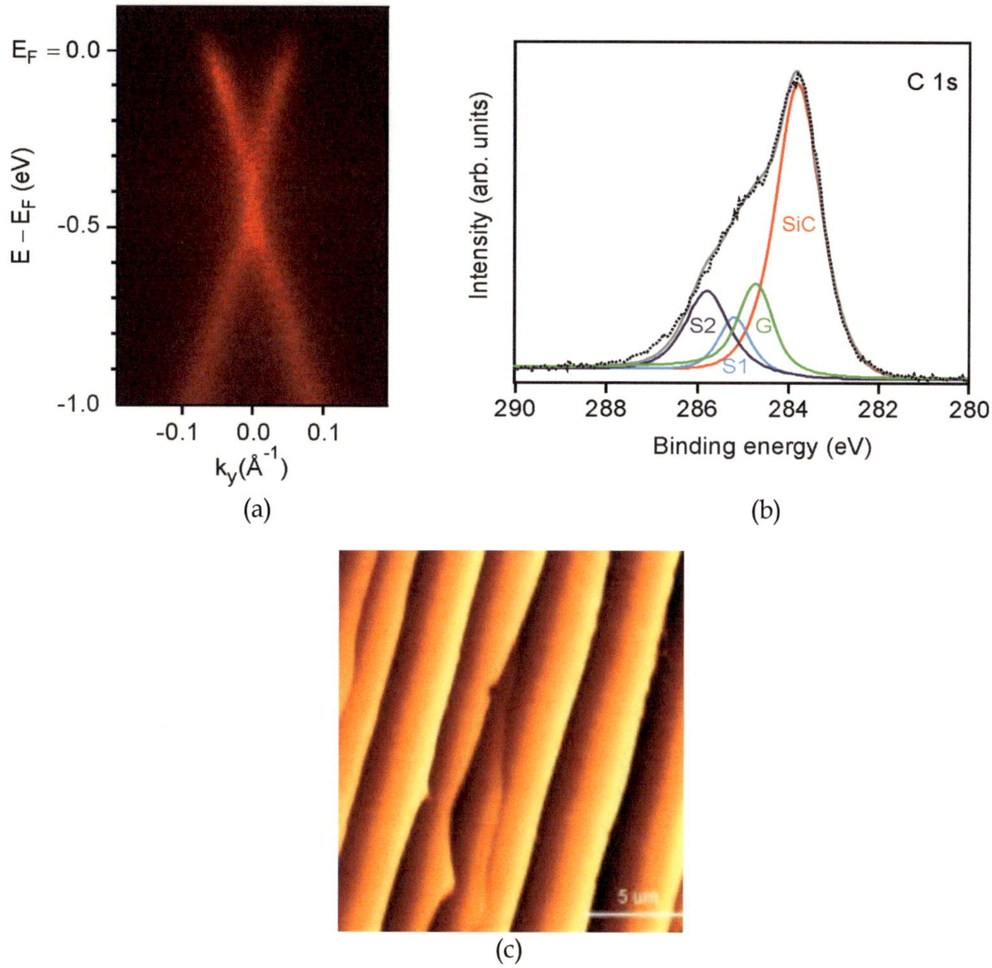

Fig. 9. ARPES (a) and XPS (b) characterization of a monolayer graphene sample. (a) Dispersion of the π-bands measured with UV excited ARPES (hν = 40.8 eV) with a display analyzer oriented for momentum scans perpendicular to the ΓK-direction of the graphene Brillouin zone. (b) C1s XPS spectrum measured using a non-monochromatic Mg Kα source, hν = 1253.6 eV, plotted as a black line and fitted components. (c) 20 μm x 20 μm AFM micrograph of epitaxial graphene on 6H-SiC (0001). Z scale -10 nm to 8 nm (Oliveros et al., 2011).

After 72 hours, for both graphene and 6H-SiC, the morphology of the HaCaT cells was similar to that on the PSt control (data not shown) with signs of cell-cell interaction and cell-substrate interaction (Fig. 10). The cells appeared to be flattened and cuboidal typical of HaCaT cells. The morphology is confirmed with AFM inspection shown in Fig. 11a & 11b where the filopodia and lamellipodia of the cells have been identified. In addition, immunofluorescence analysis of the actin cytoskeleton and the number of focal points are shown in Fig. 11c. These indicate some HaCaT cells present elongated shape while others are a more cubical. We can see the actin fibers (red) are oriented towards the focal points localization (green), indicating good surface attachment.

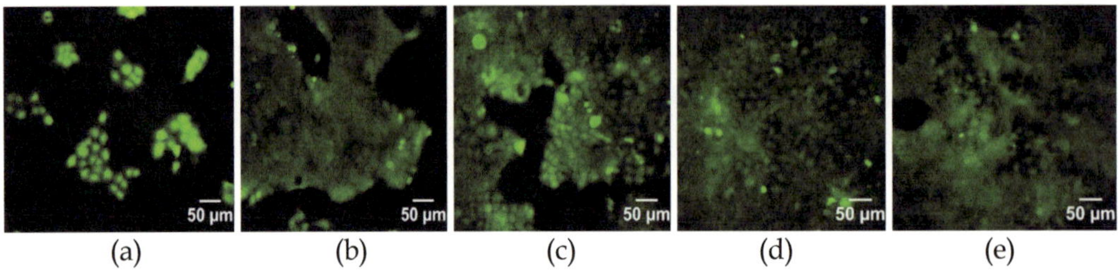

Fig. 10. Fluorescent micrographs of HaCaTs after 72 hour on a) graphene (A), b) graphene (B), c) 6H-SiC(0001), and after 120 hrs on d) 6H-SiC(0001) and e) graphene (B) (Oliveros et al., 2011).

4.3 Discussion

Certain differences were observed for cell proliferation and shape when seeded on surfaces after ethanol disinfection. For the graphene substrates from group A, as seen in Fig 10a, small islands of cells were observed compared to the monolayer that started forming on the graphene surface cleaned by method B (Fig 10b). The 6H-SiC samples also showed via optical inspection clear signs of an initial formation of a cell monolayer (see Fig 10c). It is apparent from the comparison of Figures 10a and 10b that the ethanol dip step favors a more homogeneous cell adhesion and for this reason subsequent experiments whose results are reported below were performed only on samples cleaned by using method B. It is known that HaCaTs tend to form groups of cells such as islands, and with time they start growing tighter and closer to each other and eventually form a conformal layer of cells. Consequently at a time of 120 hours optical inspection of cells plated graphene and 6H-SiC samples was performed with the intent of checking whether the cells would grow to confluence. Promisingly, as shown in Figures 10d & 10e, the 120 hrs optical inspection data showed a homogeneous monolayer of cells formed on both graphene and 6H-SiC.

On the other hand, the MTT assays provided an average value of cell viability after 72 hrs of incubation and with respect to the PSt control. The results were as follows: 17 ± 0.07 (std deviation of the mean) for graphene and 58 ± 0.05 for 6H-SiC. It should be pointed out that the lower viability values obtained for the graphene surfaces might be explained by the hydrophobic nature of the substrate. It may significantly contribute to the cell viability because the initial phase of cell attachment involves the physicochemical linkages between the cells and the surface through proteins (Akasaka et al., 2010). Despite the lower viability measured on graphene after 72 hours of incubation, the evidence of the formation of a cell monolayer on graphene substrates in a similar fashion to 6H-SiC (as in Figures 10d & 10e) after 120 hours of incubation strongly suggests the need to perform longer time MTT assays. As already discussed, because of the hydrophobic nature of the surface, the cells may adapt to it and find the right cues for increased cell proliferation over longer time spans (Akasaka et al., 2010). In addition, the cell viability on both surfaces was compared using an ANOVA test considering that the viability is sample dependent. In this case we obtained that, even though the graphene and 6H-SiC viability levels are close, the surfaces are statistically different with a p-value =0.043 (Oliveros et al., 2011).

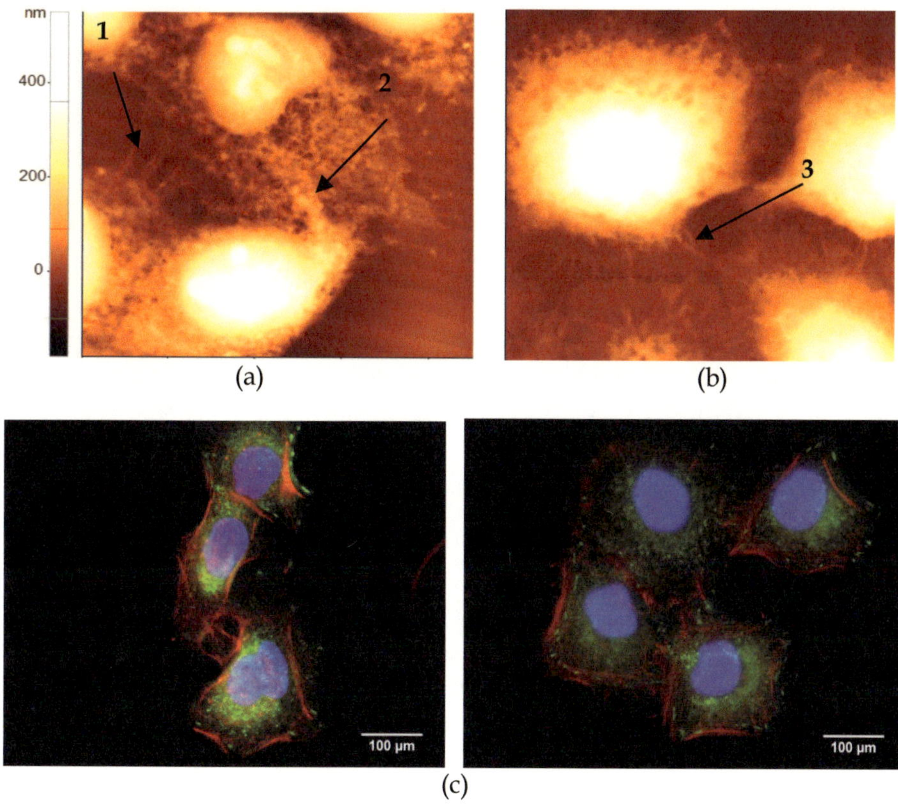

Figure 11. 45 µm x 45 µm AFM micrographs of HaCaT cells on (a) monolayer graphene and (b) H intercalated graphene. The AFM micrographs confirm the presence of 1) cell-cell interaction and 2) evidence of lamellipodia and 3) filopodia. (c) Composite images actin (red), focal points (green) and cell nuclei (blue) on epitaxial graphene (Oliveros et al., 2011).

4.4 Conclusion

In this paper we have reported preliminary methods and result for testing the in vitro biocompatibility of epitaxial graphene on (0001) 6H-SiC through the cellular interactions of HaCaT cells with these surfaces. We have compared the cell viability and cell morphology of these surfaces. Two different cleaning procedures were employed on the graphene surfaces tested. The optical inspection results after 72 hours of cell incubation suggest that the ethanol sterilization step is required in order to have a more homogeneous and enhanced cell adhesion on graphene surfaces. The results obtained from MTT assays after the same incubation time (i.e., 72 hours) evidence of cell viability almost 3 times higher for 6H-SiC than for graphene surfaces. However, the optical inspection performed after 5 days of incubation shows that cells grow in a similar trend on graphene as they do on 6H-SiC. Hence, it is possible to speculate that the viability values obtained after 3 days of incubation might be due to the initial process of surface recognition by the cell and later activation of the appropriate mechanisms for proliferation. Additional MTT assays and optical inspection over longer incubation times must be performed before giving a final answer regarding the in vitro biocompatibility level of graphene. Also, studies pertaining to the cytoskeleton organization (e.g. actin cytoskeleton) on these surfaces or the determination of the number of contact sites (e.g. vinculin staining) could give better insight into the process of cell adhesion and proliferation on graphene.

5. Conclusion

The results of this work have shown that SiC and graphene could potentially become excellent materials for use in biomedical implants. As these materials can be opaque due to the substrates they are grown on, we have shown a method that involves AFM to study the morphology and pseudopodia extensions of cells on their surfaces. In combination with techniques that measure viability, the AFM can be an excellent tool for investigating whole cells interacting on surfaces. Combining the whole cell AFM investigation with previously developed AFM techniques of protein investigation on surfaces, one could more fully understand the cell to substrate interactions and model methods to manipulate them to improve implantable biomedical devices in the future.

6. Acknowledgment

The authors wish to thank: Florida Center of Excellence for Biomolecular Identification & Targeted Therapeutics at USF for the financial support to perform this work; S. Afroz at USF for thermal annealing; Leigh West of the USF FCoE BiTT center for his assistance with fluorescence imaging; K. Emtsev of Max Planck Institute help with the preparation of graphene samples; M. Jaroszeski of USF Engineering for cell culturing.

7. References

Agarwal, S., Zhou, X. Z., Ye, F., He, Q. Y., Chen, G. C. K., Soo, J., Boey, F., Zhang, H. & Chen, P. (2010). Interfacing Live Cells with Nanocarbon Substrates. *Langmuir*, Vol. 26, No. 4, (Feb. 16, 2010), pp. 2244-2247, ISSN 0743-7463.

Akasaka, T., Yokoyama, A., Matsuoka, M., Hashimoto, T. & Watari, F. (2010). Thin films of single-walled carbon nanotubes promote human osteoblastic cells (Saos-2) proliferation in low serum concentrations. *Materials Science and Engineering C*, Vol. 30, No. 3, pp. 391-399, ISSN 0928-4931.

Bergkvist, M., Carlsson, J. & Oscarsson, S. (2003). Surface-dependent conformations of human plasma fibronectin adsorbed to silica, mica, and hydrophobic surfaces, studied with use of Atomic Force Microscopy. *Journal of Biomedical Materials Research Part A*, Vol. 64A, No. 2, (Feb 1, 2003), pp. 349-356, ISSN 0021-9304.

Birchall, J. D. & Chappell, J. S. (1988). The Chemistry of Aluminum and Silicon in Relation to Alzheimers-Disease. *Clinical Chemistry*, Vol. 34, No. 2, (Feb., 1988), pp. 265-267, ISSN 0009-9147.

Booth, M. J., Ju, R. & Wilson, T. (2008). Spectral confocal reflection microscopy using a white light source. *Journal of the European Optical Society*, Vol. 3, No. 1, (Aug. 20, 2008), pp. 08026-1-6, ISSN 1990-2573.

Boppart, S. A., Wheeler, B. C. & Wallace, C. S. (1992). A Flexible Perforated Microelectrode Array for Extended Neural Recordings. *IEEE Transactions on Biomedical Engineering*, Vol. 39, No. 1, (Jan., 1992), pp. 37-42, ISSN 0018-9294.

Carlisle, E. M. (1986). Silicon as an Essential Trace-Element in Animal Nutrition, In: *Ciba Foundation Symposia 121 - Silicon Biochemistry*, Evered, D. & O'connor, M. (eds.), pp. 123-139, John Wiley & Sons, Ltd., ISBN 0300-5208, Chichester, UK.

Catellani, A. & Cicero, G. (2007). Modifications of cubic SiC surfaces studied by ab initio simulations: from gas adsorption to organic functionalization. *Journal of Physics D - Applied Physics*, Vol. 40, No. 20, (Oct 21, 2007), pp. 6215-6224, ISSN 0022-3727.

Chen, H., Muller, M. B., Gilmore, K. J., Wallace, G. G. & Li, D. (2008). Mechanically strong, electrically conductive, and biocompatible graphene paper. *Advanced Materials*, Vol. 20, No. 18, (Sep. 17, 2008), pp. 3557-3561, ISSN 0935-9648.

Clark, P., Britland, S. & Connolly, P. (1993). Growth Cone Guidance and Neuron Morphology on Micropatterned Laminin Surfaces. *Journal of Cell Science*, Vol. 105, No. 1, (May 1, 1993), pp. 203-212, ISSN 0021-9533.

Coletti, C., Jaroszeski, M. J., Pallaoro, A., Hoff, A. M., Iannotta, S. & Saddow, S. E. (2007). Biocompatibility and wettability of crystalline SiC and Si surfaces, *Proceedings of IEEE Engineering in Medicine and Biology Society*, ISBN 1557-170X, Lyon, FR, 22 - 26 Aug., 2007

Coletti, C., Riedl, C., Lee, D. S., Krauss, B., Patthey, L., Von Klitzing, K., Smet, J. H. & Starke, U. (2010). Charge neutrality and band-gap tuning of epitaxial graphene on SiC by molecular doping. *Physical Review B*, Vol. 81, No., pp. 235401-1- 235401-8.

Dan, N. (2003). The effect of charge regulation on cell adhesion to substrates: salt-induced repulsion. *Colloids and Surfaces B-Biointerfaces*, Vol. 27, No. 1, (Jan., 2003), pp. 41-47, ISSN 0927-7765.

Donoghue, J. P. (2008). Bridging the brain to the world: a perspective on neural interface systems. *Neuron*, Vol. 60, No. 3, (Nov. 6, 2008), pp. 511-521, ISSN 1097-4199 (Electronic); 0896-6273 (Linking).

Easley Iv, C. A., Brown, C. M., Horwitz, A. F. & Tombes, R. M. (2008). CaMK-II promotes focal adhesion turnover and cell motility by inducing tyrosine dephosphorylation of FAK and paxillin. *Cell Motility and the Cytoskeleton*, Vol. 65, No. 8, (Aug., 2008), pp. 662-674, ISSN 0886-1544.

Emtsev, K. V., Bostwick, A., Horn, K., Jobst, J., Kellogg, G. L., Ley, L., Mcchesney, J. L., Ohta, T., Reshanov, S. A., Rohrl, J., Rotenberg, E., Schmid, A. K., Waldmann, D., Weber, H. B. & Seyller, T. (2009). Towards wafer-size graphene layers by atmospheric pressure graphitization of silicon carbide. *Nature Materials*, Vol. 8, No. 3, (Mar., 2009), pp. 203-207, ISSN 1476-1122.

Faucheux, N., Schweiss, R., Lutzow, K., Werner, C. & Groth, T. (2004). Self-assembled monolayers with different terminating groups as model substrates for cell adhesion studies. *Biomaterials*, Vol. 25, No. 14, (Jun., 2004), pp. 2721-2730, ISSN 0142-9612.

Fawcett, J. W. & Asher, R. A. (1999). The glial scar and central nervous system repair. *Brain Research Bulletin*, Vol. 49, No. 6, (May 14, 1999), pp. 377-391, ISSN 0361-9230.

Fine, E. G., Valentini, R. F., Bellamkonda, R. & Aebischer, P. (1991). Improved Nerve Regeneration through Piezoelectric Vinylidenefluoride-Trifluoroethylene Copolymer Guidance Channels. *Biomaterials*, Vol. 12, No. 8, (Oct., 1991), pp. 775-780, ISSN 0142-9612.

Frame, M. C., Fincham, V. J., Carragher, N. O. & Wyke, J. A. (2002). v-Src's hold over actin and cell adhesions. *Nature Reviews Molecular Cell Biology*, Vol. 3, No. 4, (Apr., 2002), pp. 233-245, ISSN 1471-0072.

Frewin, C. L., Coletti, C., Riedl, C., Starke, U. & Saddow, S. E. (2009a). A Comprehensive Study of Hydrogen Etching on the Major SiC Polytypes and Crystal Orientations. *Materials Science Forum*, Vol. 615-617, No. -, (Mar., 2009), pp. 589 - 592.

Frewin, C. L., Jaroszeski, M., Weeber, E., Muffly, K. E., Kumar, A., Peters, M., Oliveros, A. & Saddow, S. E. (2009b). Atomic force microscopy analysis of central nervous system cell morphology on silicon carbide and diamond substrates. *Journal of Molecular Recognition*, Vol. 22, No. 5, (Sep-Oct., 2009), pp. 380-388, ISSN 0952-3499.

Geim, A. K. & Novoselov, K. S. (2007). The rise of graphene. *Nature Materials*, Vol. 6, No. 3, (Mar., 2007), pp. 183-191, ISSN 1476-1122.

Gordon-Weeks, P. R. (2004). Microtubules and growth cone function. *Journal of Neurobiology*, Vol. 58, No. 1, (Jan., 2004), pp. 70-83, ISSN 0022-3034.

Hench, L. L. & Wilson, J. (1986). Biocompatibility of silicates for medical use, In: *Ciba Foundation Symposium 121 - Silicon Biochemistry*, Evered, D. & O'connor, M. (eds.), pp. 231–253, John Wiley & Sons, ISBN 0300-5208 Chichester, UK.

ISO-10993-1 (2009), Biological evaluation of medical devices Part 1: Evaluation and testing, International Standards Orginization, Geneva, Switzerland.

ISO-10993-5 (2009), Biological evaluation of medical devices Part 5: Tests for in vitro cytotoxicity, International Standards Orginization, Geniva, Switzerland.

ISO-10993-6 (2007), Biological evaluation of medical devices Part 6: Tests for local effects after implantation, International Standards Orginization, Geneva, Switzerland.

Iwata, H. & Arima, Y. (2007). Effects of surface functional groups on protein adsorption and subsequent cell adhesion using self-assembled monolayers. *Journal of Materials Chemistry*, Vol. 17, No. 38, pp. 4079-4087, ISSN 0959-9428.

Juliano, R. L. & Haskill, S. (1993). Signal transduction from the extra cellular matrix. *Journal of Cell Biology*, Vol. 120, No. 3, (Feb. 1,), pp. 577-585, ISSN 0021-9525.

Kalbac, M., Kalbacova, M., Broz, A. & Kong, J. (2010). Graphene substrates promote adherence of human osteoblasts and mesenchymal stromal cells. *Carbon*, Vol. 48, No. 15, (Dec., 2010), pp. 4323-4329, ISSN 0008-6223.

Kalnins, U., Erglis, A., Dinne, I., Kumsars, I. & Jegere, S. (2002). Clinical outcomes of silicon carbide coated stents in patients with coronary artery disease. *Medical Science Monitor*, Vol. 8, No. 2, (Feb. 23, 2002), pp. PI16-20, ISSN 1234-1010.

Kapur, R. & Rudolph, A. S. (1998). Cellular and cytoskeleton morphology and strength of adhesion of cells on self-assembled monolayers of organosilanes. *Experimental Cell Research*, Vol. 244, No. 1, (Oct. 10, 1998), pp. 275-285, ISSN 0014-4827.

Kim, K. H., Cho, J. S., Choi, D. J. & Koh, S. K. (2001). Hydrophilic group formation and cell culturing on polystyrene Petri-dish modified by ion-assisted reaction. *Nuclear Instruments & Methods in Physics Research Section B*, Vol. 175-177, No. -, (Apr., 2001), pp. 542-547, ISSN 0168-583X.

Kordina, O. & Saddow, S. E. (2004). Silicon carbide overview, In: *Advances in Silicon Carbide Processing and Applications*, Saddow, S. E. & Agarwal, A. (eds.), pp. 2–3,7–8,18, Artech House, Inc., ISBN 1580537405, Boston, MA, U.S.A.

Kumar, A., Ahmed, I. & Vedawyas, M. (2000). Growth of diamond films on Ti-6Al-4V substrates and determination of residual stresses using Raman spectroscopy. *Journal of Vacuum Science & Technology a-Vacuum Surfaces and Films*, Vol. 18, No. 5, (Sep. 2000), pp. 2486 – 2492, ISSN 0734-2101.

Kumari, T. V., Vasudev, U., Kumar, A. & Menon, B. (2002). Cell surface interactions in the study of biocompatibility. *Trends in Biomaterials & Artificial Organs*, Vol. 15, No. 2, pp. 37-41.

Lee, K. K., He, J. P., Singh, A., Massia, S., Ehteshami, G., Kim, B. & Raupp, G. (2004). Polyimide-based intracortical neural implant with improved structural stiffness. *Journal of Micromechanics and Microengineering*, Vol. 14, No. 1, (Jan., 2004), pp. 32-37, ISSN 0960-1317.

Lee, M. H., Brassb, D. A., Morris, R., Composto, R. J. & Ducheyne, P. (2005). The effect of non-specific interactions on cellular adhesion using model surfaces. *Biomaterials*, Vol. 26, No. 14, (July 20, 2004), pp. 1721-1730, ISSN 0142-9612.

Levitan, I. B. & Kaczmarek, L. K. (2002). *The Neuron - Cell and Molecular Biology* (3), Oxford University Press:, ISBN 0-19-514523-2, New York, New York.

Li, X., Wang, X., Bondokov, R., Morris, J., An, Y. H. & Sudarshan, T. S. (2005). Micro/nanoscale mechanical and tribological characterization of SiC for orthopedic applications. *Journal of Biomedical Materials Research Part B: Applied Biomaterials*, Vol. 72, No. 2, (Feb. 15, 2005), pp. 353–361, ISSN 1552-4973.

Linford, M. R. & Chidsey, C. E. D. (1993). Alkyl Monolayers Covalently Bonded to Silicon Surfaces. *Journal of the American Chemical Society*, Vol. 115, No. 26, (Dec. 29, 1993), pp. 12631-12632, ISSN 0002-7863.

Locke, C., Kravchenko, G., Waters, P., Reddy, J. D., Du, K., Volinsky, A. A., Frewin, C. L. & Saddow, S. E. (2009). 3C-SiC Films on Si for MEMS Applications: Mechanical Properties. *Material Science Forum*, Vol. 615-617, No. -, pp. 633-636.

Low, S. P., Williams, K. A., Canham, L. T. & Voelcker, N. H. (2006). Evaluation of mammalian cell adhesion on surface-modified porous silicon. *Biomaterials*, Vol. 27, No. 26, (Sep., 2006), pp. 4538-4546, ISSN 0142-9612.

Makohliso, S. A., Valentini, R. F. & Aebischer, P. (1993). Magnitude and Polarity of a Fluoroethylene Propylene Electret Substrate Charge Influences Neurite Outgrowth in-Vitro. *Journal of Biomedical Materials Research*, Vol. 27, No. 8, (Aug., 1993), pp. 1075-1085, ISSN 0021-9304.

Mcclary, K. B., Ugarova, T. & Grainger, D. W. (2000). Modulating fibroblast adhesion, spreading, and proliferation using self-assembled monolayer films of alkylthiolates on gold. *Biomedical Materials Research*, Vol. 50, No. 3, (Jun. 5, 2000), pp. 428-439, ISSN 0021-9304.

Miyamoto, S., Akiyama, S. K. & Yamada, K. M. (1995). Synergistic roles form receptor occupancy and aggregation in integrin transmembrane function. *Science*, Vol. 267, No. 5199, (Feb. 10, 1995), pp. 883–885.

Mosmann, T. (1983). Rapid colorimetric assay for cellular growth and survival: application to proliferation and cytotoxicity assays. *Journal of Immunological Methods*, Vol. 65, No. 1-2, (Dec. 16, 1983), pp. 55-63, ISSN 0022-1759.

Mrksich, M., Chen, C. S., Xia, Y., Dike, L. E., Ingber, D. E. & Whitesides, G. M. (1996). Controlling cell attachment on contoured surfaces with self-assembled monolayers of alkanethiolates on gold. *Proceedings of the National Academy of Sciences of the United States of America*, Vol. 93, No. 20, (Oct. 1, 1996), pp. 10775-8, ISSN 0027-8424.

Mrksich, M. & Whitesides, G. M. (1996). Using self-assembled monolayers to understand the interactions of man-made surfaces with proteins and cells. *Annual review of biophysics and biomolecular structure*, Vol. 25, No. -, (Jun., 1996), pp. 55-78, ISSN 1056-8700.

Novoselov, K. S., Schedin, F., Geim, A. K., Morozov, S. V., Hill, E. W., Blake, P. & Katsnelson, M. I. (2007). Detection of individual gas molecules adsorbed on graphene. *Nature Materials*, Vol. 6, No. 9, (Sep., 2007), pp. 652-655, ISSN 1476-1122.

Oliveros, A., Coletti, C., Frewin, C. L., Locke, C., Starke, U. & Saddow, S. E. (2011). Cellular Interactions on Epitaxial Graphene on SiC (0001) Substrates. *Material Science Forum*, Vol. 679-680, No. -, pp. 831-834.

Oliveros, A., Schoell, S. J., Frewin, C., Hoeb, M., Stutzmann, M., Sharp, I. D. & Saddow, S. E. (2009). Biocompatibility Assessment of SiC Surfaces After Functionalization with Self Assembled Organic Monolayers *Materials Research Society Symposium Proceedings*, Vol. 1235, No. -, pp. 1235-RR03-43-48.

Ostrovskaya, L., Perevertailo, V., Ralchenko, V., Saveliev, A. & Zhuravlev, V. (2007). Wettability of nanocrystalline diamond films. *Diamond and Related Materials*, Vol. 16, No. 12, (Dec., 2007), pp. 2109-2113, ISSN 0925-9635.

Ostuni, E., Yan, L. & Whitesides, G. M. (1999). The interaction of proteins and cells with self-assembled monolayers of alkanethiolates on gold and silver. *Colloids and Surfaces B-Biointerfaces*, Vol. 15, No. 1, (Aug. 31, 1999), pp. 3-30, ISSN 0927-7765.

Polikov, V. S., Tresco, P. A. & Reichert, W. M. (2005). Response of brain tissue to chronically implanted neural electrodes. *Journal of Neuroscience Methods*, Vol. 148, No. 1, (Aug. 8, 2005), pp. 1-18, ISSN 0165-0270.

Pumera, M. (2009). Electrochemistry of Graphene: New Horizons for Sensing and Energy Storage. *Chemical Record*, Vol. 9, No. 4, (Sep. 8, 2009), pp. 211-223, ISSN 1527-8999.

Reyes, M., Shishkin, Y., Harvey, S. & Saddow, S. E. (2006). Development of a high-growth rate 3C-SiC on Si CVD process. *Materials Research Society Symposium Proceedings*, Vol. 911, No. -, pp. 79–84.

Richards, R. G. (1996). The effect of surface roughness on fibroblast adhesion in vitro. *Injury*, Vol. 27 Suppl 3, No., (Jan. 1, 1996), pp. SC38-43, ISSN 0020-1383.

Riedl, C., Coletti, C., Iwasaki, T., Zakharov, A. A. & Starke, U. (2009). Quasi-Free-Standing Epitaxial Graphene on SiC Obtained by Hydrogen Intercalation. *Physical Review Letters*, Vol. 103, No. 24, (Dec. 11, 2009), pp. 1-4, ISSN 0031-9007.

Rosenbloom, A. J., Sipe, D. M., Shishkin, Y., Ke, Y., Devaty R. P. & Choyke, W. J. (2004). Nanoporus SiC: A Candidate Semi-Permeable Material for Biomedical Applications. *Biomedical Microdevices*, Vol. 6, No. 4, (Dec., 2004), pp. 261-267, ISSN 1387-2176.

Rouhi, A. M. (1999). Contemporary biomaterials. *Chemical & Engineering News*, Vol. 77, No. 3, (Jan. 18, 1999), pp. 51–63, ISSN 0009-2347.

Rousche, P. J. & Normann, R. A. (1998). Chronic recording capability of the Utah Intracortical Electrode Array in cat sensory cortex. *Journal of Neuroscience Methods*, Vol. 82, No. 1, (Jul. 1,1998), pp. 1-15, ISSN 0165-0270.

Rousche, P. J., Pellinen, D. S., Pivin, D. P., Williams, J. C., Vetter, R. J. & Kipke, D. R. (2001). Flexible polyimide-based intracortical electrode arrays with bioactive capability. *IEEE Transactions on Biomedical Engineering*, Vol. 48, No. 3, (Mar., 2001), pp. 361-371, ISSN 0018-9294.

Schoell, S. J., Hoeb, M., Sharp, I. D., Steins, W., Eickhoff, M., Stutzmann, M. & Brandt, M. S. (2008). Functionalization of 6H-SiC surfaces with organosilanes. *Applied Physics Letters*, Vol. 92, No. 15, (Apr. 14, 2008), pp. 92-94, ISSN 0003-6951.

Sharp, I. D., Schoell, S. J., Hoeb, M., Brandt, M. S. & Stutzmann, M. (2008). Electronic properties of self-assembled alkyl monolayers on Ge surfaces. *Applied Physics Letters*, Vol. 92, No. 92-94, (Jun 2, 2008), pp. -, ISSN 0003-6951.

Sklodowaka, A., Wozniak, M. & Matlakowska, R. (1999). The method of contact angle measurements and estimation of work of adhesion in bioleaching of metals. *Biological Procedures Online*, Vol. 1, No. -, (Apr. 29, 1999), pp. 114-121, ISSN 1480-9222.

Stenger, D. A., Pike, C. J., Hickman, J. J. & Cotman, C. W. (1993). Surface determinants of neuronal survival and growth on self-assembled monolayers in culture. *Brain Research*, Vol. 630, No. 1-2, (Dec. 10, 1993), pp. 136-47, ISSN 0006-8993.

Stichel, C. C. & Müller, H. W. (1998). The CNS lesion scar: new vistas on an old regeneration barrier. *Cell and Tissue Research*, Vol. 294, No. 1, (Oct., 1998), pp. 1-9, ISSN 0302-766X.

Stutzmann, M., Garrido, J. A., Eickhoff, M. & Brandt, M. S. (2006). Direct biofunctionalization of semiconductors: A survey. *Physica Status Solidi a-Applications and Materials Science*, Vol. 203, No. 14, (Nov., 2006), pp. 3424-3437, ISSN 0031-8965.

Tiefenauer, L., Sorribas, H., Braun, D., Leder, L. & Sonderegger, P. (2001). Adhesion proteins for a tight neuron-electrode contact. *Journal of Neuroscience Methods*, Vol. 104, No. 2, (Jan. 15, 2001), pp. 133-141, ISSN 0165-0270.

Tresco, P. A., Webb, K. & Hlady, V. (1998). Relative importance of surface wettability and charged functional groups on NIH 3T3 fibroblast attachment, spreading, and cytoskeletal organization. *Journal of Biomedical Materials Research*, Vol. 41, No. 3, (Sep. 5, 1998), pp. 422-430, ISSN 0021-9304.

Underwood, P. A., Steele, J. G. & Dalton, B. A. (1993). Effects of polystyrene surface chemistry on the biological activity of solid phase fibronectin and vitronectin, analyzed with monoclonal antibodies. *Journal of Cell Science*, Vol. 104, No. -, (Mar. 1, 1993), pp. 793-803, ISSN 0021-9533.

Vahlberg, C., Yazdi, G. R., Petoral Jr., R. M., Syväjärvi, M., Uvdal, K., Lloyd-Spetz, A., Yakimova, R. & Khranovsky, V. (2005). Surface engineering of functional materials for Biosensors, *Proceedings of IEEE Sensors*, ISBN 0-7803-9056-3, Irvine, CA, USA, Oct. 30-Nov. 3, 2005.

Van Damme, M., Tiglias, J., Nemat, N. & Preston, B. (1994). Determination of cell charge content at the surface of cells using a colloid titration technique. *Analytical Biochemistry*, Vol. 223, No. 1, (Nov. 15,1994), pp. 62-70, ISSN 0003-2697.

Wang, S., Zhang, Y., Abidi, N. & Cabrales, L. (2009). Wettability and surface free energy of graphene films. *Langmuir*, Vol. 25, No. 18, (Sep. 15, 2009), pp. 11078-11081, ISSN 0743-7463.

Williams, D. F. (2008). On the mechanisms of biocompatibility. *Biomaterials*, Vol. 29, No. 20, (Jul., 2008), pp. 2941-2953, ISSN 0142-9612.

Williams, J. C., Rennaker, R. L. & Kipke, D. R. (1999). Long-term neural recording characteristics of wire microelectrode arrays implanted in cerebral cortex. *Brain Research Protocols*, Vol. 4, No. 3, (Dec., 1999), pp. 303-313, ISSN 1385-299X.

Yakimova, R., Petoral, R. M., Yazdi, G. R., Vahlberg, C., Spetz, A. L. & Uvdal, K. (2007). Surface functionalization and biomedical applications based on SiC. *Journal of Physics D-Applied Physics*, Vol. 40, No. 20, (Oct. 21, 2007), pp. 6435-6442, ISSN 0022-3727.

Yang, W. R., Ratinac, K. R., Ringer, S. P., Thordarson, P., Gooding, J. J. & Braet, F. (2010). Carbon Nanomaterials in Biosensors: Should You Use Nanotubes or Graphene? *Angewandte Chemie-International Edition*, Vol. 49, No. 12, (Feb. 24, 2010), pp. 2114-2138, ISSN 1433-7851.

15

The Transversal Stiffness of Skeletal Muscle Fibers and Cardiomyocytes in Control and After Simulated Microgravity

Irina V. Ogneva and Igor B. Ushakov
State Scientific Center of Russian Federation Institute of Biomedical Problems
Russian Academy of Sciences
Russia

1. Introduction

The relevance of a problem of studying of mechanical characteristics of muscle fibers is stipulated by the huge number of diseases such as myopathies and myodystrophies leading to the significant change in activity of muscle cells. Moreover, the decreasing in functional properties of a muscle system is one of the main medical problems preventing the long-lasting space mission. The same reason complicates the course and prolongs the terms of readaptation period in some neurological and traumatological diseases.

Generally, the muscle fiber is a 3D mechanical structure in which the force transmission is performed both in longitudinal and transverse directions (Bloch & Gonzalez-Serratos, 2003). The structural features of a muscle fiber provide the efficacy of such transmission, whether the muscle fiber is a cell structure extended longitudinally with contractile apparatus formed by myofibrils and occupying the most part of cell volume. In general, the mechanical characteristics of a muscle fiber are determined by structural and functional interaction of three compartments with principally different mechanical properties: myofibrillar apparatus, extra-sarcomeric cytoskeleton (costameres) and sarcolemma with cortical cytoskeleton.

The flexible, or viscoelastic properties are generally implicated under the mechanical characteristics of one or another biological structure. In relation to a muscle fiber, the stiffness (that is analogue to the spring stiffness, in N/m) and the Young's modulus (in Pa) in both longitudinal (with deformation along the predominated axis) and transversal directions (with deformation in direction perpendicular to the main direction axis) are determined most often. Obviously, such two parameters are interconnected and are the integral parts of fiber stiffness. When measuring the longitudinal stiffness by compression-tension, the transversal structures contributes to the damping of deformation due to their own elastic properties. Similarly, in case of significant deformation in transversal direction, the contribution of the stiffness of the myofibrillar apparatus is present in the transversal stiffness value.

Atomic force microscopy (AFM) is one of the most informative methods used to obtain the information on transversal stiffness of both the myofibrillar apparatus and sarcolemma together with related costameres. The determination of characteristics is usually performed in contact mode in liquid measuring the force curves, and then using of solution of the Hertz contact problem, the Young's modulus and transverse rigidity is calculated. The fluctuation of indentation depth when evaluating the force curves allows estimation the stiffness of a complete fiber and sarcolemma as well.

1.1 Calculation of transversal stiffness and Young's modulus of a sample by force curves

Calculating the stiffness parameters of a sample using the data from atomic force microscopy is a dimensional contact problem. The contact stiffness to be calculated is the ratio of force to vertical movement. When the cantilever tip is conical, vertical movement can be determined quite easily, and the force can be calculated using the cantilever's deflection. Solving such contact problem that has many possible modifications (such as Sneddon's modification (Sneddon, 1965), Hertz contact problem (Hertz, 1882)) enables calculating the Young's modulus of the material. It should be noted that the section of the cantilever tip in most cases is not strictly conical, but rather a little rounded at the end. This is why determining the contact area of the cantilever and the sample is a key issue.

There are a number of works investigating these issues, but one of the first publications concerning mechanical properties of muscle fibers (Mathur et al., 2001) list formulas to determine the Young's modulus for different types of cantilevers that are quite correct from the mechanical point of view:

$$E = \frac{1 - v^2}{\pi} \cdot \frac{kd}{\varphi(\delta)}, \tag{1}$$

where k is cantilever stiffness, d is cantilever deflection, v is Poisson's ratio, $\varphi(\delta)$ is the function characterizing the dependency of the cantilever indentation δ on its geometrical parameters.

The stiffness of cantilever k when the probes supplied by the manufacturer have a range of stiffness values can be determined either by calibrating using a cantilever with a known stiffness by reading the force curves on a known stiff surface (e.g. glass), or calculated theoretically by measuring the resonance frequency of cantilever oscillations. Poisson's ratio v for each material is determined experimentally. In most cases, it equals 0.5 for cells. Thus, Mathur et al. (2001), believed that loss of liquid in the examined muscle fibers and endothelium cells is insignificant, and, along with a number of other researchers (Radmacher et al., 1996; Shin & Athanasiou, 1999; Weisenhorn et al., 1993), assumed that the cell is not compressible and used $v = 0.5$. Collinsworth et al. (2002) used the same value to determine the stiffness C2C12 of myoblasts in mice.

For a cantilever whose tip is conical with an axis parallel to axis z, the function $\varphi(\delta)$ may be determined as (Mathur et al., 2001):

$$\varphi(\delta) = \delta^2 \left[\frac{2\mathrm{tg}(\alpha)}{\pi^2} \right], \tag{2}$$

where δ is the indentation depth, α is half of the cone angle of the cantilever tip. The stiffness modulus is then as follows:

$$E = \frac{\pi\left(1 - v^2\right)}{2\mathrm{tg}\alpha} \cdot \frac{kd}{\delta^2}, \tag{3}$$

For a rounded cantilever, the function $\varphi(\delta)$ is as follows (Mathur et al., 2001):

$$\varphi(\delta) = \frac{2}{\pi}\left[a\delta - \frac{a^2}{2\mathrm{tg}\alpha}\left(\frac{\pi}{2} - \arcsin\left(\frac{b}{a}\right)\right) - \frac{a^3}{3R} + \sqrt{a^2 - b^2}\left(\frac{b}{2\mathrm{tg}\alpha} + \frac{a^2 - b^2}{3R}\right)\right], \tag{4}$$

where R is the rounding radius of the cantilever tip, $b = R\cos\alpha$, a is the contact radius determined from the following equation:

$$\delta + \frac{a}{R}\left(\sqrt{a^2 - b^2} - a\right) - \frac{a}{\mathrm{tg}\alpha}\left(\frac{\pi}{2} - \arcsin\left(\frac{b}{a}\right)\right) = 0. \tag{5}$$

It should be noted that the last formula or modifications thereof are most often used for calculations, assuming that the vertical section of the cantilever tip is conical. For instance, Defranchi et al. (2005) used the following formula in their research:

$$E = \frac{\sqrt{\pi}\left(1 - v^2\right)}{2} \cdot \frac{S}{\sqrt{A}}, \tag{6}$$

where S is the transversal stiffness of the sample determined as the slope of the force curve, A is the contact area.

1.2 The transversal stiffness of intact muscle fibers and sarcolemma

Mathur et al. (2001) obtained some of the first data about the mechanical properties of intact muscle fibers of the skeletal and cardiac muscle compared to endothelium cells using the AFM in liquid. The main working hypothesis of the research was that the stiffness model and viscosity of these three cell types will be different due to various structures and functional roles. Experiments were conducted using the fibers of a rabbit's cardiac muscle, C2C12 of the myoblast of adult C3H mice, and cells of the endothelium of HUVEC (Human Umbilical Venous Cord Endothelial Cell). The authors demonstrated that the stiffness modulus of endothelial cells was E=6.8±0.4 kPa near the core, E=3.3±0.2 kPa on the cell body and E=1.4±0.1 kPa near the end of the cell. Unlike the endothelium, the cardiac and skeletal muscles did not demonstrate any systematic changes of the stiffness modulus depending on the place of the contact point between the cantilever and the surface. For cardiac muscle cells, the Young's modulus was E=100.3±10.7 kPa, while for skeletal muscle cells it was E=24.7±3.5 kPa. Thus, the most rigid and, consequently, the most resisting to deformation are fibers of the cardiac muscle, which, in the opinion of the authors, is due to its constant rhythmical activity.

Defranchi et al. (2005) conducted experiments to study the structure and transversal stiffness of sarcolemma of fully differentiated muscle fibers under various conditions. The experiments were conducted with muscle fibers of skeletal muscles of CD1 mice, both in the culture and dried in the air. In order to obtain information about the sarcolemma structure, the authors used the semi-contact mode which enabled obtaining more informative images due to the lack of damage of sarcolemma by the cantilever. The authors demonstrated that AFM images show the convexity of sarcolemma (similar convexity was shown in our experiments with the soleus muscle of rat - see Fig. 2) and suggested that they are due to the presence of costamer near the Z-disk. In order to prove that, one of the costamer's proteins, α-actinin-2, was linked with fluorescent spheric antibodies 500 nm in diameter, which permits discovering them with the AFM. By comparing the optical and structural images, the authors have confirmed their hypothesis. Moreover, they have managed to see open T-tubules stretched along the Z-disks. Mechanical properties were measured in the contact mode, and the maximum forced applied to the membrane was 1 nN, while the indentation depth was between several hundred up to 1000 nm. The values of the stiffness modulus listed in the paper was E=61±5 kPa.

The data of the Defranchi et al. (2005) indicated the stiffness modulus exceed by almost 2.5 times the results of Mathur et al. (2001). This may be due to Defranchi et al. using fully differentiated cells in their research, while Mathur et al. used myoblasts. Moreover, Lieber et al. (2004) showed that old rats (30 months) had the Young's modulus of cardiac myocytes of 42.5±1.0 kPa, while younger rats (4 months) it was reliably lower, at 35.1±0.7 kPa. Such difference in the mechanical properties of muscle fibers and cardiac myocytes at different stages of development may denote that the ontogenetic development of the expression of proteins forming the structural basis of transversal stiffness is uneven. This issue was studied by Collinsworth et al. (2002). They studied the mechanical properties of muscle cells at various stages, from myocytes up to muscle fibers, and discovered significant increase of the Young's modulus on the 8th day after the differentiation began. Thus, for non-differentiated myoblasts, the stiffness modulus was E=11.5±1.3 kPa, while on the 8th to 10th day of differentiation it was E=45.3±4.0 kPa. The viscosity estimated using the hysteresis formed at the forward and backward movement of the cantilever when reading the force curves did not change during the differentiation. The authors' suggestion that changes in the stiffness modulus and the formation of tubules are related was not confirmed by experiments, because after colchicine treatment, the Young's modulus and the viscosity of muscle cells did not change. However, treatment with cytochalasin D resulted in significant reduction of the stiffness modulus, while the viscosity remained unchanged. For that reason, the authors link changes in the stiffness properties of muscle cells during differentiation with the development of the actin-myosin system. It should be noted that Collinsworth et al. did not analyze the contribution of the extra-sarcomeric cytoskeleton to the transversal stiffness of muscle fibers, although treatment with cytochalasin D could cause destruction of the cortical layer of actin filaments.

1.3 The transversal stiffness of myofibrillar apparatus

The contractile apparatus of muscle fiber has mechanical properties that are essentially different from sarcolemma linked with costameres, since it has another structure. E.g. Collinsworth et al. (2002) suggested that the biggest contribution to transversal stiffness is mainly from transversal bridges between actin and myosin filaments. The analysis of mechanical properties of myofibrillar bundles and separate myofibrils under various conditions (active and passive contraction, relaxation) may clarify this issue.

In order to obtain demembranized fibers, strong detergents like Triton-X100 are used, which destroy not only the sarcolemma but the sarcoplasmatic reticulum as well. Some myofibrils are obtained from demembranized fibers by way of homogenization.

Nyland & Maughan (2000) studied bundles of myofibrils of the flight musle of Drosophila, using rigor solution (without ATP), activating solution (pCa 4.5) and relaxing solution (pCa 8.0). The selected method of studying the mechanical properties was AFM in contact mode with indentation depth of 10 nm. The authors have obtained the following results: in rigor solution: transversal stiffness 10.3±5.0 pN/nm, Young's modulus 94±41 kPa; in the activating solution: transversal stiffness 5.9±3.1 pN/nm, Young's modulus 55±29 kPa; in the relaxing solution: transversal stiffness 4.4±2.0 pN/nm, Young's modulus: 40±17 kPa. The authors link such difference in stiffness to the transversal "flexibility" of the myosin molecule, assuming that myosin heads may be at a different angle to the actin thread which, consequently, leads to different transversal stiffness. It should be noted, however, that authors do not provide any information about the validity of differences between the obtained values of transversal stiffness and Young's modulus under different conditions.

Zhu et al. (2009) analyzed bundles of myofibrils from the left ventricle of cows. The authors have demonstrated that the transversal stiffness near the Z-disk in the relaxed state is 18±2.5 pN/nm (Young's modulus: 115±12 kPa); in the area of crossing of actin and myosin filaments: 6±1 pN/nm (52±8 kPa); in the area of M-band: 11±0.5 pN/nm (90±11 kPa). The values in the same areas in rigor state were as follows: for Z-disk: 25±2 pN/nm (98±10); in the area of crossing of actin and myosin filaments: 10±1 pN/nm (42±4 kPa); in the area of the M-band: 17±0.5 pN/nm (65±7 kPa).

Unlike Nyland & Maughan (2000) and Zhu et al. (2009), Akiyama et al. (2006) studied the structure and transversal stiffness of individual myofibrils rather than bundles cut out of muscle fibers of the cardiac and skeletal muscles of young rabbits and newborn rats. The method of study of the transversal stiffness was the same, with the difference that the indentation depth was 25-30 nm. Studies of the structure of individual myofibrils showed that they are approximately 1 μm in diameter, and the sarcomere length is about 2 μm. The transversal stiffness was studied in the relaxing and rigor solutions; the change of stiffness was monitored after myofibrils were treated with calpain and tripsin. The Z-line of myofibrils of skeletal muscles in the rigor solution was 100 nm wide and had the stiffness value of 7.7 pN/nm, while the same values for the cardiac muscle were 320 nm and 25.8 pN/nm. The stiffness of the myofibril of the cardiac muscle in rigor solution around the M-band which was about 200 nm wide was 11 pN/nm. The paper does not provide any data about the stiffness of myofibrils of skeletal muscles near the M-band, because it could not be identified using the AFM image of the surface. In the relaxing solution, the stiffness of myofibrils of skeletal muscles was quite homogeneous and was 3 pN/nm on average, versus the myofibrils of the cardiac muscle, where the stiffness varied between 4 and 11 pN/nm. Using the Hertz model, the authors have calculated the Young's modulus for individual myofibrils that was 61 kPa for skeletal muscles and 145 kPa for the cardiac muscle; in the relaxing stage, it was 5 kPa for myofibrils of skeletal muscles and 61 kPa for the cardiac muscle. In order to identify the mechanisms causing such values of transversal stiffness, the authors have treated myofibrils in the rigor stage first with calpain and then with tripsin. with calpain, the transversal stiffness of the myofibrils of the cardiac muscle near the Z-line quickly (2 or 3 minutes) fell from 21 pN/nm to 11 pN/nm, or to 2 pN/nm for the skeletal muscle, and did not change over time. Several minutes after the tripsin treatment began, the transversal stiffness of the Z-line of myofibrils of the skeletal muscle was 3 pN/nm and 12 pN/nm for the cardiac muscle, but it then continued to decrease to 5 pN/nm. The authors link this kind of change in transversal stiffness to calpain quickly destroying two main structural proteins of the Z-disk, α-actinin-2 and titin, and it occurs much faster for skeletal myofibrils than for cardiac myofibrils. Unlike calpain, tripsin first hydrolyzes titin, while α-actinin-2 is subject to a much slower degradation.

1.4 Muscle fibers under simulated microgravity

According to the few existing sources regarding the reaction of skeletal muscle cells to gravitational unloading, one of the first events is the accumulation of calcium ions demonstrated for the soleus muscle as early as after two days of antiorthostatic suspension of rear limbs of mice (Ingalls et al., 1999, 2001). In our paper, we have shown that the accumulated calcium ions in fibers of the soleus muscle rat and Mongolian gerbil peak as early as one day after the gravitational unloading, and for the medial head of the gastrocnemius muscle and tibialis anterior muscle the peak was somewhat later, on the seventh day of antiorthostatic suspension (Ogneva et al., 2009). The increase of the basal level of calcium ions may cause activation of calpains (Enns et al., 2007; Altaeva et al., 2010) and subsequent destruction of muscle fiber. However, the ways of such accumulation remain unknown. It may occur via the L-channels, but mechanically sensitive channels, such as trp-channels, may also have something to do with it. In any case, the operation of channels built into the membrane depends on the condition of sarcolemma itself and the condition of the cytoskeleton linked to it. Moreover, it can be suggested that the mechanical properties of cardiac myocytes will change in a different way compared to fibers of skeletal muscles, since the load on the cardiac muscle under the microgravity conditions increases, while the load on the skeletal muscles of hind limbs decreases.

It is difficult to directly evaluate the native condition of the cytoskeleton of muscle fibers under the membrane. But determining its mechanical properties, namely, the transversal stiffness may help in the analysis of its structural changes.

Moreover, complex sarcomeric structure of muscle fiber suggests that the transversal stiffness of various areas of sarcolemma and the contraction apparatus, namely the Z-disk, M-band and the area between them will be different. The differentiation of the stiffness values is especially interesting in connection with, for example, the signaling functions of various costamere proteins, possibly depending on its structure.

We have not been able to find any data about the scale of changes of the transversal stiffness of fibers of either skeletal or cardiac muscles under the conditions of gravitational unloading. The formation processes of the adaptation pattern of the mechanical properties of muscle fibers under the conditions of gravitational unloading should depend, first of all, on the level of nervous activation. It can be suggested that changes in the nervous activation will lead to changes in the properties of the contraction apparatus itself, which will provide an adequate response to microgravity conditions.

2. Materials and methods

The object of the research was the soleus muscle (Sol), the medial gastrocnemius muscle (MG) and the tibialis anterior muscle (TA) of rat and Mongolian gerbil, as well as the left ventriculum of rat. The rat is often used in research, unlike the gerbils who started to be used more often again due to the continued missions of Russian biosatellites in 2007 after the FOTON-3 mission (September 2007, Russia). In space biology, the Mongolian gerbil (*Meriones unguiculatus*) is used as an object of experimental research. Gerbils have a longer Henle's loop compared to other mammals, which enables nearly complete reabsorption of water in kidneys (Robinson, 1959). For this reason, gerbils are very convenient to study the effect of parameters of water-salt metabolism on the resistivity of various functions of the organism under the conditions of microgravity.

To simulate the gravitational unloading conditions in rodents, antiorthostatic suspension was used according to the Ilyin-Novikov method as amended by Morey-Holton E. et al. (2005). The duration of gravitational unloading for rat and Mongolian gerbils was 1, 3, 7 and 12/14 days. Each group contained 7 animals. The average body masses in each group of each animal were reliably similar. All procedures with animals were approved by the biomedical ethics committee of the State Scientific Center of Russia Institute of Biomedical Problems of the Russian Academy of Sciences.

2.1 Sample preparation

The skeletal muscle was cut from tendon to tendon and, for the purpose of partial destruction of the cell membrane, was treated according to the chemical skinning method described earlier in Stevens et al. (1993). Cardiac myocytes were obtained using the standard method (Zhu et al., 2009), but at first without using Triton X-100. Before the experiments, samples were stored at -20^{0}C in a buffer containing equal percentage (by volume) of relaxing solution R (20 mM MOPS, 170 mM of potassium propionate, 2.5 mM of magnesium acetate, 5 mM of K_2EGTA, 2.5 mM of ATP) and glycerol. On the day of the experiment, the samples were transferred to solution R where single glycerinated muscle fibers were singled out.

In order to obtain demembranized cells, single glycerinated muscle fibers in the R solution were incubated with the Triton X-100 detergent with the final concentration of 2% vol. within 12 hours at +4^{0}C. Such concentration of the detergent used and the long incubation time enable completely removing the membranes of muscle fibers to analyze only the myofibrillar apparatus. After treatment with the detergent, the obtained demembranized fibers were cleaned in the R solution.

In order to measure the transversal stiffness, the obtained fibers were fixed on the bottom of the liquid cell of the atomic force microscope, attaching their tips with special Fluka shellac wax-free glue (Sigma). Depending on the series of the experiments, the cell was filled either with the relaxing solution R or activating solution A (20 mM of MOPS, 172 mM of potassium propionate, 2.38 mM of magnesium acetate, 5 mM of CaEGTA, 2.5 mM of ATF), or with the rigor solution Rg (20 mM of MOPS, 170 mM of potassium propionate, 2.5 mM of magnesium acetate, 5 mM of K_2EGTA). All contractions of the fiber were isometric, since the tips of the fibers were fixed. All experiments were conducted at +16^{0}C.

2.2 Atomic force microscopy

The method of measurements has been described earlier in details (Ogneva et al., 2010). Measurements of transversal stiffness of both glycerinated and demembranized fibers were conducted using the Solver-P47-Pro™ platform (NT-MDT, Russia). The stiffness (N/m) for each cantilever was adjusted using the resonance position.

Work in the liquid was performed with soft cantilevers with the stiffness coefficient of about 0.05 N/m. The contact mode was used to obtain the image and to measure the transversal stiffness. Radius r_c of the tip of all cantilevers used was assumed to be 10 nm.

AFM images were used to estimate the length of sarcomeres and to identify the Z-disk and the M-band. The length of the sarcomere was understood as the distance between two adjacent convexities that were deemed a Z-disk.

Mechanical properties of muscle fibers were determined by first obtaining a calibration force curve on the glass to calculate the cantilever deflection conversion coefficient to convert it from the units of current into the units of length, a (m/A). Then, the force curves in the points of interest of the fiber were read, obtaining the ratio y(x), where y is the measured cantilever deviation (in A), and x is the generalized indentation depth (in m). Then, the real indentation depth of the fiber and the force applied to it were identified using the following formulae:

$$h_s = x - y \cdot a\,, \tag{7}$$

$$F_s = y \cdot a \cdot k_c\,, \tag{8}$$

where h_s is the real indentation depth (m), F_s is the real force applied to fiber (N), k_c is the cantilever stiffness coefficient (N/m).

Then, at the indentation depth of 150 nm, the change of the applied force was determined and the stiffness of the sample was determined as:

$$k_s = \frac{F_s}{h_s}\,. \tag{9}$$

Then, the curve $F_s(h_s)$ was drawn and approximated with the following dependency reflecting the solution of the Hertz contact problem for the rounded tip of the cantilever in order to discover the generalized stiffness modulus b ($N/m^{3/2}$):

$$F_s = b h_s^{\frac{3}{2}}\,. \tag{10}$$

The Young's modulus was calculated using the formula:

$$E_s = \frac{3b\left(1-\mu_s^{\,2}\right)}{4r_c^{\frac{1}{2}}}\,, \tag{11}$$

where E_s is the Young's modulus (Pa); μ_s is the Poisson's ratio. Assuming that the cell is not compressible, it is usually assumed that the Poisson's ratio is 0.5 (Collinsworth et al.,

2002; Mathur et al., 2001; Radmacher et al., 1996; Shin & Athanasiou, 1999; Weisenhorn et al., 1993). An example of such processing is provided in Figure 1.

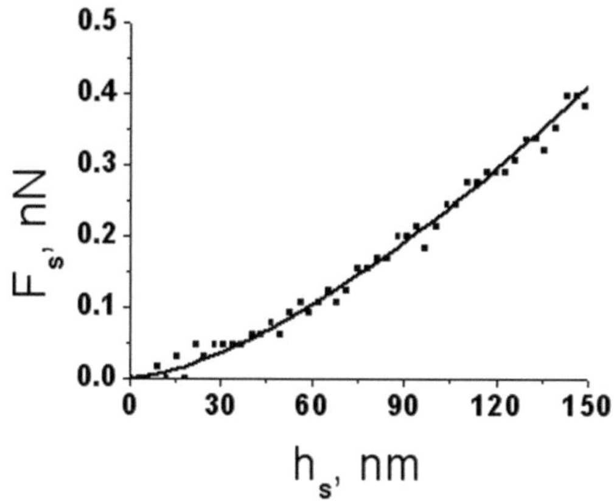

Fig. 1. Sample force-distance curve obtained at Z-disk projection on relaxed permeabilized fiber, showing a typical dependency of the applied force on the depth of indentation. Squares show experimental points, line represents the least-square fit to *Eq*. 9 (Young's modulus 38.5 kPa, apparent transversal stiffness 2.72 pN/nm at 150 nm indentation).

The above results were processed in an ad hoc program for MatLab 6.5 (The MathWorks, Natick, MA). The results obtained during the experiment were statistically processed with standard methods implemented in Microsoft Excel and Origin 6.0. The data was represented as M±m, where M is the average value of the estimated parameter and m is the standard average value error. At least 31 measurements were made to obtain each average value.

3. Results

3.1 Analysis of structure of sarcolemma surface and contractile apparatus of muscle fibers

The results in the following section 3.1 were described in details earlier (Ogneva, 2010). The analysis of striation of glycerinated muscle fibers in the relaxing solution shows that near the Z-line and the M-band the fiber is thicker compared to the surface of the semi-sarcomere, however, it is more prominent near the Z-line (Fig. 2). This kind of surface of muscle fiber near the Z-line is due to the sub-membrane structure, the costamere that links the membrane of muscle fiber and the contractile apparatus. Similarly, it can be assumed that some structure also exists near the M-band, linked to the membrane and forming a convexity similar to costamere near the Z-line.

This assumption is confirmed by the data obtained from the fiber treated with Triton, where the Z-line, M-band and semi-sarcomere surface are nearly the same in height (Fig. 3).

3.2 The transversal stiffness of skeletal muscle fibers

3.2.1 Rat

The results in the following section 3.2.1 were described in details earlier (Ogneva, 2010).

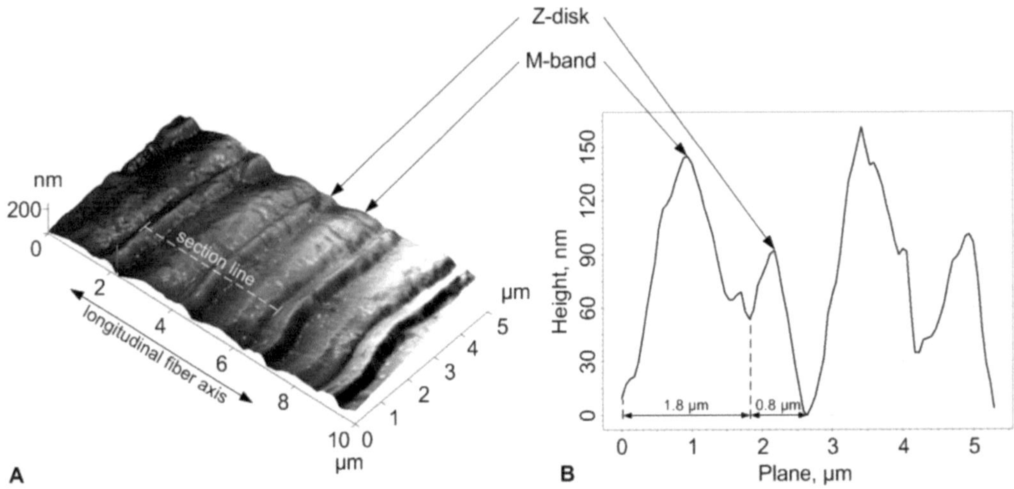

Fig. 2. 3D AFM area scan (*A*) and a surface profile (*B*) along a section line shown in *A* of a permeabilized fiber from rat soleus muscle in relaxed state. There two kinds of humps on a surface profile. One of them correspond to the A-bands (1.8 µm in length) with the M-bands in the middle. Other humps correspond to the I-bands (0.8 µm in length) with the Z-disks in the middle. (Ogneva, 2010)

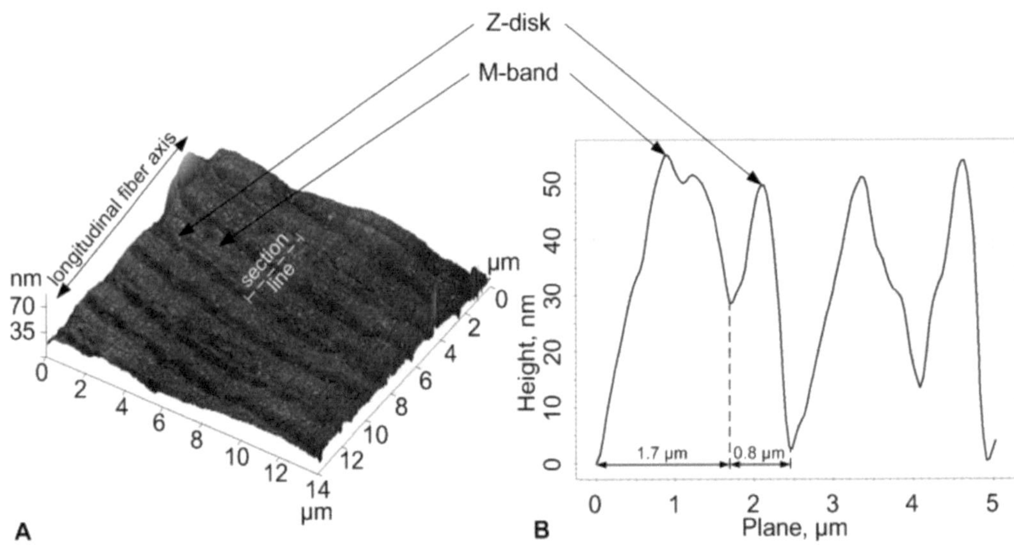

Fig. 3. 3D AFM area scan (A) and a surface profile (B) along a section line of Triton-treated muscle fiber in relaxed state. After Triton X-100 treatment the height of the Z-disk and M-band humps decreases compared to those in Fig. 2. (Ogneva, 2010)

3.2.1.1 Sol

The changes of transversal stiffness at various are as of the contractile apparatus in the course of gravitational unloading is provided in Table 1. In the control group, the transversal stiffness of the contractile apparatus of fibers of the soleus muscle near the semi-sarcomere, i.e. between the Z-disk and the M-band increases in the sequence relaxation-activation-rigor. The increase of this parameter is reliable both from relaxation to activation and from activation to rigor. This situation does not change after one day of gravitational unloading. However, in three days, the stiffness of the contractile apparatus reliably decreases near the semi-sarcomere both in the relaxed and in the activated/rigor states compared to similar states in the control group. This decrease is even more prominent seven days after antiorthostatic suspension. The minimum stiffness value compared to the control level is reached 12 days after the gravitational unloading. Nevertheless, after three, seven and twelve days of suspension, the stiffness of the semi-sarcomere when contraction is activated does reliably increase, just like in the rigor state compared to the activated calcium.

State / Group	Relaxed	Activated (pCa=4.2)	Rigor
Transversal stiffness of the half-sarcomere area $k_{\perp ca}$			
Control	2.92±0.16	5.30±0.11$^{@}$	7.22±0.13$^{@/\$}$
1-HS	2.79±0.17	5.44±0.21$^{@}$	6.98±0.17$^{@/\$}$
3-HS	1.90±0.10*	2.84±0.22$^{*/@}$	5.55±0.29$^{*/@/\$}$
7-HS	1.35±0.12*	2.10±0.15$^{*/@}$	4.35±0.21$^{*/@/\$}$
12-HS	0.93±0.14*	1.92±0.12$^{*/@}$	3.42±0.17$^{*/@/\$}$
Transversal stiffness of the M-band area $k_{\perp Ml}$			
Control	3.68±0.09	7.91±0.29$^{@}$	10.32±0.17$^{@/\$}$
1-HS	3.46±0.11	7.23±0.29$^{@}$	9.6±0.3$^{@/\$}$
3-HS	3.01±0.20*	4.1±0.1$^{*/@}$	7.27±0.28$^{*/@/\$}$
7-HS	2.95±0.29*	3.80±0.21$^{*/@}$	6.02±0.27$^{*/@/\$}$
12-HS	1.82±0.13*	2.80±0.21$^{*/@}$	5.3±0.3$^{*/@/\$}$
Transversal stiffness of the Z-disk area $k_{\perp Zd}$			
Control	8.21±0.23	11.27±0.27$^{@}$	12.92±0.23$^{@/\$}$
1-HS	7.82±0.11	11.10±0.23$^{@}$	10.83±0.17$^{@/\$}$
3-HS	3.22±0.15*	7.24±0.13$^{*/@}$	8.42±0.15$^{*/@/\$}$
7-HS	2.48±0.17*	4.31±0.23$^{*/@}$	5.29±0.13$^{*/@/\$}$
12-HS	2.12±0.09*	3.45±0.23$^{*/@}$	4.63±0.15$^{*/@/\$}$

Table 1. Transversal stiffness (pN/nm) of isolated rat's Triton-treated *Sol* muscle fibers in liquid in relaxed, calcium activated (pCa=4.2) and rigor states under gravitational unloading. * - $p<0.05$ as compared to the analogous state of the group «Control», $^{@}$ - $p<0.05$ as compared to the relaxed state at the same group, $^{\$}$ - $p<0.05$ as compared to the activated state at the same group. (Ogneva, 2010)

Near the M-band, the stiffness of the contractile apparatus of fibers of the soleus muscle is higher than the stiffness of the semi-sarcomere. The trends of gravitational unloading described for the area of the semi-sarcomere are also valid for the M-band, although its stiffness in activation and rigor stages does not increase as much as in the semi-sarcomere.

The transversal stiffness of the Z-disk is significantly higher than in the semi-sarcomere and the M-band. It also, just like described above, increases during activation and rigor, although less intensively. Furthermore, the changes of the transversal stiffness of the Z-disk in the course of gravitational unloading are the same as after three days of suspension. However, these changes are much more prominent than in the area of the semi-sarcomere and the M-band.

The transversal stiffness of various segments of glycerynized fibers of the soleus muscle of rat (Table 2) in the control group increases during the activation of contraction compared to the relaxed state and when transitioning to rigor compared to the activated state. However, the intensity of this increase is not as significant as in demembranated fiber, which is especially prominent when the stiffness of sarcolemma slightly increases between the projections of the Z-disk and M-band when contraction is activated compared to the increase of stiffness near the semi-sarcomere in a similar situation. It should be noted that in the relaxed state, the stiffness of this part of sarcolemma and the semi-sarcomere are comparable. When contraction is activated, the stiffness of sarcolemma in the projections of the Z-disk and M-band are increased more considerably; moreover, in the relaxed state, the stiffness values of this type of muscle fiber is significantly lower than of the Z-disk and M-band of the contraction apparatus.

State / Group	Relaxed	Activated (pCa=4.2)	Rigor
Transversal stiffness of sarcolemma between the M-band and Z-disk projections $k_{\perp s}$			
Control	3.05±0.03	3.19±0.06@	3.6±0.09@/$
1-HS	1.25±0.07*	1.38±0.09*	1.49±0.08*/@
3-HS	0.78±0.08*	0.87±0.12*	0.99±0.13*
7-HS	0.43±0.06*	0.54±0.04*	0.56±0.04*
12-HS	0.84±0.08*	1.01±0.14*	0.91±0.06*
Transversal stiffness of sarcolemma at the M-band projection $k_{\perp Mls}$			
Control	1.98±0.07	2.65±0.14@	3.02±0.11@/$
1-HS	1.89±0.11*	2.5±0.3*/@	3.09±0.15*/@/$
3-HS	1.77±0.08*	2.16±0.11*/@	2.68±0.14*/@
7-HS	1.05±0.12*	1.16±0.16*	1.38±0.17*
12-HS	1.08±0.09*	1.48±0.17*/@	1.92±0.16*/@/$
Transversal stiffness of sarcolemma at the Z-disk projection $k_{\perp Zds}$			
Control	3.08±0.14	3.42±0.21@	3.92±0.13@/$
1-HS	2.21±0.22*	2.84±0.16*/@	3.13±0.21*/@
3-HS	1.13±0.12*	1.53±0.14*/@	1.93±0.18*/@
7-HS	0.91±0.05*	1.21±0.11*/@	1.31±0.09*/@
12-HS	1.32±0.12*	1.83±0.13*/@	2.01±0.12*/@

Table 2. Transversal stiffness (pN/nm) of isolated rat's permeabilized *Sol* muscle fibers in liquid in relaxed, calcium activated (pCa=4.2) and rigor states under gravitational unloading. * - p<0.05 as compared to the analogous state of the group «Control», @ - p<0.05 as compared to the relaxed state at the same group, $ - p<0.05 as compared to the activated state at the same group. (Ogneva, 2010)

After one day of gravitational unloading, the stiffness of all parts of sarcolemma both in the relaxed and activated state is decreased compared to the similar state in the control group, reaching the minimum after seven days of suspension and tending to increase by the twelfth day of gravitational unloading. However, when the contraction is activated and in rigor the stiffness of sarcolemma between the projections of the Z-disk and the M-band is reliably similar as early as after one day of gravitational unloading. A similar situation may take place up to the twelfth day of antiorthostatic suspension. The transversal stiffness of the sarcolemma in the area of the projection of the Z-disk and the M-band is increased when the contraction is activated during the gravitational unloading, although not as significantly as in the control group.

3.2.1.2 MG

The transversal stiffness of various areas of the contractile apparatus of fibers of the medial gastrocnemius muscle (Table 3) is almost twice as low as the same values for fibers of the soleus muscle in the relaxed, activated and rigor states. However, the increase of transversal stiffness in the sequence semi-sarcomere - M-band - Z-disk takes places just like in the fibers of the soleus muscle.

State / Group	Relaxed	Activated (pCa=4.2)	Rigor
Transversal stiffness of the half-sarcomere area $k_{\perp ca}$			
Control	1.56±0.16	2.25±0.18$^{@}$	3.43±0.23$^{@/\$}$
1-HS	2.80±0.13*	3.65±0.29$^{*/@}$	4.17±0.22$^{*/@/\$}$
3-HS	2.38±0.14*	2.90±0.17$^{@}$	3.57±0.19$^{@/\$}$
7-HS	2.07±0.12	2.46±0.15$^{@}$	3.47±0.24$^{@/\$}$
12-HS	1.65±0.06	2.56±0.12$^{@}$	3.42±0.20$^{@/\$}$
Transversal stiffness of the M-band area $k_{\perp Ml}$			
Control	2.54±0.16	3.74±0.19$^{@}$	4.80±0.27$^{@/\$}$
1-HS	4.12±0.21*	5.08±0.24$^{*/@}$	6.52±0.19$^{*/@/\$}$
3-HS	2.98±0.25	3.60±0.15$^{@}$	5.69±0.13$^{@/\$}$
7-HS	2.72±0.14	3.39±0.26$^{@}$	5.50±0.28$^{@/\$}$
12-HS	2.22±0.18	3.47±0.14$^{@}$	6.01±0.26$^{@/\$}$
Transversal stiffness of the Z-disk area $k_{\perp Zd}$			
Control	3.87±0.29	5.94±0.22$^{@}$	7.54±0.24$^{@/\$}$
1-HS	5.7±0.3*	7.7±0.4$^{*/@}$	9.7±0.5$^{*/@/\$}$
3-HS	4.9±0.5*	6.8±0.4$^{*/@}$	8.0±0.6$^{@/\$}$
7-HS	3.80±0.14	5.5±0.6$^{@}$	7.3±0.3$^{@/\$}$
12-HS	3.51±0.19	5.7±0.6$^{@}$	7.2±0.5$^{@/\$}$

Table 3. Transversal stiffness (pN/nm) of isolated rat's Triton-treated *MG* muscle fibers in liquid in relaxed, calcium activated (pCa=4.2) and rigor states under gravitational unloading. * - p<0.05 as compared to the analogous state of the group «Control», $^{@}$ - p<0.05 as compared to the relaxed state at the same group, $^{\$}$ - p<0.05 as compared to the activated state at the same group. (Ogneva, 2010)

During the gravitational unloading, except early stages, the transversal stiffness values of the semi-sarcomere, Z-disk and M-band do not show any reliable changes in all of the studied states. At early stages (one day and three days), there is a reliable increase of the transversal stiffness of the semi-sarcomere and the Z-disk, which is more pronounced during the first day of suspension. Moreover, the increase of transversal stiffness of the M-band takes place only during the first day.

Unlike the contractile apparatus, the transversal stiffness of the sarcolemma (Table 4) in the area between the projections of the Z-disk and the M-band starts to decrease as early as after one day of gravitational unloading and continues to decrease during the whole suspension period. The stiffness of the sarcolemma during activation and rigor increases in the control group after one day of functional unloading, but after three days, there are no changes in the stiffness of this segment of the sarcolemma when contraction is activated and when transitioning to the rigor state compared to the stiffness in the relaxed state. The transversal stiffness of the sarcolemma in the M-band projection increases during the first day of gravitational unloading both in the relaxed and in the activated state compared to the fibers of the control group in a similar state, although there are no reliable differences between the relaxed and activated state. Seven days after the unloading, the stiffness values in different states are not different from the control group. A similar situation occurs in sarcolemma in the area of the Z-disk projection. However, after 12 days of suspension, the transversal stiffness of this part of sarcolemma reliably decreases compared to the control group.

State / Group	Relaxed	Activated (pCa=4.2)	Rigor
Transversal stiffness of sarcolemma between the M-band and Z-disk projections $k_{\perp s}$			
Control	2.87±0.12	3.01±0.21@	3.26±0.14@/$
1-HS	2.21±0.08*	2.38±0.09*/@	2.69±0.24*/@
3-HS	2.12±0.10*	2.34±0.17*	2.27±0.14*
7-HS	1.91±0.09*	2.11±0.11*	2.32±0.11*
12-HS	2.11±0.13*	2.29±0.18*	2.08±0.13*
Transversal stiffness of sarcolemma at the M-band projection $k_{\perp MIs}$			
Control	1.53±0.07	1.87±0.13@	2.21±0.16@/$
1-HS	2.12±0.09*	2.31±0.14*	2.55±0.13*/@
3-HS	1.75±0.15	1.95±0.14*	2.43±0.13*/@/$
7-HS	1.57±0.09	1.73±0.11@	2.13±0.16@/$
12-HS	1.26±0.12	1.64±0.11@	2.01±0.19@/$
Transversal stiffness of sarcolemma at the Z-disk projection $k_{\perp Zds}$			
Control	2.24±0.18	2.74±0.25@	3.17±0.14@/$
1-HS	2.91±0.11*	3.12±0.19*	3.47±0.26*/@
3-HS	2.69±0.27	3.14±0.21@	3.38±0.13@
7-HS	2.25±0.13	2.7±0.3@	3.12±0.21@
12-HS	1.84±0.08*	2.17±0.26*	2.35±0.19*

Table 4. Transversal stiffness (pN/nm) of isolated rat's permeabilized *MG* muscle fibers in liquid in relaxed, calcium activated (pCa=4.2) and rigor states under gravitational unloading. * - $p<0.05$ as compared to the analogous state of the group «Control», @ - $p<0.05$ as compared to the relaxed state at the same group, $ - $p<0.05$ as compared to the activated state at the same group. (Ogneva, 2010)

3.2.1.3 TA

The transversal stiffness of various segments of the contractile apparatus of fibers of the tibialis anterior muscle (Table 5) when activating the contraction and transitioning to the rigor state changes just like that of the soleus muscle in the control group.

State / Group	Relaxed	Activated (pCa=4.2)	Rigor
Transversal stiffness of the half-sarcomere area $k_{\perp ca}$			
Control	2.13±0.18	4.12±0.26$^{@}$	5.1±0.3$^{@/\$}$
1-HS	4.37±0.27*	5.7±0.3$^{*/@}$	7.4±0.3$^{*/@/\$}$
3-HS	3.87±0.11*	5.22±0.28$^{*/@}$	6.2±0.4$^{*/@/\$}$
7-HS	3.33±0.08*	5.24±0.26$^{*/@}$	6.02±0.21$^{*/@/\$}$
12-HS	2.93±0.07*	5.11±0.22$^{*/@}$	6.13±0.29$^{*/@/\$}$
Transversal stiffness of the M-band area $k_{\perp Ml}$			
Control	2.23±0.27	6.3±0.4$^{@}$	7.7±0.4$^{@/\$}$
1-HS	5.25±0.21*	8.4±0.6$^{*/@}$	11.6±0.5$^{*/@/\$}$
3-HS	4.41±0.29*	7.90±0.24$^{*/@}$	8.63±0.29$^{*/@/\$}$
7-HS	3.93±0.28*	7.15±0.26$^{*/@}$	8.42±0.28$^{*/@/\$}$
12-HS	3.23±0.25*	7.48±0.29$^{*/@}$	8.9±0.4$^{*/@/\$}$
Transversal stiffness of the Z-disk area $k_{\perp Zd}$			
Control	6.52±0.23	8.9±0.6$^{@}$	10.6±0.7$^{@/\$}$
1-HS	8.1±0.5*	10.3±0.3$^{*/@}$	14.7±0.5$^{*/@/\$}$
3-HS	8.2±0.4*	9.7±0.7$^{*/@}$	11.8±0.6$^{*/@/\$}$
7-HS	7.7±0.4	9.5±0.4$^{@}$	11.4±0.3$^{@/\$}$
12-HS	6.9±0.5	9.2±0.5$^{@}$	11.5±0.3$^{@/\$}$

Table 5. Transversal stiffness (pN/nm) of isolated rat's Triton-treated *TA* muscle fibers in liquid in relaxed, calcium activated (pCa=4.2) and rigor states under gravitational unloading. * - p<0.05 as compared to the analogous state of the group «Control», $^{@}$ - p<0.05 as compared to the relaxed state at the same group, $^{\$}$ - p<0.05 as compared to the activated state at the same group. (Ogneva, 2010)

However, after one day of gravitational unloading, the transversal stiffness near the semi-sarcomere significantly increases and then starts decreasing, although it fails to reach the control group values and still remains increased by the twelfth day, not only in the relaxed, but in the activated and rigor state as well. A similar situation is observed at the M-band of the contractile apparatus. The stiffness of the Z-disk exceeds the control level after one day and after three days of gravitational disuse, but by the seventh day the values are practically not different from the control values.

The transversal stiffness of the sarcolemma (Table 6) between the Z-disk and M-band projections does not change when contraction is activated and in rigor, unlike the soleus muscle. In the course of gravitational unloading, the stiffness of this part of sarcolemma reliably decreases one day after the antiorthostatic suspension, returning to the control value after 7 days of gravitational unloading. At the same time, the transversal stiffness of the sarcolemma at the M-band projection does not change during the suspension, although there is no difference between the values in the activated and rigor states. The increase of the transversal stiffness of the sarcolemma at the Z-disk projection is observed after three and seven days of functional unloading, while by the twelfth day the values return to the control level.

State / Group	Relaxed	Activated (pCa=4.2)	Rigor
Transversal stiffness of sarcolemma between the M-band and Z-disk projections $k_{\perp s}$			
Control	3.56±0.28	3.21±0.21	3.19±0.20
1-HS	2.46±0.13*	2.31±0.11*	2.26±0.14*
3-HS	2.86±0.27	2.93±0.26	3.01±0.16
7-HS	3.95±0.18	4.01±0.12	3.84±0.19
12-HS	4.03±0.21	3.58±0.17	3.64±0.16
Transversal stiffness of sarcolemma at the M-band projection $k_{\perp MIs}$			
Control	1.43±0.26	2.45±0.25@	2.78±0.09@
1-HS	2.14±0.27	2.55±0.3@	2.98±0.14@
3-HS	2.21±0.19	2.83±0.27@	3.04±0.23@
7-HS	2.18±0.23	2.93±0.29@	3.17±0.28@
12-HS	2.01±0.18	3.14±0.21@	3.25±0.22@
Transversal stiffness of sarcolemma at the Z-disk projection $k_{\perp Zds}$			
Control	2.98±0.29	3.47±0.23	3.71±0.13@
1-HS	3.45±0.26	3.76±0.25	4.13±0.18@
3-HS	3.81±0.24*	4.31±0.23*	4.41±0.28*
7-HS	3.71±0.27*	4.14±0.23*	4.28±0.18*
12-HS	3.37±0.26	3.88±0.25	4.12±0.24

Table 6. Transversal stiffness (pN/nm) of isolated rat's permeabilized *TA* muscle fibers in liquid in relaxed, calcium activated (pCa=4.2) and rigor states under gravitational unloading. * - $p<0.05$ as compared to the analogous state of the group «Control», @ - $p<0.05$ as compared to the relaxed state at the same group, $ - $p<0.05$ as compared to the activated state at the same group. (Ogneva, 2010)

3.2.2 Mongolian gerbil

3.2.2.1 Sol

Changes of the transversal stiffness of the contractile apparatus (Table 7) are similar to those of rat, but occur on the seventh, rather than on the third day of gravitational unloading. The reduction of stiffness of the contractile apparatus occurs in sync between all of its segments, but just like in rats, it is more prominent at the Z-disk. The trend of increasing stiffness as a result of activation of contraction and rigor persists at all stages of the gravitational unloading. At the same time, the depth of stiffness changes in Mongloian gerbil is not as considerable as in rats.

Group \ State	Relaxed	Activated (pCa=4.2)	Rigor
Transversal stiffness of the half-sarcomere area $k_{\perp ca}$			
Control	2.3±0.4	5.5±0.7$^{@}$	7.8±0.4$^{@/\$}$
1-HS	2.40±0.15	5.2±0.3$^{@}$	7.6±0.5$^{@/\$}$
3-HS	2.21±0.18	4.8±0.5$^{@}$	6.5±0.3$^{@/\$}$
7-HS	1.53±0.14*	3.6±0.5$^{*/@}$	4.3±0.3$^{*/@/\$}$
12-HS	1.18±0.04*	2.30±0.13$^{*/@}$	2.61±0.12$^{*/@/\$}$
Transversal stiffness of the M-band area $k_{\perp Ml}$			
Control	4.6±0.6	7.8±0.6$^{@}$	12.6±0.6$^{@/\$}$
1-HS	4.5±0.7	7.1±0.6$^{@}$	11.3±0.7$^{@/\$}$
3-HS	4.7±0.5	6.5±0.3$^{@}$	9.4±0.8$^{@/\$}$
7-HS	2.96±0.25*	5.2±0.4$^{*/@}$	6.3±0.7$^{*/@/\$}$
12-HS	1.9±0.3*	2.50±0.27$^{*/@}$	3.8±0.4$^{*/@/\$}$
Transversal stiffness of the Z-disk area $k_{\perp Zd}$			
Control	7.4±0.9	11.4±1.5$^{@}$	15.4±0.9$^{@/\$}$
1-HS	7.1±0.6	10.8±0.4$^{@}$	13.3±2.1$^{@/\$}$
3-HS	6.3±0.5	9.2±0.8$^{@}$	13.6±1.8$^{@/\$}$
7-HS	3.15±0.29*	5.2±0.6$^{*/@}$	7.0±0.6$^{*/@/\$}$
12-HS	2.6±0.3*	3.6±0.4$^{*/@}$	4.2±0.5$^{*/@/\$}$

Table 7. Transversal stiffness (pN/nm) of isolated gerbil's Triton-treated *Sol* muscle fibers in liquid in relaxed, calcium activated (pCa=4.2) and rigor states under gravitational unloading. * - $p<0.05$ as compared to the analogous state of the group «Control», $^{@}$ - $p<0.05$ as compared to the relaxed state at the same group, $^{\$}$ - $p<0.05$ as compared to the activated state at the same group.

The transversal stiffness of various segments of the sarcolemma (Table 8) of fibers of the soleus muscle of the Mongolian gerbil changes much earlier than the transversal stiffness of the contractile apparatus, one day after the gravitational unloading begins. Furthermore, while the effect of increased stiffness of the sarcolemma at the Z-disk projection and M-band in case of activation of contraction remains for the control group after one day of suspension, subsequently, with increased duration of hypokinesia, this trend was not observed.

3.2.2.2 MG

Changes in the transversal stiffness of some segments of the contractile apparatus of fibers of the gastrocnemius muscle of the Mongolian gerbil (Table 9) are similar to those of rats, but are considerably less prominent, although reliable. Thus, the increase of stiffness of the contractile apparatus between the Z-disk and the M-band occurs one day after the gravitational unloading, just like in rats. However, in rats, this parameter returns to the control value by the seventh day of suspension, but as early as by the third day in gerbils. Increase of stiffness of the Z-disk and the M-band is also reliable only in the first day of hypokinesia, while on the third day the transversal stiffness is not different from the control value.

Group \ State	Relaxed	Activated (pCa=4.2)	Rigor
Transversal stiffness of sarcolemma between the M-band and Z-disk projections $k_{\perp s}$			
Control	1.82±0.08	1.83±0.11	1.94±0.13
1-HS	1.34±0.09*	1.47±0.25*	1.33±0.21*
3-HS	0.98±0.08*	1.06±0.22*	1.01±0.25*
7-HS	0.76±0.08*	0.81±0.19*	0.95±0.21*
12-HS	0.13±0.14*	0.15±0.08*	0.13±0.21*
Transversal stiffness of sarcolemma at the M-band projection $k_{\perp Mls}$			
Control	1.76±0.11	2.13±0.12@	2.42±0.11@/$
1-HS	1.79±0.13	2.05±0.23	2.35±0.17@
3-HS	1.47±0.15*	1.59±0.21*	1.68±0.15*
7-HS	1.29±0.15*	1.62±0.22*	1.76±0.24*
12-HS	0.39±0.03*	0.41±0.04*	0.43±0.03*
Transversal stiffness of sarcolemma at the Z-disk projection $k_{\perp Zds}$			
Control	2.39±0.18	2.76±0.14@	3.12±0.12@/$
1-HS	2.01±0.12*	2.32±0.13@	2.53±0.16*/@
3-HS	1.53±0.29*	1.72±0.23*	1.87±0.19*
7-HS	1.63±0.23*	2.01±0.22*	2.34±0.24*
12-HS	0.49±0.06*	0.55±0.07*	0.52±0.07*

Table 8. Transversal stiffness (pN/nm) of isolated gerbil's permeabilized *Sol* muscle fibers in liquid in relaxed, calcium activated (pCa=4.2) and rigor states under gravitational unloading. * - $p<0.05$ as compared to the analogous state of the group «Control», @ - $p<0.05$ as compared to the relaxed state at the same group, $ - $p<0.05$ as compared to the activated state at the same group.

Group \ State	Relaxed	Activated (pCa=4.2)	Rigor
Transversal stiffness of the half-sarcomere area $k_{\perp ca}$			
Control	1.67±0.14	2.35±0.19@	4.5±0.3@/$
1-HS	2.71±0.15*	3.32±0.26*/@	5.7±0.4*/@/$
3-HS	2.04±0.21	3.09±0.27@	5.03±0.24@/$
7-HS	1.64±0.13	2.84±0.27@	4.9±0.3@/$
12-HS	1.42±0.22	2.41±0.22@	4.76±0.18@/$
Transversal stiffness of the M-band area $k_{\perp Ml}$			
Control	2.68±0.24	3.6±0.3@	5.4±0.3@/$
1-HS	4.11±0.14*	4.93±0.29*/@	6.10±0.29*/@/$
3-HS	2.64±0.28	3.64±0.26@	5.70±0.23@/$
7-HS	2.60±0.27	3.81±0.23@	5.40±0.27@/$
12-HS	2.4±0.3	3.92±0.27@	5.19±0.29@/$
Transversal stiffness of the Z-disk area $k_{\perp Zd}$			
Control	4.03±0.23	6.1±0.3@	9.5±0.4@/$
1-HS	5.4±0.6*	7.04±0.27@	11.3±0.7@/$

Group \ State	Relaxed	Activated (pCa=4.2)	Rigor
3-HS	5.11±0.29	6.3±0.3$^{@}$	8.9±0.5$^{@/\$}$
7-HS	4.4±0.4	5.9±0.6$^{@}$	9.7±0.6$^{@/\$}$
12-HS	4.3±0.3	6.20±0.29$^{@}$	9.3±0.5$^{@/\$}$

Table 9. Transversal stiffness (pN/nm) of isolated gerbil's Triton-treated *MG* muscle fibers in liquid in relaxed, calcium activated (pCa=4.2) and rigor states under gravitational unloading. * - p<0.05 as compared to the analogous state of the group «Control», $^{@}$ - p<0.05 as compared to the relaxed state at the same group, $^{\$}$ - p<0.05 as compared to the activated state at the same group.

The transversal stiffness of the sarcolemma (Table 10) between the Z-disk and M-band projections is only decreased relative to the control level during the first day of unloading, but does not differ from the control values afterwards. An increase of the transversal stiffness is observed from the first up to the seventh day of unloading near the sarcolemma at the Z-disk projection in Mongolian gerbils, unlike in rats; there were no significant changes at the M-band at any stage of suspension. Furthermore, the transversal stiffness of the sarcolemma at the Z-disk projection reliably increases by the activation compared to the relaxed state within the unloading of any studied length, while after seven days of suspension a difference between the activated and rigor state is also observed.

Group \ State	Relaxed	Activated (pCa=4.2)	Rigor
Transversal stiffness of sarcolemma between the M-band and Z-disk projections $k_{\perp s}$			
Control	1.54±0.21	1.60±0.11	1.79±0.13
1-HS	1.08±0.09*	1.29±0.08*$^{/@}$	1.51±0.12*$^{/@/\$}$
3-HS	1.43±0.15	1.63±0.13	1.71±0.19
7-HS	1.34±0.14	1.45±0.09	1.52±0.11
12-HS	1.13±0.17	1.28±0.13	1.39±0.19
Transversal stiffness of sarcolemma at the M-band projection $k_{\perp Mls}$			
Control	1.33±0.13	1.62±0.12$^{@}$	1.84±0.15$^{@}$
1-HS	1.39±0.21	1.41±0.13	1.52±0.19
3-HS	1.53±0.11	1.71±0.12	1.95±0.15
7-HS	1.34±0.15	1.53±0.12	1.88±0.16
12-HS	1.02±0.11	1.17±0.08	1.32±0.12
Transversal stiffness of sarcolemma at the Z-disk projection $k_{\perp Zds}$			
Control	1.86±0.11	2.27±0.09$^{@}$	2.62±0.07$^{@/\$}$
1-HS	2.11±0.09*	2.44±0.13$^{@}$	2.68±0.19$^{@}$
3-HS	2.48±0.11*	2.91±0.12*$^{/@}$	3.12±0.09*$^{/@}$
7-HS	2.15±0.14*	2.61±0.18$^{@}$	2.89±0.19$^{@/\$}$
12-HS	1.71±0.11	2.05±0.07$^{@}$	2.31±0.09$^{@/\$}$

Table 10. Transversal stiffness (pN/nm) of isolated gerbil's permeabilized *MG* muscle fibers in liquid in relaxed, calcium activated (pCa=4.2) and rigor states under gravitational unloading. * - p<0.05 as compared to the analogous state of the group «Control», $^{@}$ - p<0.05 as compared to the relaxed state at the same group, $^{\$}$ - p<0.05 as compared to the activated state at the same group.

3.2.2.3 TA

The values of transversal stiffness of various parts of the contractile apparatus of fibers of the tibialis anterior muscle of the Mongolian gerbil (Table 11) are practically the same as those of rat (Table 5). The changes appearing during the gravitational unloading, just like for the soleus muscle and the medial gastrocnemius muscle, are not so prominent and are smoothed faster. The increase of stiffness of the contractile apparatus between the Z-disk and the M-band observed after one day of gravitational unloading begins to decrease by the third day, and the value of the parameter in question is the same as the control value 12 days after the suspension begins. Similar differences in the unloading trends are observed at the Z-disk, however, its transversal stiffness differs from the control group only in the relaxed state, while after the activation of contraction and in rigor there are no reliable differences compared to the control values in similar states. The transversal stiffness of the M-band, unlike the area of the semi-sarcomere and Z-disk, increases compared to the control value one day after the gravitational unloading begins, but the differences disappear after three days.

The transversal stiffness of the sarcolemma (Table 12) changes similarly to changes in the stiffness of the contractile apparatus. However, there are no changes in the transversal stiffness of the segment of the membrane between the projections of the Z-disk and the

Group \ State	Relaxed	Activated (pCa=4.2)	Rigor
Transversal stiffness of the half-sarcomere area $k_{\perp ca}$			
Control	2.56±0.22	3.90±0.26$^{@}$	5.7±0.3$^{@/\$}$
1-HS	4.52±0.26*	5.50±0.28$^{*/@}$	9.6±0.5$^{*/@/\$}$
3-HS	3.40±0.21*	5.06±0.23$^{*/@}$	8.1±0.5$^{*/@/\$}$
7-HS	3.26±0.26*	4.12±0.14$^{@}$	7.7±0.3$^{*/@/\$}$
12-HS	2.94±0.20	4.01±0.28$^{@}$	6.9±0.5$^{@/\$}$
Transversal stiffness of the M-band area $k_{\perp Ml}$			
Control	2.8±0.6	6.4±0.3$^{@}$	8.1±0.5$^{@/\$}$
1-HS	4.7±0.4*	8.1±0.4$^{*/@}$	11.9±0.4$^{*/@/\$}$
3-HS	3.3±0.4	7.78±0.29$^{@}$	9.6±0.5$^{@/\$}$
7-HS	3.1±0.3	7.32±0.25$^{@}$	8.5±0.5$^{@/\$}$
12-HS	2.8±0.3	6.70±0.20$^{@}$	8.4±0.6$^{@/\$}$
Transversal stiffness of the Z-disk area $k_{\perp Zd}$			
Control	5.9±0.3	8.3±0.9$^{@}$	12.6±0.5$^{@/\$}$
1-HS	8.3±0.5*	10.9±0.5$^{*/@}$	14.6±0.8$^{*/@/\$}$
3-HS	7.9±0.4*	9.8±0.5$^{@}$	13.8±0.8$^{@/\$}$
7-HS	7.6±0.3*	9.2±0.5$^{@}$	12.6±0.7$^{@/\$}$
12-HS	7.1±0.4*	8.6±0.4$^{@}$	12.9±0.9$^{@/\$}$

Table 11. Transversal stiffness (pN/nm) of isolated gerbil's Triton-treated *TA* muscle fibers in liquid in relaxed, calcium activated (pCa=4.2) and rigor states under gravitational unloading. * - p<0.05 as compared to the analogous state of the group «Control», @ - p<0.05 as compared to the relaxed state at the same group, $ - p<0.05 as compared to the activated state at the same group.

State / Group	Relaxed	Activated (pCa=4.2)	Rigor
Transversal stiffness of sarcolemma between the M-band and Z-disk projections $k_{\perp s}$			
Control	2.51±0.08	2.32±0.09	2.68±0.17
1-HS	2.11±0.12*	1.94±0.11*	2.06±0.17*
3-HS	2.01±0.13*	1.72±0.19*	1.45±0.27*
7-HS	2.15±0.19	1.76±0.23	1.81±0.26
12-HS	2.18±0.12	1.94±0.11	2.01±0.18
Transversal stiffness of sarcolemma at the M-band projection $k_{\perp MIs}$			
Control	1.61±0.17	2.45±0.11$^{@}$	2.63±0.22$^{@}$
1-HS	2.11±0.08*	2.62±0.17$^{@}$	2.92±0.19$^{@}$
3-HS	1.83±0.06	2.75±0.19$^{@}$	3.04±0.23$^{@/\$}$
7-HS	1.93±0.18	2.95±0.19$^{@}$	3.12±0.22$^{@/\$}$
12-HS	1.56±0.09	2.37±0.11$^{@}$	2.51±0.13$^{@}$
Transversal stiffness of sarcolemma at the Z-disk projection $k_{\perp Zds}$			
Control	2.65±0.07	3.12±0.13$^{@}$	3.64±0.12$^{@/\$}$
1-HS	3.05±0.12*	3.46±0.17$^{*/@}$	3.65±0.13$^{@}$
3-HS	3.22±0.08*	3.54±0.09$^{*/@}$	3.81±0.14$^{@}$
7-HS	3.35±0.13*	3.66±0.14$^{*/@}$	3.98±0.15$^{@/\$}$
12-HS	2.74±0.08	3.01±0.13$^{@}$	3.27±0.11$^{@/\$}$

Table 12. Transversal stiffness (pN/nm) of isolated gerbil's permeabilized *TA* muscle fibers in liquid in relaxed, calcium activated (pCa=4.2) and rigor states under gravitational unloading. * - p<0.05 as compared to the analogous state of the group «Control», $^{@}$ - p<0.05 as compared to the relaxed state at the same group, $^{\$}$ - p<0.05 as compared to the activated state at the same group.

M-band when the contraction is activated both in the control group and during the gravitational unloading. At the same time, the transversal stiffness of the membrane in the projection of the Z-disk and the M-band increases when the contraction is activated and, in some cases, even in rigor, compared to the activated state. The changes of transversal stiffness at various areas of the sarcolemma in the course of gravitational unloading are uneven. Thus, the stiffness in the area between the Z-disk and the M-band decreases after one and three days since the start of gravitational unloading; at the M-band projection it increases after one day and only in the relaxed state; at the Z-disk projection the transversal stiffness is increased relative to the control level after one day of suspension and up to the seventh day of suspension.

3.3 The transversal stiffness of the rat's left ventricular cardiomyocytes

In the control group (Table 13), the transversal stiffness of the contractile apparatus of fibers of the left ventricle of rat near the semi-sarcomere, i.e. between the Z-disk and the M-band increased in the sequence relaxation-activation-rigor. This value increased reliably from relaxation to activation. This situation did not change after one day of antiorthostatic suspension. However, in three days, the stiffness of the contractile apparatus reliably increased near the semi-sarcomere both in the relaxed and in the activated/rigor states compared to similar states in the control group. This increase was even more prominent seven days after antiorthostatic suspension. Nevertheless, during the antiorthostatic suspension and during activation of contraction, the stiffness of the semi-sarcomere reliably decreased compared to the relaxed state.

Group \ State	Relaxed	Activated (pCa=4.2)	Rigor
Transversal stiffness of the half-sarcomere area $k_{\perp ca}$			
Control	7.1±0.4	11.0±0.5@	13.2±0.5@
1-HS	6.8±0.3	10.3±0.3@	12.9±0.3@
3-HS	8.2±0.3*	13.8±0.4*/@	14.7±0.3*/@
7-HS	8.9±0.3*	13.5±0.3*/@	15.3±0.3*/@
14-HS	8.7±0.4*	13.6±0.4*/@	15.6±0.4*/@
Transversal stiffness of the M-band area $k_{\perp Ml}$			
Control	9.9±0.6	15.0±0.6@	16.4±0.5@
1-HS	8.9±0.5	14.1±0.4@	15.8±0.5@
3-HS	9.3±0.5	14.8±0.6@	16.3±0.5@
7-HS	10.6±0.4	14.9±0.5@	16.5±0.8@
14-HS	9.8±0.5	14.2±0.6@	15.7±0.3@
Transversal stiffness of the Z-disk area $k_{\perp Zd}$			
Control	16.0±1.3	22.5±1.5@	24.5±0.9@
1-HS	15.4±0.6	21.6±0.3@	24.8±0.6@
3-HS	15.9±0.6	23.4±0.7@	26.1±1.3@
7-HS	15.9±0.5	21.7±0.3@	25.9±0.6@
14-HS	15.8±0.8	21.9±0.9@	22.9±0.7@

Table 13. Transversal stiffness (pN/nm) of isolated rat's Triton-treated left ventricular myocytes in liquid in relaxed, calcium activated (pCa=4.2) and rigor states under gravitational unloading. * - p<0.05 as compared to the analogous state of the group «Control», @ - p<0.05 as compared to the relaxed state at the same group, $ - p<0.05 as compared to the activated state at the same group.

At the M-band, the stiffness of the contractile apparatus of fibers of the left ventricular of rat was higher than the stiffness of the semi-sarcomere. During the anti-orthostatic suspension, the transversal stiffness of the M-band did not change. The transversal stiffness of the Z-disk is significantly higher than in the semi-sarcomere and the M-band. It also, just like described above, increased during activation and rigor. The trends of changes in the transversal stiffness of the Z-disk were similar to those for the M-band. The transversal stiffness of various segments of glycerinated fibers of the left ventricular of rat (Table 14) in the control group increased during the activation of contraction and in rigor compared to the relaxed state.

After one day of antiorthostatic suspension, the transversal stiffness of the sarcolemma between the Z-disk and M-band projections in the relaxed state reliably increased relative to the control values, but did not differ from the control values in the activated and rigor states. After three days of suspension, the transversal stiffness of the sarcolemma increased even more and continued to increase up to the 14th day, and it reliably differed from the control value in the relaxed, activated and rigor states. Moreover, after 14 days of suspension, the transversal stiffness values of this area during activation and in rigor did not reliably differ from the values in the relaxed state. The transversal stiffness of the sarcolemma in the M-band projection in the relaxed state reliably increased compared to the control levels by the 3rd day of suspension and subsequently increased up to the 14th day. The transversal stiffness values in this area in the activated and rigor states did not differ from the control level. The transversal stiffness of sarcolemma in the Z-disk projection reliably increased only by the 14th day of suspension.

State / Group	Relaxed	Activated (pCa=4.2)	Rigor
Transversal stiffness of sarcolemma between the M-band and Z-disk projections $k_{\perp s}$			
Control	4.03±0.11	9.1±0.4@	9.67±0.24@
1-HS	4.80±0.22*	9.5±0.5@	10.1±0.3@
3-HS	6.22±0.29*	10.2±0.3*/@	10.8±0.4*/@
7-HS	7.79±0.12*	10.5±0.3*/@	13.3±0.4*/@
14-HS	12.3±0.4*	12.9±0.4*	13.3±0.3*/@
Transversal stiffness of sarcolemma at the M-band projection $k_{\perp MIs}$			
Control	2.85±0.12	6.8±0.5@	7.4±0.6@
1-HS	2.68±0.17	6.6±0.3@	7.0±0.3@
3-HS	3.77±0.25*	6.7±0.4@	7.7±0.5@
7-HS	5.79±0.19*	6.9±0.3@	7.9±0.3@
14-HS	7.55±0.13*	7.9±0.6*	9.4±0.3*/@
Transversal stiffness of sarcolemma at the Z-disk projection $k_{\perp Zds}$			
Control	10.0±0.3	14.5±1.2@	15.3±0.5@
1-HS	10.7±0.8	15.4±0.3@	16.3±0.5@
3-HS	10.6±0.3	14.8±0.3@	15.2±0.7@
7-HS	10.4±0.3	11.9±0.3@	16.5±0.3@
14-HS	17.2±0.4*	17.9±0.4*	18.2±0.5*/@

Table 14. Transversal stiffness (pN/nm) of isolated rat's permeabilized left ventricular myocytes in liquid in relaxed, calcium activated (pCa=4.2) and rigor states under gravitational unloading. * - p<0.05 as compared to the analogous state of the group «Control», @ - p<0.05 as compared to the relaxed state at the same group, $ - p<0.05 as compared to the activated state at the same group.

4. Discussion

The obtained experimental data shows that during simulate microgravity, the stiffness of various parts of muscle fiber in various skeletal muscles, and the cardiac muscle varies in different ways. The results of changes of transversal stiffness of various skeletal muscles of rat were discussed earlier (Ogneva, 2010). Thus, the stiffness of the contractile apparatus of the relaxed soleus muscle of rat does not change relative to the control value on the first day of gravitational unloading. By the 3rd day, the stiffness of the Z-disk of relaxed fiber significantly decreases, reaching its lowest level, and remains the same for the rest of the suspension period. As we showed earlier, after one day of gravitational unloading, the fibers of the soleus muscle of rat and Mongolian gerbil increase the basal content of calcium ions (Ogneva et al., 2009). This may lead to activation of calcium-dependent proteases, the calpains (Enns et al., 2007). The structure of the Z-disk includes a number of proteins that are substrates of calpains (Sanger & Sanger, 2008). It is their destruction that may lead to early reduction of stiffness of the Z-disk as observed in the experiments. At the same time, the changes of stiffness of the Z-disk in the activated state are not so prominent: the decrease is smoother, although the difference in stiffness between the activated and rigor condition significantly decreases. The stiffness values of the M-band and the semi-sarcomere slowly decrease starting from the end of the 3rd day and reach their minimum level only by the 12th day. In the activated state, though, these changes of the M-band and the semi-sarcomere develop much faster. This effect may be due to several reasons. First of all, titin and nebulin, the proteins of the contractile apparatus, are also substrates of calpains, and their destruction is observed by the seventh day of functional unloading (Goto et al., 2003; Kasper & Xun, 2000; Shenkman et al., 2004). Second of all, the decrease of the basal number of closed bridges may also lead to a decrease in the transversal stiffness of the contractile apparatus both in the relaxed and in the activated state. The reduction of the basal number of bridges is also evidenced by various data about the reduction of the calcium sensitivity of muscle fibers, which also reflects the number of closed transversal bridges during the gravitational unloading. Thus, by the seventh day of hypokinesia, a decrease of pCa0 (McDonald & Fitts, 1995) is observed, reflecting the concentration of calcium at which the muscle fiber starts significantly contracting, being initiated by a certain number of closed transversal bridges. By the way, it may also cause reduction of stiffness in the activated state, because pCa50 also decreases during the gravitational unloading (McDonald & Fitts, 1995). The possibility of closing of transversal bridges is affected by a number of factors, including the efficiency of transfer of tension in the longitudinal direction, requiring coordination of closing of bridges in adjacent sarcomeres, mobility of myosin heads, and inter-filament distance (lattice spacing). The first of these factors may be reduced due to calcium-dependent degradation of titin (see above) and destruction of the Z-disk. The mobility of myosin heads is more likely to increase as a result of the increase in the phosphorilation of light myosin chains (Stewart et al., 2009), which is helped by the increase of the general level of activity of phosphokinase in the course of the gravitational unloading (Barton, 2006). Moreover, the increase of the basal concentration of calcium also helps the increase of the possibility of formation of transversal bridges, although the calcium sensitivity of "quick" isoforms of myosin is lower, and the reliable slow-to-fast shift is observed as early as by the seventh day of the unloading (Booth & Kelso, 1973; Caiozzo et al. 1996; Desplanches et al. 1990). The effect of changes of the lattice spacing on the transversal stiffness was shown by Xu et al. (1993) and Ranatunga et al. (1990), in experiments with osmotic agents. But the question is whether the lattice spacing is changed during the gravitational unloading. We can only suppose that the destruction of the Z-disk and M-band may cause an increase of the lattice spacing. This suggestion is confirmed by the fact that other changes develop somewhat later, namely by the 7th day of unloading, while the decrease of the stiffness of the Z-disk and contractile apparatus is observed by the 3rd day of hypokinesia.

At the same time, reliable decrease of the transversal stiffness of the sarcolemma is observed as early as by the first day of gravitational unloading. Similarly to the results of Costa et al. (2006) obtained using human aortic cells, it can be suggested that such changes are related to the destruction of the sub-membrane actin cytoskeleton, which is consistent with the data of

Collinsworth et al. (2002). This destruction may be related either to the destruction of actin fillaments or dissociation of actin-binding proteins, particularly the alpha-actinin-1, alpha-actinin-4, filamin, and Arp-proteins. A change of actin content under gravitational unloading was observed on non-muscle cells (Infanger et al., 2007; Rijken et al., 1992), which may confirm the destruction of cortical cytoskeleton, and this may be the reason for the reduction of transversal stiffness of the sarcolemma. Changes near the costamere are observed in rats after one day of unloading, but by the 12th day of suspension, this value restores. The reduction of costamere stiffness may be related to its destruction as a result of loss of desmin, the key protein of costamere enabling the transfer of tension from the contractile apparatus to the sarcolemma (Capetanaki et al., 2007; Ervasti, 2003). Desmin is a substrate of a specific calcium-dependent proteolysis system, the calpain system. Enns et al. (2007) demonstrated that desmin content in the mixture of the soleus and gastrocnemius muscle significantly decreases by the third day and is almost completely restored by the ninth day. Chopard et al. (2005) demonstrated that in case of long-term antiorthostatic suspension of rats, desmin content in the fibers of the soleus muscle is not changed. The experimental data obtained by us earlier show that the desmin content in fibers of the soleus muscle reduces one day after the suspension, reliably decreases after three days and reaches the minimum after seven days; in twelve days, the desmin content in the soleus muscle is not different from the control value (Ogneva, 2010).

The situation is different when studying the fibers of the medial gastrocnemius muscle and the tibialis anterior muscle. By the first day of gravitational unloading, the stiffness of the contractile apparatus of relaxed fibers of these muscles reliably increases, and it does so much more in the area of the semi-sarcomere than at the Z-disk. Then, in the course of unloading, the stiffness of the contractile apparatus of fibers of the gastrocnemius muscle returns to the control level, while in fibers of the tibialis anterior muscle it remains above the original values. Basing on the explanations of changes in the stiffness of the contractile apparatus of the soleus muscle, it can be assumed that during the first day of gravitational unloading, either the mobility of myosin heads increases, or the lattice spacing decreases. The changes are implemented in the area of semi-sarcomere, since the changes of stiffness of the Z-disk and the M-band are not so prominent. The change of the lattice spacing in this case might only be caused by a change in physical and chemical factors that remained constant during the experiment. This is why we may suggest that the increase of the stiffness of fibers of the gastrocnemius muscle and tibialis anterior muscle is caused by an increase of mobility of myosin heads due to possible increase of the general phosphorylation level in the cells observed during the gravitational unloading (Barton, 2006).

The transversal stiffness of the sarcolemma of fibers of both muscles, just like those of the soleus muscle reliably decreases by the first day of gravitational unloading, which, similarly to fibers of the soleus muscle, may be related to the destruction of the cortical cytoskeleton. Nevertheless, after seven days of unloading, the transversal stiffness of the sarcolemma of fibers of the gastrocnemius muscle increases and reaches the control values, while that of fibers of the tibialis anterior muscle even somewhat exceeds the control level. The stiffness of the costamere of fibers of the gastrocnemius muscle and the tibialis anterior muscle somewhat increases after three and seven days of suspension, but returns to the original values by the 12th day, which suggests another trend of changes of desmin content compared to the soleus muscle. Desmin content in fibers of the gastrocnemius muscle remains almost unchanged during the gravitational unloading, and is only slightly increased by the seventh day of suspension, while in the tibialis anterior muscle it reliably increases by the first day of gravitational unloading, peaks on the third day, and then somewhat decreases, but remains reliably higher than the control level (Ogneva, 2010).

Changes in the stiffness of fibers of the Mongolian gerbil during the gravitational unloading are similar to those of the rat, although they are less prominent and either occur later or the changes are smoothed out earlier. Our previous data (Ogneva et al., 2009) confirm a significantly higher original intra-cell ionized calcium content in rats compared to gerbils; as early as 1 day after the gravitational unloading begins, both animals show an increase of calcium content by 2.8 and 4.5 times respectively in fibers of the soleus muscle. It is possible that the originally lower calcium ion content in the muscle fiber of gerbils compared to rats, and possibly higher osmolarity of their interstitial environment confirm that they have a higher electrochemical gradient for calcium ions on the membrane of the muscle fiber in the normal state, which, for example, may mean another level of activation of the calpain system. Desmin content in slow and fast muscles in the control group correspond to the same parameters in rats (our unpublished data). Nevertheless, it should be noted that stiffness of the sarcolemma, costamere and costamere-like structure of fibers of all studied muscles, especially the soleus muscle, is higher in Mongolian gerbils than in rats.

At the same time, changes of the transversal stiffness of cardiac myocytes were opposite. Some knowledge has accumulated that confirms changes of the contractile activity and conductivity of the myocard in space flight of humans and animals (Bungo et al., 1985; Goldstein et al., 1992). At the same time, the structural and functional basis of such changes, mainly implemented on the cell level, has almost not been studied (Xiong et al., 2003). The data we obtained confirms that as a result of simulated microgravity, the transversal stiffness of the contractile apparatus of cardiac myocytes in the area of transversal bridges is increased similarly to the contractile apparatus of fibers of the tibialis anterior muscle. At the same time, transversal stiffness of the sarcolemma of cardiac myocytes considerably increases at the earliest stages of simulated microgravity.

By comparing the results obtained with fibers of skeletal muscles and cardiac myocytes using atomic force microscopy, we may propose the following suggestions about the reaction of muscle fibers to changes of external mechanical conditions. The decrease of nervous activation, like in *Sol* (Alford et al., 1987) causes a decrease of stiffness of the contractile apparatus of fibers of skeletal muscles, possible due to changes in the efficiency of transfer of tension in the longitudinal direction due to changes in the lattice spacing. An increase of activity, like in *TA* (Alford et al., 1987), and increase of the load, like in the cardiac muscle, may lead to the prevalence of factors increasing the mobility of myosin heads. Moreover, there is a direct proportional dependence between the level of activation and content of desmin as a protein ensuring transfer of tension from the contractile apparatus to the sarcolemma.

The level of activity does not affect the studied structural and functional properties of the sarcolemma. Apparently, the direct decrease of load as a mechanical factor affecting any cell may cause a decrease of stiffness of the cell membrane, as it occurs in the tibialis anterior muscle under the conditions of antiorthostatic suspension. The increase of load under these conditions, which is typical for the cardiac muscle, causes an increase of the transversal stiffness of cardiac myocytes. The mechanism of change of the transversal stiffness of the cell membrane (reduction if the load reduces and increase if the load increases) is apparently related to restructuring of the cortical cytoskeleton. This may, for example, modulate the activity of membrane channels, signal paths connected with membrane proteins and be of key importance in launching processes ensuring mechanical sensitivity of cells, possibly not only those of muscles.

5. Acknowledgment

The authors express gratitude to all employees of myology laboratory of SSC RF - IBMP RAS. The work was supported by the program of the fundamental research SSC RF - IBMP RAS as well as by RFBR grant 10-04-00106-a.

6. References

Akiyama, N.; Ohnuki, Y.; Kunioka, Y.; Saeki, Y. & Yamada, T. (2006). Transverse stiffness of myofibrils of skeletal and cardiac muscles studied by atomic force microscopy. *Journal of physiological sciences*, Vol.56, pp. 145–151.

Alford, E.K.; Roy, R.R.; Hodgson, J.A. & Edgerton, V.R. (1987). Electromyography of rat soleus, medial gastrocnemius and tibialis anterior during hind limb suspension. *Experimental neurology*, Vol.96, pp. 635–649.

Altaeva, E.G.; Lysenko, L.A.; Kantserova, N.P.; Nemova, N.N. & Shenkman, B.S. (2010). The basal calcium level in fibers of the rat soleus muscle under gravitational unloading: the mechanisms of its increase and the role in calpain activation. *Doklady biological sciences : proceedings of the Academy of Sciences of the USSR, Biological sciences sections / translated from Russian*, Vol.433, pp. 241–243.

Barton, E.R. (2006) Impact of sarcoglycan complex on mechanical signal transduction in murine skeletal muscle. *American journal of physiology. Cell physiology*, Vol.290, pp. 411–419.

Bloch, R.J. & Gonzalez-Serratos, H. (2003). Lateral force transmission across costameres in skeletal muscle. *Exercise and sport sciences reviews*, Vol.31, pp. 73–78.

Booth, F.W. & Kelso J.R. (1973). Effect of hind-limb immobilization on contractile and histochemical properties of skeletal muscle. *Pflügers Archiv : European journal of physiology*, Vol.342, pp. 231–238.

Bungo, M.W.; Charles, J.B. & Jonson P.C. Jr. (1985). Cardiovascular deconditioning during space flight and the use of saline as a countermeasure to orthostatic intolerance. *Aviation, space, and environmental medicine*, Vol.56, No. 10, pp. 985–990.

Caiozzo, V.J.; Haddad, F.; Baker, M.J.; Herrick, R.E.; Prietto, N. & Baldwin K.M. (1996). Microgravity-induced transformations of myosin isoforms and contractile properties of skeletal muscle. *Journal of applied physiology*, Vol.81, pp. 123–132.

Capetanaki, Y.; Bloch, R.J.; Kouloumenta, A.; Mavroidis, M. & Psarras, S. Muscle intermediate filaments and their links to membranes and membranous organells. *Experimental cell research*, Vol.313, pp. 2063–2076.

Chopard, A.; Arrighi, N.; Carnino, A. & Marini, J.F. (2005). Changes in dysferlin, proteins from dystrophin glycoprotein complex, costameres, and cytoskeleton in human soleus and vastus lateralis muscles after a long-term bedrest with or without exercise. *The FASEB journal : official publication of the Federation of American Societies for Experimental Biology*, Vol.19, pp. 1722–1724.

Collinsworth, A.M.; Zhang, S.; Kraus, W.E. & Truskey G.A. (2002). Apparent elastic modulus and hysteresis of skeletal muscle cells throughout differentiation. *American journal of physiology. Cell physiology*, Vol.283, pp. 1219–1227.

Costa, K.D.; Sim, A.J. & Yin F.C. (2006). Non-Hertzian approach to analyzing mechanical properties of endothelial cells probed by atomic force microscopy. *Journal of biomechanical engineering*, Vol.128, pp. 176–184.

Defranchi, E.; Bonaccurso, E.; Tedesco, M.; Canato, M.; Pavan, E.; Raiteri, R. & Reggiani, C. (2005). Imaging and elasticity measurements of the sarcolemma of fully differentiated skeletal muscle fibres. *Microscopy research and technique*, Vol.67, pp. 27–35.

Desplanches, D.; Mayet, M.H.; Ilyina-Kakueva, E.I.; Sempore, B. & Flandrois, R. Skeletal muscle adaptation in rats flown on Cosmos 1667. *Journal of applied physiology*, Vol.68, pp. 48–52.

Enns, D.L.; Raastad, T.; Ugelstad, I.; Belcastro, A.N. (2007). Calpain/calpastatin activities and substrate depletion patterns during hindlimb unweighting and reweighting in skeletal muscle. *European journal of applied physiology*, Vol.100, pp. 445–455.

Ervasti, J.M. (2003). Costameres: the Achilles' Heel of Herculean muscle. *Journal of biological chemistry*, Vol.278, pp. 13591–13594.

Goldstein, M.A.; Edwards, R.J. & Schroeter, J.P. (1992). Cardiac morphology after conditions of microgravity during COSMOS 2044. *Journal of applied physiology*, Vol.73, 2 Suppl, pp. 94S - 100S.

Goto, K.; Okuyama, R.; Honda, M.; Uchida, H.; Akema, T.; Ohira, Y. & Yoshioka, T. (2003). Profiles of connectin (titin) in atrophied soleus muscle induced by unloading of rats. *Journal of applied physiology*, Vol.94, pp. 897–902.

Hertz, H. (1882). Ueber die Beruhrung fester alastischer Korper. *Reine Angew Mathematik*, Vol.92, pp. 156-171.

Infanger, M.; Ulbrich, C.; Baatout, S.; Wehland, M.; Kreutz, R.; Bauer, J.; Grosse, J.; Vadrucci, S.; Cogoli, A.; Derradji, H.; Neefs, M.; Kusters, S.; Spain, M.; Paul, M. & Grimm, D. Modeled gravitational unloading induced downregulation of endothelin-1 in human endothelial cells. *Journal of cellular biochemistry*, Vol.101, pp. 1439–1455.

Ingalls, C.P.; Warren, G.L. & Armstrong, R.B. (1999). Intracellular Ca2+ transients in mouse soleus muscle after hindlimb unloading. *Journal of applied physiology*, Vol.87, pp. 386–390.

Ingalls, C.P.; Wenke, J.C. & Armstrong, R.B. (2001). Time course changes in [Ca2+]i, force and protein content in hindlimb-suspended mouse soleus muscles. *Aviation, space, and environmental medicine*, Vol.72, pp. 471- 476.

Kasper, C.E. & Xun, L. (2000). Expression of titin in skeletal muscle varies with hind-limb unloading. *Biological research for nursing*, Vol.2, pp. 107–115.

Lieber et, S.C.; Aurby, N.; Pain, J.; Diaz, G.; Kim, S.J. & Vatner, S.F. (2004). Aging increases stiffness of cardiac myocytes measured by atomic force microscopy nanoindentation. *American journal of physiology. Heart and circulatory physiology*, Vol.287, No.2, pp. H645–H651.

Mathur, A.B.; Collinsworth, A.M.; Reichert, W.M.; Kraus, W.E. & Truskey, G.A. (2001). Endothelial, cardiac muscle and skeletal muscle exhibit different viscous and elastic properties as determined by atomic force microscopy. *Journal of biomechanics*, Vol.34, pp. 1545–1553.

McDonald, K.S. & Fitts, R.H. (1995). Effect of hindlimb unloading on rat soleus fiber force, stiffness, and calcium sensitivity. *Journal of applied physiology*, Vol.79, pp. 1796-1802.

Morey-Holton, E.; Globus, R.K.; Kaplansky, A. & Durnova, G. (2005). The hindlimb unloading rat model: literature overview, technique update and comparison with space flight data. *Advances in space biology and medicine*, Vol.10, pp. 7-40.

Nyland, L.R. & Maughan, D.W. (2000). Morphology and transverse stiffness of Drosophila myofibrils measured by atomic force microscopy. *Biophysical journal*, Vol.78, pp. 1490-1497.

Ogneva, I.V.; Kurushin, V.A.; Altaeva, E.G.; Ponomareva, E.V. & Shenkman, B.S. (2009). Effect of short-time gravitational unloading on rat and Mongolian gerbil muscles. *Journal of muscle research and cell motility*, Vol.30, pp. 261-265.

Ogneva, I.V.; Lebedev, D.V. & Shenkman, B.S. (2010). Transversal stiffness and Young's modulus of single fibers from rat soleus muscle probed by atomic force microscopy. *Biophysical journal*, Vol.98, pp. 418-424.

Ogneva, I.V. (2010). The transversal stiffness of fibers and the desmin content in the leg muscles of rats under gravitational unloading of various duration. *Journal of applied physiology*, Vol.109, pp. 1702-1709.

Radmacher, M.; Fritz, M.; Kacher, C.M.; Cleveland, J.P. & Hansma, P.K. (1996). Measuring the viscoelastic properties of human platelets with atomic force microscope. *Biophysical journal*, Vol.70, No.1, pp. 556-557.

Ranatunga, K.W.; Fortune, N.S. & Geeves, M.A. (1990). Hydrostatic compression in glycerinated rabbit muscle fibers. *Biophysical journal*, Vol.58, pp. 1401-1410.

Rijken, P.J.; de Groot R.P.; Kruijer, W.; de Laat, S.W.; Verkleij, A.J. & Boonstra, J. (1992). Identification of specific gravity sensitive signal transduction pathways in human A431 carcinoma cells. *Advances in space research : the official journal of the Committee on Space Research (COSPAR)*, Vol.12, pp. 145-152.

Robinson, P.F. (1959). Metabolism of the Gerbil, Meriones Unguiculatus. *Science*, Vol.130, pp. 502-503.

Sanger, J.M. & Sanger, J.W. (2008). The dynamic Z band of striated muscle cells. *Science signaling [electronic resource]*, Vol.1, pp. 37-39.

Shenkman, B.S.; Litvinova, K.S.; Nemirovskaya, T.L.; Podlubnaya, Z.A.; Vikhlyantsev, I.M. & Kozlovskaya, I.B. (2004). Afferent and peripheral control of muscle fiber properties during gravitational unloading. *Journal of gravitational physiology : a journal of the International Society for Gravitational Physiology*, Vol.11, pp. 111-114.

Shin, D. & Athanasiou, K. (1999). Cytoindentation for obtaining cell biomechanical properties. *Journal of orthopaedic research : official publication of the Orthopaedic Research Society*, Vol.17, No.6, pp. 880-890.

Sneddon, I.N. (1965). The relation between load and penetration in the axisymmetric boussinesq problem for a punch of arbitrary profile. *International journal of engineering science*, Vol.3, pp. 47-57.

Stevens, L.; Holy, X. & Mounier, Y. (1993). Functional adaptation of different rat skeletal muscles to weightlessness. *American journal of physiology*, Vol.264, pp. 770-776.

Stewart, M.; Franks-Skiba, K. & Cooke, R. (2009). Myosin regulatory light chain phosphorylation inhibits shortening velocities of skeletal muscle fibers in the presence of the myosin inhibitor blebbistatin. *Journal of muscle research and cell motility*, Vol.30, pp. 17-27.

Weisenhorn, A.L.; Khorsandi, M.; Kasas, S.; Gotzos, V. & Butt, H.J. (1993). Deformation and height anomaly of soft surfaces studied with an AFM. *Nanotechnology*, Vol.4, pp. 106–113.

Xiong, J.; Li, Y. & Nie, J. (2003). Effects of simulated microgravity on nitric oxide level in cardiac myocytes and its mechanism. *Science in China. Series C, Life sciences / Chinese Academy of Sciences*, Vol. 46. № 3. pp 302–309.

Xu, S.; Brenner, B. & Yu, L.C. (1993). State-dependent radial elasticity of attached cross-bridges in single skinned fibres of rabbit psoas muscle. *Journal of physiology*, Vol.465, pp. 749–765.

Zhu, J.; Sabharwal, T.; Kalyanasundaram, A.; Guo, L. & Wang, G. (2009). Topographic mapping and compression elasticity analysis of skinned cardiac muscle fibers in vitro with atomic force microscopy and nanoindentation. *Journal of biomechanics*, Vol.42, No.13, pp. 2143–2150.